A Practitioner's Guide Functional Medicine Lab Values: Foundations of Health Testing

Part 1 of 4:
Base-Level Blood Labs, Cardiometabolic, & Nutrition

Covers foundational lab testing for general health assessment, including **CBC, CMP, nutrient levels**, and **cardiometabolic** markers.

Dr. Brandy Zachary, D.C., IFMCP, FMACP
with foreword by Dr. Nick Sidhu, M.D., ABIM, ABOM, ABAARM

Also by author:

A Practitioner's Guide to Mastering Functional Medicine Lab Values - Gut & Digestion Insights:
(Part 2 of 4) Advanced Testing for Gastrointestinal Health

A Practitioner's Guide to Mastering Functional Medicine Lab Values - Hormonal Health & Balance:
(Part 3 of 4) Panels for Reproductive, Adrenal, and Thyroid Function

A Practitioner's Guide to Mastering Functional Medicine Lab Values - Metabolic Health & Toxin Testing: (Part 4 of 4) Autoimmunity, Toxins, and Advanced Metabolic Markers

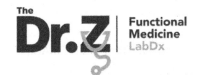

The Dr. Z Functional Medicine LabDX, LLC
Sheridan, WY 82801

A Practitioner's Guide to Mastering Functional Medicine Lab Values Foundations of Health Testing
(Part 1 of 4) Base-Level Blood Labs, Cardiometabolic, & Nutrition

© 2025 by Dr. Brandy Zachary, DC, IFMCP, FMACP
All rights reserved. This book or parts thereof may not be reproduced in any form, stored in any retrieval system, or transmitted in any form by any means—electronic, mechanical, photocopy, recording, or otherwise—without prior written permission of the publisher, except as provided by United States of America copyright law and fair use. For permission requests, write to the publisher "Attention: Permissions Coordinator," at the address below.

Book Cover Design by ebooklaunch.com
Editing by Sharon Strahan, IFMCP, FMACC, Clinical Nutritionist (BSc Dietetics, BSc Nutritional Medicine) and Lorri Kercher MSN, CRNP, FMACP, AFMCP
Book formatting by Angelica Tandoc

1st Edition 2025

ISBN 979-8-9924008-0-9 (hardback)
ISBN 979-8-9924008-1-6 (paperback)

Library of Congress Control Number - LCCN: 2025900613

Warning - Disclaimer
Dr. Brandy Zachary, DC, IFMCP, FMACP and Functional Medicine LabDX have designed this book to provide information in regards to the subject matter covered. It is sold with the understanding that the publisher and the author is not liable for the misconception or misuse of information provided. The purpose of this book is to educate. It is not intended as a substitute for medical diagnosis or treatment, nor intended as a substitute for medical counseling. Information in this book should not be construed as a treatment or diagnosis or promise of a cure or outcome for any medical condition. The interpretation and use is intended to support the practitioner's knowledge of lab markers. It should be considered as adjunctive support to other diagnostic medical procedures and every practitioner needs to make their own clinical decisions and operate within their scope of practice applicable to all local, state, and federal regulatory laws.

Publisher's Cataloging-in-Publication Data

Names: Zachary, Brandy, author. | Sidhu, Nick, foreword author.
Title: A practitioner's guide to mastering functional medicine lab values : foundations of health testing (part 1 of 4) base-level blood labs, cardiometabolic, & nutrition / Dr. Brandy Zachary, D.C., IFMCP, FMACP; with foreword by Dr. Nick Sidhu, M.D., ABIM, ABOM, ABAARM.
Description: Includes bibliographical references. | Sheridan, WY: The Dr. Z Functional Medicine LabDX, LLC, 2025.
Identifiers: LCCN: 2025900613 | ISBN: 979-8-9924008-0-9 (hardcover) | 979-8-9924008-1-6 (paperback)
Subjects: LCSH Reference values (Medicine)--Handbooks, manuals, etc. | Reference values (Medicine)--Interpretation. | Diagnosis, Laboratory--Handbooks, manuals, etc. | Functional medicine. | BISAC MEDICAL / Laboratory Medicine | MEDICAL / Reference | HEALTH & FITNESS / Diet & Nutrition / Nutrition | HEALTH & FITNESS / Reference
Classification: LCC RB37 .Z33 2025 | DDC 616.07/56--dc23

For information about special pricing for bulk purchases, sales promotions, fundraising, and educational needs contact The Dr. Z Functional Medicine LabDX, LLC at **team@thedrzlabdx.com** or 1-307-291-9885.

Visit the author's website at **www.TheDrZ.com**.

Printed in the United States of America.

The Dr. Z is a registered trademark of Dr. Brandy Zachary, DC, IFMCP, FMACP.

Published by The Dr. Z Functional Medicine LabDX, LLC
30 N Gould St #37288
Sheridan, WY 37288
www.TheDrZ.com/LabDX

Advance praise for the textbook series:

A Practitioner's Guide to Mastering Functional Medicine Lab Values

This guide simplifies lab data, enabling practitioners to uncover root causes with speed and precision. With essential labs like CBC, CMP, nutrient levels and cardiometabolic markers, it's a must-have for delivering effective, personalized care. — **Dr. Cathy Swain-Jones, MD, FACOG of Women's Hormone Wellness**

If you are a practitioner and interpreting labs daily - this resource MUST be at your disposal. No more searching PubMed and multiple supplement resources for hours. This resource brings it ALL together in one efficient and user-friendly space — **Tara Sayer, RN, BSN, MSCN, IFMP, CNSc of Perspective Health Iowa**

LabDx helps me to see any deviations on the foundational blood labs, because it looks at functional lab ranges, not the disease-based conventional lab ranges, which are often blind to trouble spots emerging, before the onset of true disease. LabDx also makes smart recommendations about diet, lifestyle and supplements that are appropriate to consider for the patient. — **Dr. Juliana Nahas MD, FMACP of Cedars Functional Medicine LLC**

Every Doctor of Chiropractic needs this book whether you are doing functional medicine or want to help your patients with targeted supplement protocols based on labs. This book truly is a game changer and can set your clinical expertise to the next level. — **Dr. Angela Davenport DC, FMACP of Davenport Healing and Functional Medicine**

Functional medicine aims to treat the whole person, and LabDX's comprehensive lab tests give practitioners a full picture of a patient's health, making it easier to create tailored treatment plans. — **Alvaro Berrios, FNP-BC, FMACP of Restore Your Health Functional Medicine**

This textbook is an essential guide that bridges the gap between conventional reference ranges and optimal ranges, empowering you to identify and address imbalances early. It has been a fundamental resource in supporting my patients who might otherwise be dismissed as "normal". — **Dr. Breanne Kallonen, ND**

This textbook is a game-changer for functional lab analysis, breaking down what labs really mean—not just "everything looks good." It transformed how I care for my patients, with one patient so impressed she decided to bring her husband next and share a testimonial about finally getting the answers no doctor had provided. It's a must-have for anyone serious about making a real impact in patient care. — **Dr. Phylicia Harris, DNP, FNP-C, FMACP of Functionally Balanced Health, PLLC**

LabDX has been a lifeline in my practice, enabling me to guide women over 40 through the complexities of midlife health with clarity. This textbook isn't just a resource—it's a bridge to deeper client connections and lasting results, making it indispensable for functional medicine practitioners committed to transforming lives. — **Martine Chin FMACC, CNP, IHP2, HPH of MC Wellness Hub**

This LabDX textbook series has completely changed the way I practice functional medicine. It's hands-down the most practical and easy-to-use reference I've ever come across. I've been in practice for 28 years, and this book has helped me simplify complex lab data, create more personalized care plans, and get better results for my patients. Honestly, it's a total game-changer—if you work with functional medicine labs, you need this on your desk. — **Jessica Farrone APRN, FNP, FMACP of Alpha Health and Wellness**

Everything I need to analyze functional labs is right here—clear, concise, and incredibly useful for both new learners and seasoned practitioners. — **Cari Caraway, MSN, FNP-C, FMACP of Florida Functional Med**

Understanding the functional labs made the entire world of Functional Medicine open up right before my eyes. — **Kimberly Wiest CRNA, FMACP of The Living Well Solutions**

Every functional medicine provider needs this book because understanding blood work and stool testing is essential to uncovering the root cause of persistent health issues. This resource simplifies interpreting functional lab values and equips you to create effective, results-driven care plans with confidence. It's a must-have tool for transforming patient outcomes and accelerating progress. — **Kacie M. Proctor, FNP-C, FMACP of Kacie Proctor Functional Medicine**

This guide has been an absolute game-changer for me as a new functional medicine nurse practitioner! It's opened my eyes to deeper insights in lab results, helping me uncover the root causes of my patients' concerns with confidence. Thanks to this resource, I've been able to create personalized, impactful care plans that truly transform my patients' health and lives! — **Kimberly B. Jones, FNP-C, FMACP of The Drip Lounge**

Every holistic doctor needs a copy of this amazing lab manual on their desk - because lab work isn't really going to make sense - or change - without nutritional markers changing. I've been in practice since 1997 & this resource is a genuine life raft in the sea of murky lab values… a true game changer. — **Dr. Julie Montgomery DNH of Holistic Therapy Services**

All tests are not 100%. Listen to the patient and ask yourself: Does this add up? — **Alissa McDivitt FNP-C, M.S., IFMCP of Spark Vital Health**

This guide completely transformed the way I approach hormone labs and Dutch tests. It connects the dots between lab markers and underlying conditions, making every report actionable. Having this guide has been like adding an expert mentor to my team. — **Lizette Reyes FMACC, CFNC, CBHC of Divinely Integrated Functional Health**

This textbook is an essential tool for any health professional working with chronic conditions and metabolic imbalances. It truly revolutionizes how we assess and treat underlying toxicity, making it a game-changer in improving patient outcomes. — **Dr Lori Bouchard, BHSc. ND of Dr Inside Health Clinic (Ontario) & Nature Doctors (Manitoba)**

As a nurse practitioner with years of experience decoding complex labs, I can confidently say this guide is a game-changer. Every healthcare professional—and anyone serious about understanding their health—needs this resource in their toolkit. It takes the guesswork out of lab interpretation, bridging the gap between numbers on a page and actionable diagnoses. This isn't just a book; it's an essential guide for anyone ready to move beyond "normal" and into optimal health. — **Paula J. Pretty, MSN, FNP-C, FMACP of A Balanced You**

Table of Contents

Dedication i
Foreword ii
Introduction iv
How to Use This Book vii
    The Complete Textbook Series vii
    Understanding Lab Ranges: Traditional vs. Functional/Optimal vii
    Navigating This Book viii
    Using This Book with LabDX Software viii
    Clinical Application and Approach viii
    Explanation of Icons ix

Base Level Health 1

CBC with Differential (Complete Blood Count) 3
    White Blood Cell Count (WBC) 3
    Red Blood Cell Count (RBC) 5
    Hemoglobin 7
    Hematocrit 8
    Mean Corpuscular Volume (MCV) 9
    Mean Corpuscular Hemoglobin (MCH) 11
    Mean Corpuscular Hemoglobin Concentration (MCHC) 12
    Red Blood Cell Distribution Width (RDW) 14
    Platelets 16
    Mean Platelet Volume (MPV) 17
    Neutrophils 19
    Lymphocytes 21
    Monocytes 22
    Eosinophils 23
    Basophils 25

CMP (Comprehensive Metabolic Panel) 27
    Glucose - Fasting 27
    Glucose - Non-Fasting 29
    Hemoglobin A1C 32
    Uric Acid 34
    BUN (Blood Urea Nitrogen) 37
    Creatinine 40
    eGFR (non-African American) 42
    eGFR (African American) 42
    Sodium 43
    Potassium 44
    Chloride 46
    Carbon Dioxide (CO_2) 48
    Calcium 50
    Phosphorus 52
    Magnesium 55
    Protein, Total 57
    Albumin 59
    Globulin 62
    Bilirubin, Total 65
    Bilirubin - Direct 67
    Bilirubin - Indirect 69
    Alkaline Phosphatase (ALP) 71
    Lactate Dehydrogenase (LDH) 73

Aspartate amino-transferase (AST) (SGOT)	75
Alanine amino-transferase (ALT) (SGPT)	78
Gamma-glutamyl transferase (GGT)	80

Metabolites 83
Choline	83
Inositol	83
Carnitine	84
Methylmalonic Acid (MMA)	85

Electrolytes 87
Sodium	87
Potassium	88

Amino Acids 89
Asparagine	89
Glutamine	90
Serine	91

Iron Panel 93
Total Iron Binding Capacity (TIBC)	93
Unsaturated Iron Binding Capacity (UIBC)	94
Iron, Serum	96
Iron Saturation (Transferrin Saturation - TSAT)	98
Ferritin, Serum	100

Anemia Panel 103
Total Iron Binding Capacity (TIBC)	103
Unsaturated Iron Binding Capacity (UIBC)	105
Iron, Serum	106
Iron Saturation (Transferrin Saturation - TSAT)	108
Ferritin, Serum	110
Hemoglobin	112
Hematocrit	113

Urinalysis 115
Specific Gravity	115
pH	116
Urine Color	118
WBC Esterase	119
Protein	120
Glucose	121
Ketones	122
Occult Blood (Microscopic Blood)	124
Bilirubin	125
Urobilinogen, Semi-Quantitative	127
Nitrite, Urine	128

Cardiometabolic *131*

Lipid Panel 133
CVD health — Commentary	133
Cholesterol	135
Triglycerides	138
HDL Cholesterol	141
LDL Cholesterol	143
Homocysteine	145
C-Reactive Protein (hsCRP)	147
Fibrinogen Activity	148

Inflammation Panel 151
C-Reactive Protein (hs-CRP)	151

- Lp-PLA2 152
- MPO (Myeloperoxidase) 153
- Oxidized LDL (OxLDL) 155
- Oxidized Phospholipids (OxPL-apoB) 156
- Erythrocyte Sedimentation Rate (ESR) 158

Advanced Heart Markers 161
- C-Reactive Protein (hs-CRP) 161
- Small Dense LDL Cholesterol (sdLDL-C) 162
- LDL-p 165
- HDL-p 167
- Lp(a) 169
- ApoA-I 171
- ApoB 174

Fatty Acids 179
- EPA (Eicosapentaenoic acid) 179
- DPA (Docosapentanoic acid) 180
- DHA (Docosahexanoic acid) 181
- Total Omega-3 182
- LA (Linolenic Acid) 183
- Total Omega-6 184
- Omega-3 Index 185

Sugar Panel 187
- Glucose - Fasting 187
- Glucose - Non-Fasting 189
- Hemoglobin A1C 191
- Fasting Insulin 194
- C-Peptide 196
- Adiponectin 199
- Homeostasis Model of Insulin Resistance (HOMA-IR) 201
- Leptin 203

Thyroid 205
- TSH (Thyroid Stimulating Hormone) 205
- Thyroxine (T4), Total 207
- T3 (Triiodothyronine), Total 209
- T4, Free (Direct) 212
- T3, Free, Serum 215
- TPO Thyroid Peroxidase 218
- TGAb Thyroglobulin Antibody 220
- T3 Uptake 222
- Reverse T3 224
- Free Thyroxine Index (FTI or T7) 227
- Thyroxine Binding Globulin (TBG) 229

Nutrient 233

Vitamins 235
- Vitamin A (Retinol) 235
- Vitamin B1 (Thiamin) 236
- Vitamin B2 (Riboflavin) 236
- Vitamin B3 (Niacin) 237
- Vitamin B5 (Pantothenic Acid) 238
- Vitamin B6 (Pyridoxine) 239
- Vitamin B9 (Folate) 240
- Vitamin B12 (Cobalamin) 241
- Vitamin C (Ascorbic Acid) 242
- Vitamin D3 243
- Vitamin D, 25-OH 244

Vitamin E 245
Vitamin K1 246
Vitamin K2 247

Minerals 249
Calcium 249
Manganese 251
Zinc 251
Copper 253
Chromium 254
Iron 255
Magnesium 256
Copper to Zinc Ratio 257

Antioxidants 259
Coenzyme Q10 259
Cysteine 260
Glutathione 261
Selenium 263

Vibrant Micronutrient 265
Lymphocyte Count (Cellular) 265
Neutrophil Count (Cellular) 267
WBC (Cellular) 268
AA (Arachidonic acid) (Cellular) 270
AA/EPA Ratio (Cellular) 271
DHA (Cellular) 273
DPA (Cellular) 274
EPA (Cellular) 275
LA (Linoleic acid) (Cellular) 277
Omega-3 Index (Cellular) 278
Total Omega-3 (Cellular) 279
Total Omega-6 (Cellular) 281
Arginine (Serum) 283
Asparagine (Serum) 284
Asparagine (Cellular) 286
Citrulline (Serum) 288
Glutamine (Serum) 289
Isoleucine (Serum) 291
Leucine (Serum) 292
Serine (Serum) 295
Valine (Serum) 296
Calcium (Serum) 298
Calcium (Cellular) 301
Chromium (Serum) 303
Copper (Serum) 305
Copper (Cellular) 307
Copper to Zinc Ratio (Serum) 308
Iron (Serum) 311
Iron (Cellular) 313
Magnesium (Serum) 316
Magnesium (Cellular) 319
Manganese (Serum) 322
Manganese (Cellular) 323
Zinc (Serum) 325
Zinc (Cellular) 326
Carnitine (Serum) 328
Carnitine (Cellular) 331
Choline (Serum) 334
Choline (Cellular) 336

Inositol (Serum) 338
Inositol (Cellular) 339
MMA (Methylmalonic Acid) (Serum) 340
Coenzyme Q10 (Serum) 341
Coenzyme Q10 (Cellular) 343
Cysteine (Serum) 346
Cysteine (Cellular) 348
Glutathione (Cellular) 350
Selenium (Serum) 351
Selenium (Cellular) 352
Folate (Serum) 353
Folate (Cellular) 355
Vitamin A (Serum) 357
Vitamin A (Cellular) 358
Vitamin B1 (Serum) 360
Vitamin B1 (Cellular) 361
Vitamin B12 (Serum) 362
Vitamin B12 (Cellular) 365
Vitamin B2 (Serum) 368
Vitamin B2 (Cellular) 370
Vitamin B3 (Serum) 371
Vitamin B3 (Cellular) 374
Vitamin B5 (Serum) 377
Vitamin B5 (Cellular) 379
Vitamin B6 (Serum) 380
Vitamin B6 (Cellular) 382
Vitamin C (Serum) 384
Vitamin C (Cellular) 386
Vitamin D, 25-OH (Serum) 388
Vitamin D3 (Serum) 390
Vitamin D3 (Cellular) 392
Vitamin E (Serum) 394
Vitamin E (Cellular) 397
Vitamin K1 (Serum) 399
Vitamin K1 (Cellular) 400
Vitamin K2 (Serum) 401
Vitamin K2 (Cellular) 403
Potassium (Serum) 404
Sodium (Serum) 406

Bibliography **407**

Research Articles **408**

Lab Companies **436**

Books **437**

Trainings/Teachers/Seminars **438**

Other digital source material **439**

Drug-Nutrient Interactions and Depletions resources **443**

Unit Conversion Links **444**

Additional Resources **445**

Frequently Ordered Blood Panels: Traditional and Optimal Ranges **446**
CBC with Differential 446
CMP (Comprehensive Metabolic Panel) 447
Lipids 448

- Thyroid 448
- Anemia 449

Blood Lab Markers: Common Patterns 450

Examples of Using Lab Analysis by Functional Medicine Practitioners 455

How Do I Become a Functional Medicine Practitioner? 465
- What is Functional Medicine? 465
- The History of Functional Medicine 466
- Functional Medicine Practitioner Eligibility 466
- Why Doctors, Nurses, PAs, & DCs Are Switching to Functional Medicine 467
- How to Choose the Right Functional Medicine Training for You 468
- Trainings and Certifications in Functional Medicine 469

How Do I Find a Functional Medicine Practitioner? 473

Acknowledgements 476

About the Author 477

Dedication

To all the patients who feel like crap but are told their labs look "normal"—this is for you. May you find the answers you deserve and the care you need.

To those brave enough to keep searching, even when the path is unclear—your courage inspires change.

To the incredible practitioners who take the time to dig deeper, challenge the status quo, and continually invest in their learning—your dedication transforms lives.

To my amazing and devoted team at The Dr, Z Functional Medicine Academy and LabDX – thank you for fighting daily to make an impact on healthcare worldwide.

And to my family—your unwavering support and encouragement make it all possible, even as you tolerate (and sometimes even join in) my obsession with data, information, and answers.

This book is for all of you.

Foreword

In the rapidly evolving landscape of modern medicine, practitioners are continually seeking tools that bridge the gap between symptom-focused care and true root-cause resolution. For those of us practicing functional medicine, this quest is both a professional commitment and a deeply personal journey. As a board-certified physician in Internal Medicine, Obesity Medicine, and Anti-Aging and Regenerative Medicine, and as the owner and medical director of the Advanced Medical and Weight Loss Center in Alpharetta, GA, I've had the privilege of witnessing firsthand how the integration of functional lab analysis transforms the clinical decision-making process, offering clarity where there was once confusion and empowering both practitioners and patients with actionable insights.

Functional lab analysis is, in essence, the cornerstone of a personalized approach to health. Traditional lab markers, while invaluable, often provide only a limited snapshot of a patient's health. They are designed to detect disease thresholds, which means many individuals fall through the cracks—their results are labeled "normal," yet they feel far from well. Functional lab markers, on the other hand, expand this view. They allow us to assess patterns, trends, and subtle imbalances long before they manifest as overt disease. This proactive, systems-based approach is what sets functional medicine apart and enables us to practice true preventive care.

In my own clinical experience, the difference between traditional and functional lab analysis is profound. I remember the early days of my practice when I relied solely on conventional lab work. Patients would come to me with complex, chronic conditions that defied simple categorization. The labs would tell me they were "fine," yet their stories said otherwise. Frustrated, I began to explore beyond the boundaries of standard testing, seeking answers in nutrient levels, hormonal rhythms, and inflammatory markers that traditional labs often overlook. This shift was nothing short of revolutionary. Suddenly, I was able to connect the dots between a patient's symptoms and their underlying biochemical individuality. The results were often life-changing—not just for my patients, but for me as a clinician.

Dr. Z's LabDX system embodies this transformative potential. This comprehensive, systematic approach to functional lab interpretation is more than a tool; it is a roadmap for practitioners who are committed to excellence. Having had the privilege of participating in Dr. Z's mentorship program, I've seen how this framework not only enhances clinical confidence but also fosters a deeper understanding of the interplay between lab results and patient outcomes. Dr. Z's ability to distill complex concepts into actionable strategies is unmatched, and this textbook is a testament to her dedication to empowering practitioners to deliver exceptional care.

One of the most remarkable aspects of the LabDX system is its emphasis on clinical applicability. This is not a dry academic resource filled with abstract theories. It is a hands-on guide designed to help you immediately implement functional lab analysis into your practice. Whether you are a seasoned functional medicine veteran or just beginning your journey, the principles and protocols outlined in this book will resonate with you. They are practical, actionable, and grounded in real-world clinical success. This textbook is your ally in that process, a trusted resource that will guide you through the complexities of functional lab data with clarity and precision.

For the seasoned practitioner, Dr. Z's LabDX system will deepen your expertise and expand your toolkit. It is a resource that challenges you to think more critically, to dig deeper, and to refine your skills. Even as someone who has spent years in the field, I found myself learning new nuances and approaches that have enhanced my practice. This speaks to the depth and breadth of knowledge encapsulated in this work.

The publication of this book marks a significant milestone for the functional medicine community. It is a call to action for all of us to elevate our practice, to bridge the divide between conventional and functional paradigms, and to lead the way in transforming healthcare. As you read and apply the insights from this textbook, remember that you are part of a larger movement—one that is redefining what is possible in medicine.

In closing, I want to extend my heartfelt gratitude to Dr. Z for her tireless dedication to advancing the field of functional medicine. Her mentorship, vision, and unwavering commitment to excellence are evident in every chapter of this book. To my fellow practitioners, I encourage you to embrace this resource with curiosity and enthusiasm. The knowledge within these pages has the power to elevate your practice and, more importantly, to change lives—beginning with your own.

Here's to the journey ahead and the countless patients who will benefit from your commitment to healing. The future of medicine is functional, and it starts with us.

Dr. Nick Sidhu, M.D. ABIM, ABOM, ABAARM
Owner/Medical Director
Advanced Medical & Weight Loss Center in Alpharetta, Ga

Introduction

I'm a terrible judge of time, and that's how this whole thing got started.

I like speed. I want to move quickly, assess information with synapses rapidly firing, and act decisively.

Then life came to a halt.

I woke up sick one day and didn't know how I got there.

I had a lot to lose and wanted this solved yesterday, so I was a "very good patient" and did everything I was told. It didn't work and I just got sicker.

Relegated to 8 prescriptions, frequent hospital visits, 7 specialists that either did not talk to one another or could not agree, and then declared permanently disabled by US Social Security Administration - it became clear that I had to find a different way out and it was on me to figure it out.

It took longer than I thought it would.

Over 3 years of seeking out specialists of every kind, reading extensive research, reactivating my own DC license so I could order my own labs.

I finally returned to the land of the living. Quite a bit battered, more than a little broken, confidence nowhere to be found - but I was determined. What I had learned, I felt everyone should have access to. So I started a little clinic focused on serving patients with functional medicine.

That issue with time, it found me once again.

My first patient, I spent 10 hours pouring over my exam findings, the numerous labs, checking contraindications, and putting together the pieces of the puzzle. I learned a lot but I knew I could not build a practice this way. It wouldn't be sustainable. How could I speed up this analysis process?

I saw another practitioner had made an excel sheet of just a few basic blood labs and said "great, this will help, can I have a copy?" "Sure," he said, "for $5,000."

I wasn't in a position to pay that at the time. I was just coming up for air and launching my own practice. I was a single mom and the toll of the last 3 years of sickness had barely started to roll off of me. I decided I would make it myself and was determined to get it done that weekend.

About 6 weeks later it was completed. I spent every minute of December and the holidays working on this. Would this be worth all the time I had put into it? I really wondered…

It was 75 blood markers that blended all the textbooks, research articles, and coursework I could find on the subject into one functional spreadsheet grid. My very first patient helped me with the formulas to pull the data so I could quickly enter in lab values and get my answers in minutes instead of hours.

That first tool was 850 pieces of data and I used it on thousands of patient's labs. It was invaluable.

My practice launched and expanded quickly as patients responded well to my blend of functional medicine and nutritional analysis plus traditional medicine referrals and co-management. We used chiropractic, physical therapy, acupuncture, massage, medical devices, herbal medicine, an organic chef, biological dentistry, functional optometry, energy medicine, integrative psychotherapy and psychiatry referrals as needed.

I had local PCPs sending me challenging cases and some patients flying in or traveling long distances. It was a busy time and the learning never stopped. My love of labs grew and my repertoire expanded. I found myself wishing I had all the advanced lab answers as easily accessible, but it was nowhere to be found - I still spent a lot of time pouring over clinical reference guides and research.

When a colleague offered me $5k for just my spreadsheet of blood markers (the same number coming back around years later), I decided to make a digital software tool so other practitioners could benefit as I had.

Ahhh…that sense of time though. My old nemesis.

I budgeted $12,000 over 3 months and hired my first software developer. This was a lot of money for me at the time and it was a leap of faith into an industry I knew nothing about. If I was going to do this however, I wanted a comprehensive stool test and a urinalysis and SIBO breath testing and a DUTCH test and some of my other favorite labs.

After 4 years, $100,000, and my second software developer - it was ready. That's a long time and it was a lot of money for this single mama.

Several times I thought of quitting.

There would be a blood lab analysis tool that would surface and I would think - "Well, they did it, so I don't have to." But, they never did it right. They used the wrong marker ranges, or overcomplicated the reports, and they never did more than blood markers.

So I persisted.

I found some help along the way. By now that 850 pieces of data was tens of thousands of pieces of data - it was overwhelming! I needed some fellow geeks who loved labs to help and I found them in colleagues through IFM (Institute for Functional Medicine).

Life changed over the years it took to get to this point. After 15 years as a single mama, I fell in love and remarried, later moving to the Caribbean coast.

I taught all types of practitioners everything from clinical care and complex cases to marketing and practice growth. I had even started my own school, the Functional Medicine Academy with a robust and full education system.

At the point that the first LabDX software app was beta launched with 25 tests in 2023, I was counting on my team of staff members and our many practitioner clients to help test the software. It was amazing and scary and thrilling and tedious and… So. Much. Data.

We made it so you could pull markers from different tests (ex. Urinalysis, serum hormones, stool tests, saliva tests, autoimmune and toxicity panels) into one PDF for the patient. No more endless hours of charting, you could upload it right into your EMR, and we white-labeled it for each private practice.

We pulled together data that had never been in one place before. Check the 37 pages of references to see why - it was a Herculean effort. Every relevant lab clinical guide, white paper, PubMed article, lab textbook, coursework, and clinical experience were considered.

I have funded this project that started with just me 9 years ago into a 30+ member staff with no less than 3-5 staff members (or more!) working on LabDX daily for the last 1.5 years. In a way, we are just getting started.

At the point that I said "we're going to take the LabDX software and put out a textbook" we had over 60 labs in the online tool. That 1 textbook became 4 - just so you could lift it.

Yes, this has been a labor of love.

Where does the willingness, determination, and perseverance for such a project come from?

That desire for answers.

Whether it was a patient who "felt like crap but told their labs are fine", or a disabling immunodeficiency, or a chronic infection masquerading as a mental health condition - I believe there is a reason for every symptom.

I believe one of the most valuable questions we can ask is "why?" And the more we ask it, the closer we get to that root cause issue - because when we find that - then healing can begin.

My intention is that these 4 textbooks intrigue and excite your love of lab work.

That you begin to look deeper and beyond merely a disease model, but also asking why, how, when, and where? To look at the whole body functionally, to see the connections, and to really partner with that patient to make the necessary lifestyle changes.

Seeing early signs of dysfunction before a diagnosable condition is a game changer.

Understanding genetics, methylation, immune complexes, and the microbiome is becoming a standard requirement.

My hope is that these textbooks and/or the LabDX software tool will assist you so you can move quickly, assess information with synapses rapidly firing, and act decisively.

Thank you for your dedication to your patients and your ongoing education. We need more practitioners like you.

With gratitude,

Dr. Z

How to Use This Book

This textbook, *A Practitioner's Guide to Mastering Functional Medicine Lab Values: Foundations of Health Testing (Part 1 of 4)*, is the first in a four-part series designed to provide Functional Medicine professionals with a detailed framework for interpreting lab values and implementing effective care plans. Together, the series spans over 60 lab panels, offering a comprehensive guide to functional lab testing across multiple domains of health.

The Complete Textbook Series

To provide the full scope of lab analysis, this series is divided into four specialized volumes:

1. **Foundations of Health Testing (Part 1 of 4): Base-Level Blood Labs, Cardiometabolic, & Nutrition**
   Covers foundational blood panels such as CBC, CMP, lipid profiles, nutrient levels, and cardiometabolic markers.

2. **Gut & Digestion Insights (Part 2 of 4): Advanced Testing for Gastrointestinal Health**
   Explores GI health markers, including stool analysis, leaky gut indicators, and microbiome diversity.

3. **Hormonal Health & Balance (Part 3 of 4): Panels for Reproductive, Adrenal, and Thyroid Function**
   Focuses on endocrine function, including sex hormones, adrenal markers, and thyroid panels.

4. **Metabolic Health & Toxin Testing (Part 4 of 4): Autoimmunity, Toxins, and Advanced Metabolic Markers**
   Includes testing for advanced metabolic markers, toxin exposures, and autoimmune conditions.

Each book is an essential resource on its own, but together, they provide a full-spectrum understanding of functional lab testing.

Understanding Lab Ranges: Traditional vs. Functional/Optimal

A key principle of Functional Medicine is the difference between traditional lab ranges and functional or optimal ranges.

- **Traditional Lab Ranges**: Derived from a statistical average of a population, traditional ranges include 80-95% of individuals, often reflecting averages influenced by widespread chronic disease. These ranges focus on diagnosing pathology, with results flagged as high or low only when severe imbalances are present.

- **Functional/Optimal Ranges**: These narrower ranges reflect physiological balance and optimal function, possibly helping identify imbalances before disease develops. Functional ranges allow practitioners to detect the subtle dysfunctions traditional ranges overlook, focusing on restoring balance and addressing root causes rather than managing symptoms alone.

For example, a traditional range might deem a value "normal" because it falls within statistical averages, even if it's far from optimal for health. Functional Medicine practitioners, however, use tighter ranges to uncover issues earlier, enabling proactive interventions like nutritional support or further testing.

It is also worth noting that traditional and functional/optimal ranges may vary from lab to lab and they may even use different units of measure from other labs. The recommendations for a marker will still be valid. We have added a section on online unit conversion tools for your information in the Bibliography section of this book.

Navigating This Book

Markers are organized into clearly defined sections to make this textbook easy to use in both clinical and educational settings:

- **Marker Description**: An overview of what the test measures and its clinical significance.
- **Range(s)**: Includes both traditional reference ranges and functional or optimal ranges, where applicable.
- **Information About the Test Result**: Insights into high or low values and what they indicate.
- **Therapeutic Insights**: Clinical strategies for addressing abnormalities.
- **Supplements or Medications**: Suggested interventions listed by ingredient names for flexibility.
- **Special Information**: Highlights noteworthy details or unique considerations.
- **Warnings and Alerts**: Identifies risks or cases that require referral to a specialist.

Icons are used throughout the book to quickly identify these sections. Refer to the **Explanation of Icons** at the end of this section for more information.

Using This Book with LabDX Software

This textbook is a static, printed resource designed for reference and invaluable whether on your desk or in the exam room. For real-time updates, supplementation by brand name/dosage, and expanded functionality, the LabDX software is an indispensable tool.

Clinical Application and Approach

Functional Medicine often requires a stepwise and individualized approach. Poor health develops gradually, with dysfunction often building upon existing imbalances. Addressing health concerns effectively means prioritizing the most pressing issues first, resolving those, and then progressing to address additional imbalances.

This textbook is not intended to serve as a "shopping list" of supplements or treatments. Instead, it is a resource to help practitioners craft personalized care plans based on the unique needs, symptoms, and priorities of each patient.

If a specific lab test isn't covered in this volume, refer to the other books in the series or cross-reference markers included in this textbook. Functional markers frequently overlap across panels, and the clinical insights offered here for that specific marker remain relevant even if it's not the exact lab panel.

Explanation of Icons

 Detailed Information — Provides detailed information about the results of the test for a specific marker.

 Therapeutic Insights — Represents therapeutic insights that can guide personalized treatment or lifestyle changes.

 Supplements/Medications — Indicates supplements or medications that might be considered to address deficiencies or imbalances.

 Key Knowledge — Highlights key knowledge, important facts, or noteworthy information related to the test or marker.

 Warnings — Warns of potential risks or important considerations to keep in mind.

Critical Alerts — Signals critical alerts that require immediate attention or further investigation.

By studying this textbook and the full series, you'll gain a deeper understanding of lab interpretation and the tools to transform patient care. Combine this knowledge with LabDX software for the most comprehensive approach to Functional Medicine lab analysis.

Base Level Health

Blood

CBC with differential (Complete Blood Count)

CMP (Comprehensive Metabolic Panel)

Metabolites

Electrolytes

Amino Acids

Iron Panel

Anemia Panel

Urine

Urinalysis

Get LabDx Online Here:

CBC with Differential (Complete Blood Count)

This test measures the specifics of your white blood cell count, plus all your other blood cell levels, including red blood cells and platelets.

White Blood Cell Count (WBC)

White blood cells (WBCs), or leukocytes, are essential for immune defense, acting as phagocytes to engulf bacteria, fungi, and viruses.

Key Facts:
- WBCs make up about 1% of blood in healthy adults.
- Lifespan: 13–20 days, after which they are broken down by the lymphatic system.
- Regulated by the endocrine system; levels can rise with stress, while effectiveness can be impaired by elevated blood sugar.

Normal Range	3.4 – 10.8 x10³/µL
Optimal Range	5.0 – 7.5 x10³/µL

If LOW or < 5 x10³/µL:

Possible conditions include chronic viral or bacterial infections, pancreatic insufficiency, bone marrow insufficiency, B12/B6/folate (B9) anemias, nutrient deficiencies, and chronic intestinal parasites.

- Support immune function and adrenal system.
- Dietary Recommendations: Include foods rich in nutrients supportive of immune function, such as carrots, red/yellow/orange vegetables, dark leafy greens, garlic, kale, almonds, and chicken.

Immune Support:
- Echinacea angustifolia
- Astragalus membranaceus
- Elderberry Extract (Sambucus nigra)
- Andrographis paniculate
- Green Tea Extract
- Arabinogalactan (larch tree)
- Lauric Acid
- Cordyceps mushroom
- Shiitake mushroom
- Maitake mushroom
- Reishi mushroom
- Beta 1,3 Glucans
- Vitamin A
- Vitamin D3
- Vitamin E
- Vitamin K2
- Wild cherry bark
- Ginger
- Lovage (Levisticum officinale)
- Wild Cherry Extract

Digestive Support:
- Digestive enzymes
- Betaine HCl
- Ox Bile
- L-taurine
- Gentian extract
- Dandelion extract
- Fennel
- Amylase
- Protease SP
- Protease
- Diastase
- Lactase
- Glucoamylase
- Alpha-galactosidase

CBC WITH DIFFERENTIAL (COMPLETE BLOOD COUNT)

- Beta-glucanase
- Acid protease
- Phytase
- Cellulase
- Hemicellulase
- Invertase
- Lipase
- Bromelain
- Papain
- Pepsin
- Triphala (Emblica officinalis, Terminalia bellirica, Terminalia chebula)
- Magnesium Hydroxide
- Mastic Gum
- DGL (Deglycyrrhizinated Licorice)
- Methylmethionine Sulfonium Chloride (MMSC)
- Zinc L-Carnosine
- Vitamin C
- Berberine
- Ginger
- Bismuth

Nutritional Support:
- Vitamin B12
- Vitamin B9 (folate)
- Vitamin B6

If **HIGH** or > 7.5 x10³/μL:

Potential indicators include acute viral or bacterial infections, stress, a diet high in refined foods, intestinal parasites, and neoplasms.

Support immune and adrenal systems.

Anti-inflammatory Support:
- Phytocannabinoids
- Hemp Flower Extract
- Hemp Seed Oil
- Palmitoylethanolamide (PEA)
- Omega-3 Fatty Acids (Fish Oil)
- Vitamin D3
- Curcumin
- Green Tea Extract (Epigallocatechin Gallate (EGCG))
- Trans Resveratrol
- Quercetin
- Nettle (Urtica dioica)
- Pro-Resolving Mediators (PRMs): 18-HEPE (18-hydroxy eicosapentaenoic acid), 17-HDHA (17-hydroxy docosahexaenoic acid), 14-HDHA (14-hydroxy docosahexaenoic acid)

Stress Support:
- Gamma-Aminobutyric acid (GABA)
- L-theanine
- 5-HTP
- Phosphatidylserine
- Chamomile
- Inositol
- Taurine
- Magnesium
- Vitamin B6
- Vitamin B12

Red Blood Cell Count (RBC)

Red blood cells (erythrocytes) circulate in the blood, carrying oxygen throughout the body. The bone marrow regulates red blood cell production to maintain stable levels.

Key Facts:
- Primary oxygen carrier to tissues
- Produced at a rate of 2.4 million per second
- 25 trillion RBCs in bloodstream, circulate in 20 seconds, lifespan of 100-120 days, filtered by the spleen

MALE	
Normal Range	$4.2 - 5.8 \times 10^6/\mu L$
Optimal Range	$4.2 - 4.9 \times 10^6/\mu L$

FEMALE	
Normal Range	$3.8 - 5.1 \times 10^6/\mu L$
Optimal Range	$3.9 - 4.5 \times 10^6/\mu L$

If LOW or < $4.2 \times 10^6/\mu L$ (Male) or $3.9 \times 10^6/\mu L$ (Female):

Possible conditions include anemia, chronic liver or kidney dysfunction, free radical damage, blood loss, and Vitamin C deficiency.

- Blood sugar balancing diet:
- For each meal select: 1 protein, 1-2 carbs & 1 fat. Optional 1 starchy carb at dinner.
- Follow the same format for snacks just make them smaller in portion size.
- Eat 2x as many veggies as fruits (ok to skip fruit if sugar-sensitive).
- Drink your water away from meals & get half your body weight in ounces each day.
- Eat every few hours for those dealing with adrenal issues or blood sugar balancing issues
- don't go longer than 4 hours without a meal or snack but try to work your way up to four hours between meals (To go longer in a healthy manner, look at adding more fat; for some gut health issues like SIBO/SIFO 4-5 hours between meals is ideal.)
- Mix cooked and raw veggies (skip raw if dealing with digestive issues)
- Prioritize your organic items by 1. Fats, 2. Protein 3. Produce (look at EWG.org for "Dirty Dozen" & "Clean Fifteen")
- Suggested increase in protein and red meat intake
- Nutritional supplementation with iron, folate (B9), B12, and B6
- Monitor for signs of bleeding or anemia

Iron Support:
- Iron, ferrous bisglycinate

Nutritional Support:
- Vitamin C
- Vitamin B12
- Vitamin B9 (folate)
- Vitamin B6

Digestive Support:
- Digestive enzymes
- Betaine HCl
- Ox Bile
- L-taurine
- Gentian extract
- Dandelion extract
- Fennel
- Amylase

CBC WITH DIFFERENTIAL (COMPLETE BLOOD COUNT)

- Protease SP
- Protease
- Diastase
- Lactase
- Glucoamylase
- Alpha-galactosidase
- Beta-glucanase
- Acid protease
- Phytase
- Cellulase
- Hemicellulase
- Invertase
- Lipase
- Bromelain
- Papain
- Pepsin
- Triphala (Emblica officinalis, Terminalia bellirica, Terminalia chebula)
- Magnesium Hydroxide
- Mastic Gum
- DGL (Deglycyrrhizinated Licorice)
- Methylmethionine Sulfonium Chloride (MMSC)
- Zinc L-Carnosine
- Vitamin C
- Berberine
- Ginger
- Bismuth

If HIGH or > 4.9x10^6/μL (Male) or > 4.5x10^6/μL (Female):

Potential indicators include dehydration, asthma or respiratory distress, or polycythemia.

- Consider respiratory support for blood and cellular oxygenation
- Suggest saltwater for rehydration

Electrolyte Support:
- Potassium
- Sodium
- Chloride
- Magnesium
- Magnesium Bisglycinate
- Vitamin C
- Zinc

Anti-inflammatory Support
- Phytocannabinoids
- Hemp Flower Extract
- Hemp Seed Oil
- Palmitoylethanolamide (PEA)
- Omega-3 Fatty Acids (Fish Oil)
- Pro-Resolving Mediators (PRMs): 18-HEPE (18-hydroxy eicosapentaenoic acid), 17-HDHA (17-hydroxy docosahexaenoic acid), 14-HDHA (14-hydroxy docosahexaenoic acid)
- Vitamin D3
- Curcumin
- Green Tea Extract (Epigallocatechin Gallate (EGCG))
- Trans Resveratrol
- Quercetin
- Nettle (Urtica dioica)

CBC WITH DIFFERENTIAL (COMPLETE BLOOD COUNT)

Hemoglobin

Hemoglobin (Hg) is a red blood cell protein that carries oxygen from the lungs to the body. It is a key marker for identifying anemia (low levels) and dehydration (high levels).

Key Facts:
- Primary oxygen carrier to tissues
- Produced at a rate of 2.4 million per second
- 25 trillion RBCs in bloodstream, circulate in 20 seconds, lifespan of 100-120 days, filtered by the spleen

MALE	
Normal Range	11.1 – 15.9 g/dL
Optimal Range	14 – 15 g/dL

FEMALE	
Normal Range	11.1 – 15.9 g/dL
Optimal Range	13.5 – 14.5 g/dL

If LOW or < 14 g/dL (Male) or 13.5 g/dL (Female):

Possible conditions include iron deficiency anemia, folate (B9) / B12 anemia, nutritional deficiencies (Vitamin C and others), bone marrow deficiencies, intestinal parasites, internal bleeding, and B6 or copper anemia.

Suggested diet high in iron-rich protein, including liver.

Iron Support:
- Iron, ferrous bisglycinate

Nutritional Support:
- Vitamin C
- Vitamin B12
- Vitamin B9 (folate)
- Vitamin B6

Digestive Support:
- Digestive enzymes
- Betaine HCl
- Ox Bile
- L-taurine
- Gentian extract
- Dandelion extract
- Fennel
- Amylase
- Protease SP
- Protease
- Diastase
- Lactase
- Glucoamylase
- Alpha-galactosidase
- Beta-glucanase
- Acid protease
- Phytase
- Cellulase
- Hemicellulase
- Invertase
- Lipase
- Bromelain
- Papain
- Pepsin
- Triphala (Emblica officinalis, Terminalia bellirica, Terminalia chebula)
- Magnesium Hydroxide
- Mastic Gum
- DGL (Deglycyrrhizinated Licorice)
- Methylmethionine Sulfonium Chloride (MMSC)

- Zinc L-Carnosine
- Vitamin C
- Berberine
- Ginger
- Bismuth

If HIGH or > 15 g/dL (Male) or > 14.5 g/dL (Female):

Possible indicators include dehydration, elevated testosterone, polycythemia vera, adrenal dysfunction, respiratory distress or asthma, and spleen hypofunction.

Increase fluid intake or add salt water to address dehydration.

Electrolyte Support:
- Potassium
- Sodium
- Chloride
- Magnesium
- Magnesium Bisglycinate
- Vitamin C
- Zinc

Hematocrit

Hematocrit (HCT) represents the proportion of blood, by volume, that contains red blood cells (RBCs) as opposed to plasma, and it's expressed as a percentage. It is useful in assessing the severity (but not type) of anemia and polycythemia.

Key Facts:
- Typical HCT is around 45% for men and 40% for women
- Typically about three times the hemoglobin concentration
- Indicates the blood's capability of delivering oxygen to cells

MALE	
Normal Range	34 – 46.6%
Optimal Range	40 – 48%

FEMALE	
Normal Range	34 – 46.6%
Optimal Range	37 – 44%

If LOW or < 40% (Male) or < 37% (Female):

Possible conditions include iron deficiency anemia, folate (B9) / B12 anemia, nutritional deficiencies (Vitamin C and others), bone marrow deficiencies, intestinal parasites, internal bleeding, and B6 or copper anemia.

Suggested diet high in iron-rich protein, including liver.

Iron Support:
- Iron, ferrous bisglycinate

Nutritional Support:
- Vitamin C
- Vitamin B12
- Vitamin B9 (folate)
- Vitamin B6

CBC WITH DIFFERENTIAL (COMPLETE BLOOD COUNT)

Digestive Support:
- Digestive enzymes
- Betaine HCl
- Ox Bile
- L-taurine
- Gentian extract
- Dandelion extract
- Fennel
- Amylase
- Protease SP
- Protease
- Diastase
- Lactase
- Glucoamylase
- Alpha-galactosidase
- Beta-glucanase
- Acid protease
- Phytase
- Cellulase
- Hemicellulase
- Invertase
- Lipase
- Bromelain
- Papain
- Pepsin
- Triphala (Emblica officinalis, Terminalia bellirica, Terminalia chebula)
- Magnesium Hydroxide
- Mastic Gum
- DGL (Deglycyrrhizinated Licorice)
- Methylmethionine Sulfonium Chloride (MMSC)
- Zinc L-Carnosine
- Vitamin C
- Berberine
- Ginger
- Bismuth

If HIGH or > 48% (Male) or > 44% (Female):

Possible conditions include various types of anemia (iron, folate (B9) / B12, copper, B6 deficiencies), nutrient deficiencies, increased RBC breakdown by the spleen, bone marrow insufficiency, and blood loss.

Important to exclude potential sources of blood loss, such as gastrointestinal bleeding, hemorrhoids, menstrual cycles, or fibroids

Electrolyte Support:
- Potassium
- Sodium
- Chloride
- Magnesium
- Magnesium Bisglycinate
- Vitamin C
- Zinc

Mean Corpuscular Volume (MCV)

Mean Corpuscular Volume (MCV) is a measure of the average size of each red blood cell (RBC), indicating if RBCs are of normal, small, or enlarged size.

Normal Range	79 – 97 fL
Optimal Range	82.0 – 89.9 fL

If LOW or < 82.0 fL:

Possible conditions include iron deficiency anemia, gastrointestinal or menstrual blood loss, intestinal parasites, rheumatoid arthritis, and heavy metal exposure.

CBC WITH DIFFERENTIAL (COMPLETE BLOOD COUNT)

 Confirm iron deficiency and investigate the underlying cause.

 Iron Support:
- Iron, ferrous bisglycinate

Nutritional Support:
- Vitamin C

Digestive Support:
- Digestive enzymes
- Betaine HCl
- Ox Bile
- L-taurine
- Gentian extract
- Dandelion extract
- Fennel
- Amylase
- Protease SP
- Protease
- Diastase
- Lactase
- Glucoamylase
- Alpha-galactosidase
- Beta-glucanase
- Acid protease
- Phytase
- Cellulase
- Hemicellulase
- Invertase
- Lipase
- Bromelain
- Papain
- Pepsin
- Triphala (Emblica officinalis, Terminalia bellirica, Terminalia chebula)
- Magnesium Hydroxide
- Mastic Gum
- DGL (Deglycyrrhizinated Licorice)
- Methylmethionine Sulfonium Chloride (MMSC)
- Zinc L-Carnosine
- Vitamin C
- Berberine
- Ginger
- Bismuth

If **HIGH** or > 89.9 fL:

 Potential indicators include folate (B9) / B12 deficiency anemia, hypochlorhydria (low stomach acid), and pernicious anemia.

 Focus on supporting gastric hydrochloric acid (HCL) and small intestine (SI) function.

 Nutritional Support:
- Vitamin B12
- Vitamin B9 (folate)
- Vitamin B6

Digestive Support:
- Digestive enzymes
- Betaine HCl
- Ox Bile
- L-taurine
- Gentian extract
- Dandelion extract
- Fennel
- Amylase
- Protease SP
- Protease
- Diastase
- Lactase
- Glucoamylase
- Alpha-galactosidase

- Beta-glucanase
- Acid protease
- Phytase
- Cellulase
- Hemicellulase
- Invertase
- Lipase
- Bromelain
- Papain
- Pepsin
- Triphala (Emblica officinalis, Terminalia bellirica, Terminalia chebula)
- Magnesium Hydroxide
- Mastic Gum
- DGL (Deglycyrrhizinated Licorice)
- Methylmethionine Sulfonium Chloride (MMSC)
- Zinc L-Carnosine
- Vitamin C
- Berberine
- Ginger
- Bismuth

Mean Corpuscular Hemoglobin (MCH)

Mean Corpuscular Hemoglobin (MCH) measures the average amount of hemoglobin inside a single red blood cell (RBC), reflecting the weight of hemoglobin in each RBC.

Normal Range	26.6 – 33 pg
Optimal Range	28.0 – 31.9 pg

If LOW or < 28 pg:

Possible conditions include iron deficiency anemia, B6 deficiency anemia, rheumatoid arthritis, and intestinal parasites.

Confirm iron deficiency and investigate the underlying cause.

Iron Support:
- Iron, ferrous bisglycinate

Nutritional Support:
- Vitamin C
- Vitamin B6

Digestive Support:
- Digestive enzymes
- Betaine HCl
- Ox Bile
- L-taurine
- Gentian extract
- Dandelion extract
- Fennel
- Amylase
- Protease SP
- Protease
- Diastase
- Lactase
- Glucoamylase
- Alpha-galactosidase
- Beta-glucanase
- Acid protease
- Phytase
- Cellulase
- Hemicellulase
- Invertase
- Lipase
- Bromelain
- Papain
- Pepsin

- Triphala (Emblica officinalis, Terminalia bellirica, Terminalia chebula)
- Magnesium Hydroxide
- Mastic Gum
- DGL (Deglycyrrhizinated Licorice)
- Methylmethionine Sulfonium Chloride (MMSC)
- Zinc L-Carnosine
- Vitamin C
- Berberine
- Ginger
- Bismuth

If **HIGH** or > 31.9 pg:

Potential indicators include folate (B9) / B12 deficiency anemia, hypochlorhydria (low stomach acid), and pernicious anemia.

Focus on supporting gastric hydrochloric acid (HCL) and small intestine (SI) function. Refer to MCV for additional context.

Nutritional Support:
- Vitamin B12
- Vitamin B9 (folate)

Digestive Support:
- Digestive enzymes
- Betaine HCl
- Ox Bile
- L-taurine
- Gentian extract
- Dandelion extract
- Fennel
- Amylase
- Protease SP
- Protease
- Diastase
- Lactase
- Glucoamylase
- Alpha-galactosidase
- Beta-glucanase
- Acid protease
- Phytase
- Cellulase
- Hemicellulase
- Invertase
- Lipase
- Bromelain
- Papain
- Pepsin
- Triphala (Emblica officinalis, Terminalia bellirica, Terminalia chebula)
- Magnesium Hydroxide
- Mastic Gum
- DGL (Deglycyrrhizinated Licorice)
- Methylmethionine Sulfonium Chloride (MMSC)
- Zinc L-Carnosine
- Vitamin C
- Berberine
- Ginger
- Bismuth

Mean Corpuscular Hemoglobin Concentration (MCHC)

Mean Corpuscular Hemoglobin Concentration (MCHC) measures the average concentration of hemoglobin in red blood cells (RBCs), relative to the size of the cells. It is a sensitive test for iron-deficiency anemia, calculated using hematocrit (HCT) and hemoglobin (Hg) values.

Normal Range	31.5 – 37 g/dL
Optimal Range	32.0 – 35.0 g/dL

CBC WITH DIFFERENTIAL (COMPLETE BLOOD COUNT)

If **LOW** or < 32 g/dL:

Possible conditions include iron deficiency anemia, B6 deficiency anemia, rheumatoid arthritis, and intestinal parasites.

Confirm iron deficiency and identify the underlying cause.

Iron Support:
- Iron, ferrous bisglycinate

Nutritional Support:
- Vitamin C
- Vitamin B6

Digestive Support:
- Digestive enzymes
- Betaine HCl
- Ox Bile
- L-taurine
- Gentian extract
- Dandelion extract
- Fennel
- Amylase
- Protease SP
- Protease
- Diastase
- Lactase
- Glucoamylase
- Alpha-galactosidase
- Beta-glucanase
- Acid protease
- Phytase
- Cellulase
- Hemicellulase
- Invertase
- Lipase
- Bromelain
- Papain
- Pepsin
- Triphala (Emblica officinalis, Terminalia bellirica, Terminalia chebula)
- Magnesium Hydroxide
- Mastic Gum
- DGL (Deglycyrrhizinated Licorice)
- Methylmethionine Sulfonium Chloride (MMSC)
- Zinc L-Carnosine
- Vitamin C
- Berberine
- Ginger
- Bismuth

If **HIGH** or > 35 g/dL:

Potential indicators include folate (B9) / B12 deficiency anemia, hypochlorhydria (low stomach acid), and pernicious anemia.

Focus on supporting gastric hydrochloric acid (HCL) and small intestine (SI) function. Refer to MCV for additional context.

Nutritional Support:
- Vitamin B12
- Vitamin B9 (folate)

Digestive Support:
- Digestive enzymes
- Betaine HCl
- Ox Bile
- L-taurine
- Gentian extract
- Dandelion extract
- Fennel
- Amylase
- Protease SP
- Protease

- Diastase
- Lactase
- Glucoamylase
- Alpha-galactosidase
- Beta-glucanase
- Acid protease
- Phytase
- Cellulase
- Hemicellulase
- Invertase
- Lipase
- Bromelain
- Papain
- Pepsin

- Triphala (Emblica officinalis, Terminalia bellirica, Terminalia chebula)
- Magnesium Hydroxide
- Mastic Gum
- DGL (Deglycyrrhizinated Licorice)
- Methylmethionine Sulfonium Chloride (MMSC)
- Zinc L-Carnosine
- Vitamin C
- Berberine
- Ginger
- Bismuth

Red Blood Cell Distribution Width (RDW)

Red Blood Cell Distribution Width (RDW) is a measure of the size variability of circulating red blood cells (RBCs), reflecting the consistency in RBC size.

Normal Range	12.3 – 15.4%
Optimal Range	12.0 – 13.0%

If LOW or < 12%:

 Possible conditions include post-hemorrhagic anemia.

 Recommended diet high in iron-rich protein, including liver. Consider supplemental iron and digestive support.

Iron Support:
- Iron, ferrous bisglycinate

Nutritional Support:
- Vitamin C

Digestive Support:
- Digestive enzymes
- Betaine HCl
- Ox Bile
- L-taurine
- Gentian extract
- Dandelion extract
- Fennel
- Amylase
- Protease SP
- Protease
- Diastase
- Lactase
- Glucoamylase
- Alpha-galactosidase
- Beta-glucanase
- Acid protease
- Phytase
- Cellulase
- Hemicellulase
- Invertase
- Lipase
- Bromelain
- Papain
- Pepsin

CBC WITH DIFFERENTIAL (COMPLETE BLOOD COUNT)

- Triphala (Emblica officinalis, Terminalia bellirica, Terminalia chebula)
- Magnesium Hydroxide
- Mastic Gum
- DGL (Deglycyrrhizinated Licorice)
- Methylmethionine Sulfonium Chloride (MMSC)
- Zinc L-Carnosine
- Vitamin C
- Berberine
- Ginger
- Bismuth

If **HIGH** or **> 13%**:

Potential indicators include folate (B9) / B12 deficiency anemia, iron-deficiency anemia, and pernicious anemia (due to decreased intrinsic factor and inability to absorb B12).

Suggested protocol includes folate (B9), B12, Iron and Digestive Support

Iron Support:
- Iron, ferrous bisglycinate

Nutritional Support:
- Vitamin B12
- Vitamin B9 (folate)

Digestive Support:
- Digestive enzymes
- Betaine HCl
- Ox Bile
- L-taurine
- Gentian extract
- Dandelion extract
- Fennel
- Amylase
- Protease SP
- Protease
- Diastase
- Lactase
- Glucoamylase
- Alpha-galactosidase
- Beta-glucanase
- Acid protease
- Phytase
- Cellulase
- Hemicellulase
- Invertase
- Lipase
- Bromelain
- Papain
- Pepsin
- Triphala (Emblica officinalis, Terminalia bellirica, Terminalia chebula)
- Magnesium Hydroxide
- Mastic Gum
- DGL (Deglycyrrhizinated Licorice)
- Methylmethionine Sulfonium Chloride (MMSC)
- Zinc L-Carnosine
- Vitamin C
- Berberine
- Ginger
- Bismuth

CBC WITH DIFFERENTIAL (COMPLETE BLOOD COUNT)

Platelets

Platelets are small cells in the blood essential for normal blood clotting, with a primary function of stopping bleeding.

Normal Range	155 – 379 x10³/µL
Optimal Range	185 – 385 x10³/µL

If LOW or < 185 x10³/µL:

 Potential conditions include inflammation, atherosclerosis, excessive oxidative stress, and neoplasm.

 If value is ≤150, refer out for further evaluation.
Consider dietary and lifestyle interventions to support immune function:

Diet Considerations:
- Emphasize foods high in essential micronutrients (e.g., zinc, Vitamin D, Vitamin C, omega-3s, and high-quality protein).
- Encourage reducing dietary sugar and alcohol, optimizing omega-3s for anti-inflammatory support, and increasing protein intake as needed (RDA: 0.8 g/kg of body weight).

Lifestyle Interventions:
- Promote sleep hygiene for restorative rest, stress management techniques (e.g., meditation, breath work), and balanced physical activity.

 Immune Support:
- Echinacea angustifolia
- Astragalus membranaceus
- Elderberry Extract (Sambucus nigra)
- Andrographis paniculate
- Green Tea Extract
- Arabinogalactan (larch tree)
- Lauric Acid
- Cordyceps mushroom
- Shiitake mushroom
- Maitake mushroom
- Reishi mushroom
- Beta 1,3 Glucans
- Vitamin A
- Vitamin D3
- Vitamin E
- Vitamin K2
- Wild cherry bark
- Ginger
- Lovage (Levisticum officinale)
- Wild Cherry Extract

Antioxidants:
- Acerola Extract (Malpighia glabra)
- Grape Seed Extract (Vitis vinifera)
- Curcumin
- Garlic (Allium sativum)
- Ginkgo Extract (Ginkgo biloba)
- Quercetin
- Rutin
- Clove (Syzygium aromaticum)
- Allspice (Pimenta dioica)
- Sweet Basil (Ocimum basilicum)
- Sage (Salvia officinalis)
- Rosemary Extract (Rosmarinus officinalis)
- Lutein
- Lycopene
- Trans Resveratrol
- Vitamin A
- Vitamin E
- L-glutathione
- NAC (N-Acetyl-L-Cysteine)
- Broccoli Powder Extract
- Sulforaphane
- Olive Leaf Extract (Olea europaea)

CBC WITH DIFFERENTIAL (COMPLETE BLOOD COUNT)

- Bergamot
- Red Grape Powder
- Alpha Lipoic Acid
- Taurine
- MVM (Multi-vitamin/mineral)
- Glutathione (reduced)

If **HIGH** or > 385 x10³/μL:

Potential conditions include inflammation, atherosclerosis, excessive oxidative stress, and neoplasm.

Obesity can be a possible contributor to platelet aggregation. [PMID: 18385810]

Anti-inflammatory Support
- Phytocannabinoids
- Hemp Flower Extract
- Hemp Seed Oil
- Palmitoylethanolamide (PEA)
- Omega-3 Fatty Acids (Fish Oil)
- Pro-Resolving Mediators (PRMs): 18-HEPE (18-hydroxy eicosapentaenoic acid), 17-HDHA (17-hydroxy docosahexaenoic acid), 14-HDHA (14-hydroxy docosahexaenoic acid)
- Vitamin D3
- Curcumin
- Green Tea Extract (Epigallocatechin Gallate (EGCG))
- Trans Resveratrol
- Quercetin
- Nettle (Urtica dioica)

Antioxidants:
- Acerola Extract (Malpighia glabra)
- Grape Seed Extract (Vitis vinifera)
- Curcumin
- Garlic (Allium sativum)
- Ginkgo Extract (Ginkgo biloba)
- Quercetin
- Rutin
- Clove (Syzygium aromaticum)
- Allspice (Pimenta dioica)
- Sweet Basil (Ocimum basilicum)
- Sage (Salvia officinalis)
- Rosemary Extract (Rosmarinus officinalis)
- Lutein
- Lycopene
- Trans Resveratrol
- Vitamin A
- Vitamin E
- L-glutathione
- NAC (N-Acetyl-L-Cysteine)
- Broccoli Powder Extract
- Sulforaphane
- Olive Leaf Extract (Olea europaea)
- Bergamot
- Red Grape Powder
- Alpha Lipoic Acid
- Taurine
- MVM (Multi-vitamin/mineral)
- Glutathione (reduced)

Mean Platelet Volume (MPV)

Mean Platelet Volume (MPV) measures the average size of platelets, with variations indicating different risks related to clotting and platelet production.

Normal Range	7.5 - 11.5 fL
Optimal Range	7.5 - 8.2 fL

CBC WITH DIFFERENTIAL (COMPLETE BLOOD COUNT)

If **LOW** or < 7.5 fL:

 Low MPV may indicate a bleeding disorder due to the presence of smaller, older platelets, possibly linked to conditions affecting platelet production in the bone marrow.

Dietary Considerations:
- Emphasize foods high in essential micronutrients (e.g., zinc, Vitamin D, Vitamin C, omega-3s, and high-quality protein).
- Encourage reducing dietary sugar and alcohol, and optimizing omega-3s for anti-inflammatory support.
- Lifestyle Interventions:
- Promote sleep hygiene for restorative rest, stress management techniques (e.g., meditation, breath work), and balanced physical activity.

Immune Support:
- Echinacea angustifolia
- Astragalus membranaceus
- Elderberry Extract (Sambucus nigra)
- Andrographis paniculate
- Green Tea Extract
- Arabinogalactan (larch tree)
- Lauric Acid
- Cordyceps mushroom
- Shiitake mushroom
- Maitake mushroom
- Reishi mushroom
- Beta 1,3 Glucans
- Vitamin A
- Vitamin D3
- Vitamin E
- Vitamin K2
- Wild cherry bark
- Ginger
- Lovage (Levisticum officinale)
- Wild Cherry Extract

If **HIGH** or > 8.2 fL:

 High MPV may increase the risk for heart attack or stroke due to larger, younger platelets. It may result from rapid platelet production by the bone marrow and can be associated with conditions like immune thrombocytopenic purpura (ITP), genetic mutations, or cancer.

Additional insights:
- Low platelet count + high MPV: Indicates platelet destruction due to antibodies, infection, or toxins.
- High platelet count + high MPV: Often due to genetic mutations or bone marrow disorders.
- Normal platelet count + high MPV: May indicate conditions like hyperthyroidism or chronic myelogenous leukemia (CML).

Regular strenuous physical activity (e.g., endurance training) may also increase MPV.

Dietary Guidelines:
- Reduce sodium, limit alcohol, minimize dietary sugar, and optimize omega-3 intake for anti-inflammatory support.
- Fatty fish: SMASH (salmon, mackerel, anchovy, sardine, herring)

Lifestyle Modifications:
- Focus on weight management and increase physical activity.

Anti-inflammatory Support:
- Phytocannabinoids
- Hemp Flower Extract
- Hemp Seed Oil
- Palmitoylethanolamide (PEA)
- Omega-3 Fatty Acids (Fish Oil)
- Vitamin D3
- Curcumin
- Green Tea Extract (Epigallocatechin Gallate (EGCG))
- Trans Resveratrol
- Quercetin
- Nettle (Urtica dioica)
- Pro-Resolving Mediators (PRMs): 18-HEPE (18-hydroxy eicosapentaenoic acid), 17-HDHA (17-hydroxy docosahexaenoic acid), 14-HDHA (14-hydroxy docosahexaenoic acid)

Antioxidants:
- Acerola Extract (Malpighia glabra)
- Grape Seed Extract (Vitis vinifera)
- Curcumin
- Garlic (Allium sativum)
- Ginkgo Extract (Ginkgo biloba)
- Quercetin
- Rutin
- Clove (Syzygium aromaticum)
- Allspice (Pimenta dioica)
- Sweet Basil (Ocimum basilicum)
- Sage (Salvia officinalis)
- Rosemary Extract (Rosmarinus officinalis)
- Lutein
- Lycopene
- Trans Resveratrol
- Vitamin A
- Vitamin E
- L-glutathione
- NAC (N-Acetyl-L-Cysteine)
- Broccoli Powder Extract
- Sulforaphane
- Olive Leaf Extract (Olea europaea)
- Bergamot
- Red Grape Powder
- Alpha Lipoic Acid
- Taurine
- MVM (Multi-vitamin/mineral)
- Glutathione (reduced)

Neutrophils

Neutrophils are the most abundant type of white blood cell in healthy adults and serve as the body's primary defense against bacterial, viral, and fungal infections.

Key Facts:
- Make up 60–70% of WBCs
- Lifespan of approximately 8 days
- First responders to infection, react to inflammation, and digest bacteria

Normal Range	4.0 – 7.4 x10³/µL	40% – 60%
Optimal Range	4.0 – 6.0 x10³/µL	40% – 60%

If **LOW** or < 4.0 x10³/µL:

Possible conditions include chronic viral or bacterial infections, pancreatic insufficiency, bone marrow insufficiency, B12/B6/folate (B9) anemias, nutrient deficiencies, and chronic intestinal parasites.

Support immune function and include a protocol with B9/B12.

CBC WITH DIFFERENTIAL (COMPLETE BLOOD COUNT)

Immune Support:
- Echinacea angustifolia
- Astragalus membranaceus
- Elderberry Extract (Sambucus nigra)
- Andrographis paniculate
- Green Tea Extract
- Arabinogalactan (larch tree)
- Lauric Acid
- Cordyceps mushroom
- Shiitake mushroom
- Maitake mushroom
- Reishi mushroom
- Beta 1,3 Glucans
- Vitamin A
- Vitamin D3
- Vitamin E
- Vitamin K2
- Wild cherry bark
- Ginger
- Lovage (Levisticum officinale)
- Wild Cherry Extract

Digestive Support
- Digestive enzymes
- Betaine HCl, Pepsin
- Ox Bile
- Taurine

Nutritional support
- Vitamin B9 (folate)
- Vitamin B12
- Vitamin B6

If **HIGH** or > 6.0 x10³/µL:

Potential indicators include acute bacterial, viral, or fungal infections, inflammation, leaky gut, emotional or physical stress, and intestinal parasites. High neutrophil levels can also be due to physiological stress, rigorous exercise, smoking, and chronic leukemia.

Consider protocols for vitamin C, PMGs (protomorphogens), adrenal support, bacterial response, and enzyme support. Anti-inflammatory and gut health protocols may be beneficial.

Anti-inflammatory Support:
- Phytocannabinoids
- Hemp Flower Extract
- Hemp Seed Oil
- Palmitoylethanolamide (PEA)
- Omega-3 Fatty Acids (Fish Oil)
- Vitamin D3
- Curcumin
- Green Tea Extract (Epigallocatechin Gallate (EGCG))
- Trans Resveratrol
- Quercetin
- Nettle (Urtica dioica)
- Pro-Resolving Mediators (PRMs): 18-HEPE (18-hydroxy eicosapentaenoic acid), 17-HDHA (17-hydroxy docosahexaenoic acid), 14-HDHA (14-hydroxy docosahexaenoic acid)

Stress Support:
- Gamma-Aminobutyric acid (GABA)
- L-theanine
- 5-HTP
- Phosphatidylserine
- Chamomile
- Inositol
- Taurine
- Magnesium
- Vitamin B6
- Vitamin B12

Lymphocytes

Lymphocytes, a type of white blood cell, play a critical role in the immune system. They include B-cells, T-cells, and natural killer cells, which are essential for adaptive immunity and immune defense.

Key Facts:
- Represent 20–40% of total white blood cells.
- Lymphocytes identify and eliminate foreign pathogens like bacteria and viruses and help attack tumor cells.

Normal Range	1.4 – 4.6 x10³/µL	24% – 44%
Optimal Range	2.4 – 4.4 x10³/µL	24% – 44%

If LOW or < 2.4 x10³/µL:

Potential conditions include chronic viral or bacterial infections, bone marrow insufficiency, oxidative stress, autoimmune disorders, bone marrow damage, and immune deficiency.

Immune support is recommended.

Immune Support:
- Echinacea angustifolia
- Astragalus membranaceus
- Elderberry Extract (Sambucus nigra)
- Andrographis paniculate
- Green Tea Extract
- Arabinogalactan (larch tree)
- Lauric Acid
- Cordyceps mushroom
- Shiitake mushroom
- Maitake mushroom
- Reishi mushroom
- Beta 1,3 Glucans
- Vitamin A
- Vitamin D3
- Vitamin E
- Vitamin K2
- Wild cherry bark
- Ginger
- Lovage (Levisticum officinale)
- Wild Cherry Extract

If HIGH or > 4.4 x10³/µL:

Potential indicators include acute viral or bacterial infections, parasitic infections, inflammation, compromised detox pathways, and overall toxicity. High lymphocyte levels are often seen in response to acute viral infections and some bacterial infections.

Support immune function, build natural defense mechanisms, and consider anti-inflammatory and gut-healing protocols, as well as anti-parasitic support if necessary.

Immune Support:
- Echinacea angustifolia
- Astragalus membranaceus
- Elderberry Extract (Sambucus nigra)
- Andrographis paniculate
- Green Tea Extract
- Arabinogalactan (larch tree)
- Lauric Acid
- Cordyceps mushroom
- Shiitake mushroom
- Maitake mushroom
- Reishi mushroom
- Beta 1,3 Glucans

- Vitamin A
- Vitamin D3
- Vitamin E
- Vitamin K2

Anti-inflammatory Support:
- Phytocannabinoids
- Hemp Flower Extract
- Hemp Seed Oil
- Palmitoylethanolamide (PEA)
- Omega-3 Fatty Acids (Fish Oil)
- docosahexaenoic acid), 14-HDHA (14-hydroxy docosahexaenoic acid)
- Vitamin D3
- Curcumin

Antimicrobial Agents:
- Oregano Oil (Origanum vulgare)
- Garlic
- Tribulus terrestris
- Magnesium Caprylate
- Berberine
- Bearberry Extract (Arctostaphylos uva-ursi)

Gut & Immune Support:
- Serum-Derived Bovine Immunoglobulin Concentrate
- Immunoglobulin G
- N-Acetyl-D-Glucosamine
- Colostrum
- Protein Powder
- Mixed Amino Acids
- Zinc L-Carnosine
- L-Glutamine
- Citrus Pectin
- Deglycyrrhizinated Licorice Extract (DGL)
- Aloe Vera

- Wild cherry bark
- Ginger
- Lovage (Levisticum officinale)
- Wild Cherry Extract

- Green Tea Extract (Epigallocatechin Gallate (EGCG))
- Trans Resveratrol
- Quercetin
- Nettle (Urtica dioica)
- Pro-Resolving Mediators (PRMs): 18-HEPE (18-hydroxy eicosapentaenoic acid), 17-HDHA (17-hydroxy

- Black Walnut Powder (Juglans nigra)
- Barberry Extract (Berberis spp.)
- Artemisia (wormwood)
- Purified Silver
- Alpha Lipoic Acid

- Slippery Elm
- Mucin
- Chamomile Extract
- Marshmallow
- Okra
- Cat's Claw
- Methylsulfonylmethane (MSM)
- Quercetin
- Prune Powder
- Aloe Vera Leaf Gel Extract
- Apple Pectin
- Iron
- Glucosamine HCl

Monocytes

Monocytes are large white blood cells that engulf bacteria and other foreign particles. They make up 2–8% of total WBCs. Once in the tissues, monocytes mature into macrophages, which are scavenger cells that remove dead cells and destroy invasive microorganisms.

Normal Range	0.4 – 1.2 x10³/µL	0% – 7%
Optimal Range	0.4 – 0.7 x10³/µL	0% – 7%

CBC WITH DIFFERENTIAL (COMPLETE BLOOD COUNT)

If LOW or < 0.4 x10³/µL:

 Low monocyte levels, known as monocytopenia, can result from bone marrow damage, bone marrow failure, or conditions like hairy-cell leukemia.

 Anti-inflammatory support is recommended.

 Anti-inflammatory Support:
- Phytocannabinoids
- Hemp Flower Extract
- Hemp Seed Oil
- Palmitoylethanolamide (PEA)
- Omega-3 Fatty Acids (Fish Oil)
- Vitamin D3
- Curcumin
- Green Tea Extract (Epigallocatechin Gallate (EGCG))
- Trans Resveratrol
- Quercetin
- Nettle (Urtica dioica)
- Pro-Resolving Mediators (PRMs): 18-HEPE (18-hydroxy eicosapentaenoic acid), 17-HDHA (17-hydroxy docosahexaenoic acid), 14-HDHA (14-hydroxy docosahexaenoic acid)

If HIGH or > 0.7 x10³/µL:

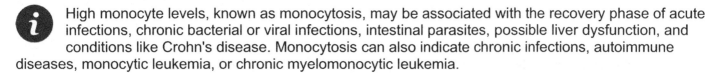 High monocyte levels, known as monocytosis, may be associated with the recovery phase of acute infections, chronic bacterial or viral infections, intestinal parasites, possible liver dysfunction, and conditions like Crohn's disease. Monocytosis can also indicate chronic infections, autoimmune diseases, monocytic leukemia, or chronic myelomonocytic leukemia.

 Immune support is recommended until further cause identification.

 Immune Support:
- Echinacea angustifolia
- Astragalus membranaceus
- Elderberry Extract (Sambucus nigra)
- Andrographis paniculate
- Green Tea Extract
- Arabinogalactan (larch tree)
- Lauric Acid
- Cordyceps mushroom
- Shiitake mushroom
- Maitake mushroom
- Reishi mushroom
- Beta 1,3 Glucans
- Vitamin A
- Vitamin D3
- Vitamin E
- Vitamin K2
- Wild cherry bark
- Ginger
- Lovage (Levisticum officinale)
- Wild Cherry Extract

Eosinophils

Eosinophils are white blood cells that respond to infections caused by parasites and play a role in allergic reactions. They help regulate immune responses and inflammation. Eosinophils are primarily found in tissues rather than the blood, and elevated levels indicate immune activity in tissues.

Normal Range	0 – 0.5 x10³/µL	0% – 3%
Optimal Range	< 0.5 x10E3/µL	0% – 3%

CBC WITH DIFFERENTIAL (COMPLETE BLOOD COUNT)

If HIGH or > 0.5 x10³/µL:

 High eosinophil levels, known as eosinophilia, can be associated with intestinal parasites, food or environmental allergies, skin disorders, and systemic infections. Other causes include asthma, allergies, drug reactions, inflammatory disorders, and certain cancers.
Eosinophils release histamine, serotonin, and heparin, which influence the immune system.

 Consider protocols for parasite and GI cleansing, and address food allergies if indicated.

Immune Support:
- Echinacea angustifolia
- Astragalus membranaceus
- Elderberry Extract (Sambucus nigra)
- Andrographis paniculate
- Green Tea Extract
- Arabinogalactan (larch tree)
- Lauric Acid
- Cordyceps mushroom
- Shiitake mushroom
- Maitake mushroom
- Reishi mushroom
- Beta 1,3 Glucans
- Vitamin A
- Vitamin D3
- Vitamin E
- Vitamin K2
- Wild cherry bark
- Ginger
- Lovage (Levisticum officinale)
- Wild Cherry Extract

Anti-inflammatory Support:
- Phytocannabinoids
- Hemp Flower Extract
- Hemp Seed Oil
- Palmitoylethanolamide (PEA)
- Omega-3 Fatty Acids (Fish Oil)
- docosahexaenoic acid), 14-HDHA (14-hydroxy docosahexaenoic acid)
- Vitamin D3
- Curcumin
- Green Tea Extract (Epigallocatechin Gallate (EGCG))
- Trans Resveratrol
- Quercetin
- Nettle (Urtica dioica)
- Pro-Resolving Mediators (PRMs): 18-HEPE (18-hydroxy eicosapentaenoic acid), 17-HDHA (17-hydroxy

Antimicrobial Agents:
- Oregano Oil (Origanum vulgare)
- Garlic
- Tribulus terrestris
- Magnesium Caprylate
- Berberine
- Bearberry Extract (Arctostaphylos uva-ursi)
- Black Walnut Powder (Juglans nigra)
- Barberry Extract (Berberis spp.)
- Artemisia (wormwood)
- Purified Silver
- Alpha Lipoic Acid

Gut & Immune Support:
- Serum-Derived Bovine Immunoglobulin Concentrate
- Immunoglobulin G
- N-Acetyl-D-Glucosamine
- Colostrum
- Protein Powder
- Mixed Amino Acids
- Zinc L-Carnosine
- L-Glutamine
- Citrus Pectin
- Deglycyrrhizinated Licorice Extract (DGL)
- Aloe Vera
- Slippery Elm
- Mucin
- Chamomile Extract
- Marshmallow
- Okra

- Cat's Claw
- Methylsulfonylmethane (MSM)
- Quercetin
- Prune Powder
- Aloe Vera Leaf Gel Extract
- Apple Pectin
- Iron
- Glucosamine HCl

Basophils

Basophils are white blood cells involved in allergic responses and inflammation control. They release histamine, which increases blood flow to tissues, and heparin to prevent blood clotting too quickly. Basophils, while less than 1% of circulating WBCs, are the largest mature WBC and aid in phagocytosis, engulfing pathogens. They help regulate eosinophil levels and respond to allergens.

Normal Range	0 - 0.3 x10³/µL	0% – 1%
Optimal Range	< 0.3 x10³/µL	0% – 1%

If HIGH or > 0.3 x10E3/µL:

High eosinophil levels, known as eosinophilia, can be associated with intestinal parasites, food or environmental allergies, skin disorders, and systemic infections. Other causes include asthma, allergies, drug reactions, inflammatory disorders, and certain cancers.
Eosinophils release histamine, serotonin, and heparin, which influence the immune system.

Consider protocols for parasite and GI cleansing, and address food allergies if indicated.

Immune Support:
- Echinacea angustifolia
- Astragalus membranaceus
- Elderberry Extract (Sambucus nigra)
- Andrographis paniculate
- Green Tea Extract
- Arabinogalactan (larch tree)
- Lauric Acid
- Cordyceps mushroom
- Shiitake mushroom
- Maitake mushroom
- Reishi mushroom
- Beta 1,3 Glucans
- Vitamin A
- Vitamin D3
- Vitamin E
- Vitamin K2
- Wild cherry bark
- Ginger
- Lovage (Levisticum officinale)
- Wild Cherry Extract

Anti-inflammatory Support:
- Phytocannabinoids
- Hemp Flower Extract
- Hemp Seed Oil
- Palmitoylethanolamide (PEA)
- Omega-3 Fatty Acids (Fish Oil)
- docosahexaenoic acid), 14-HDHA (14-hydroxy docosahexaenoic acid)
- Vitamin D3
- Curcumin
- Green Tea Extract (Epigallocatechin Gallate (EGCG))
- Trans Resveratrol
- Quercetin
- Nettle (Urtica dioica)
- Pro-Resolving Mediators (PRMs): 18-HEPE (18-hydroxy eicosapentaenoic acid), 17-HDHA (17-hydroxy

Histamine Support:
- Vitamin C
- Nettle
- Quercetin
- Sodium Bicarbonate
- Potassium Bicarbonate
- Guduchi (Tinospora cordifolia)

Thyroid Support:
- N-Acetyl-L-Tyrosine
- American Ginseng (Panax quinquefolius)
- Forskolin (Coleus forskohlii)
- Iodine
- Chromium
- Zinc
- Selenium
- Copper
- Manganese
- Vitamin A
- Vitamin B2
- Potassium Iodide
- Myo-Inositol

Antimicrobial Agents:
- Oregano Oil (Origanum vulgare)
- Garlic
- Tribulus terrestris
- Magnesium Caprylate
- Berberine
- Bearberry Extract (Arctostaphylos uva-ursi)
- Black Walnut Powder (Juglans nigra)
- Barberry Extract (Berberis spp.)
- Artemisia (wormwood)
- Purified Silver
- Alpha Lipoic Acid

Gut & Immune Support:
- Serum-Derived Bovine Immunoglobulin Concentrate
- Immunoglobulin G
- N-Acetyl-D-Glucosamine
- Colostrum
- Protein Powder
- Mixed Amino Acids
- Zinc L-Carnosine
- L-Glutamine
- Citrus Pectin
- Deglycyrrhizinated Licorice Extract (DGL)
- Aloe Vera
- Slippery Elm
- Mucin
- Chamomile Extract
- Marshmallow
- Okra
- Cat's Claw
- Methylsulfonylmethane (MSM)
- Quercetin
- Prune Powder
- Aloe Vera Leaf Gel Extract
- Apple Pectin
- Iron
- Glucosamine HCl

CMP (Comprehensive Metabolic Panel)

A comprehensive metabolic panel (CMP) is a blood sample test that measures 18 different markers in your blood. It provides important information about your body's chemical balance and metabolism (how your body transforms the food you eat into energy).

Glucose - Fasting

Fasting glucose provides insight into blood sugar regulation, a complex process involving the pancreas (insulin/glucagon), adrenal glands (cortisol), and liver (gluconeogenesis). Imbalances may arise from issues like poor glycogen storage or breakdown in the liver, hormone imbalances (e.g., cortisol, estrogen), receptor insensitivity, or insufficient insulin production from pancreatic beta cells. Stable blood sugar is critical for a healthy immune response.

Normal Range	65 – 99 mg/dL
Optimal Range	80 – 100 mg/dL

If LOW or < 80 mg/dL:

 Possible causes include reactive hypoglycemia, impaired liver glycogen storage, excessive insulin, adrenal or thyroid hypofunction, high-dose salicylates, protein malnutrition, or liver dysfunction.

 Consider increasing protein and fat intake, monitor glucose handling throughout the day, and consider additional blood sugar-related testing.

Manage stress with relaxation techniques, avoid stimulants, ensure regular balanced exercise with high-intensity intervals, stay hydrated, avoid alcohol and smoking, and maintain adequate sleep.

Eat several small meals throughout the day, include healthy fats and proteins, avoid refined carbs, increase dietary fiber, consume omega-3-rich foods, and aim for 9 servings of vegetables/fruits daily.

 Glucose Metabolism Support:

- Magnesium
- Zinc
- Selenium
- Manganese
- Chromium
- Molybdenum
- Potassium Iodide
- Taurine
- Carnosine
- R-Lipoic Acid
- Vitamin A
- Vitamin D3
- Vitamin E
- Vitamin K1
- Benfotiamine (Fat-Soluble Vitamin B1)
- Vitamin B1
- Vitamin B2
- Vitamin B3
- Vitamin B5
- Vitamin B6
- Vitamin B7 (Biotin)
- Vitamin B9 (Folate)
- Vitamin B12
- Vitamin C
- Berberine
- Fenugreek
- Gymnema sylvestre
- Banaba (Lagerstroemia speciosa)
- Kudzu (Pueraria lobata)
- Cinnamon
- Inositol (as Myo and D-Chiro)
- Alpha Lipoic Acid
- MVM (Multi-vitamin/mineral)

Adrenal Support:
- gamma-Aminobutyric Acid (GABA)
- Eleutherococcus senticosus
- American Ginseng
- Ashwagandha
- Rhodiola
- Licorice
- Vitamin B2
- Vitamin B5
- Vitamin B6
- Vitamin C
- N-Acetyl-L-Tyrosine
- Phosphatidylserine
- Valerian
- Passion Flower
- Lemon Balm
- Chamomile
- L-theanine
- 5-HTP
- Melatonin
- Rhodiola rosea
- Pyrroloquinoline Quinone (PQQ)
- Taurine
- Vitamin B1
- Vitamin B12
- Magnesium Malate
- Magnesium Taurinate
- Magnesium Glycinate

If **HIGH** or > 100 mg/dL:

Elevated glucose levels may suggest insulin resistance, early-stage diabetes, metabolic syndrome, or issues like liver congestion, thiamine (B1) deficiency, stress, or pancreatitis.

Support for glucose metabolism, anti-inflammatory, and antioxidant supplements are recommended, along with lifestyle and dietary adjustments to enhance insulin sensitivity.

Reduce stress, maintain regular physical activity, incorporate high-intensity interval training, and practice daily relaxation.

Focus on a protein-rich breakfast, low-glycemic foods, balanced meals, and avoid high-sugar snacks and beverages. Incorporate omega-3 fats, low-glycemic vegetables and fruits, and antioxidant-rich herbs and spices.

Glucose Metabolism Support:
- Magnesium
- Zinc
- Selenium
- Manganese
- Chromium
- Molybdenum
- Potassium Iodide
- Taurine
- Carnosine
- R-Lipoic Acid
- Vitamin A
- Vitamin D3
- Vitamin E
- Vitamin K1
- Benfotiamine (Fat-Soluble Vitamin B1)
- Vitamin B1
- Vitamin B2
- Vitamin B3
- Vitamin B5
- Vitamin B6
- Vitamin B7 (Biotin)
- Vitamin B9 (Folate)
- Vitamin B12
- Vitamin C
- Berberine
- Fenugreek
- Gymnema sylvestre
- Banaba (Lagerstroemia speciosa)
- Kudzu (Pueraria lobata)
- Cinnamon
- Inositol (as Myo and D-Chiro)
- Alpha Lipoic Acid
- MVM (Multi-vitamin/mineral)

CMP (COMPREHENSIVE METABOLIC PANEL)

Anti-inflammatory Support:
- Phytocannabinoids
- Hemp Flower Extract
- Hemp Seed Oil
- Palmitoylethanolamide (PEA)
- Omega-3 Fatty Acids (Fish Oil)
- docosahexaenoic acid), 14-HDHA (14-hydroxy docosahexaenoic acid)
- Vitamin D3
- Curcumin
- Green Tea Extract (Epigallocatechin Gallate (EGCG))
- Trans Resveratrol
- Quercetin
- Nettle (Urtica dioica)
- Pro-Resolving Mediators (PRMs): 18-HEPE (18-hydroxy eicosapentaenoic acid), 17-HDHA (17-hydroxy

High Dose Probiotics:
- Multi-strain probiotic blend
- Saccharomyces boulardii
- Beta Glucans
- Lactobacillus plantarum strain L-137 (HK L-137)
- Xylooligosaccharide (XOS)

Antioxidant Support:
- Acerola Extract (Malpighia glabra)
- Grape Seed Extract (Vitis vinifera)
- Curcumin
- Garlic (Allium sativum)
- Ginkgo Extract (Ginkgo biloba)
- Quercetin
- Rutin
- Clove (Syzygium aromaticum)
- Allspice (Pimenta dioica)
- Sweet Basil (Ocimum basilicum)
- Sage (Salvia officinalis)
- Rosemary Extract (Rosmarinus officinalis)
- Lutein
- Lycopene
- Trans Resveratrol
- Vitamin A
- Vitamin E
- L-glutathione
- NAC (N-Acetyl-L-Cysteine)
- Broccoli Powder Extract
- Sulforaphane
- Olive Leaf Extract (Olea europaea)
- Bergamot
- Red Grape Powder
- Alpha Lipoic Acid
- Taurine
- MVM (Multi-vitamin/mineral)
- Glutathione (reduced)

Glucose - Non-Fasting

Non-fasting glucose levels offer insight into blood sugar balance influenced by the pancreas (insulin/glucagon), adrenal glands (cortisol), and liver (gluconeogenesis). Deviations can result from glycogen storage or breakdown issues in the liver, hormone imbalances (e.g., cortisol, estrogen), receptor insensitivity, or poor insulin production from pancreatic beta cells. Blood sugar stability is essential for coordinated immune response and overall health.

Normal Range	65 – 125 mg/dL
Optimal Range	80 – 125 mg/dL

CMP (COMPREHENSIVE METABOLIC PANEL)

If **LOW** or **< 80 mg/dL:**

 Low non-fasting glucose may suggest reactive hypoglycemia, impaired glycogen storage in the liver, excessive insulin, adrenal or thyroid hypofunction, high-dose salicylates, protein malnutrition, or liver dysfunction.

 Increase protein and fat intake, monitor glucose response at various intervals, and consider chromium GTF to enhance insulin action.

Avoid stressful situations, engage in regular balanced exercise with high-intensity intervals, avoid stimulants, alcohol, and smoking, and ensure hydration and sufficient sleep.

Increase dietary fiber, eat small balanced meals, avoid refined carbs, consume omega-3-rich foods, and aim for 9 servings of vegetables/fruits daily.

 Glucose Metabolism Support:
- Magnesium
- Zinc
- Selenium
- Manganese
- Chromium
- Molybdenum
- Potassium Iodide
- Taurine
- Carnosine
- R-Lipoic Acid
- Vitamin A
- Vitamin D3
- Vitamin E
- Vitamin K1
- Benfotiamine (Fat-Soluble Vitamin B1)
- Vitamin B1
- Vitamin B2
- Vitamin B3
- Vitamin B5
- Vitamin B6
- Vitamin B7 (Biotin)
- Vitamin B9 (Folate)
- Vitamin B12
- Vitamin C
- Berberine
- Fenugreek
- Gymnema sylvestre
- Banaba (Lagerstroemia speciosa)
- Kudzu (Pueraria lobata)
- Cinnamon
- Inositol (as Myo and D-Chiro)
- Alpha Lipoic Acid
- MVM (Multi-vitamin/mineral)

Adrenal Support:
- gamma-Aminobutyric Acid (GABA)
- Eleutherococcus senticosus
- American Ginseng
- Ashwagandha
- Rhodiola
- Licorice
- Vitamin B2
- Vitamin B5
- Vitamin B6
- Vitamin C
- N-Acetyl-L-Tyrosine
- Phosphatidylserine
- Valerian
- Passion Flower
- Lemon Balm
- Chamomile
- L-theanine
- 5-HTP
- Melatonin
- Rhodiola rosea
- Pyrroloquinoline Quinone (PQQ)
- Taurine
- Vitamin B1
- Vitamin B12
- Magnesium Malate
- Magnesium Taurinate
- Magnesium Glycinate

CMP (COMPREHENSIVE METABOLIC PANEL)

If HIGH or > 125 mg/dL:

 Elevated non-fasting glucose levels may indicate insulin resistance, early-stage diabetes, metabolic syndrome, or factors like liver congestion, B1 deficiency, stress, pancreatitis, or corticosteroid medication use.

 Support for glucose metabolism, anti-inflammatory, and antioxidant supplements is recommended, with dietary and lifestyle modifications to improve insulin sensitivity.

Reduce stress, avoid a sedentary lifestyle, incorporate high-intensity interval training, and focus on hydration and relaxation practices.

Eat a high-protein breakfast, consume low-glycemic foods, avoid high-sugar snacks and beverages, include omega-3-rich fats, low-glycemic vegetables and fruits, and antioxidant-rich herbs and spices.

Glucose Metabolism Support:
- Magnesium
- Zinc
- Selenium
- Manganese
- Chromium
- Molybdenum
- Potassium Iodide
- Taurine
- Carnosine
- R-Lipoic Acid
- Vitamin A
- Vitamin D3
- Vitamin E
- Vitamin K1
- Benfotiamine (Fat-Soluble Vitamin B1)
- Vitamin B1
- Vitamin B2
- Vitamin B3
- Vitamin B5
- Vitamin B6
- Vitamin B7 (Biotin)
- Vitamin B9 (Folate)
- Vitamin B12
- Vitamin C
- Berberine
- Fenugreek
- Gymnema sylvestre
- Banaba (Lagerstroemia speciosa)
- Kudzu (Pueraria lobata)
- Cinnamon
- Inositol (as Myo and D-Chiro)
- Alpha Lipoic Acid
- MVM (Multi-vitamin/mineral)

Anti-inflammatory Support:
- Phytocannabinoids
- Hemp Flower Extract
- Hemp Seed Oil
- Palmitoylethanolamide (PEA)
- Omega-3 Fatty Acids (Fish Oil)
- docosahexaenoic acid), 14-HDHA (14-hydroxy docosahexaenoic acid)
- Vitamin D3
- Curcumin
- Green Tea Extract (Epigallocatechin Gallate (EGCG))
- Trans Resveratrol
- Quercetin
- Nettle (Urtica dioica)
- Pro-Resolving Mediators (PRMs): 18-HEPE (18-hydroxy eicosapentaenoic acid), 17-HDHA (17-hydroxy

High Dose Probiotics:
- Multi-strain probiotic blend
- Saccharomyces boulardii
- Beta Glucans
- Lactobacillus plantarum strain L-137 (HK L-137)
- Xylooligosaccharide (XOS)

Antioxidant Support:
- Acerola Extract (Malpighia glabra)
- Grape Seed Extract (Vitis vinifera)
- Curcumin
- Garlic (Allium sativum)

- Ginkgo Extract (Ginkgo biloba)
- Quercetin
- Rutin
- Clove (Syzygium aromaticum)
- Allspice (Pimenta dioica)
- Sweet Basil (Ocimum basilicum)
- Sage (Salvia officinalis)
- Rosemary Extract (Rosmarinus officinalis)
- Lutein
- Lycopene
- Trans Resveratrol
- Vitamin A
- Vitamin E
- L-glutathione
- NAC (N-Acetyl-L-Cysteine)
- Broccoli Powder Extract
- Sulforaphane
- Olive Leaf Extract (Olea europaea)
- Bergamot
- Red Grape Powder
- Alpha Lipoic Acid
- Taurine
- MVM (Multi-vitamin/mineral)
- Glutathione (reduced)

Hemoglobin A1C

Hemoglobin A1C (HbA1C) measures the glycosylation of red blood cells over a 3-4 month period and is a key diabetes risk marker. Glycohemoglobin levels are directly proportional to blood glucose levels over this period. Elevated HbA1C indicates hyperglycemia and can impair immune function.

Normal Range	4.8 – 5.7%
Optimal Range	4.1 – 5.3%

If LOW or < 4.1%:

Low HbA1C may indicate hypoglycemia, liver storage dysfunction, or excessive insulin. Patterns may show associations with low fasting glucose and HbA1C.

Increase protein and fat intake, check glucose handling throughout the day, and consider chromium GTF to enhance insulin action.

Minimize stress, avoid stimulants, engage in regular balanced exercise with resistance training, ensure adequate sleep, and stay well-hydrated.

Increase dietary fiber, eat balanced small meals, avoid refined carbs, incorporate omega-3s, and aim for 9 servings of vegetables/fruits daily.

Glucose Metabolism Support:
- Magnesium
- Zinc
- Selenium
- Manganese
- Chromium
- Molybdenum
- Potassium Iodide
- Taurine
- Carnosine
- R-Lipoic Acid
- Vitamin A
- Vitamin D3
- Vitamin E
- Vitamin K1
- Benfotiamine (Fat-Soluble Vitamin B1)
- Vitamin B1
- Vitamin B2
- Vitamin B3
- Vitamin B5
- Vitamin B6
- Vitamin B7 (Biotin)
- Vitamin B9 (Folate)
- Vitamin B12
- Vitamin C

- Berberine
- Fenugreek
- Gymnema sylvestre
- Banaba (Lagerstroemia speciosa)
- Kudzu (Pueraria lobata)
- Cinnamon
- Inositol (as Myo and D-Chiro)
- Alpha Lipoic Acid
- MVM (Multi-vitamin/mineral)

Adrenal Support:
- gamma-Aminobutyric Acid (GABA)
- Eleutherococcus senticosus
- American Ginseng
- Ashwagandha
- Rhodiola
- Licorice
- Vitamin B2
- Vitamin B5
- Vitamin B6
- Vitamin C
- N-Acetyl-L-Tyrosine
- Phosphatidylserine
- Valerian
- Passion Flower
- Lemon Balm
- Chamomile
- L-theanine
- 5-HTP
- Melatonin
- Rhodiola rosea
- Pyrroloquinoline Quinone (PQQ)
- Taurine
- Vitamin B1
- Vitamin B12
- Magnesium Malate
- Magnesium Taurinate
- Magnesium Glycinate

If **HIGH** or > 5.3%:

 Elevated HbA1C may suggest insulin resistance, diabetes, or metabolic dysfunction. Early detection of insulin resistance is possible through elevated fasting insulin, even before HbA1C levels rise.

 Focus on glucose metabolism support, anti-inflammatory and antioxidant supplements, and lifestyle modifications to improve insulin sensitivity.

Manage stress, maintain an active lifestyle, consider high-intensity interval training, and practice daily relaxation techniques.

Emphasize a high-protein breakfast, consume low-glycemic foods, limit high-sugar snacks, incorporate omega-3s, and use antioxidant-rich herbs and spices.

 Glucose Metabolism Support:
- Magnesium
- Zinc
- Selenium
- Manganese
- Chromium
- Molybdenum
- Potassium Iodide
- Taurine
- Carnosine
- R-Lipoic Acid
- Vitamin A
- Vitamin D3
- Vitamin E
- Vitamin K1
- Benfotiamine (Fat-Soluble Vitamin B1)
- Vitamin B1
- Vitamin B2
- Vitamin B3
- Vitamin B5
- Vitamin B6
- Vitamin B7 (Biotin)
- Vitamin B9 (Folate)
- Vitamin B12
- Vitamin C
- Berberine
- Fenugreek
- Gymnema sylvestre
- Banaba (Lagerstroemia speciosa)
- Kudzu (Pueraria lobata)
- Cinnamon

- Inositol (as Myo and D-Chiro)
- Alpha Lipoic Acid

Anti-inflammatory Support:
- Phytocannabinoids
- Hemp Flower Extract
- Hemp Seed Oil
- Palmitoylethanolamide (PEA)
- Omega-3 Fatty Acids (Fish Oil)
- docosahexaenoic acid), 14-HDHA (14-hydroxy docosahexaenoic acid)
- Vitamin D3
- Curcumin

High Dose Probiotics:
- Multi-strain probiotic blend
- Saccharomyces boulardii
- Beta Glucans

Antioxidant Support:
- Acerola Extract (Malpighia glabra)
- Grape Seed Extract (Vitis vinifera)
- Curcumin
- Garlic (Allium sativum)
- Ginkgo Extract (Ginkgo biloba)
- Quercetin
- Rutin
- Clove (Syzygium aromaticum)
- Allspice (Pimenta dioica)
- Sweet Basil (Ocimum basilicum)
- Sage (Salvia officinalis)
- Rosemary Extract (Rosmarinus officinalis)
- Lutein
- Lycopene

- MVM (Multi-vitamin/mineral)

- Green Tea Extract (Epigallocatechin Gallate (EGCG))
- Trans Resveratrol
- Quercetin
- Nettle (Urtica dioica)
- Pro-Resolving Mediators (PRMs): 18-HEPE (18-hydroxy eicosapentaenoic acid), 17-HDHA (17-hydroxy

- Lactobacillus plantarum strain L-137 (HK L-137)
- Xylooligosaccharide (XOS)

- Trans Resveratrol
- Vitamin A
- Vitamin E
- L-glutathione
- NAC (N-Acetyl-L-Cysteine)
- Broccoli Powder Extract
- Sulforaphane
- Olive Leaf Extract (Olea europaea)
- Bergamot
- Red Grape Powder
- Alpha Lipoic Acid
- Taurine
- MVM (Multi-vitamin/mineral)
- Glutathione (reduced)

Uric Acid

Uric acid is the end-product of purine, nucleic acid, and nucleoprotein metabolism. It can increase due to overproduction or decreased excretion, which may contribute to conditions such as gout and kidney stones. Elevated uric acid is an early marker for potential gout and may signal liver or kidney issues. Levels may reflect cellular turnover, detoxification issues, or metabolic disturbances in the body.

Normal Range	2.5 – 6.8 mg/dL
Optimal Range	3.0 – 5.5 mg/dL

If **LOW** or < 3.0 mg/dL:

Low uric acid may suggest detoxification issues, potential deficiencies (molybdenum, B12, folate), and conditions like B12/folate anemia or copper deficiency.

CMP (COMPREHENSIVE METABOLIC PANEL)

Typically measured to assess risks for gout, renal failure, or metabolic inflammation.

 Support liver and kidney function and consider further urinalysis to investigate detoxification status.

Nutritional Support:
- Vitamin B9 (folate)
- Vitamin B12
- Vitamin B6
- Molybdenum

Liver Support:
- Milk Thistle
- L-methionine
- Taurine
- Inositol
- Ox Bile
- Artichoke
- Beet Powder
- Vitamin A
- Vitamin B6
- Vitamin B12
- Plant protein powder with MVM (multi-vitamin/mineral)
- L-glutathione
- N-Acetyl-L-Cysteine (NAC)
- Quercetin
- Methylsulfonylmethane (MSM)
- Sodium Sulfate
- Green Tea Extract
- Reishi
- Cordyceps
- Chinese Skullcap
- Schisandra
- Burdock Extract
- Phosphatidylcholine

Digestive Support:
- Digestive enzymes
- Betaine HCl
- Ox Bile
- L-taurine
- Gentian extract
- Dandelion extract
- Fennel
- Amylase
- Protease SP
- Protease
- Diastase
- Lactase
- Glucoamylase
- Alpha-galactosidase
- Beta-glucanase
- Acid protease
- Phytase
- Cellulase
- Hemicellulase
- Invertase
- Lipase
- Bromelain
- Papain
- Pepsin
- Triphala (Emblica officinalis, Terminalia bellirica, Terminalia chebula)
- Magnesium Hydroxide
- Mastic Gum
- DGL (Deglycyrrhizinated Licorice)
- Methylmethionine Sulfonium Chloride (MMSC)
- Zinc L-Carnosine
- Vitamin C
- Berberine
- Ginger
- Bismuth

If **HIGH** or > 5.5 mg/dL:

 Elevated uric acid levels are linked to gout, kidney dysfunction, liver issues, and oxidative stress. It's an indicator of potential inflammation and metabolic imbalance.

CMP (COMPREHENSIVE METABOLIC PANEL)

High levels may reflect dehydration, renal dysfunction, tissue breakdown, or a high intake of purines and fructose.

Avoid purine-rich foods and refined sugars; increase hydration and monitor for potential risk factors.

Lifestyle Recommendations:
- Prioritize weight management, regular physical activity, and proper hydration.
- Limit alcohol, especially beer, and avoid smoking. Moderate coffee may be beneficial.
- Avoid high-purine foods (e.g., organ meats, shellfish) and refined sugars.
- Increase intake of fiber, magnesium, and potassium; consider tart or black cherry juice for anti-inflammatory support.
- Use healthy oils (olive, coconut, avocado) and avoid vegetable and industrial seed oils.

Urinary Support:
- D-Mannose
- Cranberry (Vaccinium macrocarpon)
- Bearberry (Arctostaphylos uva ursi)
- Hibiscus (Hibiscus sabdaria)
- Nettle (Urtica spp.)
- Aloe Vera
- Parsley Powder (Petroselinum crispum)
- Horsetail (Equisetum spp.)
- Vitamin B6
- L-Carnitine
- Acetyl-L-Carnitine
- Champignon (Agaricus bisporus)
- Cordyceps (Cordyceps sinensis)
- Poria (Poria cocos)
- American Ginseng
- Astragalus (Astragalus membranaceus)
- Belleric Myrobalan (Terminalia bellerica)
- Tart Cherry (Prunus cerasus)

Glucose Metabolism Support:
- Magnesium
- Zinc
- Selenium
- Manganese
- Chromium
- Molybdenum
- Potassium Iodide
- Taurine
- Carnosine
- R-Lipoic Acid
- Vitamin A
- Vitamin D3
- Vitamin E
- Vitamin K1
- Benfotiamine (Fat-Soluble Vitamin B1)
- Vitamin B1
- Vitamin B2
- Vitamin B3
- Vitamin B5
- Vitamin B6
- Vitamin B7 (Biotin)
- Vitamin B9 (Folate)
- Vitamin B12
- Vitamin C
- Berberine
- Fenugreek
- Gymnema sylvestre
- Banaba (Lagerstroemia speciosa)
- Kudzu (Pueraria lobata)
- Cinnamon
- Inositol (as Myo and D-Chiro)
- Alpha Lipoic Acid
- MVM (Multi-vitamin/mineral)

Nutritional Support:
- Vitamin B9 (folate)

Anti-inflammatory Support:
- Phytocannabinoids
- Hemp Flower Extract
- Hemp Seed Oil
- Palmitoylethanolamide (PEA)
- Omega-3 Fatty Acids (Fish Oil)
- docosahexaenoic acid), 14-HDHA (14-hydroxy docosahexaenoic acid)
- Vitamin D3

- Curcumin
- Green Tea Extract (Epigallocatechin Gallate (EGCG))
- Trans Resveratrol
- Quercetin

Antioxidants:
- Acerola Extract (Malpighia glabra)
- Grape Seed Extract (Vitis vinifera)
- Curcumin
- Garlic (Allium sativum)
- Ginkgo Extract (Ginkgo biloba)
- Quercetin
- Rutin
- Clove (Syzygium aromaticum)
- Allspice (Pimenta dioica)
- Sweet Basil (Ocimum basilicum)
- Sage (Salvia officinalis)
- Rosemary Extract (Rosmarinus officinalis)
- Lutein
- Lycopene

Intestinal Hyperpermeability Support:
- Colostrum
- Serum-Derived Bovine Immunoglobulin Concentrate
- Immunoglobulin G
- N-Acetyl-D-Glucosamine
- Zinc L-Carnosine
- L-Glutamine
- Citrus Pectin
- Deglycyrrhizinated Licorice Extract (DGL)
- Aloe Vera
- Slippery Elm
- Mucin
- Chamomile Extract
- Marshmallow
- Okra
- Cat's Claw
- Methylsulfonylmethane (MSM)
- Nettle (Urtica dioica)
- Pro-Resolving Mediators (PRMs): 18-HEPE (18-hydroxy eicosapentaenoic acid), 17-HDHA (17-hydroxy

- Trans Resveratrol
- Vitamin A
- Vitamin E
- L-glutathione
- NAC (N-Acetyl-L-Cysteine)
- Broccoli Powder Extract
- Sulforaphane
- Olive Leaf Extract (Olea europaea)
- Bergamot
- Red Grape Powder
- Alpha Lipoic Acid
- Taurine
- MVM (Multi-vitamin/mineral)
- Glutathione (reduced)

- Quercetin
- Prune Powder
- Aloe Vera Leaf Gel Extract
- Apple Pectin
- Iron
- Glucosamine HCl
- Protein Powder
- Mixed Amino Acids
- Glycine
- Mastic Gum
- Methylmethionine Sulfonium Chloride (MMSC)
- Vitamin C
- Berberine
- Ginger
- Bismuth
- Alpha Lipoic Acid

BUN (Blood Urea Nitrogen)

Blood Urea Nitrogen (BUN), also known as "Urea," is a waste product formed by the liver during protein metabolism. BUN is primarily excreted by the kidneys and serves as a marker of kidney function, particularly useful if other kidney markers are normal. Gut bacteria can release ammonia, which converts into urea, contributing to increased BUN levels. The BUN level reflects both protein metabolism efficiency and kidney health.

CMP (COMPREHENSIVE METABOLIC PANEL)

Normal Range	8 – 27 mg/dL
Optimal Range	10 – 16 mg/dL

If LOW or < 10 mg/dL:

Low BUN may indicate issues with protein metabolism or absorption, possibly due to low protein intake, malabsorption, or conditions affecting liver and kidney function, including "leaky gut."

Support protein digestion and absorption, and address potential digestive or liver issues.

Protein Source:
- Protein Powder
- Mixed Amino Acids
- Dairy-Free, Plant-Based Protein Powder
- Whey-Based Protein Powder

Digestive Support:
- Digestive enzymes
- Betaine HCl
- Ox Bile
- L-taurine
- Gentian extract
- Dandelion extract
- Fennel
- Amylase
- Protease SP
- Protease
- Diastase
- Lactase
- Glucoamylase
- Alpha-galactosidase
- Beta-glucanase
- Acid protease
- Phytase
- Cellulase
- Hemicellulase
- Invertase
- Lipase
- Bromelain
- Papain
- Pepsin
- Triphala (Emblica officinalis, Terminalia bellirica, Terminalia chebula)
- Magnesium Hydroxide
- Mastic Gum
- DGL (Deglycyrrhizinated Licorice)
- Methylmethionine Sulfonium Chloride (MMSC)
- Zinc L-Carnosine
- Vitamin C
- Berberine
- Ginger
- Bismuth

Kidney Support:
- Champignon (Agaricus bisporus)
- Cordyceps (Cordyceps sinensis)
- Poria (Poria cocos)
- American Ginseng (Panax quinquefolius)
- Astragalus (Astragalus membranaceus)

Liver Support:
- Milk Thistle
- L-methionine
- Taurine
- Inositol
- Ox Bile
- Artichoke
- Beet Powder
- Vitamin A
- Vitamin B6
- Vitamin B12
- Plant protein powder with MVM (multi-vitamin/mineral)

CMP (COMPREHENSIVE METABOLIC PANEL)

- L-glutathione
- N-Acetyl-L-Cysteine (NAC)
- Quercetin
- Methylsulfonylmethane (MSM)
- Sodium Sulfate
- Green Tea Extract
- Reishi
- Cordyceps
- Chinese Skullcap
- Schisandra
- Burdock Extract
- Phosphatidylcholine

Intestinal Hyperpermeability Support:
- Colostrum
- Serum-Derived Bovine Immunoglobulin Concentrate
- Immunoglobulin G
- N-Acetyl-D-Glucosamine
- Zinc L-Carnosine
- L-Glutamine
- Citrus Pectin
- Deglycyrrhizinated Licorice Extract (DGL)
- Aloe Vera
- Slippery Elm
- Mucin
- Chamomile Extract
- Marshmallow
- Okra
- Cat's Claw
- Methylsulfonylmethane (MSM)
- Quercetin
- Prune Powder
- Aloe Vera Leaf Gel Extract
- Apple Pectin
- Iron
- Glucosamine HCl
- Protein Powder
- Mixed Amino Acids
- Glycine
- Mastic Gum
- Methylmethionine Sulfonium Chloride (MMSC)
- Vitamin C
- Berberine
- Ginger
- Bismuth
- Alpha Lipoic Acid

If **HIGH** or **> 16 mg/dL:**

Elevated BUN levels may indicate kidney strain, dehydration, high protein intake, or dysbiosis. It may also reflect metabolic disturbance or inflammatory states in the body.

Support kidney function, ensure adequate hydration, and consider dysbiosis (gut bacteria imbalance) as a potential factor. Adjust dietary protein intake as necessary.

Kidney Support:
- Champignon (Agaricus bisporus)
- Cordyceps (Cordyceps sinensis)
- Poria (Poria cocos)
- American Ginseng (Panax quinquefolius)
- Astragalus (Astragalus membranaceus)

Digestive Support:
- Digestive enzymes
- Betaine HCl
- Ox Bile
- L-taurine
- Gentian extract
- Dandelion extract
- Fennel
- Amylase
- Protease SP
- Protease
- Diastase
- Lactase
- Glucoamylase
- Alpha-galactosidase
- Beta-glucanase
- Acid protease
- Phytase
- Cellulase

CMP (COMPREHENSIVE METABOLIC PANEL)

- Hemicellulase
- Invertase
- Lipase
- Bromelain
- Papain
- Pepsin
- Triphala (Emblica officinalis, Terminalia bellirica, Terminalia chebula)
- Magnesium Hydroxide
- Mastic Gum
- DGL (Deglycyrrhizinated Licorice)
- Methylmethionine Sulfonium Chloride (MMSC)
- Zinc L-Carnosine
- Vitamin C
- Berberine
- Ginger
- Bismuth

High Dose Probiotics:
- Multi-strain probiotic blend
- Saccharomyces boulardii
- Beta Glucans
- Lactobacillus plantarum strain L-137 (HK L-137)
- Xylooligosaccharide (XOS)

Antimicrobial Agents:
- Oregano Oil (Origanum vulgare)
- Garlic
- Tribulus terrestris
- Magnesium Caprylate
- Berberine
- Bearberry Extract (Arctostaphylos uva-ursi)
- Black Walnut Powder (Juglans nigra)
- Barberry Extract (Berberis spp.)
- Artemisia (wormwood)
- Purified Silver
- Alpha Lipoic Acid

Adrenal Support:
- gamma-Aminobutyric Acid (GABA)
- Eleutherococcus senticosus
- American Ginseng
- Ashwagandha
- Rhodiola
- Licorice
- Vitamin B2
- Vitamin B5
- Vitamin B6
- Vitamin C
- N-Acetyl-L-Tyrosine
- Phosphatidylserine
- Valerian
- Passion Flower
- Lemon Balm
- Chamomile
- L-theanine
- 5-HTP
- Melatonin
- Rhodiola rosea
- Pyrroloquinoline Quinone (PQQ)
- Taurine
- Vitamin B1
- Vitamin B12
- Magnesium Malate
- Magnesium Taurinate
- Magnesium Glycinate

Creatinine

Creatinine is a byproduct of muscle breakdown that occurs during muscle contraction. The kidneys filter it from the blood, making creatinine levels a useful indicator of kidney function, particularly when evaluated with BUN. Elevated levels may reflect kidney strain, while low levels can indicate low muscle mass or insufficient dietary protein.

Normal Range	0.57 – 1.00 mg/dL
Optimal Range	0.8 – 1.0 mg/dL

CMP (COMPREHENSIVE METABOLIC PANEL)

If LOW or < 0.8 mg/dL:

Low creatinine may indicate low protein intake, muscle atrophy, or the need for enhanced physical activity.

Consider a higher protein diet and regular exercise (30 minutes, HIIT, 3x/week) to support muscle growth and creatinine production.

Protein Source:
- Protein Powder
- Mixed Amino Acids
- Dairy-Free, Plant-Based Protein Powder
- Whey-Based Protein Powder

Digestive Support:
- Digestive enzymes
- Betaine HCl
- Ox Bile
- L-taurine
- Gentian extract
- Dandelion extract
- Fennel
- Amylase
- Protease SP
- Protease
- Diastase
- Lactase
- Glucoamylase
- Alpha-galactosidase
- Beta-glucanase
- Acid protease
- Phytase
- Cellulase
- Hemicellulase
- Invertase
- Lipase
- Bromelain
- Papain
- Pepsin
- Triphala (Emblica officinalis, Terminalia bellirica, Terminalia chebula)
- Magnesium Hydroxide
- Mastic Gum
- DGL (Deglycyrrhizinated Licorice)
- Methylmethionine Sulfonium Chloride (MMSC)
- Zinc L-Carnosine
- Vitamin C
- Berberine
- Ginger
- Bismuth

If HIGH or > 16 mg/dL:

Consider kidney insufficiency.
Also consider BPH, Urinary Tract congestion/dysfunction (male or female), and cardio disease.

Support kidney function, ensure adequate hydration, and consider dysbiosis (gut bacteria imbalance) as a potential factor. Adjust dietary protein intake as necessary.

Kidney Support:
- Champignon (Agaricus bisporus)
- Cordyceps (Cordyceps sinensis)
- Poria (Poria cocos)
- American Ginseng (Panax quinquefolius)
- Astragalus (Astragalus membranaceus)

Circulatory Support:
- L-Arginine

eGFR (non-African American)

Estimated Glomerular Filtration Rate (eGFR) is a measure of kidney function and screens for early kidney damage. Calculated using creatinine levels along with factors such as age, sex, and race, eGFR is a key indicator in monitoring kidney health, particularly in patients with known Chronic Kidney Disease (CKD), diabetes, or hypertension. Ideal values are 90+ mL/min/1.73 m², with values <15 indicating kidney failure.

Normal Range	> 59 mL/min/1.73 m²
Optimal Range	> 90 mL/min/ 1.73 m²

If LOW or < 59 mL/min/1.73 m²:

A low eGFR may indicate kidney damage or distress. Patients with eGFR <40 should be referred to a medical professional for further evaluation.

Support kidney function and evaluate lifestyle and dietary factors that may impact kidney health. Monitoring creatinine, BUN, and other markers can provide additional insights.

Kidney Support:
- Champignon (Agaricus bisporus)
- Cordyceps (Cordyceps sinensis)
- Poria (Poria cocos)
- American Ginseng (Panax quinquefolius)
- Astragalus (Astragalus membranaceus)

Circulatory Support:
- L-Arginine

eGFR (African American)

Estimated Glomerular Filtration Rate (eGFR) for African Americans is an important screening tool for early kidney damage. It is calculated based on creatinine levels along with factors like age, sex, and race. eGFR, along with creatinine and BUN, is used to monitor kidney function in patients with known Chronic Kidney Disease (CKD), diabetes (DM), or high blood pressure (HBP). Ideal eGFR levels are 90+ mL/min/1.73 m², with values below 15 indicating kidney failure.

Normal Range	> 59 mL/min/1.73 m²
Optimal Range	> 90 mL/min/ 1.73 m²

If LOW or < 59 mL/min/1.73 m²:

A low eGFR may suggest kidney damage or distress. If eGFR falls below 40, a referral to a healthcare provider is recommended for further assessment.

To support kidney function, consider lifestyle and dietary modifications to protect against further decline. Regular monitoring of related markers (creatinine, BUN) is advised for comprehensive kidney health evaluation.

Kidney Support:
- Champignon (Agaricus bisporus)
- Cordyceps (Cordyceps sinensis)
- Poria (Poria cocos)
- American Ginseng (Panax quinquefolius)
- Astragalus (Astragalus membranaceus)

Circulatory Support:
- L-Arginine

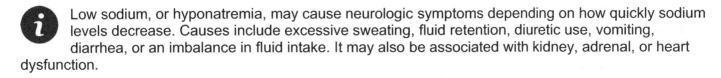

Sodium

Sodium is a primary extracellular mineral crucial for maintaining osmotic pressure and acid-base balance in plasma. It works closely with potassium via the Na/K pump and is controlled primarily by adrenal cortex hormones (aldosterone). Sodium also plays a significant role in nerve impulse transmission, renal function, cardiac performance, and adrenal function.

Normal Range	134 - 144 mEq/L
Optimal Range	135 - 142 mEq/L

If **LOW** or < 135 mEq/L:

Low sodium, or hyponatremia, may cause neurologic symptoms depending on how quickly sodium levels decrease. Causes include excessive sweating, fluid retention, diuretic use, vomiting, diarrhea, or an imbalance in fluid intake. It may also be associated with kidney, adrenal, or heart dysfunction.

Potential Causes:
- Conditions: Addison's disease, fluid overload (edema), kidney or heart issues.
- Symptoms: Weakness, confusion, seizures (in severe cases).

Increase sodium intake through dietary adjustments and support adrenal and kidney health as needed.

Kidney Support:
- Champignon (Agaricus bisporus)
- Cordyceps (Cordyceps sinensis)
- Poria (Poria cocos)
- American Ginseng (Panax quinquefolius)
- Astragalus (Astragalus membranaceus)

Electrolyte Support:
- Potassium
- Sodium
- Chloride
- Magnesium
- Magnesium Bisglycinate
- Vitamin C
- Zinc

Adrenal Support:
- gamma-Aminobutyric Acid (GABA)
- Eleutherococcus senticosus
- American Ginseng
- Ashwagandha

- Rhodiola
- Licorice
- Vitamin B2
- Vitamin B5
- Vitamin B6
- Vitamin C
- N-Acetyl-L-Tyrosine
- Phosphatidylserine
- Valerian
- Passion Flower
- Lemon Balm
- Chamomile

- L-theanine
- 5-HTP
- Melatonin
- Rhodiola rosea
- Pyrroloquinoline Quinone (PQQ)
- Taurine
- Vitamin B1
- Vitamin B12
- Magnesium Malate
- Magnesium Taurinate
- Magnesium Glycinate

If **HIGH** or **> 142 mEq/L:**

Elevated sodium, or hypernatremia, can result from dehydration, high sodium intake, or adrenal stress. Additional causes include kidney dysfunction, diabetes insipidus, or Cushing's syndrome.

Potential Causes:
- Conditions: Kidney disease, dehydration, Cushing's syndrome.
- Symptoms: Thirst, confusion, restlessness, fatigue.

Monitor sodium intake, increase hydration, and avoid processed foods high in sodium.

Kidney Support:
- Champignon (Agaricus bisporus)
- Cordyceps (Cordyceps sinensis)
- Poria (Poria cocos)
- American Ginseng (Panax quinquefolius)
- Astragalus (Astragalus membranaceus)

Electrolyte Support:
- Potassium
- Sodium
- Chloride
- Magnesium

- Magnesium Bisglycinate
- Vitamin C
- Zinc

Potassium

Potassium is essential for nerve conduction, muscle function, maintaining osmotic pressure, and balancing cellular transport via the sodium-potassium pump. It supports heart function in coordination with calcium and magnesium and is regulated by adrenal hormones to maintain precise levels in the body. Potassium is the primary intracellular electrolyte, working closely with sodium for optimal function.

Normal Range	3.5 - 5.2 mEq/L
Optimal Range	4.0 - 4.5 mEq/L

CMP (COMPREHENSIVE METABOLIC PANEL)

If **LOW** or < 135 mEq/L:

Low potassium, or hypokalemia, may cause symptoms like muscle weakness, cramps, and irregular heartbeat. It may result from inadequate dietary intake, dehydration, or conditions such as Cushing syndrome or excessive use of diuretics.

Potential Causes:
- Conditions: Cushing's syndrome, diuretic use, adrenal hyperactivity, excessive licorice intake, dehydration.
- Symptoms: Fatigue, muscle cramps, arrhythmias.

Increase dietary potassium with foods such as green leafy vegetables, coconut water, bananas, yams, and avocados. Support hydration and kidney health.

Kidney Support:
- Champignon (Agaricus bisporus)
- Cordyceps (Cordyceps sinensis)
- Poria (Poria cocos)
- American Ginseng (Panax quinquefolius)
- Astragalus (Astragalus membranaceus)

Electrolyte Support:
- Potassium
- Sodium
- Chloride
- Magnesium
- Magnesium Bisglycinate
- Vitamin C
- Zinc

If **HIGH** or > 142 mEq/L:

Elevated potassium, or hyperkalemia, may occur due to kidney disease, dehydration, or overconsumption of potassium. In severe cases, high potassium can cause EKG changes or arrhythmias..

Potential Causes:
- Conditions: Kidney disease, diabetes, Addison's disease, tissue injury, metabolic acidosis.
- Symptoms: Irregular heartbeat, muscle fatigue.

Monitor potassium intake, increase water and salt water intake, and support kidney and adrenal function as needed.

Alkalizing Support:
- Vitamin C, Calcium ascorbate, Magnesium ascorbate, Potassium ascorbate
- Quercetin, Hesperidin, Rutin
- Potassium Bicarbonate, Potassium Glycinate

Kidney Support:
- Champignon (Agaricus bisporus)
- Cordyceps (Cordyceps sinensis)
- Poria (Poria cocos)
- American Ginseng (Panax quinquefolius)
- Astragalus (Astragalus membranaceus)

Adrenal Support:

- gamma-Aminobutyric Acid (GABA)
- Eleutherococcus senticosus
- American Ginseng
- Ashwagandha
- Rhodiola
- Licorice
- Vitamin B2
- Vitamin B5
- Vitamin B6
- Vitamin C
- N-Acetyl-L-Tyrosine
- Phosphatidylserine
- Valerian
- Passion Flower
- Lemon Balm
- Chamomile
- L-theanine
- 5-HTP
- Melatonin
- Rhodiola rosea
- Pyrroloquinoline Quinone (PQQ)
- Taurine
- Vitamin B1
- Vitamin B12
- Magnesium Malate
- Magnesium Taurinate
- Magnesium Glycinate

Electrolyte Support:
- Potassium
- Sodium
- Chloride
- Magnesium
- Magnesium Bisglycinate
- Vitamin C
- Zinc

Chloride

Chloride is crucial for maintaining acid-base balance, fluid regulation, and proper nerve transmission. It works closely with sodium and CO_2 to regulate cellular hydration and has a direct relationship with sodium. Chloride is an essential component in processes such as fluid flow across cell membranes and maintaining overall electrolyte balance.

Normal Range	97 - 108 mmol/L
Optimal Range	100 - 106 mmol/L

If LOW or < 100 mmol/L:

Low chloride levels, or hypochloremia, may suggest issues such as adrenal hypofunction, GI or kidney dysfunction, or excessive loss of chloride due to factors like sweating or laxative use. Symptoms can include dehydration and acid-base imbalances.

Potential Causes:
- Conditions: Adrenal hypofunction (Addison disease), hypochlorhydria (low stomach acid), chronic lung disease, metabolic alkalosis, excessive sweating, or heart failure.
- Symptoms: Fatigue, muscle cramps, dehydration.

Support chloride levels through electrolytes, hydration, and adrenal support if needed. Check kidney function and monitor for blood sugar fluctuations.

Adrenal Support:
- gamma-Aminobutyric Acid (GABA)
- Eleutherococcus senticosus
- American Ginseng
- Ashwagandha
- Rhodiola
- Licorice
- Vitamin B2
- Vitamin B5

- Vitamin B6
- Vitamin C
- N-Acetyl-L-Tyrosine
- Phosphatidylserine
- Valerian
- Passion Flower
- Lemon Balm
- Chamomile
- L-theanine
- 5-HTP
- Melatonin
- Rhodiola rosea
- Pyrroloquinoline Quinone (PQQ)
- Taurine
- Vitamin B1
- Vitamin B12
- Magnesium Malate
- Magnesium Taurinate
- Magnesium Glycinate

Kidney Support:
- Champignon (Agaricus bisporus)
- Cordyceps (Cordyceps sinensis)
- Poria (Poria cocos)
- American Ginseng (Panax quinquefolius)
- Astragalus (Astragalus membranaceus)

Electrolyte Support:
- Potassium
- Sodium
- Chloride
- Magnesium
- Magnesium Bisglycinate
- Vitamin C
- Zinc

If **HIGH** or > 106 mmol/L:

Elevated chloride, or hyperchloremia, may indicate dehydration, excessive salt intake, or metabolic acidosis. Symptoms may include fatigue, dehydration, and acid-base imbalances.

Potential Causes:
- Conditions: Dehydration, hyperadrenal activity, high sodium intake, kidney dysfunction, diabetes insipidus, Cushing's syndrome.
- Symptoms: Nausea, fatigue, dehydration.

Focus on hydration, support alkalization, and balance electrolyte intake. Monitor for metabolic acidosis and kidney function as needed.

Alkalizing Support:
- Vitamin C, Calcium ascorbate, Magnesium ascorbate, Potassium ascorbate
- Quercetin, Hesperidin, Rutin
- Potassium Bicarbonate, Potassium Glycinate

Electrolyte Support:
- Potassium
- Sodium
- Chloride
- Magnesium
- Magnesium Bisglycinate
- Vitamin C
- Zinc

CMP (COMPREHENSIVE METABOLIC PANEL)

Carbon Dioxide (CO_2)

Carbon dioxide (CO_2) in blood represents bicarbonate, a primary buffer that helps maintain pH balance. CO_2 levels in blood reflect kidney function in acid-base balance, rather than the respiratory CO_2 managed by the lungs. CO_2 primarily assists in neutralizing acids and is tightly regulated by kidney activity.

Normal Range	19 - 28 mmol/L
Optimal Range	21 - 26 mmol/L

If LOW or < 21 mmol/L:

Low CO_2 levels may indicate metabolic acidosis, respiratory alkalosis, or challenges in maintaining acid-base balance due to nutritional or kidney factors.

Potential Causes:
- Conditions: Metabolic acidosis (e.g., chronic vomiting, low potassium, hypoventilation), respiratory alkalosis (e.g., lung conditions like asthma), thiamine (B1) deficiency.
- Symptoms: Fatigue, rapid breathing, low blood pH.

Consider bicarbonate, citrate, and alkaline minerals to support pH balance. Evaluate kidney and lung health, along with dietary adjustments for increased alkalization.

Kidney Support:
- Champignon (Agaricus bisporus)
- Cordyceps (Cordyceps sinensis)
- Poria (Poria cocos)
- American Ginseng (Panax quinquefolius)
- Astragalus (Astragalus membranaceus)

Alkalizing Support:
- Vitamin C, Calcium ascorbate, Magnesium ascorbate, Potassium ascorbate
- Quercetin, Hesperidin, Rutin
- Potassium Bicarbonate, Potassium Glycinate

Electrolyte Support:
- Potassium
- Sodium
- Chloride
- Magnesium
- Magnesium Bisglycinate
- Vitamin C
- Zinc

Antioxidant Support:
- Acerola Extract (Malpighia glabra)
- Grape Seed Extract (Vitis vinifera)
- Curcumin
- Garlic (Allium sativum)
- Ginkgo Extract (Ginkgo biloba)
- Quercetin
- Rutin
- Clove (Syzygium aromaticum)
- Allspice (Pimenta dioica)
- Sweet Basil (Ocimum basilicum)
- Sage (Salvia officinalis)
- Rosemary Extract (Rosmarinus officinalis)
- Lutein
- Lycopene
- Trans Resveratrol
- Vitamin A
- Vitamin E
- L-glutathione
- NAC (N-Acetyl-L-Cysteine)

- Broccoli Powder Extract
- Sulforaphane
- Olive Leaf Extract (Olea europaea)
- Bergamot
- Red Grape Powder
- Alpha Lipoic Acid
- Taurine
- MVM (Multi-vitamin/mineral)
- Glutathione (reduced)

Stress Support:
- Phosphatidylserine

If **HIGH** or **> 26 mmol/L:**

Elevated CO_2 levels may suggest metabolic alkalosis or respiratory acidosis. Higher CO_2 could also reflect challenges in acid production or retention and may result from certain medications or imbalances in electrolyte or protein levels.

Potential Causes:
- Conditions: Metabolic alkalosis (e.g., from prolonged vomiting or diuretic use), respiratory acidosis (e.g., lung diseases like asthma or pulmonary hypertension), hyperadrenal activity, hypochlorhydria (low stomach acid).
- Symptoms: Muscle twitching, confusion, decreased respiration rate.

Focus on balancing dietary acids, supporting kidney and digestive function, and potentially reducing any acid-reducing medications.

Digestive Support:
- Digestive enzymes

Electrolyte Support:
- Potassium
- Sodium
- Chloride
- Magnesium
- Magnesium Bisglycinate
- Vitamin C
- Zinc

Antioxidant Support:
- Acerola Extract (Malpighia glabra)
- Grape Seed Extract (Vitis vinifera)
- Curcumin
- Garlic (Allium sativum)
- Ginkgo Extract (Ginkgo biloba)
- Quercetin
- Rutin
- Clove (Syzygium aromaticum)
- Allspice (Pimenta dioica)
- Sweet Basil (Ocimum basilicum)
- Sage (Salvia officinalis)
- Rosemary Extract (Rosmarinus officinalis)
- Lutein
- Lycopene
- Trans Resveratrol
- Vitamin A
- Vitamin E
- L-glutathione
- NAC (N-Acetyl-L-Cysteine)
- Broccoli Powder Extract
- Sulforaphane
- Olive Leaf Extract (Olea europaea)
- Bergamot
- Red Grape Powder
- Alpha Lipoic Acid
- Taurine
- MVM (Multi-vitamin/mineral)
- Glutathione (reduced)

Stress Support:
- Phosphatidylserine

Anti-inflammatory Support:
- Phytocannabinoids
- Hemp Flower Extract
- Hemp Seed Oil
- Palmitoylethanolamide (PEA)
- Omega-3 Fatty Acids (Fish Oil)
- docosahexaenoic acid), 14-HDHA (14-hydroxy docosahexaenoic acid)
- Vitamin D3
- Curcumin
- Green Tea Extract (Epigallocatechin Gallate (EGCG))
- Trans Resveratrol
- Quercetin
- Nettle (Urtica dioica)
- Pro-Resolving Mediators (PRMs): 18-HEPE (18-hydroxy eicosapentaenoic acid), 17-HDHA (17-hydroxy

Calcium

Calcium is primarily stored in bones and teeth, with blood levels tightly regulated to support muscle contraction, nerve transmission, and blood clotting. Calcium absorption depends on stomach acid, phosphate, and magnesium, and it is regulated by vitamin D and parathyroid hormone (PTH). Calcium plays a role in inflammation and tissue repair. Deficiency is rare but may arise due to inadequate cofactors.

Normal Range	8.6 - 10.2 mg/dL
Optimal Range	9.2 - 10.0 mg/dL

If LOW or < 9.2 mg/dL:

Low calcium levels, or hypocalcemia, can present as muscle cramps, spasms, or tingling. Often linked to factors like poor absorption, low vitamin D, and hypoparathyroidism.

Potential Causes:
- Conditions: Hypochlorhydria (low stomach acid), malabsorption, vitamin D deficiency, hypoparathyroidism.
- Symptoms: Muscle cramps, spasms, tingling.

Ensure adequate fat digestion, vitamin D levels, and parathyroid function. Consider supporting calcium levels through dietary sources and supplements.

Digestive Support:
- Digestive enzymes
- Betaine HCl
- Ox Bile
- L-taurine
- Gentian extract
- Dandelion extract
- Fennel
- Amylase
- Protease SP
- Protease
- Diastase
- Lactase
- Glucoamylase
- Alpha-galactosidase
- Beta-glucanase
- Acid protease
- Phytase
- Cellulase
- Hemicellulase
- Invertase
- Lipase
- Bromelain
- Papain
- Pepsin
- Triphala (Emblica officinalis, Terminalia bellirica, Terminalia chebula)
- Magnesium Hydroxide
- Mastic Gum
- DGL (Deglycyrrhizinated Licorice)

CMP (COMPREHENSIVE METABOLIC PANEL)

- Methylmethionine Sulfonium Chloride (MMSC)
- Zinc L-Carnosine
- Vitamin C
- Berberine
- Ginger
- Bismuth

Protein Source:
- Protein Powder
- Mixed Amino Acids
- Dairy-Free, Plant-Based Protein Powder
- Whey-Based Protein Powder

Bone Health Support:
- Calcium Malate
- Vitamin D3
- Trans-Geranylgeraniol
- Calcium
- Magnesium
- Zinc
- Copper
- Manganese
- Boron
- Vitamin E
- Vitamin K1
- Vitamin K2
- Vitamin C
- Vitamin A
- Omega-3 Fatty Acids (Fish Oil)
- Genistein
- Magnesium Citrate
- Magnesium Taurinate
- Magnesium Glycinate
- Magnesium Malate

Vitamin D Support:
- Vitamins D3, K2

Intestinal Support:
- Zinc L-Carnosine
- N-Acetyl-D-Glucosamine
- Citrus Pectin
- Deglycyrrhizinated Licorice Extract (DGL)
- Slippery Elm, Mucin, Chamomile Extract, Marshmallow, Okra
- Cat's Claw
- Methylsulfonylmethane (MSM)
- Quercetin
- Prune Powder
- L-Glutamine
- Aloe Vera

Liver Support:
- Milk Thistle
- L-methionine
- Taurine
- Inositol
- Ox Bile
- Artichoke
- Beet Powder
- Vitamin A
- Vitamin B6
- Vitamin B12
- Plant protein powder with MVM (multi-vitamin/mineral)
- L-glutathione
- N-Acetyl-L-Cysteine (NAC)
- Quercetin
- Methylsulfonylmethane (MSM)
- Sodium Sulfate
- Green Tea Extract
- Reishi
- Cordyceps
- Chinese Skullcap
- Schisandra
- Burdock Extract
- Phosphatidylcholine

CMP (COMPREHENSIVE METABOLIC PANEL)

If **HIGH** or > 10.0 mg/dL:

Elevated calcium levels, or hypercalcemia, may present symptoms like fatigue, loss of appetite, nausea, constipation, or increased thirst.

Potential Causes:
- Conditions: Hyperparathyroidism, excessive vitamin D intake, hypothyroid, certain cancers, dehydration, or prolonged immobilization.
- Symptoms: Fatigue, appetite loss, nausea, constipation, thirst.

Check for potential hyperparathyroidism, high vitamin D intake, and assess kidney and adrenal function. Consider dietary adjustments to reduce calcium intake if needed.

Bone Health Support:
- Calcium Malate
- Vitamin D3
- Trans-Geranylgeraniol
- Calcium
- Magnesium
- Zinc
- Copper
- Manganese
- Boron
- Vitamin E

- Vitamin K1
- Vitamin K2
- Vitamin C
- Vitamin A
- Omega-3 Fatty Acids (Fish Oil)
- Genistein
- Magnesium Citrate
- Magnesium Taurinate
- Magnesium Glycinate
- Magnesium Malate

Alkalizing Support:
- Vitamin C, Calcium ascorbate, Magnesium ascorbate, Potassium ascorbate
- Quercetin, Hesperidin, Rutin
- Potassium Bicarbonate, Potassium Glycinate

Phosphorus

Phosphorus is a critical mineral involved in forming muscles, red blood cells, and ATP (the cell's energy source), as well as in maintaining acid-base balance and metabolizing carbohydrates, proteins, and fats. Phosphorus levels can vary based on age, gender, physiological state (e.g., pregnancy), and vitamin D status. It is regulated in part by vitamin D and the parathyroid hormone.

Normal Range	2.5 - 4.5 mg/dL
Optimal Range	3.0 - 4.0 mg/dL

If **LOW** or < 3.0 mEq/L:

Low phosphorus levels, or hypophosphatemia, may indicate conditions like malnutrition, malabsorption, acid-base imbalance, hypercalcemia, or renal dysfunction.

Potential Causes:
- Conditions: Alcoholism, malnutrition, vitamin D deficiency, hyperparathyroidism, chronic diarrhea, or excessive antacid use.
- Symptoms: Weakness, fatigue, and muscle pain.

CMP (COMPREHENSIVE METABOLIC PANEL)

 Increase intake of phosphorus-rich foods, consider vitamin D supplementation, and support digestion to optimize absorption.

Kidney Support:
- Champignon (Agaricus bisporus)
- Cordyceps (Cordyceps sinensis)
- Poria (Poria cocos)
- American Ginseng (Panax quinquefolius)
- Astragalus (Astragalus membranaceus)

Nutritional Support:
- Phosphorus
- Vitamins D3, K1, K2

Glucose Metabolism Support:
- Magnesium
- Zinc
- Selenium
- Manganese
- Chromium
- Molybdenum
- Potassium Iodide
- Taurine
- Carnosine
- R-Lipoic Acid
- Vitamin A
- Vitamin D3
- Vitamin E
- Vitamin K1
- Benfotiamine (Fat-Soluble Vitamin B1)
- Vitamin B1
- Vitamin B2
- Vitamin B3
- Vitamin B5
- Vitamin B6
- Vitamin B7 (Biotin)
- Vitamin B9 (Folate)
- Vitamin B12
- Vitamin C
- Berberine
- Fenugreek
- Gymnema sylvestre
- Banaba (Lagerstroemia speciosa)
- Kudzu (Pueraria lobata)
- Cinnamon
- Inositol (as Myo and D-Chiro)
- Alpha Lipoic Acid
- MVM (Multi-vitamin/mineral)

Adrenal Support:
- gamma-Aminobutyric Acid (GABA)
- Eleutherococcus senticosus
- American Ginseng
- Ashwagandha
- Rhodiola
- Licorice
- Vitamin B2
- Vitamin B5
- Vitamin B6
- Vitamin C
- N-Acetyl-L-Tyrosine
- Phosphatidylserine
- Valerian
- Passion Flower
- Lemon Balm
- Chamomile
- L-theanine
- 5-HTP
- Melatonin
- Rhodiola rosea
- Pyrroloquinoline Quinone (PQQ)
- Taurine
- Vitamin B1
- Vitamin B12
- Magnesium Malate
- Magnesium Taurinate
- Magnesium Glycinate

Digestive Support:
- Digestive enzymes
- Betaine HCl
- Ox Bile
- L-taurine
- Gentian extract
- Dandelion extract

CMP (COMPREHENSIVE METABOLIC PANEL)

- Fennel
- Amylase
- Protease SP
- Protease
- Diastase
- Lactase
- Glucoamylase
- Alpha-galactosidase
- Beta-glucanase
- Acid protease
- Phytase
- Cellulase
- Hemicellulase
- Invertase
- Lipase
- Bromelain
- Papain
- Pepsin
- Triphala (Emblica officinalis, Terminalia bellirica, Terminalia chebula)
- Magnesium Hydroxide
- Mastic Gum
- DGL (Deglycyrrhizinated Licorice)
- Methylmethionine Sulfonium Chloride (MMSC)
- Zinc L-Carnosine
- Vitamin C
- Berberine
- Ginger
- Bismuth

If **HIGH** or > 4.0 mEq/L:

Elevated phosphorus levels, or hyperphosphatemia, may be linked to conditions such as renal dysfunction, hypocalcemia, or excessive phosphorus or vitamin D intake.

Potential Causes:
- Conditions: Kidney dysfunction, hypoparathyroidism, diabetic ketoacidosis, excess dietary phosphate, or vitamin D toxicity.
- Symptoms: Muscle cramps or spasms and potential impact on calcium balance.

Reduce intake of dietary phosphorus, vitamin D, and calcium. Regularly monitor kidney function.

Kidney Support:
- Champignon (Agaricus bisporus)
- Cordyceps (Cordyceps sinensis)
- Poria (Poria cocos)
- American Ginseng (Panax quinquefolius)
- Astragalus (Astragalus membranaceus)

Adrenal Support:
- gamma-Aminobutyric Acid (GABA)
- Eleutherococcus senticosus
- American Ginseng
- Ashwagandha
- Rhodiola
- Licorice
- Vitamin B2
- Vitamin B5
- Vitamin B6
- Vitamin C
- N-Acetyl-L-Tyrosine
- Phosphatidylserine
- Valerian
- Passion Flower
- Lemon Balm
- Chamomile
- L-theanine
- 5-HTP
- Melatonin
- Rhodiola rosea
- Pyrroloquinoline Quinone (PQQ)
- Taurine
- Vitamin B1
- Vitamin B12
- Magnesium Malate
- Magnesium Taurinate
- Magnesium Glycinate

Digestive Support:
- Digestive enzymes
- Betaine HCl
- Ox Bile
- L-taurine
- Gentian extract
- Dandelion extract
- Fennel
- Amylase
- Protease SP
- Protease
- Diastase
- Lactase
- Glucoamylase
- Alpha-galactosidase
- Beta-glucanase
- Acid protease
- Phytase
- Cellulase
- Hemicellulase
- Invertase
- Lipase
- Bromelain
- Papain
- Pepsin
- Triphala (Emblica officinalis, Terminalia bellirica, Terminalia chebula)
- Magnesium Hydroxide
- Mastic Gum
- DGL (Deglycyrrhizinated Licorice)
- Methylmethionine Sulfonium Chloride (MMSC)
- Zinc L-Carnosine
- Vitamin C
- Berberine
- Ginger
- Bismuth

Nutritional Support:
- Magnesium Citrate
- Calcium malate
- Vitamin D3

Magnesium

Magnesium is essential for energy production, muscle contraction, nerve function, and bone health. It plays a key role in carbohydrate and protein metabolism and is mainly stored in bones. Low magnesium levels are more common than high levels due to losses through the gastrointestinal tract, kidneys, and sweat.

Normal Range	1.88 - 2.22 mg/dL
Optimal Range	2.0 - 3.0 mg/dL

If **LOW** or < 2.0 mEq/L:

Low magnesium, or hypomagnesemia, can result from insufficient intake, increased gastrointestinal or urinary losses, or conditions like diabetes or chronic stress.

Potential Causes:
- Conditions: Kidney disease, GI disorders (Crohn's, celiac disease), excessive alcohol, high caffeine or sugar intake, or diuretic use.
- Symptoms: Muscle cramps, fatigue, and weakness.

Increase dietary magnesium through green leafy vegetables, nuts, seeds, and whole grains. Manage stress and reduce caffeine and alcohol intake.

CMP (COMPREHENSIVE METABOLIC PANEL)

Nutritional Support:
- Magnesium Citrate

Glucose Metabolism Support:
- Magnesium
- Zinc
- Selenium
- Manganese
- Chromium
- Molybdenum
- Potassium Iodide
- Taurine
- Carnosine
- R-Lipoic Acid
- Vitamin A
- Vitamin D3
- Vitamin E
- Vitamin K1
- Benfotiamine (Fat-Soluble Vitamin B1)
- Vitamin B1
- Vitamin B2
- Vitamin B3
- Vitamin B5
- Vitamin B6
- Vitamin B7 (Biotin)
- Vitamin B9 (Folate)
- Vitamin B12
- Vitamin C
- Berberine
- Fenugreek
- Gymnema sylvestre
- Banaba (Lagerstroemia speciosa)
- Kudzu (Pueraria lobata)
- Cinnamon
- Inositol (as Myo and D-Chiro)
- Alpha Lipoic Acid
- MVM (Multi-vitamin/mineral)

Adrenal Support:
- gamma-Aminobutyric Acid (GABA)
- Eleutherococcus senticosus
- American Ginseng
- Ashwagandha
- Rhodiola
- Licorice
- Vitamin B2
- Vitamin B5
- Vitamin B6
- Vitamin C
- N-Acetyl-L-Tyrosine
- Phosphatidylserine
- Valerian
- Passion Flower
- Lemon Balm
- Chamomile
- L-theanine
- 5-HTP
- Melatonin
- Rhodiola rosea
- Pyrroloquinoline Quinone (PQQ)
- Taurine
- Vitamin B1
- Vitamin B12
- Magnesium Malate
- Magnesium Taurinate
- Magnesium Glycinate

Digestive Support:
- Digestive enzymes
- Betaine HCl
- Ox Bile
- L-taurine
- Gentian extract
- Dandelion extract
- Fennel
- Amylase
- Protease SP
- Protease
- Diastase
- Lactase
- Glucoamylase
- Alpha-galactosidase
- Beta-glucanase
- Acid protease
- Phytase
- Cellulase
- Hemicellulase
- Invertase
- Lipase
- Bromelain
- Papain
- Pepsin

CMP (COMPREHENSIVE METABOLIC PANEL)

- Triphala (Emblica officinalis, Terminalia bellirica, Terminalia chebula)
- Magnesium Hydroxide
- Mastic Gum
- DGL (Deglycyrrhizinated Licorice)
- Methylmethionine Sulfonium Chloride (MMSC)
- Zinc L-Carnosine
- Vitamin C
- Berberine
- Ginger
- Bismuth

If **HIGH** or > 3.0 mEq/L:

High magnesium, or hypermagnesemia, is uncommon from dietary sources and typically results from excretion issues, kidney dysfunction, or excessive magnesium supplementation.

Potential Causes:
- Conditions: Kidney dysfunction, hyperparathyroidism, hypothyroidism, adrenal disorders (e.g., Addison's disease), dehydration, and overuse of magnesium-containing supplements.
- Symptoms: Nausea, muscle weakness, and cardiac irregularities if severe.

Avoid high magnesium foods and supplementation if not necessary. Enhance diuresis if kidney function is adequate.

Kidney Support:
- Champignon (Agaricus bisporus)
- Cordyceps (Cordyceps sinensis)
- Poria (Poria cocos)
- American Ginseng (Panax quinquefolius)
- Astragalus (Astragalus membranaceus)

Adrenal Support:
- gamma-Aminobutyric Acid (GABA)
- Eleutherococcus senticosus
- American Ginseng
- Ashwagandha
- Rhodiola
- Licorice
- Vitamin B2
- Vitamin B5
- Vitamin B6
- Vitamin C
- N-Acetyl-L-Tyrosine
- Phosphatidylserine
- Valerian
- Passion Flower
- Lemon Balm
- Chamomile
- L-theanine
- 5-HTP
- Melatonin
- Rhodiola rosea
- Pyrroloquinoline Quinone (PQQ)
- Taurine
- Vitamin B1
- Vitamin B12
- Magnesium Malate
- Magnesium Taurinate
- Magnesium Glycinate

Protein, Total

Total protein measures the combined levels of albumin and globulin in the blood, essential for metabolic activities. Albumin helps maintain fluid balance in blood vessels, while globulin supports the immune system.

CMP (COMPREHENSIVE METABOLIC PANEL)

Normal Range	6.0 - 8.5 g/dL
Optimal Range	6.9 - 7.4 g/dL

If LOW or < 6.9 g/dL:

Low total protein may indicate liver dysfunction, kidney disease, malabsorption, or protein deficiency.

Potential Causes:
- Conditions: Malnutrition, liver disease, inflammatory bowel disease, kidney disorder, or hypochlorhydria (low stomach acid).
- Symptoms: Fatigue, swelling, or immune deficiencies.

Evaluate albumin and globulin levels individually to pinpoint deficiency. Increase dietary protein and support digestive health for better absorption.

Protein Source:
- Protein Powder
- Mixed Amino Acids
- Dairy-Free, Plant-Based Protein Powder
- Whey-Based Protein Powder

Digestive Support:
- Digestive enzymes
- Betaine HCl
- Ox Bile
- L-taurine
- Gentian extract
- Dandelion extract
- Fennel
- Amylase
- Protease SP
- Protease
- Diastase
- Lactase
- Glucoamylase
- Alpha-galactosidase
- Beta-glucanase
- Acid protease
- Phytase
- Cellulase
- Hemicellulase
- Invertase
- Lipase
- Bromelain
- Papain
- Pepsin
- Triphala (Emblica officinalis, Terminalia bellirica, Terminalia chebula)
- Magnesium Hydroxide
- Mastic Gum
- DGL (Deglycyrrhizinated Licorice)
- Methylmethionine Sulfonium Chloride (MMSC)
- Zinc L-Carnosine
- Vitamin C
- Berberine
- Ginger
- Bismuth

If HIGH or > 7.4 g/dL:

High total protein levels may suggest chronic inflammation, infections, or bone marrow disorders.

Potential Causes:
- Conditions: Chronic infections (e.g., viral hepatitis, HIV), bone marrow disorders (e.g., multiple myeloma), or adrenal stress.
- Symptoms: Fatigue, weight loss, or immune irregularities.

CMP (COMPREHENSIVE METABOLIC PANEL)

 Assess individual albumin and globulin levels to identify specific elevation. Support adrenal and digestive health.

Adrenal Support:
- gamma-Aminobutyric Acid (GABA)
- Eleutherococcus senticosus
- American Ginseng
- Ashwagandha
- Rhodiola
- Licorice
- Vitamin B2
- Vitamin B5
- Vitamin B6
- Vitamin C
- N-Acetyl-L-Tyrosine
- Phosphatidylserine
- Valerian
- Passion Flower
- Lemon Balm
- Chamomile
- L-theanine
- 5-HTP
- Melatonin
- Rhodiola rosea
- Pyrroloquinoline Quinone (PQQ)
- Taurine
- Vitamin B1
- Vitamin B12
- Magnesium Malate
- Magnesium Taurinate
- Magnesium Glycinate

Digestive Support:
- Digestive enzymes
- Betaine HCl
- Ox Bile
- L-taurine
- Gentian extract
- Dandelion extract
- Fennel
- Amylase
- Protease SP
- Protease
- Diastase
- Lactase
- Glucoamylase
- Alpha-galactosidase
- Beta-glucanase
- Acid protease
- Phytase
- Cellulase
- Hemicellulase
- Invertase
- Lipase
- Bromelain
- Papain
- Pepsin
- Triphala (Emblica officinalis, Terminalia bellirica, Terminalia chebula)
- Magnesium Hydroxide
- Mastic Gum
- DGL (Deglycyrrhizinated Licorice)
- Methylmethionine Sulfonium Chloride (MMSC)
- Zinc L-Carnosine
- Vitamin C
- Berberine
- Ginger
- Bismuth

Albumin

Albumin, synthesized by the liver, is a major protein in blood plasma. It regulates plasma osmotic pressure, transports various substances, and helps maintain fluid volume within blood vessels.

Normal Range	3.6 - 4.8 g/dL
Optimal Range	4.6 - 5.0 g/dL

CMP (COMPREHENSIVE METABOLIC PANEL)

If LOW or < 4.6 g/dL:

Low albumin may be associated with liver disease, protein malnutrition, malabsorption, or chronic conditions affecting protein synthesis.

Potential Causes:
- Conditions: Chronic liver disease, kidney disease, protein malnutrition, inflammatory bowel disease, Crohn's, or Celiac disease.
- Symptoms: Fatigue, swelling, and muscle weakness.

Evaluate liver, kidney, and digestive health. Consider protein supplementation and support for improved digestion and liver function.

Protein Source:
- Protein Powder
- Mixed Amino Acids
- Dairy-Free, Plant-Based Protein Powder
- Whey-Based Protein Powder

Digestive Support:
- Digestive enzymes
- Betaine HCl
- Ox Bile
- L-taurine
- Gentian extract
- Dandelion extract
- Fennel
- Amylase
- Protease SP
- Protease
- Diastase
- Lactase
- Glucoamylase
- Alpha-galactosidase
- Beta-glucanase
- Acid protease
- Phytase
- Cellulase
- Hemicellulase
- Invertase
- Lipase
- Bromelain
- Papain
- Pepsin
- Triphala (Emblica officinalis, Terminalia bellirica, Terminalia chebula)
- Magnesium Hydroxide
- Mastic Gum
- DGL (Deglycyrrhizinated Licorice)
- Methylmethionine Sulfonium Chloride (MMSC)
- Zinc L-Carnosine
- Vitamin C
- Berberine
- Ginger
- Bismuth

Bone Health Support:
- Calcium Malate
- Vitamin D3
- Trans-Geranylgeraniol
- Calcium
- Magnesium
- Zinc
- Copper
- Manganese
- Boron
- Vitamin E
- Vitamin K1
- Vitamin K2
- Vitamin C
- Vitamin A
- Omega-3 Fatty Acids (Fish Oil)
- Genistein
- Magnesium Citrate
- Magnesium Taurinate
- Magnesium Glycinate
- Magnesium Malate

CMP (COMPREHENSIVE METABOLIC PANEL)

Anti-inflammatory Support:
- Phytocannabinoids
- Hemp Flower Extract
- Hemp Seed Oil
- Palmitoylethanolamide (PEA)
- Omega-3 Fatty Acids (Fish Oil)
- docosahexaenoic acid), 14-HDHA (14-hydroxy docosahexaenoic acid)
- Vitamin D3
- Curcumin
- Green Tea Extract (Epigallocatechin Gallate (EGCG))
- Trans Resveratrol
- Quercetin
- Nettle (Urtica dioica)
- Pro-Resolving Mediators (PRMs): 18-HEPE (18-hydroxy eicosapentaenoic acid), 17-HDHA (17-hydroxy

Liver Support:
- Milk Thistle
- L-methionine
- Taurine
- Inositol
- Ox Bile
- Artichoke
- Beet Powder
- Vitamin A
- Vitamin B6
- Vitamin B12
- Plant protein powder with MVM (multi-vitamin/mineral)
- L-glutathione
- N-Acetyl-L-Cysteine (NAC)
- Quercetin
- Methylsulfonylmethane (MSM)
- Sodium Sulfate
- Green Tea Extract
- Reishi
- Cordyceps
- Chinese Skullcap
- Schisandra
- Burdock Extract
- Phosphatidylcholine

If **HIGH** or > 5.0 g/dL:

Elevated albumin levels are often linked to dehydration, a high-protein diet, or potential thyroid or liver conditions.

Potential Causes:
- Conditions: Dehydration, high-protein diet, hypothyroidism, liver or kidney dysfunction.
- Symptoms: Often minimal with mild elevation, but dehydration-related symptoms or high protein diet effects can occur.

Support hydration and kidney function, and monitor thyroid health if related symptoms are present.

Protein Source:
- Protein Powder
- Mixed Amino Acids
- Dairy-Free, Plant-Based Protein Powder
- Whey-Based Protein Powder

Digestive Support:
- Digestive enzymes
- Betaine HCl
- Ox Bile
- L-taurine
- Gentian extract
- Dandelion extract
- Fennel
- Amylase
- Protease SP
- Protease
- Diastase
- Lactase
- Glucoamylase
- Alpha-galactosidase
- Beta-glucanase
- Acid protease

- Phytase
- Cellulase
- Hemicellulase
- Invertase
- Lipase
- Bromelain
- Papain
- Pepsin
- Triphala (Emblica officinalis, Terminalia bellirica, Terminalia chebula)
- Magnesium Hydroxide
- Mastic Gum
- DGL (Deglycyrrhizinated Licorice)
- Methylmethionine Sulfonium Chloride (MMSC)
- Zinc L-Carnosine
- Vitamin C
- Berberine
- Ginger
- Bismuth

Liver Support:
- Milk Thistle
- L-methionine
- Taurine
- Inositol
- Ox Bile
- Artichoke
- Beet Powder
- Vitamin A
- Vitamin B6
- Vitamin B12
- Plant protein powder with MVM (multi-vitamin/mineral)
- L-glutathione
- N-Acetyl-L-Cysteine (NAC)
- Quercetin
- Methylsulfonylmethane (MSM)
- Sodium Sulfate
- Green Tea Extract
- Reishi
- Cordyceps
- Chinese Skullcap
- Schisandra
- Burdock Extract
- Phosphatidylcholine

Kidney Support:
- Champignon (Agaricus bisporus)
- Cordyceps (Cordyceps sinensis)
- Poria (Poria cocos)
- American Ginseng (Panax quinquefolius)
- Astragalus (Astragalus membranaceus)

Thyroid Support:
- N-Acetyl-L-Tyrosine
- American Ginseng (Panax quinquefolius)
- Forskolin (Coleus forskohlii)
- Iodine
- Chromium
- Zinc
- Selenium
- Copper
- Manganese
- Vitamin A
- Vitamin B2
- Potassium Iodide
- Myo-Inositol

Globulin

Globulins are a diverse group of proteins with multiple functions, including immune support, enzymatic activity, and transport. They are classified into four main types: Alpha 1, Alpha 2, Beta, and Gamma globulins. Gamma globulins, largely composed of antibodies (immunoglobulins), are crucial for immune defense.

Normal Range	2.2 - 3.5 g/dL
Optimal Range	2.8 - 3.0 g/dL

CMP (COMPREHENSIVE METABOLIC PANEL)

If **LOW** or < 2.8 g/dL:

 Low globulin levels may indicate immune deficiency, liver dysfunction, GI inflammation, or poor protein digestion.

Potential Causes:
- Conditions: Hypogammaglobulinemia, liver dysfunction, nephrotic syndrome, malnutrition, congenital immune deficiency.
- Symptoms: Fatigue, frequent infections, muscle weakness.

 Focus on immune support, protein intake, and improved digestive health.

Protein Source:
- Protein Powder
- Mixed Amino Acids
- Dairy-Free, Plant-Based Protein Powder
- Whey-Based Protein Powder

Digestive Support:
- Digestive enzymes
- Betaine HCl
- Ox Bile
- L-taurine
- Gentian extract
- Dandelion extract
- Fennel
- Amylase
- Protease SP
- Protease
- Diastase
- Lactase
- Glucoamylase
- Alpha-galactosidase
- Beta-glucanase
- Acid protease
- Phytase
- Cellulase
- Hemicellulase
- Invertase
- Lipase
- Bromelain
- Papain
- Pepsin
- Triphala (Emblica officinalis, Terminalia bellirica, Terminalia chebula)
- Magnesium Hydroxide
- Mastic Gum
- DGL (Deglycyrrhizinated Licorice)
- Methylmethionine Sulfonium Chloride (MMSC)
- Zinc L-Carnosine
- Vitamin C
- Berberine
- Ginger
- Bismuth

Immune Support:
- Echinacea angustifolia
- Astragalus membranaceus
- Elderberry Extract (Sambucus nigra)
- Andrographis paniculate
- Green Tea Extract
- Arabinogalactan (larch tree)
- Lauric Acid
- Cordyceps mushroom
- Shiitake mushroom
- Maitake mushroom
- Reishi mushroom
- Beta 1,3 Glucans
- Vitamin A
- Vitamin D3
- Vitamin E
- Vitamin K2
- Wild cherry bark
- Ginger
- Lovage (Levisticum officinale)
- Wild Cherry Extract

Liver Support:
- Milk Thistle
- L-methionine
- Taurine
- Inositol
- Ox Bile
- Artichoke
- Beet Powder
- Vitamin A
- Vitamin B6
- Vitamin B12
- Plant protein powder with MVM (multi-vitamin/mineral)
- L-glutathione
- N-Acetyl-L-Cysteine (NAC)
- Quercetin
- Methylsulfonylmethane (MSM)
- Sodium Sulfate
- Green Tea Extract
- Reishi
- Cordyceps
- Chinese Skullcap
- Schisandra
- Burdock Extract
- Phosphatidylcholine

If HIGH or > 3.0 g/dL:

Elevated globulin levels may result from chronic inflammation, autoimmune conditions, or infections.

Potential Causes:
- Conditions: Chronic infections, liver disease, autoimmune conditions, multiple myeloma, Waldenström's macroglobulinemia, ulcerative colitis.
- Symptoms: Possible inflammation, joint pain, swelling, fatigue.

Support hydration and kidney function, and monitor thyroid health if related symptoms are present.

Gut Lining Support:
- Zinc L-Carnosine
- N-Acetyl-D-Glucosamine
- Citrus Pectin
- Deglycyrrhizinated Licorice Extract (DGL)
- Slippery Elm, Mucin, Chamomile Extract, Marshmallow, Okra
- Cat's Claw
- Methylsulfonylmethane (MSM)
- Quercetin
- Prune Powder
- L-Glutamine
- Aloe Vera

Anti-inflammatory Support:
- Phytocannabinoids
- Hemp Flower Extract
- Hemp Seed Oil
- Palmitoylethanolamide (PEA)
- Omega-3 Fatty Acids (Fish Oil)
- docosahexaenoic acid), 14-HDHA (14-hydroxy docosahexaenoic acid)
- Vitamin D3
- Curcumin
- Green Tea Extract (Epigallocatechin Gallate (EGCG))
- Trans Resveratrol
- Quercetin
- Nettle (Urtica dioica)
- Pro-Resolving Mediators (PRMs): 18-HEPE (18-hydroxy eicosapentaenoic acid), 17-HDHA (17-hydroxy

CBC WITH DIFFERENTIAL (COMPLETE BLOOD COUNT)

Immune Support:
- Echinacea angustifolia
- Astragalus membranaceus
- Elderberry Extract (Sambucus nigra)
- Andrographis paniculate
- Green Tea Extract
- Arabinogalactan (larch tree)
- Lauric Acid
- Cordyceps mushroom
- Shiitake mushroom
- Maitake mushroom
- Reishi mushroom
- Beta 1,3 Glucans
- Vitamin A
- Vitamin D3
- Vitamin E
- Vitamin K2
- Wild cherry bark
- Ginger
- Lovage (Levisticum officinale)
- Wild Cherry Extract

Bilirubin, Total

Total Bilirubin measures both conjugated (direct) and unconjugated (indirect) forms of bilirubin. It is a by-product of red blood cell breakdown, processed in the liver, and excreted in bile. Elevated levels may cause jaundice, indicating liver or biliary issues, while low levels can indicate spleen insufficiency or iron deficiency.

Normal Range	0.1 - 1.2 mg/dL
Optimal Range	0.5 – 0.9 mg/dL

If LOW or < 0.5 mg/dL:

Low bilirubin levels may indicate spleen insufficiency, iron deficiency anemia, or compromised digestive function, particularly with fat absorption.

Potential Causes:
- Conditions: Spleen insufficiency, iron deficiency anemia, impaired fat digestion.

Focus on liver and digestive support to enhance bilirubin processing and address iron deficiency if present.

Liver Support:
- Milk Thistle
- L-methionine
- Taurine
- Inositol
- Ox Bile
- Artichoke
- Beet Powder
- Vitamin A
- Vitamin B6
- Vitamin B12
- Plant protein powder with MVM (multi-vitamin/mineral)
- L-glutathione
- N-Acetyl-L-Cysteine (NAC)
- Quercetin
- Methylsulfonylmethane (MSM)
- Sodium Sulfate
- Green Tea Extract
- Reishi
- Cordyceps
- Chinese Skullcap
- Schisandra
- Burdock Extract
- Phosphatidylcholine

Digestive Support:
- Digestive enzymes
- Betaine HCl
- Ox Bile
- L-taurine

- Gentian extract
- Dandelion extract
- Fennel
- Amylase
- Protease SP
- Protease
- Diastase
- Lactase
- Glucoamylase
- Alpha-galactosidase
- Beta-glucanase
- Acid protease
- Phytase
- Cellulase
- Hemicellulase
- Invertase
- Lipase

- Bromelain
- Papain
- Pepsin
- Triphala (Emblica officinalis, Terminalia bellirica, Terminalia chebula)
- Magnesium Hydroxide
- Mastic Gum
- DGL (Deglycyrrhizinated Licorice)
- Methylmethionine Sulfonium Chloride (MMSC)
- Zinc L-Carnosine
- Vitamin C
- Berberine
- Ginger
- Bismuth

Iron Support:
- Iron, ferrous bisglycinate

If HIGH or > 0.9 mg/dL:

Elevated bilirubin levels may suggest liver or biliary obstruction, possibly from conditions such as hepatitis, cirrhosis, or gallstones. Prolonged high levels may result in visible jaundice.

Potential Causes:
- Conditions: Hepatitis, cirrhosis, hemolytic disease, biliary obstruction, liver cancer, or gallbladder dysfunction.
- Symptoms: Jaundice (yellowing of the skin/eyes), fatigue, dark urine, light-colored stools.

Emphasis on liver and biliary support to optimize bilirubin processing, as well as digestive aid to support fat metabolism.

Liver Support:
- Milk Thistle
- L-methionine
- Taurine
- Inositol
- Ox Bile
- Artichoke
- Beet Powder
- Vitamin A
- Vitamin B6
- Vitamin B12
- Plant protein powder with MVM (multi-vitamin/mineral)

- L-glutathione
- N-Acetyl-L-Cysteine (NAC)
- Quercetin
- Methylsulfonylmethane (MSM)
- Sodium Sulfate
- Green Tea Extract
- Reishi
- Cordyceps
- Chinese Skullcap
- Schisandra
- Burdock Extract
- Phosphatidylcholine

Digestive Support:
- Digestive enzymes
- Betaine HCl

- Ox Bile
- L-taurine

- Gentian extract
- Dandelion extract
- Fennel
- Amylase
- Protease SP
- Protease
- Diastase
- Lactase
- Glucoamylase
- Alpha-galactosidase
- Beta-glucanase
- Acid protease
- Phytase
- Cellulase
- Hemicellulase
- Invertase
- Lipase
- Bromelain
- Papain
- Pepsin
- Triphala (Emblica officinalis, Terminalia bellirica, Terminalia chebula)
- Magnesium Hydroxide
- Mastic Gum
- DGL (Deglycyrrhizinated Licorice)
- Methylmethionine Sulfonium Chloride (MMSC)
- Zinc L-Carnosine
- Vitamin C
- Berberine
- Ginger
- Bismuth

Nutritional Support:
- Mixed reds powder from fruits and vegetables

Bilirubin - Direct

Direct (conjugated) bilirubin is formed as a result of red blood cell breakdown, primarily in the spleen and bone marrow, and is processed by the liver for excretion. Conjugation makes bilirubin water-soluble, allowing for efficient elimination through bile and digestive processes. Direct bilirubin levels can indicate liver health and function in relation to red blood cell recycling and bile production.

Normal Range	0 - 0.2 mg/dL
Optimal Range	0.1 - 0.15 mg/dL

If LOW or < 0.1 mg/dL:

Low levels of direct bilirubin may suggest issues with the spleen, iron deficiency, or impaired digestion of fats, affecting bilirubin formation and processing.

Potential Causes:
- Conditions: Spleen insufficiency, iron deficiency anemia, impaired digestive ability.

Support liver and digestive health, particularly for iron metabolism and fat digestion.

Digestive Support:
- Digestive enzymes
- Betaine HCl
- Ox Bile
- L-taurine
- Gentian extract
- Dandelion extract
- Fennel
- Amylase
- Protease SP
- Protease

CMP (COMPREHENSIVE METABOLIC PANEL)

- Diastase
- Lactase
- Glucoamylase
- Alpha-galactosidase
- Beta-glucanase
- Acid protease
- Phytase
- Cellulase
- Hemicellulase
- Invertase
- Lipase
- Bromelain
- Papain
- Pepsin
- Triphala (Emblica officinalis, Terminalia bellirica, Terminalia chebula)
- Magnesium Hydroxide
- Mastic Gum
- DGL (Deglycyrrhizinated Licorice)
- Methylmethionine Sulfonium Chloride (MMSC)
- Zinc L-Carnosine
- Vitamin C
- Berberine
- Ginger
- Bismuth

Iron Support:
- Iron, ferrous bisglycinate

If **HIGH** or > 0.15 mg/dL:

Elevated direct bilirubin levels are often associated with liver dysfunction, biliary stasis, or blockage, which may result in jaundice if levels are significantly high.

Potential Causes:
- Conditions: Liver dysfunction, biliary stasis, bile duct obstruction, hepatitis, Gilbert's syndrome, anemia, oxidative stress.

Emphasize liver and biliary support to improve bilirubin processing and bile flow, as well as oxidative stress management.

Liver Support:
- Milk Thistle
- L-methionine
- Taurine
- Inositol
- Ox Bile
- Artichoke
- Beet Powder
- Vitamin A
- Vitamin B6
- Vitamin B12
- Plant protein powder with MVM (multi-vitamin/mineral)
- L-glutathione
- N-Acetyl-L-Cysteine (NAC)
- Quercetin
- Methylsulfonylmethane (MSM)
- Sodium Sulfate
- Green Tea Extract
- Reishi
- Cordyceps
- Chinese Skullcap
- Schisandra
- Burdock Extract
- Phosphatidylcholine

Digestive Support:
- Digestive enzymes
- Betaine HCl
- Ox Bile
- L-taurine
- Gentian extract
- Dandelion extract
- Fennel
- Amylase
- Protease SP
- Protease
- Diastase
- Lactase
- Glucoamylase
- Alpha-galactosidase

CMP (COMPREHENSIVE METABOLIC PANEL)

- Beta-glucanase
- Acid protease
- Phytase
- Cellulase
- Hemicellulase
- Invertase
- Lipase
- Bromelain
- Papain
- Pepsin
- Triphala (Emblica officinalis, Terminalia bellirica, Terminalia chebula)

- Magnesium Hydroxide
- Mastic Gum
- DGL (Deglycyrrhizinated Licorice)
- Methylmethionine Sulfonium Chloride (MMSC)
- Zinc L-Carnosine
- Vitamin C
- Berberine
- Ginger
- Bismuth

Nutritional Support:
- Mixed reds powder from fruits and vegetables

Bilirubin - Indirect

Indirect (unconjugated) bilirubin is the result of red blood cell breakdown in the spleen and bone marrow. This bilirubin is not water-soluble, requiring liver processing before excretion. Elevated levels of indirect bilirubin often point to increased RBC breakdown or liver dysfunction. Levels of direct and indirect bilirubin can help differentiate between liver and hemolytic disorders.

Normal Range	0.2 - 1.2 mg/dL
Optimal Range	0.4 – 0.75 mg/dL

If LOW or < 0.4 mg/dL:

Low levels of indirect bilirubin may indicate decreased red blood cell turnover, liver or spleen function impairment, or impaired fat digestion.

Potential Causes:
- Conditions: Spleen insufficiency, iron deficiency anemia, impaired digestive ability (especially fats).
- Additional Factors: Caffeine intake, barbiturate use, high doses of salicylates, penicillin use.

Support liver and digestive health to improve bilirubin processing.

Liver Support:
- Milk Thistle
- L-methionine
- Taurine
- Inositol
- Ox Bile
- Artichoke
- Beet Powder
- Vitamin A
- Vitamin B6
- Vitamin B12
- Plant protein powder with MVM (multi-vitamin/mineral)
- L-glutathione
- N-Acetyl-L-Cysteine (NAC)
- Quercetin
- Methylsulfonylmethane (MSM)
- Sodium Sulfate
- Green Tea Extract

CMP (COMPREHENSIVE METABOLIC PANEL)

- Reishi
- Cordyceps
- Chinese Skullcap

Digestive Support:
- Digestive enzymes
- Betaine HCl
- Ox Bile
- L-taurine
- Gentian extract
- Dandelion extract
- Fennel
- Amylase
- Protease SP
- Protease
- Diastase
- Lactase
- Glucoamylase
- Alpha-galactosidase
- Beta-glucanase
- Acid protease
- Phytase
- Cellulase

- Schisandra
- Burdock Extract
- Phosphatidylcholine

- Hemicellulase
- Invertase
- Lipase
- Bromelain
- Papain
- Pepsin
- Triphala (Emblica officinalis, Terminalia bellirica, Terminalia chebula)
- Magnesium Hydroxide
- Mastic Gum
- DGL (Deglycyrrhizinated Licorice)
- Methylmethionine Sulfonium Chloride (MMSC)
- Zinc L-Carnosine
- Vitamin C
- Berberine
- Ginger
- Bismuth

Iron Support:
- Iron, ferrous bisglycinate

If **HIGH** or > 0.75 mg/dL:

Elevated indirect bilirubin levels can be associated with increased red blood cell breakdown, liver dysfunction, or genetic conditions affecting bilirubin processing.

Potential Causes:
- Conditions: Liver dysfunction, biliary stasis, bile duct obstruction, oxidative stress, RBC hemolysis, hepatitis, Gilbert's syndrome, anemia.
- Genetic Factors: Rotor syndrome, Crigler-Najjar syndrome, Dubin-Johnson syndrome, Gilbert syndrome.
- Additional Factors: Hemolytic anemia, strenuous exercise, HIV medications (e.g., Atazanavir).

Liver and biliary support may help reduce elevated levels and improve bile flow.

Liver Support:
- Milk Thistle
- L-methionine
- Taurine
- Inositol
- Ox Bile
- Artichoke
- Beet Powder
- Vitamin A
- Vitamin B6

- Vitamin B12
- Plant protein powder with MVM (multi-vitamin/mineral)
- L-glutathione
- N-Acetyl-L-Cysteine (NAC)
- Quercetin
- Methylsulfonylmethane (MSM)
- Sodium Sulfate
- Green Tea Extract

- Reishi
- Cordyceps
- Chinese Skullcap

Digestive Support:
- Digestive enzymes
- Betaine HCl
- Ox Bile
- L-taurine
- Gentian extract
- Dandelion extract
- Fennel
- Amylase
- Protease SP
- Protease
- Diastase
- Lactase
- Glucoamylase
- Alpha-galactosidase
- Beta-glucanase
- Acid protease
- Phytase
- Cellulase

- Schisandra
- Burdock Extract
- Phosphatidylcholine

- Hemicellulase
- Invertase
- Lipase
- Bromelain
- Papain
- Pepsin
- Triphala (Emblica officinalis, Terminalia bellirica, Terminalia chebula)
- Magnesium Hydroxide
- Mastic Gum
- DGL (Deglycyrrhizinated Licorice)
- Methylmethionine Sulfonium Chloride (MMSC)
- Zinc L-Carnosine
- Vitamin C
- Berberine
- Ginger
- Bismuth

Nutritional Support:
- Mixed reds powder from fruits and vegetables

Alkaline Phosphatase (ALP)

Alkaline Phosphatase (ALP) is a zinc-dependent enzyme produced mainly by the liver and bones. Elevated ALP levels can indicate liver or bile duct obstruction, as well as bone-related conditions. Low levels may correlate with zinc deficiency. ALP is also pH-sensitive, requiring an alkaline environment to function effectively.

Note on Age Variations:
Children and adolescents have naturally higher ALP levels due to bone growth, with reference ranges varying by age.

Normal Range	39 - 117 IU/L
Optimal Range	70 - 100 IU/L

If LOW or < 70 IU/L:

Low ALP may indicate zinc deficiency, low dietary protein, or adrenal insufficiency.

Potential Causes:
- Deficiencies: Zinc deficiency, low protein diet, B9 deficiency.
- Additional Factors: Use of estrogen, low stomach acid (HCL).

CMP (COMPREHENSIVE METABOLIC PANEL)

 Support liver, digestion, stress response, and zinc and vitamin B status

Digestive Support:
- Digestive enzymes
- Betaine HCl
- Ox Bile
- L-taurine
- Gentian extract
- Dandelion extract
- Fennel
- Amylase
- Protease SP
- Protease
- Diastase
- Lactase
- Glucoamylase
- Alpha-galactosidase
- Beta-glucanase
- Acid protease
- Phytase
- Cellulase
- Hemicellulase
- Invertase
- Lipase
- Bromelain
- Papain
- Pepsin
- Triphala (Emblica officinalis, Terminalia bellirica, Terminalia chebula)
- Magnesium Hydroxide
- Mastic Gum
- DGL (Deglycyrrhizinated Licorice)
- Methylmethionine Sulfonium Chloride (MMSC)
- Zinc L-Carnosine
- Vitamin C
- Berberine
- Ginger
- Bismuth

Protein Source:
- Protein Powder
- Mixed Amino Acids
- Dairy-Free, Plant-Based Protein Powder
- Whey-Based Protein Powder

If HIGH or > 100 IU/L:

 Elevated ALP levels may indicate liver or biliary issues, increased bone turnover, or leaky gut syndrome.

Potential Causes:
- Conditions: Increased bone turnover, biliary obstruction, intestinal hyperpermeability (leaky gut), excessive vitamin D intake.
- Additional Factors: Liver damage, shingles (herpes zoster).

 Support liver health and gut lining integrity.

Liver Support:
- Milk Thistle
- L-methionine
- Taurine
- Inositol
- Ox Bile
- Artichoke
- Beet Powder
- Vitamin A
- Vitamin B6
- Vitamin B12
- Plant protein powder with MVM (multi-vitamin/mineral)
- L-glutathione
- N-Acetyl-L-Cysteine (NAC)
- Quercetin
- Methylsulfonylmethane (MSM)
- Sodium Sulfate
- Green Tea Extract

CMP (COMPREHENSIVE METABOLIC PANEL)

- Reishi
- Cordyceps
- Chinese Skullcap
- Schisandra
- Burdock Extract
- Phosphatidylcholine

Gut Lining Support:
- Zinc L-Carnosine
- N-Acetyl-D-Glucosamine
- Citrus Pectin
- Deglycyrrhizinated Licorice Extract (DGL)
- Slippery Elm, Mucin, Chamomile Extract, Marshmallow, Okra
- Cat's Claw
- Methylsulfonylmethane (MSM)
- Quercetin
- Prune Powder
- L-Glutamine
- Aloe Vera

Lactate Dehydrogenase (LDH)

Lactate Dehydrogenase (LDH) is an enzyme that catalyzes the conversion of pyruvate to lactate, playing a critical role in cellular energy production. Elevated LDH levels can indicate acute or chronic cell damage across multiple organs. LDH is especially useful in evaluating hepatic cellular damage and is associated with cardiac injury when elevated alongside other specific markers. Low LDH levels are rare and generally clinically insignificant.

Normal Range	120 - 240 IU/L
Optimal Range	90 - 150 IU/L

If **LOW** or **< 90 IU/L:**

 Low LDH may indicate decreased cellular activity, often associated with low thyroid or adrenal function, malnutrition, or inactivity.

Low LDH is generally not harmful and often requires no immediate action.

Potential Causes:
- Conditions: Low thyroid or adrenal function, malnutrition, inactivity.

 Support thyroid and adrenal function to promote cellular metabolism as needed.

 Thyroid Support:
- N-Acetyl-L-Tyrosine
- American Ginseng (Panax quinquefolius)
- Forskolin (Coleus forskohlii)
- Iodine
- Chromium
- Zinc
- Selenium
- Copper
- Manganese
- Vitamin A
- Vitamin B2
- Potassium Iodide
- Myo-Inositol

Adrenal Support:
- gamma-Aminobutyric Acid (GABA)
- Eleutherococcus senticosus
- American Ginseng
- Ashwagandha
- Rhodiola
- Licorice
- Vitamin B2
- Vitamin B5
- Vitamin B6
- Vitamin C
- N-Acetyl-L-Tyrosine
- Phosphatidylserine
- Valerian
- Passion Flower
- Lemon Balm
- Chamomile
- L-theanine
- 5-HTP
- Melatonin
- Rhodiola rosea
- Pyrroloquinoline Quinone (PQQ)
- Taurine
- Vitamin B1
- Vitamin B12
- Magnesium Malate
- Magnesium Taurinate
- Magnesium Glycinate

If **HIGH** or **> 150 IU/L:**

Elevated LDH is a non-specific indicator of tissue damage and may signify conditions affecting the liver, muscles, heart, kidneys, brain, or red blood cells.

Significantly elevated LDH levels may warrant additional testing, such as LDH isoenzymes, to determine the specific location of damage.

Potential Causes:
- Conditions: Hepatitis, liver congestion, pulmonary infarct, pneumonia, various anemias, skeletal muscle injury, liver or biliary dysfunction.

Support liver health and gut lining integrity.

Liver Support:
- Milk Thistle
- L-methionine
- Taurine
- Inositol
- Ox Bile
- Artichoke
- Beet Powder
- Vitamin A
- Vitamin B6
- Vitamin B12
- Plant protein powder with MVM (multi-vitamin/mineral)
- L-glutathione
- N-Acetyl-L-Cysteine (NAC)
- Quercetin
- Methylsulfonylmethane (MSM)
- Sodium Sulfate
- Green Tea Extract
- Reishi
- Cordyceps
- Chinese Skullcap
- Schisandra
- Burdock Extract
- Phosphatidylcholine

Kidney Support:
- Champignon (Agaricus bisporus)
- Cordyceps (Cordyceps sinensis)
- Poria (Poria cocos)
- American Ginseng (Panax quinquefolius)
- Astragalus (Astragalus membranaceus)

CMP (COMPREHENSIVE METABOLIC PANEL)

Cardio Support:
- Bonito Peptide Powder
- Grape seed extract (Vitis vinefera)
- PQQ (Pyrroloquinoline Quinone), Rhodiola Extract (Rhodiola rosea)
- Monostroma nitidum (seaweed) extract

Anti-inflammatory Support:
- Phytocannabinoids
- Hemp Flower Extract
- Hemp Seed Oil
- Palmitoylethanolamide (PEA)
- Omega-3 Fatty Acids (Fish Oil)
- docosahexaenoic acid), 14-HDHA (14-hydroxy docosahexaenoic acid)
- Vitamin D3
- Curcumin
- Green Tea Extract (Epigallocatechin Gallate (EGCG))
- Trans Resveratrol
- Quercetin
- Nettle (Urtica dioica)
- Pro-Resolving Mediators (PRMs): 18-HEPE (18-hydroxy eicosapentaenoic acid), 17-HDHA (17-hydroxy

Aspartate amino-transferase (AST) (SGOT)

Aspartate Aminotransferase (AST), primarily produced in muscle tissue, plays a role in energy production and is released into circulation following cellular injury or death. AST is less specific for liver issues than ALT but can indicate liver, cardiac, or skeletal muscle damage. AST is often evaluated in tandem with ALT and other liver enzymes to assess liver health or cardiovascular status. Elevated AST is common in myocardial infarction (MI) and liver damage, while lower levels can point to deficiencies or malabsorption

Normal Range	0 - 40 IU/L
Optimal Range	10 - 30 IU/L

If **LOW** or **< 10 IU/L:**

Low AST may indicate protein deficiency, malabsorption, or vitamin B6 deficiency, as well as other digestive or glandular concerns.

Potential Causes:
- Conditions: Protein deficiency, malabsorption, B6 deficiency, alcoholism, gonadal hypofunction.

Support liver and digestive health, protein intake, and B-complex vitamins, particularly B6.

Digestive Support:
- Digestive enzymes
- Betaine HCl
- Ox Bile
- L-taurine
- Gentian extract
- Dandelion extract
- Fennel
- Amylase
- Protease SP
- Protease
- Diastase
- Lactase
- Glucoamylase
- Alpha-galactosidase
- Beta-glucanase
- Acid protease
- Phytase
- Cellulase
- Hemicellulase
- Invertase

CMP (COMPREHENSIVE METABOLIC PANEL)

- Lipase
- Bromelain
- Papain
- Pepsin
- Triphala (Emblica officinalis, Terminalia bellirica, Terminalia chebula)
- Magnesium Hydroxide
- Mastic Gum
- DGL (Deglycyrrhizinated Licorice)
- Methylmethionine Sulfonium Chloride (MMSC)
- Zinc L-Carnosine
- Vitamin C
- Berberine
- Ginger
- Bismuth

Protein & Gut Support:
- Protein powder, mixed amino acids
- Zinc L-Carnosine
- N-Acetyl-D-Glucosamine
- Citrus Pectin
- Deglycyrrhizinated Licorice Extract (DGL)
- Slippery Elm, Mucin, Chamomile Extract, Marshmallow, Okra
- Cat's Claw
- Methylsulfonylmethane (MSM)
- Quercetin
- Prune Powder
- L-Glutamine
- Aloe Vera

Nutritional Support:
- Vitamin B Complex
- Vitamin B6

Liver Support:
- Milk Thistle
- L-methionine
- Taurine
- Inositol
- Ox Bile
- Artichoke
- Beet Powder
- Vitamin A
- Vitamin B6
- Vitamin B12
- Plant protein powder with MVM (multi-vitamin/mineral)
- L-glutathione
- N-Acetyl-L-Cysteine (NAC)
- Quercetin
- Methylsulfonylmethane (MSM)
- Sodium Sulfate
- Green Tea Extract
- Reishi
- Cordyceps
- Chinese Skullcap
- Schisandra
- Burdock Extract
- Phosphatidylcholine

Vessel & Gland Support:
- Diosmin (from Sweet Orange)
- Quercetin
- Gotu Kola Extract (Centella asiatica)
- Horse Chestnut Extract (Aesculus hippocastanum)
- Grape Seed Extract (Vitis vinifera)
- Vitamin C
- Broccoli Powder Extract
- Vitex Agnus Castus (Chasteberry)
- Black Cohosh
- Mustard Powder (Sinapis alba)
- Chrysin
- Trans Resveratrol
- Green Tea Extract
- Diindolylmethane (DIM)
- Calcium D-Glucarate (CDG)
- Magnesium
- Vitamin B6
- Vitamin B9 (Folate)
- Vitamin B12

CMP (COMPREHENSIVE METABOLIC PANEL)

If **HIGH** or > 30 IU/L:

Elevated AST may reflect liver dysfunction, cardiovascular concerns, pancreatitis, diabetes, or increased oxidative stress.

Potential Causes:
- Conditions: Liver dysfunction, pancreatitis, cardiovascular disease, alcohol consumption, early onset congestive heart disease, acute MI, oxidative stress.

Support antioxidant and leafy green intake for detoxification, as well as cardiovascular and glucose management support.

Nutritional Support:
- Mixed greens powder from fruits and vegetables
- Vitamin B Complex
- Vitamin B6

Vessel & Glucose Support:
- Diosmin (from Sweet Orange)
- Quercetin
- Gotu Kola Extract (Centella asiatica)
- Horse Chestnut Extract (Aesculus hippocastanum)
- Grape Seed Extract (Vitis vinifera)
- Vitamin C
- Magnesium
- Zinc
- Selenium
- Manganese
- Chromium
- Molybdenum
- Iodine
- Taurine
- Carnosine
- Inositol (as Myo and D-Chiro)
- R-Lipoic Acid
- Vitamin A
- Vitamin D
- Vitamin E
- Vitamin K
- Benfotiamine (Fat Soluble Vitamin B1)
- Vitamin B1
- Vitamin B2
- Vitamin B3
- Vitamin B5
- Vitamin B6
- Vitamin B7 (Biotin)
- Vitamin B9 (Folate)
- Vitamin B12

Antioxidant Support:
- Acerola Extract (Malpighia glabra)
- Grape Seed Extract (Vitis vinifera)
- Curcumin
- Garlic (Allium sativum)
- Ginkgo Extract (Ginkgo biloba)
- Quercetin
- Rutin
- Clove (Syzygium aromaticum)
- Allspice (Pimenta dioica)
- Sweet Basil (Ocimum basilicum)
- Sage (Salvia officinalis)
- Rosemary Extract (Rosmarinus officinalis)
- Lutein
- Lycopene
- Trans Resveratrol
- Vitamin A
- Vitamin E
- L-glutathione
- NAC (N-Acetyl-L-Cysteine)
- Broccoli Powder Extract
- Sulforaphane
- Olive Leaf Extract (Olea europaea)
- Bergamot
- Red Grape Powder
- Alpha Lipoic Acid
- Taurine
- MVM (Multi-vitamin/mineral)
- Glutathione (reduced)

Alanine amino-transferase (ALT) (SGPT)

Alanine Aminotransferase (ALT) is primarily produced in the liver and is released into the bloodstream when liver tissue is damaged. ALT levels are often evaluated to assess liver function, monitor potential liver injury, or evaluate biliary dysfunction to a lesser degree. Elevated ALT levels are more specific to liver issues than other transaminases and may indicate liver cell injury or inflammation.

Normal Range	0 - 32 IU/L
Optimal Range	10 - 30 IU/L

If LOW or < 10 IU/L:

Low ALT levels may indicate early signs of liver congestion, fatty liver disease, or nutritional deficiencies, including B6 and zinc.

Potential Causes:
- Conditions: Early-stage fatty liver, liver congestion, protein deficiency, malabsorption, alcoholism, B6 deficiency.

Support liver health, protein digestion, and nutrient intake, particularly B vitamins and zinc, to improve ALT levels.

Liver Support:
- Milk Thistle
- L-methionine
- Taurine
- Inositol
- Ox Bile
- Artichoke
- Beet Powder
- Vitamin A
- Vitamin B6
- Vitamin B12
- Plant protein powder with MVM (multi-vitamin/mineral)
- L-glutathione
- N-Acetyl-L-Cysteine (NAC)
- Quercetin
- Methylsulfonylmethane (MSM)
- Sodium Sulfate
- Green Tea Extract
- Reishi
- Cordyceps
- Chinese Skullcap
- Schisandra
- Burdock Extract
- Phosphatidylcholine

Nutritional Support:
- Vitamin B Complex
- Vitamins B6, B2
- Zinc
- Molybdenum

Digestive & Intestinal Support:
- Betaine HCl, Pepsin
- Digestive enzymes, Betaine HCl, Ox Bile
- Zinc L-Carnosine
- N-Acetyl-D-Glucosamine
- Citrus Pectin
- Deglycyrrhizinated Licorice Extract (DGL)
- Slippery Elm, Mucin, Chamomile Extract, Marshmallow, Okra

- Cat's Claw
- Methylsulfonylmethane (MSM)
- Quercetin
- Prune Powder
- L-Glutamine
- Aloe Vera

If HIGH or > 30 IU/L:

Elevated ALT often indicates liver damage or dysfunction. Chronic conditions, fatty liver, or medications can increase ALT.

Potential Causes:
- Conditions: Liver dysfunction, biliary obstruction, fatty liver, chronic or autoimmune hepatitis, cirrhosis, drug or alcohol-induced liver injury.

Prioritize liver, vascular, and immune support to address potential inflammation and damage to the liver and biliary system.

Liver Support:
- Milk Thistle
- L-methionine
- Taurine
- Inositol
- Ox Bile
- Artichoke
- Beet Powder
- Vitamin A
- Vitamin B6
- Vitamin B12
- Plant protein powder with MVM (multi-vitamin/mineral)
- L-glutathione
- N-Acetyl-L-Cysteine (NAC)
- Quercetin
- Methylsulfonylmethane (MSM)
- Sodium Sulfate
- Green Tea Extract
- Reishi
- Cordyceps
- Chinese Skullcap
- Schisandra
- Burdock Extract
- Phosphatidylcholine

Nutritional Support:
- Vitamin B Complex

Vessel Support:
- Diosmin (from Sweet Orange)
- Quercetin
- Gotu Kola Extract (Centella asiatica)
- Horse Chestnut Extract (Aesculus hippocastanum)
- Grape Seed Extract (Vitis vinifera)
- Vitamin C

CMP (COMPREHENSIVE METABOLIC PANEL)

Gamma-glutamyl transferase (GGT)

Gamma-Glutamyl Transferase (GGT) is a liver enzyme produced in the endoplasmic reticulum, primarily used to detect liver damage and assess biliary obstruction, as it will elevate early in liver or bile duct issues. Elevated GGT can also indicate excessive alcohol intake or other liver-related issues, and is associated with conditions that elevate oxidative stress.

Normal Range	1 - 70 IU/L
Optimal Range	20 - 30 IU/L

If LOW or < 20 IU/L:

Low GGT can sometimes indicate issues related to hypothyroidism or nutrient deficiencies, particularly magnesium and vitamin B6.

Potential Causes:
- Conditions: Low magnesium, hypothyroidism, hypothalamic malfunction.

Support thyroid function and address possible magnesium, B6, and zinc deficiencies to maintain GGT within optimal range.

Thyroid Support:
- N-Acetyl-L-Tyrosine
- American Ginseng (Panax quinquefolius)
- Forskolin (Coleus forskohlii)
- Iodine
- Chromium
- Zinc
- Selenium
- Copper
- Manganese
- Vitamin A
- Vitamin B2
- Potassium Iodide
- Myo-Inositol

Glandular Support:
- Glandular formulas: thyroid, pituitary, hypothalamus

Nutritional Support:
- Magnesium, Zinc, Molybdenum,
- Vitamin B2, B6
- Taurine
- Malic Acid / malate

If HIGH or > 30 IU/L:

Elevated GGT often indicates liver or biliary dysfunction, and in high values, it may suggest issues like alcohol abuse, viral hepatitis, or biliary obstruction. Moderately high GGT can correlate with oxidative stress, cardiovascular disease risk, type 2 diabetes, or fatty liver disease.

Potential Causes:
- Conditions: Viral hepatitis, alcohol abuse, trauma, biliary stasis, sepsis, cardiovascular disease, diabetes, chronic obstructive pulmonary disease.

Support liver health, reduce oxidative stress, and closely monitor for biliary obstruction or any bleeding-related complications.

Liver Support:
- Milk Thistle
- L-methionine
- Taurine
- Inositol
- Ox Bile
- Artichoke
- Beet Powder
- Vitamin A
- Vitamin B6
- Vitamin B12
- Plant protein powder with MVM (multi-vitamin/mineral)
- L-glutathione
- N-Acetyl-L-Cysteine (NAC)
- Quercetin
- Methylsulfonylmethane (MSM)
- Sodium Sulfate
- Green Tea Extract
- Reishi
- Cordyceps
- Chinese Skullcap
- Schisandra
- Burdock Extract
- Phosphatidylcholine

Metabolites

A vitamin panel helps assess a person's nutritional status and identify any deficiencies or excesses in specific vitamins.

Choline

Choline is a critical nutrient involved in methyl donation, liver health, and brain function. It converts to acetylcholine (ACh) and trimethylglycine (TMG), supporting cellular energy and liver health. Dietary sources include eggs, liver, peanuts, and cruciferous vegetables, with an Adequate Intake (AI) of 425 mg/day for women and 550 mg/day for men.

Normal Range	8.6 - 24.1 nmol/mL
Optimal Range	8.6 - 24.1 nmol/mL

If **LOW** or < 8.6 nmol/mL:

Low choline levels may affect methylation efficiency, liver health, and muscle integrity. Deficiency may lead to hepatic triglyceride accumulation and is particularly relevant for those with MTHFR gene mutations.

Dietary Sources: Increase choline intake from eggs, liver, poultry, fish, and cruciferous vegetables.
Potential Health Impact: Inadequate choline may lead to muscle damage, inefficient methylation, and increased triglyceride buildup in the liver.

Nutritional Support:
- Phosphatidylcholine

If **HIGH** or > 24.1 nmol/mL:

Elevated choline levels may arise from excessive dietary intake (meat, eggs, soybeans, etc.) or mitochondrial dysfunction in metabolic syndrome.
Metabolic Impact: High plasma choline can correlate with elevated triglycerides, glucose, body mass index (BMI), body fat, and waist circumference, potentially disrupting normal lipid metabolism.

Reduce choline intake from rich sources (e.g., eggs, liver).
Monitor metabolic markers for triglycerides, glucose, and BMI to assess potential metabolic syndrome risk factors.

Considerations for High Choline Intake:
Excessive choline consumption (>7,500 mg) may cause side effects like low blood pressure, sweating, and gastrointestinal issues.

Inositol

Inositol is essential in cellular signaling, particularly in insulin receptor activation. It supports peripheral nerve development, fat metabolism, and anti-arteriosclerotic and anti-atherogenic functions. Commonly used in treating insulin resistance and female fertility (e.g., PCOS), inositol may improve insulin sensitivity and glycemic control at doses of 2-4 g/day, while doses for psychiatric support (e.g., anxiety, OCD) range from 12-18 g/day.

Normal Range	20.3 - 50.6 nmol/mL
Optimal Range	20.3 - 50.6 nmol/mL

If **LOW** or **< 20.3 nmol/mL**:

Low inositol levels may impact insulin sensitivity and increase the risk of metabolic-related conditions (e.g., diabetes, PCOS). Conditions like depression, anxiety, PCOS, and cardiovascular disease are linked to inositol depletion.

Dietary Sources: Boost intake of inositol-rich foods, including oranges, cantaloupe, prunes, beans, blackberries, and green beans.
Gut Health Consideration: Antibiotic use can reduce microbiome-mediated inositol release, affecting natural synthesis.

Nutritional Support:
- myo-Inositol

If **HIGH** or **> 50.6 nmol/mL**:

Elevated inositol levels can influence metabolic function and may play a role in managing conditions like metabolic syndrome. There is no established toxicity level, though high doses may cause mild gastrointestinal discomfort.

Clinical Relevance: High inositol intake has potential applications in reducing LDL-C and ApoB in metabolic syndrome and may improve markers of glycemic control.

Considerations for High Choline Intake:
Monitor for possible side effects at higher doses, such as mild gastrointestinal symptoms.

Carnitine

Carnitine is essential for lipid metabolism, energy production, and neuroprotection. It plays a key role in the antioxidant response and neurotransmitter support. Carnitine supplementation is often utilized for neuroprotective purposes and in the management of degenerative brain conditions such as Alzheimer's. Excessive dietary carnitine, however, may promote cardiovascular inflammation due to microbial conversion to trimethylamine N-oxide (TMAO).

Normal Range	16.6 - 47.1 nmol/mL
Optimal Range	16.6 - 47.1 nmol/mL

If **LOW** or **< 16.6 nmol/mL**:

Low carnitine may affect muscle metabolism, energy production, and cognitive function. This deficiency is uncommon among omnivores but more likely in vegetarians, vegans, or those with nutrient malabsorption (e.g., inflammatory bowel disease, liver dysfunction).

Dietary Sources: Increase consumption of carnitine-rich foods like red meat, eggs, and dairy.
Supplemental Support: Consider carnitine supplements to support energy production and muscle metabolism.

 Nutritional Support:
- Acetyl-L-Carnitine
- L-Carnitine

If **HIGH** or > 47.1 nmol/mL:

 Elevated carnitine may suggest an increased intake or excessive synthesis within the body. While carnitine is generally safe, high levels can be associated with increased cardiovascular risks due to conversion to TMAO by certain gut bacteria.

Clinical Relevance: Evaluate dietary sources and consider testing for gut microbial balance to check for bacteria that promote TMAO synthesis.

 Considerations for High Levels:
Monitor cardiovascular health markers if intake of red meat or supplements is high. Reduce dietary intake if necessary and assess gut health.

Methylmalonic Acid (MMA)

MMA is produced when methylmalonyl-CoA converts to succinyl-CoA, a reaction dependent on Vitamin B12. This conversion supports energy production in the Krebs cycle. MMA serves as a functional marker for Vitamin B12 status; elevated MMA indicates B12 deficiency, as insufficient B12 causes MMA accumulation.

Normal Range	≤ 0.8 nmol/mL
Optimal Range	≤ 0.8 nmol/mL

If **HIGH** or > 0.8 nmol/mL:

 Elevated MMA indicates potential Vitamin B12 deficiency, as B12 is required to convert MMA into succinyl-CoA for the Krebs cycle. Without adequate B12, MMA accumulates, potentially leading to toxic effects and symptoms of B12 deficiency.

Clinical Relevance: High MMA levels may signal a need to assess B12 levels directly and evaluate for conditions related to B12 malabsorption, such as certain types of anemia, renal insufficiency, and celiac disease.

 Consider B12 Supplementation: To support MMA conversion and address potential deficiency.

 Vitamin B12 Support:
- Vitamin B12: Methylcobalamin or Hydroxocobalamin
- For patients with malabsorption issues, consider intramuscular B12 injections per medical guidance.

Electrolytes

An electrolytes blood test is used to measure the levels of specific ions, such as sodium and potassium, within a person's bloodstream.

Sodium

Sodium is a key electrolyte essential for fluid balance, muscle contractions, and nerve signaling. Imbalances in sodium can indicate various health issues and may require dietary or hydration adjustments. Supplementation is sometimes necessary in cases of extreme fluid loss or dehydration. Sodium is commonly supplemented through dietary sources, salt tablets, or IV administration when levels are critically low.

Normal Range	136 - 145 nmol/mL
Optimal Range	136 - 145 nmol/mL

If LOW or < 136.0 nmol/mL:

Low sodium levels, or hyponatremia, can result from fluid loss due to diarrhea, vomiting, or excessive sweating, as well as from certain medications (e.g., diuretics, SSRIs, NSAIDs). Chronic low sodium can lead to adverse effects, including balance instability, cognitive deficits, and poor nutrient absorption.

Sodium loss is common when reducing processed foods, which are often high in sodium. Additionally, conditions like Addison's disease and specific medications increase the risk of sodium depletion.

Electrolyte Support:
- Potassium
- Sodium
- Chloride
- Magnesium
- Magnesium Bisglycinate
- Vitamin C
- Zinc

If HIGH or > 145.0 nmol/mL:

Elevated sodium levels often indicate dehydration or can be due to factors like diarrhea, adrenal disorders, kidney disease, or specific medications (e.g., diuretics).

Increase water intake, avoid caffeine and alcohol, and evaluate for potential underlying causes such as dehydration or kidney issues.

ELECTROLYTES

Potassium

Potassium is a vital electrolyte that regulates blood pressure, heart rhythm, and muscle contractions. It maintains fluid balance in conjunction with sodium, influencing both intracellular and extracellular fluid dynamics. Low potassium levels can lead to hypotension, muscle weakness, and bradycardia, while high levels can cause cardiac issues and may require urgent treatment. Dietary potassium is often obtained from raw, unprocessed foods, and levels are affected by fluid loss, kidney function, and certain medications.

Normal Range	3.5 - 5.5 nmol/mL
Optimal Range	3.5 - 5.5 nmol/mL

If LOW or < 3.5 nmol/mL:

 Hypokalemia may cause hypotension, muscle weakness, and a slowed heart rate. It can also impact insulin regulation, reducing carbohydrate tolerance.

Causes: Fluid loss (e.g., vomiting, diarrhea, sweating), magnesium deficiency, alcohol use, certain medications (potassium-wasting diuretics), and conditions like diabetic ketoacidosis can contribute to low potassium levels.

 Dietary Sources: High-potassium foods include bananas, avocados, sweet potatoes, leafy greens, and tomatoes. Cooking may deplete potassium content, so raw sources are preferable.

 Electrolyte Support:
- Potassium
- Sodium
- Chloride
- Magnesium
- Magnesium Bisglycinate
- Vitamin C
- Zinc

If HIGH or > 5.5 nmol/mL:

 Hyperkalemia can result in cardiac arrhythmias and, if severe, may require emergency care.

Causes: Chronic kidney disease, dehydration, injury-related blood loss, excessive potassium intake, and medications (e.g., ACE inhibitors, NSAIDs) can elevate potassium.

 Monitor potassium intake, review medications, and ensure hydration. In cases of critical elevation, EKG monitoring and treatment may be necessary.

Amino Acids

Amino acids are the building blocks of proteins and play crucial roles in various physiological processes within the body. The levels of different amino acids can provide insights into metabolic, nutritional, and genetic conditions.

Asparagine

Asparagine is a non-essential amino acid synthesized from glutamine and aspartate, crucial for brain development, function, and cellular processes. It supports DNA/RNA synthesis and the removal of ammonia, a cellular waste product. Asparagine is readily available from both plant and animal sources, and endogenous production typically prevents deficiencies. No established RDA, AI, or UL exists for asparagine, and it is not commonly supplemented due to the body's natural production capability.

Normal Range	37.8 - 131.8 nmol/mL
Optimal Range	37.8 - 131.8 nmol/mL

If LOW or < 37.8 nmol/mL:

Although asparagine deficiencies are uncommon, lower levels may theoretically impact brain function or contribute to fatigue.

Dietary Sources: Asparagine is found in foods like dairy, whey, beef, poultry, eggs, fish, seafood, asparagus, legumes, nuts, seeds, soy, and grains. Additional asparagine can be indirectly supplemented via glutamine.

Electrolyte Support:
- Potassium
- Sodium
- Chloride
- Magnesium
- Magnesium Bisglycinate
- Vitamin C
- Zinc

If HIGH or > 131.8 nmol/mL:

High dietary protein intake can elevate asparagine levels. Additionally, asparagine may be elevated in hyperammonemia to serve as a reservoir for waste nitrogen. Elevated asparagine levels can also indicate problems with purine (and therefore protein) synthesis.

Reduce L-glutamine supplements and food sources like red meat, poultry, fish, dairy, soy, quinoa, buckwheat, nuts, seeds, and beans.

Nutritional Support:
- Magnesium Citrate
- Magnesium Taurinate
- Magnesium Glycinate
- Magnesium Malate
- Zinc
- Vitamin B6
- Vitamin B complex
- MVM (Multi-vitamin/mineral)

Glutamine

Glutamine is a conditionally essential amino acid that supports immune function, gut health, and cellular repair, especially under physiological stress or muscle wasting conditions (e.g., severe infections, cancer, or trauma). It is the primary fuel source for intestinal epithelial cells and immune cells, aids nitrogen transport, and is a precursor to glutathione and nucleotides for DNA and RNA synthesis. Glutamine also helps regulate intestinal barrier function and can moderate blood glucose levels after high-carbohydrate meals. There is no established RDA, AI, or UL for glutamine, though it is commonly supplemented as L-glutamine, especially for gut health at doses of up to 10 g/day.

Normal Range	295.3 - 721.8 nmol/mL
Optimal Range	295.3 - 721.8 nmol/mL

If LOW or < 295.3 nmol/mL:

 Glutamine may be depleted under intense physiological stress, trauma, burns, or chronic endurance exercise. Deficiency is rare due to endogenous synthesis, but reduced levels can impact immune cell function and increase intestinal permeability.

 Dietary Sources: Good sources include whey, casein, milk, rice, corn, tofu, meat, and eggs.

- L-Glutamine

If HIGH or > 721.8 nmol/mL:

 There is currently no established Recommended Dietary Allowance (RDA), Adequate Intake (AI), or Upper Limit (UL) for glutamine. Glutamine is usually sold as L-glutamine, and studies in humans have examined doses ranging from 500 mg per day to 50 grams per day. Higher doses (exceeding 10 grams per day) are commonly used in treating intestinal barrier permeability.

 In some individuals, glutamine is converted more efficiently to glutamate, which can lead to a neuron-excitatory state, increased anxiety, tension headaches or migraines, and even tachycardia. If any of these symptoms occur after consuming glutamine, supplementation should be discontinued.

If glutamate seems to be the problem, consider supporting these co-factors:
- Magnesium and manganese are required for the conversion of glutamate to glutamine.
- Magnesium is also required for the conversion of glutamine to glutamate.
- Zinc and Vitamin B6 are required for the conversion of glutamate to GABA.

 Nutritional Support:
- Magnesium Citrate
- Magnesium Taurinate
- Magnesium Glycinate
- Magnesium Malate
- Manganese

- Zinc
- Vitamin B6
- Vitamin B complex
- MVM (Multi-vitamin/mineral)

AMINO ACIDS

Serine

Serine, especially in its form as D-serine, functions as a neuromodulator in the brain, supporting neural communication and cognitive processes. It enhances the action of NMDA (N-methyl-D-aspartate) receptors, which play a role in synaptic plasticity and memory formation. While serine is non-essential and synthesized from glycine in the body, it has potential benefits as a nootropic and is studied in relation to cognitive decline, addiction, and neurodegenerative conditions.

Normal Range	58.0 - 139.6 nmol/mL
Normal Range	58.0 - 139.6 nmol/mL

If **LOW** or **< 58.0 nmol/mL**:

 While deficiency is rare due to endogenous production, low serine may correlate with higher risks of cognitive decline and certain neuropsychiatric behaviors.

 Dietary Sources: Foods rich in serine include fish, meat, dairy, soybeans, spinach, kale, cauliflower, cabbage, pumpkin, banana, and beans.

- Glycine

If **HIGH** or **> 139.6 nmol/mL**:

 High dietary intake of serine-rich foods or supplementation may cause elevated levels. Low threonine levels indicate glucogenic compensation and catabolism. Supplement threonine and BCAAs.

Homocysteinemia and methylation defects may lower plasma serine levels. Vitamin B6, B12, folate, or betaine can normalize homocysteine and serine.

There's no established RDA, AL, or UL for serine supplementation or intake. Excessive supplementation may reduce cognitive decline, cocaine dependence, and schizophrenia symptoms. Phosphatidylserine, a common supplemental phospholipid containing serine, has doses of 30 mg/kg of body weight used in cognitive decline patients.

Nutrient deficiencies in cofactors needed for serine metabolism can elevate levels. Vitamin B6 and B1 have been shown to lower serine levels and other amino acids.

 Reduce dietary and supplement sources of vitamins B6, B1, B12, folate, or betaine (TMG).

Additional investigations:
- Genetic testing (methylation/folate pathways)
- Homocysteine
- Folate, B12 status

 Nutritional Support:
- Vitamin B complex
- Thiamine (Vitamin B1)
- Vitamin B6
- Biotin (Vitamin B7)
- MVM (Multi-vitamin/mineral)
- Magnesium Taurinate
- Magnesium Glycinate
- Magnesium Malate

Iron Panel

Standard Iron Panel including: TIBC, UIBC, Iron serum, Iron Saturation, Ferritin (male and female values)

Total Iron Binding Capacity (TIBC)

TIBC measures the total amount of iron-binding sites available in the blood, primarily through the protein transferrin. This test is commonly used alongside a serum iron test to assess for iron deficiency or overload. Elevated TIBC levels typically indicate iron deficiency, whereas low levels can suggest iron overload or other health issues such as liver disease or malnutrition.

Normal Range	250 - 450 µg/dL
Optimal Range	250 - 350 µg/dL

If LOW or < 250 µg/dL:

May indicate iron overload or related conditions such as hemochromatosis, liver disease, malnutrition, or nephrotic syndrome.

Check ferritin and iron levels to rule out iron overload. Evaluate recent iron intake, including supplements and use of iron cookware. Elevated iron with low TIBC may signal an early infection or inflammatory state.

Liver Support:
- Milk Thistle
- L-methionine
- Taurine
- Inositol
- Ox Bile
- Artichoke
- Beet Powder
- Vitamin A
- Vitamin B6
- Vitamin B12
- Plant protein powder with MVM (multi-vitamin/mineral)

- L-glutathione
- N-Acetyl-L-Cysteine (NAC)
- Quercetin
- Methylsulfonylmethane (MSM)
- Sodium Sulfate
- Green Tea Extract
- Reishi
- Cordyceps
- Chinese Skullcap
- Schisandra
- Burdock Extract
- Phosphatidylcholine

Kidney Support:
- Champignon (Agaricus bisporus)
- Cordyceps (Cordyceps sinensis)
- Poria (Poria cocos)
- American Ginseng (Panax quinquefolius)
- Astragalus (Astragalus membranaceus)

If HIGH or > 350 µg/dL:

Typically indicates iron deficiency, though levels may also increase during pregnancy or with oral contraceptive use. High TIBC combined with low iron often points to iron deficiency anemia.

Potential Causes:
- Conditions: Viral hepatitis, alcohol abuse, trauma, biliary stasis, sepsis, cardiovascular disease, diabetes, chronic obstructive pulmonary disease.

Assess dietary iron intake and sources, particularly for vegetarians or those with menstrual bleeding, which can affect iron levels. Vitamin C can aid absorption when taken with iron-rich foods or supplements.

Iron Support:
- Iron, ferrous bisglycinate

Nutritional Support:
- Vitamin C

Digestive Support:
- Digestive enzymes
- Betaine HCl
- Ox Bile
- L-taurine
- Gentian extract
- Dandelion extract
- Fennel
- Amylase
- Protease SP
- Protease
- Diastase
- Lactase
- Glucoamylase
- Alpha-galactosidase
- Beta-glucanase
- Acid protease
- Phytase
- Cellulase
- Hemicellulase
- Invertase
- Lipase
- Bromelain
- Papain
- Pepsin
- Triphala (Emblica officinalis, Terminalia bellirica, Terminalia chebula)
- Magnesium Hydroxide
- Mastic Gum
- DGL (Deglycyrrhizinated Licorice)
- Methylmethionine Sulfonium Chloride (MMSC)
- Zinc L-Carnosine
- Vitamin C
- Berberine
- Ginger
- Bismuth

Constipation Support (if needed):
- Triphala (Emblica officinalis
- Terminalia bellirica
- Terminalia chebula)
- Magnesium Hydroxide
- Magnesium Citrate

Unsaturated Iron Binding Capacity (UIBC)

UIBC measures the reserve capacity of transferrin, indicating how much transferrin is available to bind iron in the bloodstream. It is a valuable marker in diagnosing iron deficiency or overload and assessing overall iron transport. UIBC is commonly ordered as an alternative to TIBC and is useful in conjunction with other iron tests.

Normal Range	131 - 425 µg/dL
Optimal Range	131 - 325 µg/dL

IRON PANEL

If LOW or < 131 µg/dL:

 Low UIBC can indicate iron overload or conditions like hemochromatosis, chronic infections, or anemia types related to iron overload. It may also occur in cases of liver disease, malnutrition, or kidney issues.

 Assess potential sources of excess iron, such as supplementation or dietary factors like cooking with iron cookware. Elevated iron with low UIBC could be an early indicator of infection or inflammatory response.

 Rule out hemochromatosis if other symptoms or high iron levels are present. Consulting a healthcare provider may be necessary for further iron level management.

 Liver Support:
- Milk Thistle
- L-methionine
- Taurine
- Inositol
- Ox Bile
- Artichoke
- Beet Powder
- Vitamin A
- Vitamin B6
- Vitamin B12
- Plant protein powder with MVM (multi-vitamin/mineral)
- L-glutathione
- N-Acetyl-L-Cysteine (NAC)
- Quercetin
- Methylsulfonylmethane (MSM)
- Sodium Sulfate
- Green Tea Extract
- Reishi
- Cordyceps
- Chinese Skullcap
- Schisandra
- Burdock Extract
- Phosphatidylcholine

Kidney Support:
- Champignon (Agaricus bisporus)
- Cordyceps (Cordyceps sinensis)
- Poria (Poria cocos)
- American Ginseng (Panax quinquefolius)
- Astragalus (Astragalus membranaceus)

If HIGH or > 325 µg/dL:

 Elevated UIBC levels generally indicate iron deficiency, which may also be seen in pregnant women or with oral contraceptive use. In cases of high UIBC with low iron, iron deficiency anemia is likely.

 Evaluate dietary iron intake, particularly for those with heavy menstrual bleeding or restrictive diets (e.g., vegetarian or vegan). Enhancing vitamin C intake with iron-rich foods can support absorption. Evaluate for possible internal bleeding or hormonal influences like estrogen dominance.

 Iron Support:
- Iron, ferrous bisglycinate

Nutritional Support:
- Vitamin C

Digestive Support:
- Digestive enzymes
- Betaine HCl
- Ox Bile
- L-taurine

- Gentian extract
- Dandelion extract
- Fennel
- Amylase
- Protease SP
- Protease
- Diastase
- Lactase
- Glucoamylase
- Alpha-galactosidase
- Beta-glucanase
- Acid protease
- Phytase
- Cellulase
- Hemicellulase
- Invertase
- Lipase

- Bromelain
- Papain
- Pepsin
- Triphala (Emblica officinalis, Terminalia bellirica, Terminalia chebula)
- Magnesium Hydroxide
- Mastic Gum
- DGL (Deglycyrrhizinated Licorice)
- Methylmethionine Sulfonium Chloride (MMSC)
- Zinc L-Carnosine
- Vitamin C
- Berberine
- Ginger
- Bismuth

Constipation Support (if needed):
- Triphala (Emblica officinalis
- Terminalia bellirica
- Terminalia chebula)

- Magnesium Hydroxide
- Magnesium Citrate

Iron, Serum

Serum iron measures the amount of circulating iron in the blood, essential for hemoglobin function and oxygen transport. Serum ferritin is typically the most accurate indicator of iron status, as serum iron levels alone may not fully reflect iron metabolism or stores. Evaluating CBC, liver enzymes, BUN, and creatinine can provide a comprehensive picture when assessing iron levels.

Normal Range	27 - 159 µg/dL
Optimal Range	85 - 130 µg/dL

If LOW or < 85 µg/dL:

Low serum iron may indicate iron deficiency, commonly due to low dietary intake, increased demand, or blood loss. Iron deficiency is especially common in menstruating women, and additional factors such as dietary sources and absorption issues should be considered.

Assess dietary intake for heme (animal) vs. non-heme (plant) iron, as non-heme iron is less easily absorbed. Vitamin C can enhance iron absorption, while factors like estrogen dominance and internal bleeding may contribute to low levels.

Increased TIBC and low transferrin saturation are typical in iron deficiency anemia.

Iron Support:
- Iron, ferrous bisglycinate
- Iron Infusions: Prescribe or refer as necessary for severe deficiency

IRON PANEL

Nutritional Support:
- Vitamin C

Digestive Support:
- Digestive enzymes
- Betaine HCl
- Ox Bile
- L-taurine
- Gentian extract
- Dandelion extract
- Fennel
- Amylase
- Protease SP
- Protease
- Diastase
- Lactase
- Glucoamylase
- Alpha-galactosidase
- Beta-glucanase
- Acid protease
- Phytase
- Cellulase
- Hemicellulase
- Invertase
- Lipase
- Bromelain
- Papain
- Pepsin
- Triphala (Emblica officinalis, Terminalia bellirica, Terminalia chebula)
- Magnesium Hydroxide
- Mastic Gum
- DGL (Deglycyrrhizinated Licorice)
- Methylmethionine Sulfonium Chloride (MMSC)
- Zinc L-Carnosine
- Vitamin C
- Berberine
- Ginger
- Bismuth

Constipation Support (if needed):
- Triphala (Emblica officinalis
- Terminalia bellirica
- Terminalia chebula)
- Magnesium Hydroxide
- Magnesium Citrate

If **HIGH** or > 130 µg/dL:

Elevated serum iron levels may indicate iron overload, potentially caused by excessive supplementation, high dietary intake, or hemochromatosis. Elevated levels may also result from liver disease or chronic inflammation.

Evaluate sources of iron intake, such as supplements or cooking in iron cookware, and monitor for conditions like hemochromatosis. Elevated iron levels with low TIBC and high transferrin saturation are indicative of iron overload states.

Elevated iron with normal or high ferritin may be an early sign of infection or inflammation.

Liver Support:
- Milk Thistle
- L-methionine
- Taurine
- Inositol
- Ox Bile
- Artichoke
- Beet Powder
- Vitamin A
- Vitamin B6
- Vitamin B12
- Plant protein powder with MVM (multi-vitamin/mineral)
- L-glutathione
- N-Acetyl-L-Cysteine (NAC)
- Quercetin
- Methylsulfonylmethane (MSM)
- Sodium Sulfate
- Green Tea Extract
- Reishi
- Cordyceps

- Chinese Skullcap
- Schisandra

Kidney Support:
- Champignon (Agaricus bisporus)
- Cordyceps (Cordyceps sinensis)
- Poria (Poria cocos)
- American Ginseng (Panax quinquefolius)
- Astragalus (Astragalus membranaceus)

- Burdock Extract
- Phosphatidylcholine

Iron Saturation (Transferrin Saturation - TSAT)

Transferrin saturation (TSAT) is calculated using TIBC and serum iron levels and represents the percentage of transferrin binding sites occupied by iron. This marker is a critical indicator of iron status. In healthy individuals, about 20-40% of transferrin sites are saturated with iron. TSAT provides insights into liver health and nutrition, as transferrin production depends on liver function and protein intake.

Normal Range	15 - 55%
Optimal Range	25 - 35%

If LOW or < 25%:

Low TSAT suggests possible iron deficiency, often associated with inadequate dietary intake, absorption issues, or increased iron demand. This condition is common in menstruating women or those experiencing blood loss.

Symptoms of Low Iron:
- Fatigue, weakness
- Dizziness, headaches
- Pale skin

Evaluate dietary intake for heme vs. non-heme iron sources, as non-heme iron from plant sources is less bioavailable. Vitamin C can improve iron absorption, and underlying issues such as estrogen dominance or chronic blood loss should be assessed.

Iron Support:
- Iron, ferrous bisglycinate
- Iron Infusions: Prescribe or refer as needed for severe deficiency

Nutritional Support:
- Vitamin C

Digestive Support:
- Digestive enzymes
- Betaine HCl
- Ox Bile
- L-taurine
- Gentian extract
- Dandelion extract
- Fennel
- Amylase
- Protease SP
- Protease
- Diastase
- Lactase
- Glucoamylase
- Alpha-galactosidase
- Beta-glucanase
- Acid protease

- Phytase
- Cellulase
- Hemicellulase
- Invertase
- Lipase
- Bromelain
- Papain
- Pepsin
- Triphala (Emblica officinalis, Terminalia bellirica, Terminalia chebula)
- Magnesium Hydroxide
- Mastic Gum
- DGL (Deglycyrrhizinated Licorice)
- Methylmethionine Sulfonium Chloride (MMSC)
- Zinc L-Carnosine
- Vitamin C
- Berberine
- Ginger
- Bismuth

Constipation Support (if needed):
- Triphala (Emblica officinalis
- Terminalia bellirica
- Terminalia chebula)
- Magnesium Hydroxide
- Magnesium Citrate

If **HIGH** or **> 35%**:

Elevated TSAT may indicate iron overload, which could stem from excessive iron intake or hereditary hemochromatosis, a condition that causes the body to absorb too much iron.

Symptoms of Iron Overload:
- Joint pain
- Fatigue, weakness
- Abdominal pain
- Heart issues

Check dietary iron sources and evaluate potential iron supplements or cookware contributing to iron levels. High TSAT can indicate genetic conditions such as hemochromatosis, and elevated transferrin saturation may lead to iron deposits in tissues, causing damage.

Liver Support:
- Milk Thistle
- L-methionine
- Taurine
- Inositol
- Ox Bile
- Artichoke
- Beet Powder
- Vitamin A
- Vitamin B6
- Vitamin B12
- Plant protein powder with MVM (multi-vitamin/mineral)
- L-glutathione
- N-Acetyl-L-Cysteine (NAC)
- Quercetin
- Methylsulfonylmethane (MSM)
- Sodium Sulfate
- Green Tea Extract
- Reishi
- Cordyceps
- Chinese Skullcap
- Schisandra
- Burdock Extract
- Phosphatidylcholine

Kidney Support:
- Champignon (Agaricus bisporus)
- Cordyceps (Cordyceps sinensis)
- Poria (Poria cocos)
- American Ginseng (Panax quinquefolius)
- Astragalus (Astragalus membranaceus)

IRON PANEL

Ferritin, Serum

Ferritin is a blood protein that stores iron and releases it as needed. It's a key marker used to assess iron levels in the body and is tested to diagnose iron deficiency, iron overload, or to monitor iron support therapy. Ferritin is mainly stored in the liver, spleen, and bone marrow, and its levels reflect the amount of iron stored in the body. Commonly ordered with iron tests and TIBC.

MALE	
Normal Range	30 - 400 ng/mL
Optimal Range	33 - 236 ng/mL

FEMALE	
Normal Range	15 - 150 ng/mL
Optimal Range	40 - 122 ng/mL

If **LOW** or **< 33 ng/mL** or **< 40 ng/mL**:

Low ferritin levels suggest iron deficiency, often associated with chronic blood loss, inadequate dietary iron, or increased iron needs (e.g., during growth or pregnancy).

Associated Symptoms:
- Chronic fatigue, weakness
- Dizziness, headaches
- Pale skin, shortness of breath

Assess for possible sources of blood loss (e.g., gastrointestinal bleeding, heavy menstruation) or low dietary intake of heme iron. Low ferritin can result in symptoms such as fatigue, weakness, headaches, and shortness of breath.

Iron Support:
- Iron, ferrous bisglycinate
- Iron Infusions: Prescribe or refer as needed for severe deficiency

Nutritional Support:
- Vitamin C

Digestive Support:
- Digestive enzymes
- Betaine HCl
- Ox Bile
- L-taurine
- Gentian extract
- Dandelion extract
- Fennel
- Amylase
- Protease SP
- Protease
- Diastase
- Lactase
- Glucoamylase
- Alpha-galactosidase
- Beta-glucanase
- Acid protease
- Phytase
- Cellulase
- Hemicellulase
- Invertase
- Lipase
- Bromelain
- Papain
- Pepsin
- Triphala (Emblica officinalis, Terminalia bellirica, Terminalia chebula)
- Magnesium Hydroxide
- Mastic Gum
- DGL (Deglycyrrhizinated Licorice)
- Methylmethionine Sulfonium Chloride (MMSC)
- Zinc L-Carnosine
- Vitamin C
- Berberine
- Ginger

- Bismuth

Constipation Support (if needed):
- Triphala (Emblica officinalis
- Terminalia bellirica
- Terminalia chebula)
- Magnesium Hydroxide
- Magnesium Citrate

If HIGH or > 236 ng/mL or > 122 ng/mL:

Elevated ferritin levels may indicate iron overload, which can occur due to genetic conditions such as hereditary hemochromatosis, excessive iron supplementation, or liver disease. Accumulation of excess iron in the body can lead to tissue damage, particularly in organs such as the liver and heart.

Associated Conditions:
- Hemochromatosis, liver disease, inflammation
- Thalassemia, certain types of anemia

Check dietary iron sources and evaluate potential iron supplements or cookware contributing to iron levels. High TSAT can indicate genetic conditions such as hemochromatosis, and elevated transferrin saturation may lead to iron deposits in tissues, causing damage.

Liver Support:
- Milk Thistle
- L-methionine
- Taurine
- Inositol
- Ox Bile
- Artichoke
- Beet Powder
- Vitamin A
- Vitamin B6
- Vitamin B12
- Plant protein powder with MVM (multi-vitamin/mineral)
- L-glutathione
- N-Acetyl-L-Cysteine (NAC)
- Quercetin
- Methylsulfonylmethane (MSM)
- Sodium Sulfate
- Green Tea Extract
- Reishi
- Cordyceps
- Chinese Skullcap
- Schisandra
- Burdock Extract
- Phosphatidylcholine

Kidney Support:
- Champignon (Agaricus bisporus)
- Cordyceps (Cordyceps sinensis)
- Poria (Poria cocos)
- American Ginseng (Panax quinquefolius)
- Astragalus (Astragalus membranaceus)

Anemia Panel

Standard Anemia Panel including: All markers from an Iron Panel (TIBC, UIBC, Iron serum, Iron Saturation, Ferritin (male and female values)) plus Hemoglobin and Hematocrit (male and female values)

Total Iron Binding Capacity (TIBC)

The Total Iron Binding Capacity (TIBC) test is often used with a serum iron test to evaluate suspected iron deficiency or iron overload. TIBC reflects the total amount of iron that can be bound by proteins in the blood, primarily transferrin. TIBC indirectly indicates the availability of transferrin for iron transport, providing insight into iron status and protein binding capacity.

Normal Range	250 - 450 µg/dL
Optimal Range	250 - 350 µg/dL

If LOW or < 250 µg/dL:

Low TIBC may indicate decreased transferrin availability, which can be seen in iron overload conditions such as hemochromatosis, chronic infections, or liver disease. This could also point to inflammation, malnutrition, or kidney conditions affecting protein levels.

Additional Diagnostic Actions: Check ferritin levels and liver function tests (e.g., AST, ALT) to assess iron storage and liver health.

Check for elevated iron levels as low TIBC with high iron may signal iron overload. Evaluate any iron supplementation or potential iron sources (e.g., cooking with iron cookware).

Liver Support:
- Milk Thistle
- L-methionine
- Taurine
- Inositol
- Ox Bile
- Artichoke
- Beet Powder
- Vitamin A
- Vitamin B6
- Vitamin B12
- Plant protein powder with MVM (multi-vitamin/mineral)
- L-glutathione
- N-Acetyl-L-Cysteine (NAC)
- Quercetin
- Methylsulfonylmethane (MSM)
- Sodium Sulfate
- Green Tea Extract
- Reishi
- Cordyceps
- Chinese Skullcap
- Schisandra
- Burdock Extract
- Phosphatidylcholine

Kidney Support:
- Champignon (Agaricus bisporus)
- Cordyceps (Cordyceps sinensis)
- Poria (Poria cocos)
- American Ginseng (Panax quinquefolius)
- Astragalus (Astragalus membranaceus)

ANEMIA PANEL

If **HIGH** or > 350 µg/dL:

High TIBC may be indicative of iron deficiency, as the body produces more transferrin to increase iron-binding capacity. Common in menstruating women, iron deficiency can also be caused by low dietary iron, inadequate absorption, or chronic blood loss.

Associated Symptoms of Iron Deficiency: Fatigue, dizziness, weakness, pallor, and potential digestive complaints due to low iron.

Assess dietary iron intake, especially sources rich in heme iron, which is more easily absorbed. Vitamin C intake alongside meals can enhance iron absorption. Evaluate for heavy menstrual bleeding, internal bleeding, or estrogen dominance if relevant.

Iron Support:
- Iron, ferrous bisglycinate
- Iron Infusions: Consider referral for iron infusions if deficiency is severe

Nutritional Support:
- Vitamin C to improve iron absorption

Digestive Support:
- Digestive enzymes
- Betaine HCl
- Ox Bile
- L-taurine
- Gentian extract
- Dandelion extract
- Fennel
- Amylase
- Protease SP
- Protease
- Diastase
- Lactase
- Glucoamylase
- Alpha-galactosidase
- Beta-glucanase
- Acid protease
- Phytase
- Cellulase
- Hemicellulase
- Invertase
- Lipase
- Bromelain
- Papain
- Pepsin
- Triphala (Emblica officinalis, Terminalia bellirica, Terminalia chebula)
- Magnesium Hydroxide
- Mastic Gum
- DGL (Deglycyrrhizinated Licorice)
- Methylmethionine Sulfonium Chloride (MMSC)
- Zinc L-Carnosine
- Vitamin C
- Berberine
- Ginger
- Bismuth

Constipation Support (if needed):
- Triphala (Emblica officinalis
- Terminalia bellirica
- Terminalia chebula)
- Magnesium Hydroxide
- Magnesium Citrate

Unsaturated Iron Binding Capacity (UIBC)

The UIBC test assesses the body's ability to transport iron in the blood by measuring the transferrin available for binding. UIBC, alongside serum iron and TIBC, provides insight into iron status and is an alternative test to TIBC. Elevated UIBC may suggest iron deficiency, while a decrease may point to iron overload or other conditions.

Normal Range	131 - 425 µg/dL
Optimal Range	131 - 325 µg/dL

If LOW or < 131 µg/dL:

 Low UIBC suggests limited transferrin availability for binding iron, which may indicate iron overload (e.g., hemochromatosis), chronic infection, or conditions affecting protein levels, such as liver or kidney disease.

Additional Diagnostic Actions: Measure ferritin and assess liver function to investigate further.

 Elevated serum iron with low UIBC may suggest iron overload. Check for potential causes, including hemochromatosis, inflammation, or excess iron supplementation.

Liver Support:
- Milk Thistle
- L-methionine
- Taurine
- Inositol
- Ox Bile
- Artichoke
- Beet Powder
- Vitamin A
- Vitamin B6
- Vitamin B12
- Plant protein powder with MVM (multi-vitamin/mineral)

- L-glutathione
- N-Acetyl-L-Cysteine (NAC)
- Quercetin
- Methylsulfonylmethane (MSM)
- Sodium Sulfate
- Green Tea Extract
- Reishi
- Cordyceps
- Chinese Skullcap
- Schisandra
- Burdock Extract
- Phosphatidylcholine

Kidney Support:
- Champignon (Agaricus bisporus)
- Cordyceps (Cordyceps sinensis)
- Poria (Poria cocos)
- American Ginseng (Panax quinquefolius)
- Astragalus (Astragalus membranaceus)

If HIGH or > 325 µg/dL:

 Elevated UIBC levels suggest iron deficiency, as the body produces more transferrin to bind available iron. This is common in iron deficiency anemia, potentially due to low dietary iron, poor absorption, or blood loss.

Associated Symptoms of Iron Deficiency: Fatigue, dizziness, weakness, and pallor.

Evaluate dietary intake of iron-rich foods, especially sources of heme iron, and enhance iron absorption with vitamin C. Monitor for heavy menstrual bleeding or internal bleeding if relevant.

Iron Support:
- Iron, ferrous bisglycinate
- Iron Infusions: Consider referral for iron infusions if deficiency is severe

Nutritional Support:
- Vitamin C to improve iron absorption

Digestive Support:
- Digestive enzymes
- Betaine HCl
- Ox Bile
- L-taurine
- Gentian extract
- Dandelion extract
- Fennel
- Amylase
- Protease SP
- Protease
- Diastase
- Lactase
- Glucoamylase
- Alpha-galactosidase
- Beta-glucanase
- Acid protease
- Phytase
- Cellulase
- Hemicellulase
- Invertase
- Lipase
- Bromelain
- Papain
- Pepsin
- Triphala (Emblica officinalis, Terminalia bellirica, Terminalia chebula)
- Magnesium Hydroxide
- Mastic Gum
- DGL (Deglycyrrhizinated Licorice)
- Methylmethionine Sulfonium Chloride (MMSC)
- Zinc L-Carnosine
- Vitamin C
- Berberine
- Ginger
- Bismuth

Constipation Support (if needed):
- Triphala (Emblica officinalis
- Terminalia bellirica
- Terminalia chebula)
- Magnesium Hydroxide
- Magnesium Citrate

Iron, Serum

Serum iron is closely related to hemoglobin, as it helps transport oxygen (O_2) throughout the body. It is crucial to evaluate serum iron levels alongside ferritin and TIBC, as ferritin levels provide insight into stored iron, while TIBC reflects transferrin availability for binding iron. For the most accurate assessment of iron metabolism, ferritin levels and soluble transferrin receptors should be checked, especially in cases of inflammation.

Normal Range	27 - 159 µg/dL
Optimal Range	85 - 130 µg/dL

ANEMIA PANEL

If LOW or < 85 µg/dL:

 Low serum iron may indicate iron deficiency anemia, potentially due to insufficient dietary intake, poor absorption, blood loss, or increased physiological demand.

Common Symptoms of Low Iron: Fatigue, dizziness, weakness, headaches, and pallor.

 Evaluate dietary iron sources, particularly heme iron. Assess digestive health for iron absorption issues and rule out chronic blood loss, especially in menstruating individuals.

 Iron Support:
- Iron, ferrous bisglycinate
- Iron Infusions: Consider for severe deficiency upon referral

Nutritional Support:
- Vitamin C to enhance absorption

Digestive Support:
- Digestive enzymes
- Betaine HCl
- Ox Bile
- L-taurine
- Gentian extract
- Dandelion extract
- Fennel
- Amylase
- Protease SP
- Protease
- Diastase
- Lactase
- Glucoamylase
- Alpha-galactosidase
- Beta-glucanase
- Acid protease
- Phytase
- Cellulase
- Hemicellulase
- Invertase
- Lipase
- Bromelain
- Papain
- Pepsin
- Triphala (Emblica officinalis, Terminalia bellirica, Terminalia chebula)
- Magnesium Hydroxide
- Mastic Gum
- DGL (Deglycyrrhizinated Licorice)
- Methylmethionine Sulfonium Chloride (MMSC)
- Zinc L-Carnosine
- Vitamin C
- Berberine
- Ginger
- Bismuth

Constipation Support (if needed):
- Triphala (Emblica officinalis
- Terminalia bellirica
- Terminalia chebula)
- Magnesium Hydroxide
- Magnesium Citrate

If HIGH or > 130 µg/dL:

 Elevated serum iron may suggest iron overload, potentially from excessive supplementation, dietary intake, or conditions like hereditary hemochromatosis.

Common Symptoms of Iron Overload: Joint pain, fatigue, weight loss, abdominal pain, and darkened skin tone.

Excess iron may signal liver or kidney involvement. Check ferritin levels to confirm iron status, especially if iron overload or liver disease is suspected.

Liver Support:
- Milk Thistle
- L-methionine
- Taurine
- Inositol
- Ox Bile
- Artichoke
- Beet Powder
- Vitamin A
- Vitamin B6
- Vitamin B12
- Plant protein powder with MVM (multi-vitamin/mineral)
- L-glutathione
- N-Acetyl-L-Cysteine (NAC)
- Quercetin
- Methylsulfonylmethane (MSM)
- Sodium Sulfate
- Green Tea Extract
- Reishi
- Cordyceps
- Chinese Skullcap
- Schisandra
- Burdock Extract
- Phosphatidylcholine

Kidney Support:
- Champignon (Agaricus bisporus)
- Cordyceps (Cordyceps sinensis)
- Poria (Poria cocos)
- American Ginseng (Panax quinquefolius)
- Astragalus (Astragalus membranaceus)

Iron Saturation (Transferrin Saturation - TSAT)

Iron saturation, or transferrin saturation (TSAT), measures the percentage of transferrin (an iron-binding protein) currently bound with iron. In healthy individuals, 20-40% of transferrin sites are typically bound. Transferrin levels can decrease in cases of liver disease or low protein intake, which makes TSAT a useful indicator of both iron status and overall nutritional health.

Normal Range	15 - 55%
Optimal Range	25 - 35%

If LOW or < 25%:

 Low transferrin saturation could indicate iron deficiency, possibly due to inadequate dietary intake, absorption issues, or chronic blood loss.

Symptoms of Iron Deficiency: Fatigue, weakness, pale skin, dizziness, and headaches.

 Evaluate dietary iron sources, especially heme iron, and assess absorption, particularly for those with heavy menstrual periods or known gastrointestinal blood loss.

Iron Support:
- Iron, ferrous bisglycinate
- Iron Infusions: Consider for severe deficiency upon referral

Nutritional Support:
- Vitamin C to enhance absorption

ANEMIA PANEL

Digestive Support:
- Digestive enzymes
- Betaine HCl
- Ox Bile
- L-taurine
- Gentian extract
- Dandelion extract
- Fennel
- Amylase
- Protease SP
- Protease
- Diastase
- Lactase
- Glucoamylase
- Alpha-galactosidase
- Beta-glucanase
- Acid protease
- Phytase
- Cellulase
- Hemicellulase
- Invertase
- Lipase
- Bromelain
- Papain
- Pepsin
- Triphala (Emblica officinalis, Terminalia bellirica, Terminalia chebula)
- Magnesium Hydroxide
- Mastic Gum
- DGL (Deglycyrrhizinated Licorice)
- Methylmethionine Sulfonium Chloride (MMSC)
- Zinc L-Carnosine
- Vitamin C
- Berberine
- Ginger
- Bismuth

Constipation Support (if needed):
- Triphala (Emblica officinalis
- Terminalia bellirica
- Terminalia chebula)
- Magnesium Hydroxide
- Magnesium Citrate

If **HIGH** or **> 35%**:

 Elevated transferrin saturation can suggest iron overload, potentially due to excessive iron intake or hereditary hemochromatosis.

Symptoms of Iron Overload: Joint pain, fatigue, abdominal pain, hair loss, and heart issues.

 Excess iron may point to liver or kidney involvement; consider checking ferritin and evaluating for hemochromatosis or iron overload conditions.

Liver Support:
- Milk Thistle
- L-methionine
- Taurine
- Inositol
- Ox Bile
- Artichoke
- Beet Powder
- Vitamin A
- Vitamin B6
- Vitamin B12
- Plant protein powder with MVM (multi-vitamin/mineral)
- L-glutathione
- N-Acetyl-L-Cysteine (NAC)
- Quercetin
- Methylsulfonylmethane (MSM)
- Sodium Sulfate
- Green Tea Extract
- Reishi
- Cordyceps
- Chinese Skullcap
- Schisandra
- Burdock Extract
- Phosphatidylcholine

Kidney Support:
- Champignon (Agaricus bisporus)
- Cordyceps (Cordyceps sinensis)
- Poria (Poria cocos)
- American Ginseng (Panax quinquefolius)
- Astragalus (Astragalus membranaceus)

Ferritin, Serum

Ferritin is a cellular protein that stores iron and releases it when needed, serving as an indicator of the body's iron reserves. Testing ferritin levels helps diagnose conditions like iron deficiency anemia or iron overload. In conjunction with iron and TIBC tests, ferritin measurement provides a comprehensive view of iron status and potential inflammation.

MALE	
Normal Range	30 - 400 ng/mL
Optimal Range	33 - 236 ng/mL

FEMALE	
Normal Range	15 - 150 ng/mL
Optimal Range	40 - 122 ng/mL

If LOW or < 33ng/mL or < 40 ng/mL:

Low ferritin levels are indicative of iron deficiency, often due to low dietary intake, inadequate iron absorption, or chronic blood loss.

Symptoms of Iron Deficiency: Chronic fatigue, weakness, dizziness, pale skin, ringing in the ears, and shortness of breath.

Assess dietary intake of heme iron (animal sources) and rule out gastrointestinal blood loss or heavy menstrual bleeding. Monitor for symptoms associated with iron deficiency.

Iron Support:
- Iron, ferrous bisglycinate
- Iron Infusions: Consider for severe deficiency upon referral

Nutritional Support:
- Vitamin C to enhance absorption

Digestive Support:
- Digestive enzymes
- Betaine HCl
- Ox Bile
- L-taurine
- Gentian extract
- Dandelion extract
- Fennel
- Amylase
- Protease SP
- Protease
- Diastase
- Lactase
- Glucoamylase
- Alpha-galactosidase
- Beta-glucanase
- Acid protease
- Phytase
- Cellulase
- Hemicellulase
- Invertase
- Lipase
- Bromelain
- Papain
- Pepsin

- Triphala (Emblica officinalis, Terminalia bellirica, Terminalia chebula)
- Magnesium Hydroxide
- Mastic Gum
- DGL (Deglycyrrhizinated Licorice)
- Methylmethionine Sulfonium Chloride (MMSC)
- Zinc L-Carnosine
- Vitamin C
- Berberine
- Ginger
- Bismuth

Constipation Support (if needed):
- Triphala (Emblica officinalis
- Terminalia bellirica
- Terminalia chebula)
- Magnesium Hydroxide
- Magnesium Citrate

If **HIGH** or **> 236 ng/mL** or **> 122 ng/mL**:

Elevated ferritin may be a sign of iron overload, often seen in hemochromatosis, excessive iron intake, or inflammatory conditions.

Symptoms of Iron Overload: Joint pain, fatigue, weakness, weight loss, abdominal pain, and potential damage to organs like the liver and heart.

Check for signs of liver and kidney dysfunction. Excessive iron intake, use of iron cookware, or hereditary hemochromatosis may contribute to elevated ferritin. Correlate with other iron panel results for further evaluation.

Liver Support:
- Milk Thistle
- L-methionine
- Taurine
- Inositol
- Ox Bile
- Artichoke
- Beet Powder
- Vitamin A
- Vitamin B6
- Vitamin B12
- Plant protein powder with MVM (multi-vitamin/mineral)
- L-glutathione
- N-Acetyl-L-Cysteine (NAC)
- Quercetin
- Methylsulfonylmethane (MSM)
- Sodium Sulfate
- Green Tea Extract
- Reishi
- Cordyceps
- Chinese Skullcap
- Schisandra
- Burdock Extract
- Phosphatidylcholine

Kidney Support:
- Champignon (Agaricus bisporus)
- Cordyceps (Cordyceps sinensis)
- Poria (Poria cocos)
- American Ginseng (Panax quinquefolius)
- Astragalus (Astragalus membranaceus)

Hemoglobin

Hemoglobin (Hg) is a key red blood cell protein responsible for transporting oxygen from the lungs to tissues throughout the body. Hemoglobin levels are an important marker for assessing anemia (low) and dehydration (high).

MALE	
Normal Range	11.1 - 15.9 g/dL
Optimal Range	14 - 15 g/dL

FEMALE	
Normal Range	11.1 - 15.9 g/dL
Optimal Range	13.5 - 14.5 g/dL

If **LOW** or **< 14 g/dL** or **< 13.5 g/dL**:

Low hemoglobin may indicate iron deficiency anemia, B12 or folate deficiency, bone marrow issues, internal bleeding, or malabsorption.

Potential Causes of Low Hemoglobin:
- Iron deficiency anemia
- Vitamin B12 or folate deficiency
- Bone marrow disorders
- Gastrointestinal blood loss or malabsorption

Evaluate dietary intake of iron-rich foods (e.g., liver, red meat) and assess for underlying causes like nutrient deficiencies, parasitic infections, or internal bleeding. Monitor for symptoms such as fatigue, weakness, and pallor.

Iron Support:
- Iron, ferrous bisglycinate

Nutritional Support:
- Vitamin C
- Vitamin B9 (folate)
- Vitamin B12
- Vitamin B6

Digestive Support:
- Digestive enzymes
- Betaine HCl
- Ox Bile
- L-taurine
- Gentian extract
- Dandelion extract
- Fennel
- Amylase
- Protease SP
- Protease
- Diastase
- Lactase
- Glucoamylase
- Alpha-galactosidase
- Beta-glucanase
- Acid protease
- Phytase
- Cellulase
- Hemicellulase
- Invertase
- Lipase
- Bromelain
- Papain
- Pepsin
- Triphala (Emblica officinalis, Terminalia bellirica, Terminalia chebula)
- Magnesium Hydroxide
- Mastic Gum
- DGL (Deglycyrrhizinated Licorice)
- Methylmethionine Sulfonium Chloride (MMSC)

- Zinc L-Carnosine
- Vitamin C
- Berberine
- Ginger
- Bismuth

If HIGH or > 15 g/dL or 14.5g/dL:

Elevated hemoglobin levels may be a sign of dehydration, increased testosterone, or other conditions like polycythemia vera, respiratory issues, or adrenal dysfunction.

Potential Causes of Elevated Hemoglobin:
- Dehydration
- Increased testosterone
- Polycythemia vera
- Adrenal dysfunction

Encourage increased fluid intake and monitor for symptoms of dehydration or underlying conditions. Evaluate for potential causes such as respiratory distress or polycythemia.

Electrolyte Support:
- Potassium
- Sodium
- Chloride
- Magnesium
- Magnesium Bisglycinate
- Vitamin C
- Zinc

Hematocrit

Hematocrit (HCT) measures the proportion of blood volume composed of red blood cells (RBCs). It is expressed as a percentage and reflects the oxygen-carrying capacity of blood, aiding in the evaluation of anemia and polycythemia. Typical values are around 45% for men and 40% for women, generally about three times the hemoglobin concentration.

MALE	
Normal Range	34 - 46.6%
Optimal Range	40 - 48%

FEMALE	
Normal Range	34 - 46.6%
Optimal Range	37 - 44%

If LOW or < 40% or < 37%:

Low hematocrit levels may indicate anemia, often associated with reduced oxygen transport capacity and fatigue.

Potential Causes of Low Hemoglobin:
- Nutritional deficiencies (iron, folic acid, B12, copper, B6)
- Increased RBC breakdown by the spleen
- Bone marrow insufficiency
- Blood loss

- Assess for possible blood loss, such as gastrointestinal bleeding, hemorrhoids, or heavy menstrual periods, which can lower hematocrit.
- Check for nutrient deficiencies, including iron, folic acid, B12, B6, or copper.

- In menstruating women, heavy periods may contribute to low iron levels. Evaluate dietary intake and rule out estrogen dominance with supplements like CALCIUM D-GLUCARATE, DIM EVAIL, FEMGUARD + BALANCE, ADRENOTONE, and ADRENAL COMPLEX.

Iron Support:
- Iron, ferrous bisglycinate

Nutritional Support:
- Vitamin C
- Vitamin B9 (folate)
- Vitamin B12
- Vitamin B6

Digestive Support:
- Digestive enzymes
- Betaine HCl
- Ox Bile
- L-taurine
- Gentian extract
- Dandelion extract
- Fennel
- Amylase
- Protease SP
- Protease
- Diastase
- Lactase
- Glucoamylase
- Alpha-galactosidase
- Beta-glucanase
- Acid protease
- Phytase
- Cellulase
- Hemicellulase
- Invertase
- Lipase
- Bromelain
- Papain
- Pepsin
- Triphala (Emblica officinalis, Terminalia bellirica, Terminalia chebula)
- Magnesium Hydroxide
- Mastic Gum
- DGL (Deglycyrrhizinated Licorice)
- Methylmethionine Sulfonium Chloride (MMSC)
- Zinc L-Carnosine
- Vitamin C
- Berberine
- Ginger
- Bismuth

If **HIGH** or > 48% or > 44%:

Elevated hematocrit may suggest dehydration or conditions that increase RBC concentration, raising blood viscosity and potentially placing strain on the cardiovascular system.

Potential Causes of Elevated Hemoglobin:
- Dehydration
- Exogenous testosterone or steroid use
- Polycythemia vera (a rare blood disorder causing increased RBC production)
- Respiratory issues such as COPD

Encourage increased fluid intake to address potential dehydration.

Electrolyte Support:
- Potassium
- Sodium
- Chloride
- Magnesium
- Magnesium Bisglycinate
- Vitamin C
- Zinc

Urinalysis

The urinalysis report should be looked at as a whole and taken into context of symptom picture.   Other issues may need to be addressed, e.g. - hydration - diet - lifestyle - blood sugar balancing - immunity - liver function - gut function - hormones Additional functional tests may be advised in some cases.

Specific Gravity

Specific gravity measures urine concentration and assesses kidney function. Ideally, specific gravity should fall between 1.002 and 1.030, indicating balanced hydration and kidney function. Higher values suggest dehydration, while lower values may indicate overhydration or kidney issues.

Normal Range	1.002 - 1.030 SG
Optimal Range	1.002 - 1.030 SG

Urine specific gravity is within the optimal range, suggesting balanced hydration and proper kidney function. No further action required unless accompanied by other symptoms.

If **LOW** or **< 1.002 SG**:

Low specific gravity indicates diluted urine, potentially due to overhydration, kidney issues, or conditions such as diabetes insipidus or chronic kidney inflammation.

Potential Causes:
- Overhydration
- Kidney infection or inflammation
- Kidney failure
- Urinary tract infection (UTI)

- Overhydration or kidney function issues (e.g., inflammation, diabetes insipidus).
- Check other markers for urinary tract infections or kidney stones.

Electrolyte Support:
- Potassium
- Sodium
- Chloride
- Magnesium
- Magnesium Bisglycinate
- Vitamin C
- Zinc

Urinary Support:
- D-Mannose
- Cranberry (Vaccinium macrocarpon)
- Bearberry (Arctostaphylos uva ursi)
- Hibiscus (Hibiscus sabdaria)
- Nettle (Urtica spp.)
- Aloe Vera
- Parsley Powder (Petroselinum crispum)
- Horsetail (Equisetum spp.)
- Vitamin B6
- L-Carnitine
- Acetyl-L-Carnitine
- Champignon (Agaricus bisporus)
- Cordyceps (Cordyceps sinensis)
- Poria (Poria cocos)
- American Ginseng
- Astragalus (Astragalus membranaceus)

URINALYSIS

- Belleric Myrobalan (Terminalia bellerica)
- Tart Cherry (Prunus cerasus)

If **HIGH** or > 1.030 SG:

High specific gravity indicates concentrated urine, often due to dehydration, diarrhea, or conditions like heart failure or kidney stones.

Potential Causes:
- Dehydration, diarrhea, or vomiting
- Heart failure
- Kidney stones
- Glycosuria
- SIADH or hepatorenal syndrome

- Assess for dehydration, possible infections, or kidney stones.
- Other possible signs include glycosuria (sugar in urine) or syndrome of inappropriate antidiuretic hormone secretion (SIADH).

Electrolyte Support:
- Potassium
- Sodium
- Chloride
- Magnesium
- Magnesium Bisglycinate
- Vitamin C
- Zinc

High Dose Probiotics:
- Multi-strain probiotic blend
- Saccharomyces boulardii
- Beta Glucans
- Lactobacillus plantarum strain L-137 (HK L-137)
- Xylooligosaccharide (XOS)

Urinary Support:
- D-Mannose
- Cranberry (Vaccinium macrocarpon)
- Bearberry (Arctostaphylos uva ursi)
- Hibiscus (Hibiscus sabdaria)
- Nettle (Urtica spp.)
- Aloe Vera
- Parsley Powder (Petroselinum crispum)
- Horsetail (Equisetum spp.)
- Vitamin B6
- L-Carnitine
- Acetyl-L-Carnitine
- Champignon (Agaricus bisporus)
- Cordyceps (Cordyceps sinensis)
- Poria (Poria cocos)
- American Ginseng
- Astragalus (Astragalus membranaceus)
- Belleric Myrobalan (Terminalia bellerica)
- Tart Cherry (Prunus cerasus)

pH

Urine pH indicates the acidity or alkalinity of urine. Neutral pH is 7.0, while a typical urine pH is around 6.0. Low pH values reflect more acidic urine, while high pH values indicate alkalinity. Both extremes may be influenced by diet, hydration, metabolic status, or underlying conditions.

Normal Range	5 - 7.5
Optimal Range	5 - 7.5

URINALYSIS

Urine pH is within the optimal range, suggesting balanced acidity and alkalinity. No further action required unless accompanied by other abnormalities.

If **LOW** or **< 5:**

A low pH (more acidic urine) could result from a high-protein diet, systemic acidosis, or conditions like diabetes or dehydration. Acidic urine may create an environment conducive to kidney stones.

Potential Causes:
- Acidosis
- Dehydration
- Diabetic ketoacidosis
- Starvation
- Diarrhea
- High protein or cranberry-rich diet

- Evaluate other markers (urine and blood) to pinpoint root causes such as systemic acidosis or diabetes.
- Dietary factors like high protein or cranberry intake may contribute.

Electrolyte Support:
- Potassium
- Sodium
- Chloride
- Magnesium
- Magnesium Bisglycinate
- Vitamin C
- Zinc

Urinary Support:
- D-Mannose
- Cranberry (Vaccinium macrocarpon)
- Bearberry (Arctostaphylos uva ursi)
- Hibiscus (Hibiscus sabdaria)
- Nettle (Urtica spp.)
- Aloe Vera
- Parsley Powder (Petroselinum crispum)
- Horsetail (Equisetum spp.)
- Vitamin B6
- L-Carnitine
- Acetyl-L-Carnitine
- Champignon (Agaricus bisporus)
- Cordyceps (Cordyceps sinensis)
- Poria (Poria cocos)
- American Ginseng
- Astragalus (Astragalus membranaceus)
- Belleric Myrobalan (Terminalia bellerica)
- Tart Cherry (Prunus cerasus)

If **HIGH** or **> 7.5:**

A high pH (more alkaline urine) may be influenced by a vegetarian diet, certain medications, or a urinary tract infection. It may also reflect renal tubular acidosis or kidney issues.

Potential Causes
- UTIs
- Renal tubular acidosis
- Kidney stones
- Alkaline diet (e.g., high in vegetables or citrus fruits)
- Certain medications (e.g., acetazolamide)
- Vomiting or stomach pumping

URINALYSIS

- Assess other markers for potential UTIs or kidney stones.
- Other dietary and lifestyle factors like low carbohydrate intake or citrus fruits can increase alkalinity.

Electrolyte Support:
- Potassium
- Sodium
- Chloride
- Magnesium
- Magnesium Bisglycinate
- Vitamin C
- Zinc

Urinary Support:
- D-Mannose
- Cranberry (Vaccinium macrocarpon)
- Bearberry (Arctostaphylos uva ursi)
- Hibiscus (Hibiscus sabdaria)
- Nettle (Urtica spp.)
- Aloe Vera
- Parsley Powder (Petroselinum crispum)
- Horsetail (Equisetum spp.)
- Vitamin B6
- L-Carnitine
- Acetyl-L-Carnitine
- Champignon (Agaricus bisporus)
- Cordyceps (Cordyceps sinensis)
- Poria (Poria cocos)
- American Ginseng
- Astragalus (Astragalus membranaceus)
- Belleric Myrobalan (Terminalia bellerica)
- Tart Cherry (Prunus cerasus)

Urine Color

Urine color can vary significantly, often reflecting hydration levels, dietary intake, medication use, or underlying health conditions. Normal urine color typically ranges from pale yellow to amber. Any deviation from these shades may indicate abnormal conditions, medications, or dietary factors. This is a visual check with categories classified as Normal or Abnormal.

Normal Color Range	Straw to amber yellow
Abnormal Color Indicators	Any color outside normal range flags as ABNORMAL

If NORMAL:

The urine color is within the typical yellow spectrum, indicating likely adequate hydration and no visible abnormalities from dietary, medication, or systemic health factors.

If ABNORMAL:

Abnormal urine color may suggest specific dietary influences, medication effects, or potential health conditions affecting the urinary system, liver function, or other metabolic processes.

Color Variations and Possible Causes:
- **Colorless**: Alcohol ingestion, severe iron deficiency, or chronic interstitial nephritis.
- **White:** Potential indicators of infection, parasites, STIs, or hypoparathyroidism.
- **Orange:** Possible causes include high-carotene foods (e.g., carrot juice), riboflavin, or uric acid crystals.

- **Yellow-brown or Greenish-brown:** May indicate bilirubin presence related to liver issues or jaundice, or caused by certain medications or infections.
- **Red (straw to port wine):** Often due to diet (e.g., beets, blackberries), certain herbs (cascara, senna), or dyes; can also indicate blood presence.
- **Brown:** Potentially due to indican, phenols, certain medications (e.g., flagyl, nitrofurantoin, l-dopa), or poisoning (e.g., lysol).
- **Blue hue:** Could be related to Pseudomonas infection or rare metabolic conditions (some porphyrias).
- **Green:** Often associated with Pseudomonas infection.

Investigate abnormal color causes if persistent or unexplained by recent diet or medications.

Urinary Support:
- D-Mannose
- Cranberry (Vaccinium macrocarpon)
- Bearberry (Arctostaphylos uva ursi)
- Hibiscus (Hibiscus sabdaria)
- Nettle (Urtica spp.)
- Aloe Vera
- Parsley Powder (Petroselinum crispum)
- Horsetail (Equisetum spp.)
- Vitamin B6
- L-Carnitine
- Acetyl-L-Carnitine
- Champignon (Agaricus bisporus)
- Cordyceps (Cordyceps sinensis)
- Poria (Poria cocos)
- American Ginseng
- Astragalus (Astragalus membranaceus)
- Belleric Myrobalan (Terminalia bellerica)
- Tart Cherry (Prunus cerasus)

WBC Esterase

WBC (Leukocyte) esterase is a screening test to detect white blood cells (WBCs) in urine. A positive result can indicate the presence of WBCs, suggesting a possible urinary tract infection (UTI). If WBC esterase is positive, a microscopic examination is recommended to confirm infection and to further investigate.

Negative Result	No WBC esterase detected; no immediate indication of infection
Abnormal Result	Positive for WBC esterase, warranting further investigation for infection or inflammation

If NEGATIVE:

No leukocyte esterase detected. This is within the normal range, and no infection is indicated at this time.

If ABNORMAL:

Presence of WBC esterase suggests an increased likelihood of infection or inflammation in the urinary tract. It could indicate a UTI, kidney infection, or cystitis. A follow-up microscopic examination is recommended to confirm infection and evaluate for other markers.

Potential Causes of Positive WBC Esterase:
- **Infections:** UTIs, kidney infections, cystitis, urethritis, or prostatitis
- **Inflammation:** From kidney stones, dehydration, or retained foreign bodies

- **Additional Factors:** Possible causes could include dehydration, fever, or stress.

Examine other urine markers, assess symptoms such as flank pain for kidney stones, and rule out infections or GI issues.

High Dose Probiotics:
- Multi-strain probiotic blend
- Saccharomyces boulardii
- Beta Glucans
- Lactobacillus plantarum strain L-137 (HK L-137)
- Xylooligosaccharide (XOS)

Urinary Support:
- D-Mannose
- Cranberry (Vaccinium macrocarpon)
- Bearberry (Arctostaphylos uva ursi)
- Hibiscus (Hibiscus sabdaria)
- Nettle (Urtica spp.)
- Aloe Vera
- Parsley Powder (Petroselinum crispum)
- Horsetail (Equisetum spp.)
- Vitamin B6
- L-Carnitine
- Acetyl-L-Carnitine
- Champignon (Agaricus bisporus)
- Cordyceps (Cordyceps sinensis)
- Poria (Poria cocos)
- American Ginseng
- Astragalus (Astragalus membranaceus)
- Belleric Myrobalan (Terminalia bellerica)
- Tart Cherry (Prunus cerasus)

Antimicrobial Agents:
- Oregano Oil (Origanum vulgare)
- Garlic
- Tribulus terrestris
- Magnesium Caprylate
- Berberine
- Bearberry Extract (Arctostaphylos uva-ursi)
- Black Walnut Powder (Juglans nigra)
- Barberry Extract (Berberis spp.)
- Artemisia (wormwood)
- Purified Silver
- Alpha Lipoic Acid

Protein

The presence of protein in urine (proteinuria) can indicate kidney function and overall health status. Elevated levels may occur temporarily due to factors like infection, stress, pregnancy, diet, exercise, or cold exposure. Persistent proteinuria, however, may indicate kidney damage or disease and requires further evaluation.

Negative Result	No protein detected, indicating normal kidney function.
Positive Result	Protein detected, which may suggest kidney damage, infection, or other underlying conditions that require additional diagnostic testing.

If **NEGATIVE:**

No protein detected in the urine, indicating normal kidney function. No immediate follow-up required.

If POSITIVE:

Presence of protein suggests possible renal stress or damage. It could indicate kidney or non-renal conditions that should be investigated further.

Possible Causes of Proteinuria:
- Renal Conditions: Glomerulonephritis, nephritis, chronic urinary tract obstruction, nephrosis, malignant hypertension, polycystic kidney disease.
- Non-Renal Conditions: Acute infection, leukemia, multiple myeloma, diabetes, systemic lupus erythematosus (SLE), or toxemia in pregnancy.

Examine for additional markers, such as urinary tract infections or systemic indicators of kidney damage.

Urinary Support:
- D-Mannose
- Cranberry (Vaccinium macrocarpon)
- Bearberry (Arctostaphylos uva ursi)
- Hibiscus (Hibiscus sabdaria)
- Nettle (Urtica spp.)
- Aloe Vera
- Parsley Powder (Petroselinum crispum)
- Horsetail (Equisetum spp.)
- Vitamin B6
- L-Carnitine
- Acetyl-L-Carnitine
- Champignon (Agaricus bisporus)
- Cordyceps (Cordyceps sinensis)
- Poria (Poria cocos)
- American Ginseng
- Astragalus (Astragalus membranaceus)
- Belleric Myrobalan (Terminalia bellerica)
- Tart Cherry (Prunus cerasus)

Glucose

The presence of glucose in urine (glycosuria) is commonly associated with high blood sugar levels, typically due to diabetes. Other potential causes include renal issues, stress, infections, or certain metabolic conditions.

Negative Result	No glucose detected, indicating normal glucose handling.
Positive Result	Presence of glucose, possibly indicating diabetes or other conditions affecting glucose regulation.

If NEGATIVE:

No glucose detected in urine, suggesting normal glucose control. No follow-up needed unless clinical symptoms arise.

If POSITIVE:

Presence of glucose in the urine may indicate elevated blood glucose or renal threshold issues. Evaluate blood glucose levels and check for related markers or symptoms.

Possible Causes of Glycosuria:
- With High Blood Glucose:

- Diabetes (often with high specific gravity as well)
- Severe emotional stress
- Obesity
- Endocrine disorders
- Infections
- Without High Blood Glucose:
- Inflammatory renal disease
- Renal tubule disease
- Pregnancy
- Heavy metal poisoning
- Fanconi syndrome

Check fasting and postprandial blood glucose, HbA1c, or other markers to confirm or rule out diabetes.

Glucose Metabolism Support:
- Magnesium
- Zinc
- Selenium
- Manganese
- Chromium
- Molybdenum
- Potassium Iodide
- Taurine
- Carnosine
- R-Lipoic Acid
- Vitamin A
- Vitamin D3
- Vitamin E
- Vitamin K1
- Benfotiamine (Fat-Soluble Vitamin B1)
- Vitamin B1
- Vitamin B2
- Vitamin B3
- Vitamin B5
- Vitamin B6
- Vitamin B7 (Biotin)
- Vitamin B9 (Folate)
- Vitamin B12
- Vitamin C
- Berberine
- Fenugreek
- Gymnema sylvestre
- Banaba (Lagerstroemia speciosa)
- Kudzu (Pueraria lobata)
- Cinnamon
- Inositol (as Myo and D-Chiro)
- Alpha Lipoic Acid
- MVM (Multi-vitamin/mineral)

Ketones

Ketones are produced when the body uses fat for energy due to a lack of glucose availability. Ketone presence in urine may signal that the body is in a state of ketosis, commonly due to diabetes, starvation, or low-carbohydrate diets. Elevated ketone levels, particularly in individuals with diabetes, could indicate diabetic ketoacidosis (DKA), a serious metabolic complication.

Negative Result	No ketones detected, indicating typical glucose metabolism.
Positive Result	Ketones detected in urine, possibly indicating altered metabolic state or insufficient glucose for energy.

URINALYSIS

If NEGATIVE:

 Presence of ketones in the urine may indicate altered glucose metabolism, insufficient carbohydrate intake, dehydration, or fat metabolism due to various conditions.

If POSITIVE:

 Presence of glucose in the urine may indicate elevated blood glucose or renal threshold issues. Evaluate blood glucose levels and check for related markers or symptoms.

Possible Causes of Ketosis:
- Dietary and Metabolic Factors:
- Low-carbohydrate or high-fat/protein diets
- Starvation, fasting, or prolonged vomiting
- Pregnancy or lactation
- Blood sugar irregularities, including diabetes
- Liver or adrenal dysfunction
- Medical Conditions:
- Diabetic ketoacidosis (DKA) – potentially serious in diabetic patients
- Kidney disease or kidney failure
- Hyperthyroidism
- Adrenal hypofunction – cortisol deficiency affecting glycogen release

Assess blood glucose levels and re-evaluate ketone levels if symptoms like nausea, dehydration, or confusion arise. Check for potential dehydration or infection if ketones persist.

Electrolyte Support:
- Potassium
- Sodium
- Chloride
- Magnesium
- Magnesium Bisglycinate
- Vitamin C
- Zinc

Kidney Support:
- Champignon (Agaricus bisporus)
- Cordyceps (Cordyceps sinensis)
- Poria (Poria cocos)
- American Ginseng (Panax quinquefolius)
- Astragalus (Astragalus membranaceus)

Liver Support:
- Milk Thistle
- L-methionine
- Taurine
- Inositol
- Ox Bile
- Artichoke
- Beet Powder
- Vitamin A
- Vitamin B6
- Vitamin B12
- Plant protein powder with MVM (multi-vitamin/mineral)
- L-glutathione
- N-Acetyl-L-Cysteine (NAC)
- Quercetin
- Methylsulfonylmethane (MSM)
- Sodium Sulfate
- Green Tea Extract
- Reishi
- Cordyceps
- Chinese Skullcap
- Schisandra
- Burdock Extract
- Phosphatidylcholine

Adrenal Support:
- gamma-Aminobutyric Acid (GABA)
- Eleutherococcus senticosus
- American Ginseng
- Ashwagandha
- Rhodiola
- Licorice
- Vitamin B2
- Vitamin B5
- Vitamin B6
- Vitamin C
- N-Acetyl-L-Tyrosine
- Phosphatidylserine
- Valerian
- Passion Flower
- Lemon Balm
- Chamomile
- L-theanine
- 5-HTP
- Melatonin
- Rhodiola rosea
- Pyrroloquinoline Quinone (PQQ)
- Taurine
- Vitamin B1
- Vitamin B12
- Magnesium Malate
- Magnesium Taurinate
- Magnesium Glycinate

Occult Blood (Microscopic Blood)

Occult blood in urine may indicate a condition affecting the kidneys or urinary tract, such as infections, stones, or other potential causes. Some non-pathologic factors, like dehydration or intense exercise, can also lead to a false positive result. Persistent positive findings should prompt further evaluation.

Negative Result	No microscopic blood detected.
Positive Result	Microscopic blood present, suggesting possible urinary tract or kidney issues.

If NEGATIVE:

No microscopic blood detected. No further action required unless new symptoms arise.

If POSITIVE:

Presence of microscopic blood may suggest potential issues in the kidneys or urinary tract, including infections, stones, or other underlying conditions. Follow-up testing is recommended if symptoms persist or if underlying conditions are suspected.

Potential Causes of Hematuria:
- Urinary and Renal Conditions:
- Urinary tract infections (UTIs)
- Kidney stones
- Glomerular diseases or inflammation
- Urinary tract or kidney cancer
- Kidney trauma or oxidative stress
- Systemic conditions like lupus or hypertension
- Smoking-related effects or oxidative damage
- Non-Pathologic Causes:
- Dehydration or strenuous physical activity

Reassess if persistent or if accompanied by symptoms such as flank pain, suggesting kidney stones, or signs of infection (e.g., fever, pain during urination).

Electrolyte Support:
- Potassium
- Sodium
- Chloride
- Magnesium
- Magnesium Bisglycinate
- Vitamin C
- Zinc

Urinary Support:
- D-Mannose
- Cranberry (Vaccinium macrocarpon)
- Bearberry (Arctostaphylos uva ursi)
- Hibiscus (Hibiscus sabdaria)
- Nettle (Urtica spp.)
- Aloe Vera
- Parsley Powder (Petroselinum crispum)
- Horsetail (Equisetum spp.)
- Vitamin B6
- L-Carnitine
- Acetyl-L-Carnitine
- Champignon (Agaricus bisporus)
- Cordyceps (Cordyceps sinensis)
- Poria (Poria cocos)
- American Ginseng
- Astragalus (Astragalus membranaceus)
- Belleric Myrobalan (Terminalia bellerica)
- Tart Cherry (Prunus cerasus)

Kidney Stone Support (if stones are suspected):
- Phosphorus
- Chanca Piedra / Quebra Pedra (stone breaker) (Phyllanthus niruri)

Antioxidants and Cardiovascular Support:
- Acerola Extract (Malpighia glabra)
- Grape Seed Extract (Vitis vinifera)
- Curcumin
- Garlic (Allium sativum)
- Ginkgo Extract (Ginkgo biloba)
- Quercetin, Lutein
- Lycopene, Rutin
- Clove (Syzygium aromaticum)
- Allspice (Pimenta dioica)
- Sweet Basil (Ocimum basilicum)
- Sage (Salvia officinalis)
- Rosemary Extract (Rosmarinus officinalis)
- Trans Resveratrol
- Vitamins A, E
- NAC (N-Acetyl-L-Cysteine)
- Bonito Peptide Powder
- Grape seed extract (Vitis vinefera)

Bilirubin

Bilirubin, a liver-produced waste product from the breakdown of red blood cells, is typically not found in the urine of healthy individuals. Its presence may indicate early liver dysfunction or bile duct obstruction. Bilirubinuria (bilirubin in urine) can occur before clinical signs such as jaundice, making it an early marker of liver disease. Further tests, such as a liver panel, are usually indicated to assess liver health.

Negative Result	No bilirubin detected (normal).
Positive Result	Bilirubin detected, indicating potential liver or bile duct issues.

If NEGATIVE:

 No bilirubin detected, which is normal and indicates no immediate concerns related to liver or bile duct health.

If POSITIVE:

 Presence of bilirubin in urine suggests potential liver dysfunction or biliary obstruction, such as hepatitis, cirrhosis, or gallstones. Additional diagnostic workup, including liver function tests, is recommended to determine the underlying cause.

Potential Causes of Elevated Urine Bilirubin:
- Liver and Biliary Conditions:
- Biliary stasis or gallstones
- Infectious hepatitis
- Cirrhosis of the liver
- Liver cancer or metastatic disease
- Gilbert's syndrome (benign condition with mild jaundice)
- Heart failure or other conditions affecting blood flow to the liver
- Other Considerations:
- Oxidative stress, leading to increased red blood cell breakdown
- Protein maldigestion, affecting bile processing
- Potential issues with phase II liver detoxification

Check for liver panel markers, imaging studies if indicated, and assess for symptoms of biliary obstruction (such as jaundice, abdominal pain, or nausea).

Digestive Support:
- Digestive enzymes
- Betaine HCl
- Ox Bile
- L-taurine
- Gentian extract
- Dandelion extract
- Fennel
- Amylase
- Protease SP
- Protease
- Diastase
- Lactase
- Glucoamylase
- Alpha-galactosidase
- Beta-glucanase
- Acid protease
- Phytase
- Cellulase
- Hemicellulase
- Invertase
- Lipase
- Bromelain
- Papain
- Pepsin
- Triphala (Emblica officinalis, Terminalia bellirica, Terminalia chebula)
- Magnesium Hydroxide
- Mastic Gum
- DGL (Deglycyrrhizinated Licorice)
- Methylmethionine Sulfonium Chloride (MMSC)
- Zinc L-Carnosine
- Vitamin C
- Berberine
- Ginger
- Bismuth

Liver Support:
- Milk Thistle
- L-methionine
- Taurine
- Inositol
- Ox Bile
- Artichoke
- Beet Powder
- Vitamin A

- Vitamin B6
- Vitamin B12
- Plant protein powder with MVM (multi-vitamin/mineral)
- L-glutathione
- N-Acetyl-L-Cysteine (NAC)
- Quercetin
- Methylsulfonylmethane (MSM)
- Sodium Sulfate
- Green Tea Extract
- Reishi
- Cordyceps
- Chinese Skullcap
- Schisandra
- Burdock Extract
- Phosphatidylcholine

Antioxidant Support:
- Acerola Extract (Malpighia glabra)
- Grape Seed Extract (Vitis vinifera)
- Curcumin
- Garlic (Allium sativum)
- Ginkgo Extract (Ginkgo biloba)
- Quercetin
- Rutin
- Clove (Syzygium aromaticum)
- Allspice (Pimenta dioica)
- Sweet Basil (Ocimum basilicum)
- Sage (Salvia officinalis)
- Rosemary Extract (Rosmarinus officinalis)
- Lutein
- Lycopene
- Trans Resveratrol
- Vitamin A
- Vitamin E
- L-glutathione
- NAC (N-Acetyl-L-Cysteine)
- Broccoli Powder Extract
- Sulforaphane
- Olive Leaf Extract (Olea europaea)
- Bergamot
- Red Grape Powder
- Alpha Lipoic Acid
- Taurine
- MVM (Multi-vitamin/mineral)
- Glutathione (reduced)

Urobilinogen, Semi-Quantitative

Urobilinogen is formed by the reduction of bilirubin and is usually excreted through the urine. This test helps assess liver function and red blood cell breakdown. Deviations in urobilinogen levels may suggest conditions like liver dysfunction, biliary obstruction, or hemolytic disorders..

Normal Range	0.2 - 1.0 mg/dL

If LOW or < 0.2 mg/dL:

Low levels of urobilinogen may be due to impaired bilirubin excretion or bile duct issues, which could be indicative of conditions that limit bile flow.

Potential Causes:
- Gallstones or biliary obstruction
- Inflammation of bile ducts
- Pancreatic issues, such as pancreatic cancer

Imaging studies (e.g., ultrasound) and additional liver function tests may be warranted to investigate biliary stasis or obstruction.

Further evaluation by a healthcare provider is advised if low urobilinogen persists.

If **HIGH** or > 1.0 mg/dL:

Elevated urobilinogen levels indicate increased red blood cell breakdown or potential liver dysfunction, which could be associated with liver inflammation, infections, or biliary obstruction.

Potential Causes:
- Conditions causing red blood cell destruction (hemolytic anemia, malaria, oxidative stress)
- Liver issues (acute hepatitis, cirrhosis, biliary disease)
- Biliary obstruction or gallbladder disease

Additional liver function tests and imaging may be necessary to determine underlying liver or biliary causes.

Liver Support:
- Milk Thistle
- L-methionine
- Taurine
- Inositol
- Ox Bile
- Artichoke
- Beet Powder
- Vitamin A
- Vitamin B6
- Vitamin B12
- Plant protein powder with MVM (multi-vitamin/mineral)
- L-glutathione
- N-Acetyl-L-Cysteine (NAC)
- Quercetin
- Methylsulfonylmethane (MSM)
- Sodium Sulfate
- Green Tea Extract
- Reishi
- Cordyceps
- Chinese Skullcap
- Schisandra
- Burdock Extract
- Phosphatidylcholine

Anti-inflammatory Support:
- Phytocannabinoids
- Hemp Flower Extract
- Hemp Seed Oil
- Palmitoylethanolamide (PEA)
- Omega-3 Fatty Acids (Fish Oil)
- docosahexaenoic acid), 14-HDHA (14-hydroxy docosahexaenoic acid)
- Vitamin D3
- Curcumin
- Green Tea Extract (Epigallocatechin Gallate (EGCG))
- Trans Resveratrol
- Quercetin
- Nettle (Urtica dioica)
- Pro-Resolving Mediators (PRMs): 18-HEPE (18-hydroxy eicosapentaenoic acid), 17-HDHA (17-hydroxy

Nitrite, Urine

The presence of nitrites in urine generally indicates a bacterial infection, most commonly a urinary tract infection (UTI). Certain bacteria, especially gram-negative bacteria, convert urinary nitrates to nitrites, which are then detectable in the urine.

Negative Result	No detectable nitrites
Positive Result	Presence of nitrites suggests potential bacterial infection (e.g., UTI)

URINALYSIS

If NEGATIVE:

 A negative result indicates an absence of detectable nitrites, suggesting no bacterial infection in the urinary tract. No further action required unless symptoms persist or other abnormalities are present.

If POSITIVE:

 A positive nitrite test suggests bacterial activity in the urinary tract, likely indicating a UTI. Confirmation with a microscopic evaluation and urine culture is recommended to verify the infection and identify the bacterial strain.

Potential Causes:
- Urinary Tract Infection (UTI)
- Bacterial contamination

Urine microscopy and culture to confirm bacterial presence and determine appropriate treatment.

 Urinary Support:
- D-Mannose
- Cranberry (Vaccinium macrocarpon)
- Bearberry (Arctostaphylos uva ursi)
- Hibiscus (Hibiscus sabdaria)
- Nettle (Urtica spp.)
- Aloe Vera
- Parsley Powder (Petroselinum crispum)
- Horsetail (Equisetum spp.)
- Vitamin B6
- L-Carnitine
- Acetyl-L-Carnitine
- Champignon (Agaricus bisporus)
- Cordyceps (Cordyceps sinensis)
- Poria (Poria cocos)
- American Ginseng
- Astragalus (Astragalus membranaceus)
- Belleric Myrobalan (Terminalia bellerica)
- Tart Cherry (Prunus cerasus)

High Dose Probiotics:
- Multi-strain probiotic blend
- Saccharomyces boulardii
- Beta Glucans
- Lactobacillus plantarum strain L-137 (HK L-137)
- Xylooligosaccharide (XOS)

Antimicrobial Agents:
- Oregano Oil (Origanum vulgare)
- Garlic
- Tribulus terrestris
- Magnesium Caprylate
- Berberine
- Bearberry Extract (Arctostaphylos uva-ursi)
- Black Walnut Powder (Juglans nigra)
- Barberry Extract (Berberis spp.)
- Artemisia (wormwood)
- Purified Silver
- Alpha Lipoic Acid

Cardiometabolic

Blood

Lipid Panel

Inflammation Panel

Advanced Heart Markers

Fatty Acids

Sugar Panel

Get LabDx Online Here:

Lipid Panel

A Lipid Panel is a blood test that measures various types of lipids (fats) present in your blood. This test provides important information about your cardiovascular health and can help identify potential risks for heart disease and other metabolic conditions. In functional medicine, we view the results of this test as part of a holistic approach to understanding the body's lipid metabolism and overall well-being.

CVD health — Commentary

Cardiovascular diseases and stroke are the leading causes of death for women, accounting for one in every three women's deaths annually. This equates to approximately one woman losing their life every 80 seconds. Cardiovascular disease is more fatal to women than all types of cancer, respiratory illness, and diabetes combined. In fact, 25% of all deaths occur due to cardiovascular disease, making it the leading cause of death for both men and women.

Interestingly, nearly two-thirds (64%) of women who die suddenly of coronary heart disease have had no prior symptoms. Several risk factors contribute to the development of cardiovascular disease, including high blood pressure, high LDL cholesterol, smoking, diabetes, overweight and obesity (which is covered in FMA 5), poor diet, physical inactivity, excessive alcohol consumption, and certain lifestyle patterns.

If you have any of these risk factors, it's important to address them or seek medical attention. Some of the risk factors that may require specific management or referral include dysglycemia/insulin resistance/blood sugar balancing, dyslipidemia/elevated lipids, vascular injury, autonomic dysfunction, coagulation issues/platelet irregularity, acute or chronic immune deregulation or toxicity.

Of course, if you experience any acute signs of a heart attack or stroke, it's crucial to call 911 immediately.

ⓘ 50% of heart attacks leading to sudden death occur in patients with normal cholesterol levels. Elevated cholesterol in the arteries and plaque on the walls is a response to an underlying issue. Simply addressing cholesterol levels doesn't resolve the original problem and may lead to complications. It's crucial to address elevated cholesterol, as seen in the blood lab section, but also to understand the underlying cause and determine the type of cholesterol. Metabolic syndrome significantly increases the risk of diabetes by 9 to 30 times, with a 900 to 3000% increased risk of developing diabetes. It also doubles the risk of heart disease, or increases the risk by 200 to 400%. Genetic considerations play a vital role in this condition. The CMT gene encodes an enzyme involved in the metabolism of estrogen and catecholamines, which are neurotransmitters. A specific SNP in this gene impairs its function and increases the risk of cardiovascular disease (CVD). The MTHFR gene, which regulates the methyl cycle, a crucial metabolic process involved in neurotransmitter synthesis, genetic function, detoxification, ATP production, and more, is also affected by a SNP. This SNP/dysfunction can alter DNA and RNA expression, potentially contributing to chronic diseases, including CVD. Nutritional factors also influence the effects of statins and beta-blockers. Statins and beta-blockers reduce CoQ10 levels, decrease selenium, O3, carnitine, T3f, and melatonin. Diuretics may reduce electrolytes and essential minerals. Metformin reduces B9 (folate) and B12. ACE inhibitors/blockers decrease zinc and sodium. Statindecisionaid.mayoclinic.org is a valuable resource, particularly for documenting the standard of care for medical professionals and patients who choose not to take statins. Statins work by inhibiting HMG CoA reductase, effectively halting the production of CoQ10, cholesterol, and lowering levels of vitamin D, estrogen, progesterone, testosterone, and cortisol.

For heart health, maintaining a balanced blood sugar level and avoiding diabetes or metabolic syndrome are crucial. The Mediterranean diet, rich in monounsaturated fats (MUFA) and marine omega-3 fatty acids (DHA and EPA), is particularly beneficial for reducing the risk of cardiovascular disease (CVD).

Several lifestyle changes can significantly impact inflammation and contribute to heart health:

- Non-inflammatory diet: Emphasize foods that reduce inflammation, such as fruits, vegetables, whole grains, and healthy fats.
- Proper sleep: Ensure adequate sleep, as sleep apnea can lead to oxygen deprivation, which can be detrimental to both the heart and brain.
- Regular exercise: Incorporate high-intensity interval training (HIIT) into your routine to promote cardiovascular fitness and reduce inflammation.
- Stress management: Practice stress-reducing techniques like meditation and monitor heart rate variability (HRV) to manage stress effectively.
- Address nutritional deficiencies: Consult with a healthcare professional to identify and address any nutritional deficiencies that may be affecting your heart health.

Preventive measures to support heart health include:

- Monitor liver health.
- Maintain adrenal health.
- Quit smoking.
- Move throughout the day.
- Consider getting a pet.

Key dietary support for heart health includes:

- Non-inflammatory diet: Emphasize a diet low in sugar and starch to reduce inflammation.
- Limit canola oil and other polyunsaturated fats (PUFAs): These fats can increase inflammation, so it's best to limit their intake.
- Reduce sugar consumption: Excessive sugar intake can drive up triglyceride levels, lower immune function, convert to fat in the body, elevate insulin levels, and contribute to plaque formation in the arteries.
- Increase healthy fats: Include saturated fats in your diet, as they have been shown to have heart-protective properties.
- Limit grains or learn proper preparation techniques: Grains can contribute to inflammation, so it's best to limit their intake or learn how to prepare them in a way that reduces inflammation.
- Eat cholesterol-rich foods: Include cholesterol-rich foods in your diet, such as eggs, fish, and organ meats, as they have been shown to have heart-protective benefits.
- Egg yolks, processed foods, and a Metabolic Reset & Weight Loss program or maintenance plan are all to be avoided.
- Antioxidants and free radicals should be consumed in moderation, as should cholesterol antagonists to reduce excess cholesterol in the bloodstream.
- Vitamin and mineral deficiencies should be addressed, and random vitamin and mineral supplements, including multivitamins, should be avoided.
- Green tea can block HMG-CoA Reductase and lower cholesterol absorption.

Here are some dietary tips and caveats:
- Limit starchy foods like potatoes, pasta, bread, crackers, and rice.
- Avoid simple sugars and sugary drinks and sodas.
- Incorporate heart-healthy, anti-inflammatory snacks like blueberries, pomegranate seeds, avocados, walnuts, and pistachios.
- Avoid hydrogenated vegetable oils, trans fats, and fried foods.
- Cook with coconut and avocado oils; add olive oil to cooked foods and raw vegetables.
- Choose organic produce, organic, antibiotic-free, hormone-free, grass-fed dairy and animal products.
- Eat freshly ground flax seeds or chia seeds to increase fiber intake; eat the skin of fruits and vegetables.
- Consume adequate amounts of antioxidants and flavonoids, which can be obtained daily through 5-9 servings of organic vegetables and fruit.
- Eat garlic frequently.

Plant phenols, found in berries and nuts, are rich in antioxidants and have been linked to heart health. Antioxidant foods and supplements, such as vitamin C, quercetin, and resveratrol, help protect cells from damage caused by free radicals. Essential nutrients like D3 K2, niacinamide (B3), and B6 are crucial for maintaining healthy cholesterol levels and blood pressure. Lecithin and cholesterol antagonists regulate cholesterol levels and reduce the risk of heart disease. Numerous herbs and supplements, including hawthorn berry, motherwort, gymnema, ashwagandha, milk thistle, vitamin C, quercetin, gotu kola extract, horse chestnut, grape seed, buckwheat, omega 3 fatty acids, B vitamins, carnitine, and ginkgo extract, are known for their heart-protective properties.

Rhamnan sulfate is a specialized sulfated polysaccharide derived from the green seaweed Monostroma nitidum. It is a glycocalyx regenerating compound (GRC) that has been shown to possess anticoagulant and antithrombotic activity.

Red Yeast Rice (RYR) is a powerful supplement that is similar to statins in its ability to lower cholesterol levels. However, it is less likely to cause myopathy as a side effect, but it is still possible.

ARTEROSIL ® is a supplement that targets the endothelial glycocalyx (EG), which is a thin "gel-like" layer that coats the inside of the vascular endothelium, including every artery, vein, and capillary.

Here are some important facts about the endothelial glycocalyx:
- The EG is crucial for maintaining healthy arteries.
- It prevents cholesterol and other particles from adhering to or penetrating the endothelial wall.
- The primary contributors to the breakdown of the EG are high blood glucose, oxidative stress, and inflammation.
- Pathologies associated with impaired EG include coronary heart disease, hyperglycemia, diabetes, renal diseases, lacunar stroke, and severe trauma.

Cholesterol

Component of cell membranes, myelin sheath, bile salts, and a precursor for steroid hormones. Cholesterol serves many functions, and while elevated levels can contribute to cardiovascular (CV) risk, underlying causes should be investigated, such as increased steroid hormone production, fighting infection (acting as an antioxidant), or hypothyroidism. Cholesterol, although classified as a "lipid," does not provide energy. Primarily made in the body, it is also found in the diet as a "waxy" lipid present in all cells, contributing to hormone production, vitamin D, digestion, nerve sheath structure, and the adrenal glands and brain.

- **Production**: 25% from diet, 75% made in liver, intestines, and skin. Low dietary intake can increase liver production.
- **Functions**: Structural role in cell membranes, precursor to steroid hormones, essential for vitamin D production, bile salt precursor for fat digestion, antioxidant, and necessary for serotonin function in the brain.
- **Health Implications**: Levels <180 are linked to a 200% increase in cerebrovascular accidents, lung disease, depression, suicide, and a 300% increase in liver cancer.

Cholesterol is essential to the body because it:
- Provides cell membrane stiffness/stability.
- Acts as a precursor to steroid hormones and vitamin D.
- Is essential for bile salt formation for fat digestion.
- Serves as an antioxidant.
- Supports serotonin function, crucial for brain health.

Normal Range	100 - 199 mg/dL
Optimal Range	180 - 220 mg/dL

If **LOW** or **< 180 mg/dL**:

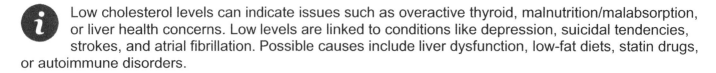

Low cholesterol levels can indicate issues such as overactive thyroid, malnutrition/malabsorption, or liver health concerns. Low levels are linked to conditions like depression, suicidal tendencies, strokes, and atrial fibrillation. Possible causes include liver dysfunction, low-fat diets, statin drugs, or autoimmune disorders.

- Support immune and digestive systems.
- Address potential malnutrition, poor pancreas/liver function, and hyperthyroidism.

Digestive Support:
- Digestive enzymes
- Betaine HCl
- Ox Bile
- L-taurine
- Gentian extract
- Dandelion extract
- Fennel
- Amylase
- Protease SP
- Protease
- Diastase
- Lactase
- Glucoamylase
- Alpha-galactosidase
- Beta-glucanase
- Acid protease
- Phytase
- Cellulase

- Hemicellulase
- Invertase
- Lipase
- Bromelain
- Papain
- Pepsin
- Triphala (Emblica officinalis, Terminalia bellirica, Terminalia chebula)
- Magnesium Hydroxide
- Mastic Gum
- DGL (Deglycyrrhizinated Licorice)
- Methylmethionine Sulfonium Chloride (MMSC)
- Zinc L-Carnosine
- Vitamin C
- Berberine
- Ginger
- Bismuth

Nutritional Support:
- Borage oil (GLA - Gamma Linolenic Acid)
- Manganese

Immune Support:
- Echinacea angustifolia
- Astragalus membranaceus
- Elderberry Extract (Sambucus nigra)
- Andrographis paniculate
- Green Tea Extract
- Arabinogalactan (larch tree)
- Lauric Acid
- Cordyceps mushroom
- Shiitake mushroom
- Maitake mushroom
- Reishi mushroom
- Beta 1,3 Glucans
- Vitamin A
- Vitamin D3
- Vitamin E
- Vitamin K2
- Wild cherry bark
- Ginger
- Lovage (Levisticum officinale)
- Wild Cherry Extract

If **HIGH** or > 220 mg/dL:

Elevated cholesterol may result from issues such as poor metabolism of fats, biliary stasis, hypothyroidism, or dietary habits high in sugars or refined carbohydrates. Elevated levels can signal a need for increased liver, biliary, or thyroid support, as well as monitoring of sugar handling.

Primary areas to address include liver and biliary health, sugar handling, and possibly thyroid and estrogen levels. Consider lowering dietary sugar and increasing intake of omega-3 fatty acids, high-dose niacin, and pantothenic acid.

Lipid Support (high):
- Red Yeast Rice (Monascus purpureus)
- Coenzyme Q10
- Sweet Orange (Citrus sinensis)
- Quercetin
- Gotu Kola (Centella asiatica)
- Horse Chestnut (Aesculus hippocastanum)
- Grape Seed Extract (Vitis vinifera)
- Vitamin C
- Plant Sterols/Stanols (Beta-Sitosterol, Campesterol, Campestanol, Sitostanol)
- Monostroma nitidum (seaweed) extract

Anti-inflammatory Support:
- Phytocannabinoids
- Hemp Flower Extract
- Hemp Seed Oil
- Palmitoylethanolamide (PEA)
- Omega-3 Fatty Acids (Fish Oil)
- docosahexaenoic acid), 14-HDHA (14-hydroxy docosahexaenoic acid)
- Vitamin D3
- Curcumin
- Green Tea Extract (Epigallocatechin Gallate (EGCG))
- Trans Resveratrol
- Quercetin
- Nettle (Urtica dioica)
- Pro-Resolving Mediators (PRMs): 18-HEPE (18-hydroxy eicosapentaenoic acid), 17-HDHA (17-hydroxy

Nutritional Support:
- Vitamins A, D, E, K

Liver Support:
- Milk Thistle
- L-methionine

- Taurine
- Inositol
- Ox Bile
- Artichoke
- Beet Powder
- Vitamin A
- Vitamin B6
- Vitamin B12
- Plant protein powder with MVM (multi-vitamin/mineral)
- L-glutathione

- N-Acetyl-L-Cysteine (NAC)
- Quercetin
- Methylsulfonylmethane (MSM)
- Sodium Sulfate
- Green Tea Extract
- Reishi
- Cordyceps
- Chinese Skullcap
- Schisandra
- Burdock Extract
- Phosphatidylcholine

Thyroid Support:
- N-Acetyl-L-Tyrosine
- American Ginseng (Panax quinquefolius)
- Forskolin (Coleus forskohlii)
- Iodine
- Chromium
- Zinc

- Selenium
- Copper
- Manganese
- Vitamin A
- Vitamin B2
- Potassium Iodide
- Myo-Inositol

Fiber Support:
- Acacia gum
- Cellulose
- Guar gum
- Cranberry seed powder
- Carrot fiber
- Inulin

- Orange fiber
- Glucomannan
- Apple pectin
- Psyllium husk
- Flax seed
- Prune powder

Triglycerides

Triglycerides are esters formed from glycerol and three chains of fatty acids (FA). They are consumed through dietary fat and are the body's primary source of energy. While triglycerides can be beneficial when used correctly, they may pose a cardiovascular risk if produced in excess by the liver from unused sugars (particularly refined/simple carbohydrates). Triglycerides differ from cholesterol, although both are classified as lipids.

- **Sources**: Dietary fats account for over 90% of triglyceride intake. Excess triglycerides are stored as adipose tissue once liver and muscle storage sites are full.
- **Transport**: Chylomicrons (largest lipoproteins) transport dietary triglycerides, while very-low-density lipoproteins (VLDL) transport those produced by the liver.
- **Functions**: Provides energy, insulation, and organ padding. Proper fat metabolism should result in triglyceride levels around half of total cholesterol.

Normal Range	0 - 149 mg/dL
Optimal Range	70 - 100 mg/dL

If LOW or < 70 mg/dL:

 Low triglycerides may indicate insufficient fat intake, liver or biliary dysfunction, protein malnutrition, autoimmune diseases, or hyperthyroidism.

LIPID PANEL

 Increase protein intake and support immune and biliary systems.
Common underlying causes include insufficient fat intake, liver biliary dysfunction, protein malnutrition, or hyperthyroidism.

 Protein Source:
- Protein Powder
- Mixed Amino Acids
- Dairy-Free, Plant-Based Protein Powder
- Whey-Based Protein Powder

Digestive Support:
- Digestive enzymes
- Betaine HCl
- Ox Bile
- L-taurine
- Gentian extract
- Dandelion extract
- Fennel
- Amylase
- Protease SP
- Protease
- Diastase
- Lactase
- Glucoamylase
- Alpha-galactosidase
- Beta-glucanase
- Acid protease
- Phytase
- Cellulase
- Hemicellulase
- Invertase
- Lipase
- Bromelain
- Papain
- Pepsin
- Triphala (Emblica officinalis, Terminalia bellirica, Terminalia chebula)
- Magnesium Hydroxide
- Mastic Gum
- DGL (Deglycyrrhizinated Licorice)
- Methylmethionine Sulfonium Chloride (MMSC)
- Zinc L-Carnosine
- Vitamin C
- Berberine
- Ginger
- Bismuth

Immune Support:
- Echinacea angustifolia
- Astragalus membranaceus
- Elderberry Extract (Sambucus nigra)
- Andrographis paniculate
- Green Tea Extract
- Arabinogalactan (larch tree)
- Lauric Acid
- Cordyceps mushroom
- Shiitake mushroom
- Maitake mushroom
- Reishi mushroom
- Beta 1,3 Glucans
- Vitamin A
- Vitamin D3
- Vitamin E
- Vitamin K2
- Wild cherry bark
- Ginger
- Lovage (Levisticum officinale)
- Wild Cherry Extract

If **HIGH** or > 100 mg/dL:

 Elevated triglycerides may signal poor fat metabolism, liver congestion, fatty liver, hypothyroidism, insulin resistance, or high intake of carbohydrates. They are often high when the diet is rich in sugars or carbs.

 Evaluate biliary function, fat metabolism, liver function, and blood sugar balance.

LIPID PANEL

Consider a high-MUFA Mediterranean diet with omega-3 fatty acids for cardiovascular risk reduction.

Lipid Support (high):
- Red Yeast Rice (Monascus purpureus)
- Coenzyme Q10
- Sweet Orange (Citrus sinensis)
- Quercetin
- Gotu Kola (Centella asiatica)
- Horse Chestnut (Aesculus hippocastanum)
- Grape Seed Extract (Vitis vinifera)
- Vitamin C
- Plant Sterols/Stanols (Beta-Sitosterol, Campesterol, Campestanol, Sitostanol)
- Monostroma nitidum (seaweed) extract

Liver Support:
- Milk Thistle
- L-methionine
- Taurine
- Inositol
- Ox Bile
- Artichoke
- Beet Powder
- Vitamin A
- Vitamin B6
- Vitamin B12
- Plant protein powder with MVM (multi-vitamin/mineral)
- L-glutathione
- N-Acetyl-L-Cysteine (NAC)
- Quercetin
- Methylsulfonylmethane (MSM)
- Sodium Sulfate
- Green Tea Extract
- Reishi
- Cordyceps
- Chinese Skullcap
- Schisandra
- Burdock Extract
- Phosphatidylcholine

Glucose Metabolism Support:
- Magnesium
- Zinc
- Selenium
- Manganese
- Chromium
- Molybdenum
- Potassium Iodide
- Taurine
- Carnosine
- R-Lipoic Acid
- Vitamin A
- Vitamin D3
- Vitamin E
- Vitamin K1
- Benfotiamine (Fat-Soluble Vitamin B1)
- Vitamin B1
- Vitamin B2
- Vitamin B3
- Vitamin B5
- Vitamin B6
- Vitamin B7 (Biotin)
- Vitamin B9 (Folate)
- Vitamin B12
- Vitamin C
- Berberine
- Fenugreek
- Gymnema sylvestre
- Banaba (Lagerstroemia speciosa)
- Kudzu (Pueraria lobata)
- Cinnamon
- Inositol (as Myo and D-Chiro)
- Alpha Lipoic Acid
- MVM (Multi-vitamin/mineral)

Thyroid Support:
- N-Acetyl-L-Tyrosine
- American Ginseng (Panax quinquefolius)
- Forskolin (Coleus forskohlii)
- Iodine
- Chromium
- Zinc
- Selenium
- Copper
- Manganese
- Vitamin A
- Vitamin B2
- Potassium Iodide
- Myo-Inositol

Nutritional Support:
- Vitamins A, D, E, K

HDL Cholesterol

HDL cholesterol is a protein carrier that transports fats from tissues to the liver, where they are processed into bile salts. HDL is produced by the liver and intestines and is inversely proportional to LDL cholesterol, making it a good indicator of cardiovascular disease (CVD) risk. Higher HDL levels are generally protective, with levels between 60-74 mg/dL indicating below-average risk for CVD.

Factors: Low-fat diets and calorie restriction may lower HDL, whereas high-fat diets can increase HDL levels.

Normal Range	> 39 mg/dL
Optimal Range	> 55 mg/dL

If **LOW** or < 55 U/L:

Low HDL levels can be associated with liver congestion, high carbohydrate intake, a sedentary lifestyle, metabolic syndrome, CVD, or oxidative stress.

Dietary recommendations: Increase healthy fats (e.g., olive oil, avocado, fatty fish) and limit simple sugars and starchy foods.
Lifestyle recommendations: Normalize weight and incorporate regular exercise.

Lipid Support (high):
- Red Yeast Rice (Monascus purpureus)
- Coenzyme Q10
- Sweet Orange (Citrus sinensis)
- Quercetin
- Gotu Kola (Centella asiatica)
- Horse Chestnut (Aesculus hippocastanum)
- Grape Seed Extract (Vitis vinifera)
- Vitamin C
- Plant Sterols/Stanols (Beta-Sitosterol, Campesterol, Campestanol, Sitostanol)
- Monostroma nitidum (seaweed) extract

Liver Support:
- Milk Thistle
- L-methionine
- Taurine
- Inositol
- Ox Bile
- Artichoke
- Beet Powder
- Vitamin A
- Vitamin B6
- Vitamin B12
- Plant protein powder with MVM (multi-vitamin/mineral)
- L-glutathione
- N-Acetyl-L-Cysteine (NAC)
- Quercetin
- Methylsulfonylmethane (MSM)
- Sodium Sulfate
- Green Tea Extract
- Reishi
- Cordyceps
- Chinese Skullcap
- Schisandra
- Burdock Extract
- Phosphatidylcholine

Glucose Metabolism Support:
- Magnesium
- Zinc
- Selenium
- Manganese
- Chromium
- Molybdenum
- Potassium Iodide
- Taurine
- Carnosine
- R-Lipoic Acid
- Vitamin A
- Vitamin D3
- Vitamin E
- Vitamin K1
- Benfotiamine (Fat-Soluble Vitamin B1)
- Vitamin B1
- Vitamin B2
- Vitamin B3
- Vitamin B5
- Vitamin B6
- Vitamin B7 (Biotin)
- Vitamin B9 (Folate)
- Vitamin B12
- Vitamin C
- Berberine
- Fenugreek
- Gymnema sylvestre
- Banaba (Lagerstroemia speciosa)
- Kudzu (Pueraria lobata)
- Cinnamon
- Inositol (as Myo and D-Chiro)
- Alpha Lipoic Acid
- MVM (Multi-vitamin/mineral)

Thyroid Support:
- N-Acetyl-L-Tyrosine
- American Ginseng (Panax quinquefolius)
- Forskolin (Coleus forskohlii)
- Iodine
- Chromium
- Zinc
- Selenium
- Copper
- Manganese
- Vitamin A
- Vitamin B2
- Potassium Iodide
- Myo-Inositol

Fiber Support:
- Acacia gum
- Cellulose
- Guar gum
- Cranberry seed powder
- Carrot fiber
- Inulin
- Orange fiber
- Glucomannan
- Apple pectin
- Psyllium husk
- Flax seed
- Prune powder

If **HIGH** or > 80 mg/dL:

High HDL levels may be due to genetics (CETP gene), hyperthyroidism, primary biliary cholangitis, alcohol use disorder, certain medications (e.g., estrogen, H2 blockers), steroid use, or autoimmune diseases.

Support immunity and manage inflammation.

Immune Support:
- Echinacea angustifolia
- Astragalus membranaceus
- Elderberry Extract (Sambucus nigra)
- Andrographis paniculate
- Green Tea Extract
- Arabinogalactan (larch tree)
- Lauric Acid
- Cordyceps mushroom
- Shiitake mushroom
- Maitake mushroom

- Reishi mushroom
- Beta 1,3 Glucans
- Vitamin A
- Vitamin D3
- Vitamin E

Anti-inflammatory Support:
- Phytocannabinoids
- Hemp Flower Extract
- Hemp Seed Oil
- Palmitoylethanolamide (PEA)
- Omega-3 Fatty Acids (Fish Oil)
- docosahexaenoic acid), 14-HDHA (14-hydroxy docosahexaenoic acid)
- Vitamin D3
- Curcumin

Glucose Metabolism Support:
- Magnesium
- Zinc
- Selenium
- Manganese
- Chromium
- Molybdenum
- Potassium Iodide
- Taurine
- Carnosine
- R-Lipoic Acid
- Vitamin A
- Vitamin D3
- Vitamin E
- Vitamin K1
- Benfotiamine (Fat-Soluble Vitamin B1)
- Vitamin B1
- Vitamin B2

- Vitamin K2
- Wild cherry bark
- Ginger
- Lovage (Levisticum officinale)
- Wild Cherry Extract

- Green Tea Extract (Epigallocatechin Gallate (EGCG))
- Trans Resveratrol
- Quercetin
- Nettle (Urtica dioica)
- Pro-Resolving Mediators (PRMs): 18-HEPE (18-hydroxy eicosapentaenoic acid), 17-HDHA (17-hydroxy

- Vitamin B3
- Vitamin B5
- Vitamin B6
- Vitamin B7 (Biotin)
- Vitamin B9 (Folate)
- Vitamin B12
- Vitamin C
- Berberine
- Fenugreek
- Gymnema sylvestre
- Banaba (Lagerstroemia speciosa)
- Kudzu (Pueraria lobata)
- Cinnamon
- Inositol (as Myo and D-Chiro)
- Alpha Lipoic Acid
- MVM (Multi-vitamin/mineral)

LDL Cholesterol

LDL cholesterol is a protein carrier that transports fats (cholesterol) from the liver to cells. LDL is often referred to as the "fire truck" while cholesterol is the "fireman," responsible for delivering necessary cholesterol where needed in the body. About 60-70% of total serum cholesterol is carried on LDL, which is produced and recycled in the liver.

LDL levels can rise in response to inflammation or dysfunction. The triglyceride/HDL ratio is ideally less than 2.0 for better cardiovascular health. The size and particle number of LDL are also important: two individuals with the same LDL number (e.g., 150) may have different cardiovascular risks depending on the LDL particle size.

Normal Range	65 - 99 mg/dL
Optimal Range	80 - 130 mg/dL

LIPID PANEL

If **LOW** or < 80 mg/dL:

 Low LDL may be associated with low Vitamin D levels, steroid hormone imbalances, the need for increased exercise, hyperthyroidism, severe liver disease, or chronic anemia.

 Support liver function and blood sugar regulation.
Encourage regular exercise, such as high-intensity interval training (HIIT).

 Nutritional Support:
- Vitamin D3, K2

Liver Support:
- Milk Thistle
- L-methionine
- Taurine
- Inositol
- Ox Bile
- Artichoke
- Beet Powder
- Vitamin A
- Vitamin B6
- Vitamin B12
- Plant protein powder with MVM (multi-vitamin/mineral)
- L-glutathione
- N-Acetyl-L-Cysteine (NAC)
- Quercetin
- Methylsulfonylmethane (MSM)
- Sodium Sulfate
- Green Tea Extract
- Reishi
- Cordyceps
- Chinese Skullcap
- Schisandra
- Burdock Extract
- Phosphatidylcholine

If **HIGH** or > 130 mg/dL:

 Elevated LDL may be due to increased carbohydrate intake, liver congestion, use of exogenous hormones, hypothyroidism, insulin resistance, or cardiovascular disease.

 Consider a ketogenic diet and support for the liver, immune, and cardiovascular systems.
For heart health, focus on blood sugar balance and avoiding metabolic syndrome.
Recommended diet: high-MUFA Mediterranean diet with marine omega-3 (DHA/EPA).

 Lipid Support (high):
- Red Yeast Rice (Monascus purpureus)
- Coenzyme Q10
- Sweet Orange (Citrus sinensis)
- Quercetin
- Gotu Kola (Centella asiatica)
- Horse Chestnut (Aesculus hippocastanum)
- Grape Seed Extract (Vitis vinifera)
- Vitamin C
- Plant Sterols/Stanols (Beta-Sitosterol, Campesterol, Campestanol, Sitostanol)
- Monostroma nitidum (seaweed) extract

Anti-inflammatory Support:
- Phytocannabinoids
- Hemp Flower Extract
- Hemp Seed Oil
- Palmitoylethanolamide (PEA)
- Omega-3 Fatty Acids (Fish Oil)
- docosahexaenoic acid), 14-HDHA (14-hydroxy docosahexaenoic acid)
- Vitamin D3
- Curcumin
- Green Tea Extract (Epigallocatechin Gallate (EGCG))
- Trans Resveratrol
- Quercetin
- Nettle (Urtica dioica)

- Pro-Resolving Mediators (PRMs): 18-HEPE (18-hydroxy eicosapentaenoic acid), 17-HDHA (17-hydroxy

Liver Support:
- Milk Thistle
- L-methionine
- Taurine
- Inositol
- Ox Bile
- Artichoke
- Beet Powder
- Vitamin A
- Vitamin B6
- Vitamin B12
- Plant protein powder with MVM (multi-vitamin/mineral)
- L-glutathione
- N-Acetyl-L-Cysteine (NAC)
- Quercetin
- Methylsulfonylmethane (MSM)
- Sodium Sulfate
- Green Tea Extract
- Reishi
- Cordyceps
- Chinese Skullcap
- Schisandra
- Burdock Extract
- Phosphatidylcholine

Thyroid Support:
- N-Acetyl-L-Tyrosine
- American Ginseng (Panax quinquefolius)
- Forskolin (Coleus forskohlii)
- Iodine
- Chromium
- Zinc
- Selenium
- Copper
- Manganese
- Vitamin A
- Vitamin B2
- Potassium Iodide
- Myo-Inositol

Fiber Support:
- Acacia gum
- Cellulose
- Guar gum
- Cranberry seed powder
- Carrot fiber
- Inulin
- Orange fiber
- Glucomannan
- Apple pectin
- Psyllium husk
- Flax seed
- Prune powder

Homocysteine

Homocysteine levels can be a useful marker for identifying potential deficiencies in vitamin B12 or folate. Elevated homocysteine may occur before a B12 deficiency becomes detectable.

Normal Range	0.0 - 15.0 µmol/L
Optimal Range	< 7.2 µmol/L

If **HIGH** or **> 7.2 µmol/L:**

Elevated homocysteine levels may indicate a need for further testing to rule out cardiovascular disease (CVD), malnutrition, anemia, or vitamin B9/B12 deficiency. In cases of suspected small intestinal bacterial overgrowth (SIBO), homocysteine may also be high.

LIPID PANEL

Lifestyle Recommendations:
- Avoid or reduce chronic stress, as it can deplete B vitamins.
- Ensure adequate sleep, manage weight, exercise daily, and avoid alcohol and smoking.
- Consider testing for B vitamin levels with a Comprehensive Metabolic Profile and monitor insulin, blood glucose, blood pressure, liver function (LFTs), glutathione (GGT), estrogen metabolites, FIGLU, MMA, and methylation SNPs if needed.

Dietary Tips and Caveats:
- Adopt a heart-healthy eating plan.
- Increase intake of B vitamin-rich foods like broccoli, asparagus, green peas, yams, avocados, bananas, oranges, meats, fish, and lentils.
- Avoid refined sugars, white flour, high-sugar beverages, and alcohol.
- Increase antioxidant-rich vegetables and fruits (5-9 servings daily).

Homocysteine Support:
- Vitamin B2
- Vitamin B6
- Vitamin B9 (Folate)
- Vitamin B12
- TMG (Trimethylglycine)
- L-Serine
- NAC (N-Acetyl-L-Cysteine)
- Vitamin B Complex
- 5-Methyltetrahydrofolate (Vitamin B9 / Folate)

Anti-inflammatory Support:
- Phytocannabinoids
- Hemp Flower Extract
- Hemp Seed Oil
- Palmitoylethanolamide (PEA)
- Omega-3 Fatty Acids (Fish Oil)
- docosahexaenoic acid), 14-HDHA (14-hydroxy docosahexaenoic acid)
- Vitamin D3
- Curcumin
- Green Tea Extract (Epigallocatechin Gallate (EGCG))
- Trans Resveratrol
- Quercetin
- Nettle (Urtica dioica)
- Pro-Resolving Mediators (PRMs): 18-HEPE (18-hydroxy eicosapentaenoic acid), 17-HDHA (17-hydroxy

Digestive Support:
- Digestive enzymes
- Betaine HCl
- Ox Bile
- L-taurine
- Gentian extract
- Dandelion extract
- Fennel
- Amylase
- Protease SP
- Protease
- Diastase
- Lactase
- Glucoamylase
- Alpha-galactosidase
- Beta-glucanase
- Acid protease
- Phytase
- Cellulase
- Hemicellulase
- Invertase
- Lipase
- Bromelain
- Papain
- Pepsin
- Triphala (Emblica officinalis, Terminalia bellirica, Terminalia chebula)
- Magnesium Hydroxide
- Mastic Gum
- DGL (Deglycyrrhizinated Licorice)
- Methylmethionine Sulfonium Chloride (MMSC)
- Zinc L-Carnosine
- Vitamin C
- Berberine
- Ginger
- Bismuth

Antioxidant Support:
- Acerola Extract (Malpighia glabra)
- Grape Seed Extract (Vitis vinifera)
- Curcumin
- Garlic (Allium sativum)
- Ginkgo Extract (Ginkgo biloba)
- Quercetin
- Rutin
- Clove (Syzygium aromaticum)
- Allspice (Pimenta dioica)
- Sweet Basil (Ocimum basilicum)
- Sage (Salvia officinalis)
- Rosemary Extract (Rosmarinus officinalis)
- Lutein
- Lycopene
- Trans Resveratrol
- Vitamin A
- Vitamin E
- L-glutathione
- NAC (N-Acetyl-L-Cysteine)
- Broccoli Powder Extract
- Sulforaphane
- Olive Leaf Extract (Olea europaea)
- Bergamot
- Red Grape Powder
- Alpha Lipoic Acid
- Taurine
- MVM (Multi-vitamin/mineral)
- Glutathione (reduced)

C-Reactive Protein (hsCRP)

C-Reactive Protein (CRP) is a protein produced by the liver in response to systemic inflammation. It acts as an acute-phase reactant and is an independent predictor of cardiovascular disease (CVD) events. The "high sensitivity" CRP (hsCRP) test is required to detect very low levels of CRP, which may indicate vascular and/or systemic inflammation. hsCRP provides independent prognostic information useful for managing and monitoring treatment protocols.

MALE	
Normal Range	0 - 3.00 mg/dL
Optimal Range	< 0.6 mg/dL

FEMALE	
Normal Range	0 - 3.00 mg/dL
Optimal Range	< 1.5 mg/dL

If **HIGH** or **> 0.6 mg/dL (Male)** or **> 1.5 mg/dL (Female)**:

Elevated hsCRP levels may indicate increased systemic or vascular inflammation, raising the risk for cardiovascular disease and events. Levels should not be measured during acute stress or infection as they may temporarily elevate. Consider a follow-up test if levels exceed 10 mg/dL to rule out infection or other inflammatory conditions.

Rule out underlying chronic inflammation (e.g., rheumatoid arthritis) or infections (e.g., periodontitis, C. pneumoniae, H. pylori, CMV), as these can elevate hsCRP and increase CVD risk.

Lifestyle Modifications:
- Improve insulin sensitivity through weight reduction and aerobic exercise.
- Avoid smoking.

Dietary Support:
- Limit simple starches, sugars, and high-glycemic foods.
- Avoid trans fats and minimize alcohol intake.
- Increase intake of omega-3 fatty acids (cold-water fish), fruits, vegetables, legumes, soluble fiber, nuts, and seeds.

LIPID PANEL

- Consume foods rich in choline and betaine (e.g., animal-based foods, whole grains, spinach, beets) to help lower CRP.

Anti-inflammatory and antioxidant support:
- Fish oils
- Vitamins C & E
- Carotenoids
- Pycnogenol
- Flavonoids
- Resveratrol
- Sea buckthorn berries.

Insulin-sensitizing agents:
- Chromium,
- Alpha-lipoic acid,
- Zinc,
- Biotin,
- Magnesium.

Fibrinogen Activity

Fibrinogen is a protein (coagulation factor) produced by the liver, essential for blood clot formation. The activity test measures how effectively fibrinogen contributes to clot formation. As an acute phase reactant, fibrinogen levels can increase with acute tissue inflammation or damage.

Normal Range	193 - 507 mg/dL
Optimal Range	200 - 300 mg/dL

If LOW or < 200 mg/dL:

Low fibrinogen activity may be associated with liver dysfunction or malnutrition, potentially impairing blood clot formation and response to injury.

Evaluate for potential malnutrition or digestive issues that may affect nutrient absorption. Support liver function and assess digestive health to ensure effective protein and enzyme processing.

Digestive Support:
- Digestive enzymes
- Betaine HCl
- Ox Bile
- L-taurine
- Gentian extract
- Dandelion extract
- Fennel
- Amylase
- Protease SP
- Protease
- Diastase
- Lactase
- Glucoamylase
- Alpha-galactosidase
- Beta-glucanase
- Acid protease
- Phytase
- Cellulase
- Hemicellulase
- Invertase
- Lipase
- Bromelain
- Papain
- Pepsin

- Triphala (Emblica officinalis, Terminalia bellirica, Terminalia chebula)
- Magnesium Hydroxide
- Mastic Gum
- DGL (Deglycyrrhizinated Licorice)
- Bismuth
- Methylmethionine Sulfonium Chloride (MMSC)
- Zinc L-Carnosine
- Vitamin C
- Berberine
- Ginger

Liver Support:
- Milk Thistle
- L-methionine
- Taurine
- Inositol
- Ox Bile
- Artichoke
- Beet Powder
- Vitamin A
- Vitamin B6
- Vitamin B12
- Plant protein powder with MVM (multi-vitamin/mineral)
- L-glutathione
- N-Acetyl-L-Cysteine (NAC)
- Quercetin
- Methylsulfonylmethane (MSM)
- Sodium Sulfate
- Green Tea Extract
- Reishi
- Cordyceps
- Chinese Skullcap
- Schisandra
- Burdock Extract
- Phosphatidylcholine

Whole Food Support:
- Mixed greens powder from fruits and vegetables
- Mixed reds powder from fruits and vegetables

If **HIGH** or **> 300 mg/dL:**

 Elevated fibrinogen activity is a non-specific marker of inflammation, indicating potential systemic inflammation that should be further assessed in relation to other inflammatory markers and clinical examination.

 Consider an inflammation protocol to address systemic inflammation and support cardiovascular health.

Anti-inflammatory Support:
- Phytocannabinoids
- Hemp Flower Extract
- Hemp Seed Oil
- Palmitoylethanolamide (PEA)
- Omega-3 Fatty Acids (Fish Oil)
- Vitamin D3
- Curcumin
- Green Tea Extract (Epigallocatechin Gallate (EGCG))
- Trans Resveratrol
- Quercetin
- Nettle (Urtica dioica)
- Pro-Resolving Mediators (PRMs): 18-HEPE (18-hydroxy eicosapentaenoic acid), 17-HDHA (17-hydroxy docosahexaenoic acid), 14-HDHA (14-hydroxy docosahexaenoic acid)

Inflammation Panel

A comprehensive assessment of various markers associated with inflammation, oxidative stress, and cardiovascular health. It focuses on identifying potential risk factors for cardiovascular disease and related conditions.

C-Reactive Protein (hs-CRP)

C-Reactive Protein (CRP) is a liver-produced protein that rises in response to systemic inflammation and serves as an acute-phase reactant. High-sensitivity CRP (hs-CRP) detects low levels of CRP and is associated with vascular inflammation. It is an independent predictor of cardiovascular disease (CVD) events and offers valuable prognostic information.

MALE	
Normal Range	0.00–3.00 mg/L
Optimal Range	0.00–0.60 mg/L

FEMALE	
Normal Range	0.00–3.00 mg/L
Optimal Range	0.00–1.50 mg/L

If HIGH or > 0.60 mg/L or > 1.50 mg/L:

Elevated hs-CRP suggests systemic inflammation, potentially from chronic conditions or infections, increasing cardiovascular risk. Consider re-testing if there are signs of temporary inflammation or infection.

Potential Causes:
- Chronic inflammation (e.g., rheumatoid arthritis)
- Infections such as periodontitis, C. pneumonia, H. pylori, or CMV
- If hs-CRP is high with lipids or suspected cardiac issues, consider additional cardiac markers.

Lifestyle Modifications:
- Insulin Sensitivity: Weight reduction, aerobic exercise
- Avoid smoking, high-glycemic foods, trans fats, and limit alcohol intake
- Diet: Emphasize omega-3 fatty acids (cold-water fish), fruits, vegetables, legumes, soluble fiber, nuts, seeds
- Choline/Betaine-Rich Foods: Animal-based foods, whole grains, spinach, beets

Anti-inflammatory Support:
- Phytocannabinoids
- Hemp Flower Extract
- Hemp Seed Oil
- Palmitoylethanolamide (PEA)
- Omega-3 Fatty Acids (Fish Oil)
- Vitamin D3
- Curcumin
- Green Tea Extract (Epigallocatechin Gallate (EGCG))
- Trans Resveratrol
- Quercetin
- Nettle (Urtica dioica)
- Pro-Resolving Mediators (PRMs): 18-HEPE (18-hydroxy eicosapentaenoic acid), 17-HDHA (17-hydroxy docosahexaenoic acid), 14-HDHA (14-hydroxy docosahexaenoic acid)

Antioxidants:
- Acerola Extract (Malpighia glabra)
- Grape Seed Extract (Vitis vinifera)
- Curcumin
- Garlic (Allium sativum)

- Ginkgo Extract (Ginkgo biloba)
- Quercetin
- Rutin
- Clove (Syzygium aromaticum)
- Allspice (Pimenta dioica)
- Sweet Basil (Ocimum basilicum)
- Sage (Salvia officinalis)
- Rosemary Extract (Rosmarinus officinalis)
- Lutein
- Lycopene
- Trans Resveratrol
- Vitamin A
- Vitamin E
- L-glutathione
- NAC (N-Acetyl-L-Cysteine)
- Broccoli Powder Extract
- Sulforaphane
- Olive Leaf Extract (Olea europaea)
- Bergamot
- Red Grape Powder
- Alpha Lipoic Acid
- Taurine
- MVM (Multi-vitamin/mineral)
- Glutathione (reduced)

Lipid Support (high):
- Red Yeast Rice (Monascus purpureus)
- Coenzyme Q10
- Sweet Orange (Citrus sinensis)
- Quercetin
- Gotu Kola (Centella asiatica)
- Horse Chestnut (Aesculus hippocastanum)
- Grape Seed Extract (Vitis vinifera)
- Vitamin C
- Plant Sterols/Stanols (Beta-Sitosterol, Campesterol, Campestanol, Sitostanol)
- Monostroma nitidum (seaweed) extract

Lp-PLA2

Lp-PLA2 is an enzyme produced by immune cells like monocytes and macrophages that contributes to the breakdown of phospholipids. Elevated Lp-PLA2 levels indicate the presence of soft, active plaque, which is a marker for unstable and active inflammation within the arteries. This marker helps predict the risk for cardiovascular events such as coronary heart disease and stroke, independently of LDL-C levels and other inflammatory markers.

Normal Range	0 - 123 nmol/min/mL

If HIGH or > 123 nmol/min/mL:

Elevated Lp-PLA2 levels indicate an increased risk for active plaque formation, which can heighten the risk for cardiovascular events such as coronary heart disease or stroke.

Risk Considerations:
- Elevated levels are associated with a 2-fold increased risk for coronary events and stroke.
- High Lp-PLA2 levels suggest the presence of soft, potentially unstable plaque rather than stable calcified plaque.

Lifestyle & Dietary Recommendations:
- Diet & Exercise: Emphasize a balanced diet, regular physical activity, and weight management as necessary.
- Blood Pressure Support: Maintain healthy blood pressure through dietary choices, lifestyle changes, and supplementary measures.
- Avoid Smoking and Manage Stress Levels

INFLAMMATION PANEL

Anti-inflammatory Support:
- Phytocannabinoids
- Hemp Flower Extract
- Hemp Seed Oil
- Palmitoylethanolamide (PEA)
- Omega-3 Fatty Acids (Fish Oil)
- Vitamin D3
- Curcumin
- Green Tea Extract (Epigallocatechin Gallate (EGCG))
- Trans Resveratrol
- Quercetin
- Nettle (Urtica dioica)
- Pro-Resolving Mediators (PRMs): 18-HEPE (18-hydroxy eicosapentaenoic acid), 17-HDHA (17-hydroxy docosahexaenoic acid), 14-HDHA (14-hydroxy docosahexaenoic acid)

Antioxidants:
- Acerola Extract (Malpighia glabra)
- Grape Seed Extract (Vitis vinifera)
- Curcumin
- Garlic (Allium sativum)
- Ginkgo Extract (Ginkgo biloba)
- Quercetin
- Rutin
- Clove (Syzygium aromaticum)
- Allspice (Pimenta dioica)
- Sweet Basil (Ocimum basilicum)
- Sage (Salvia officinalis)
- Rosemary Extract (Rosmarinus officinalis)
- Lutein
- Lycopene
- Trans Resveratrol
- Vitamin A
- Vitamin E
- L-glutathione
- NAC (N-Acetyl-L-Cysteine)
- Broccoli Powder Extract
- Sulforaphane
- Olive Leaf Extract (Olea europaea)
- Bergamot
- Red Grape Powder
- Alpha Lipoic Acid
- Taurine
- MVM (Multi-vitamin/mineral)
- Glutathione (reduced)

Lipid Support (high):
- Red Yeast Rice (Monascus purpureus)
- Coenzyme Q10
- Sweet Orange (Citrus sinensis)
- Quercetin
- Gotu Kola (Centella asiatica)
- Horse Chestnut (Aesculus hippocastanum)
- Grape Seed Extract (Vitis vinifera)
- Vitamin C
- Plant Sterols/Stanols (Beta-Sitosterol, Campesterol, Campestanol, Sitostanol)
- Monostroma nitidum (seaweed) extract

MPO (Myeloperoxidase)

MPO is an enzyme produced by white blood cells (neutrophils and monocytes) that can indicate inflammation and instability of plaque within the arterial walls. High MPO levels are associated with an increased risk of cardiovascular events, such as plaque rupture, due to the enzyme's role in lipid peroxidation, HDL dysfunction, and nitric oxide depletion. Monitoring MPO can be especially valuable for those with known cardiovascular risk factors or symptoms like chest pain.

Normal Range	< 470 pmol/L

If MODERATE RISK or 470 – 539 pmol/L:

Elevated MPO indicates an increased likelihood of arterial inflammation and growing plaque formation. At moderate levels, MPO is associated with a greater risk for near-term cardiovascular events. Further cardiovascular evaluation may be recommended.

- **CVD Assessment:** Consider additional cardiovascular testing such as stress testing and physical exam.
- **Lifestyle Modifications**: Support cardiovascular health with diet and exercise improvements.
- **Medication Considerations:** Statins, beta-blockers, and ACE inhibitors may be beneficial; monitor liver function with statins or Red Yeast Rice (RYR) use.

Anti-inflammatory Support:
- Phytocannabinoids
- Hemp Flower Extract
- Hemp Seed Oil
- Palmitoylethanolamide (PEA)
- Omega-3 Fatty Acids (Fish Oil)
- Vitamin D3
- Curcumin
- Green Tea Extract (Epigallocatechin Gallate (EGCG))
- Trans Resveratrol
- Quercetin
- Nettle (Urtica dioica)
- Pro-Resolving Mediators (PRMs): 18-HEPE (18-hydroxy eicosapentaenoic acid), 17-HDHA (17-hydroxy docosahexaenoic acid), 14-HDHA (14-hydroxy docosahexaenoic acid)

Antioxidants:
- Acerola Extract (Malpighia glabra)
- Grape Seed Extract (Vitis vinifera)
- Curcumin
- Garlic (Allium sativum)
- Ginkgo Extract (Ginkgo biloba)
- Quercetin
- Rutin
- Clove (Syzygium aromaticum)
- Allspice (Pimenta dioica)
- Sweet Basil (Ocimum basilicum)
- Sage (Salvia officinalis)
- Rosemary Extract (Rosmarinus officinalis)
- Lutein
- Lycopene
- Trans Resveratrol
- Vitamin A
- Vitamin E
- L-glutathione
- NAC (N-Acetyl-L-Cysteine)
- Broccoli Powder Extract
- Sulforaphane
- Olive Leaf Extract (Olea europaea)
- Bergamot
- Red Grape Powder
- Alpha Lipoic Acid
- Taurine
- MVM (Multi-vitamin/mineral)
- Glutathione (reduced)

If **HIGH RISK** or **> 539 pmol/L:**

E Significantly elevated MPO levels indicate an increased risk of a near-term cardiovascular event and may reflect active arterial inflammation or unstable plaque. High MPO levels, especially when combined with elevated hs-CRP or Lp-PLA2, are predictive of major cardiac events in the short term.

- **Comprehensive CVD Management:** Evaluate all cardiovascular risk factors and consider advanced cardiovascular screening.
- **Medications:** Statins, beta-blockers, and ACE inhibitors, as clinically appropriate, may reduce MPO and associated risks.
- **Lifestyle & Dietary Support:** Diet low in trans fats, increased physical activity, and stress management are advised.

INFLAMMATION PANEL

Anti-inflammatory Support:
- Phytocannabinoids
- Hemp Flower Extract
- Hemp Seed Oil
- Palmitoylethanolamide (PEA)
- Omega-3 Fatty Acids (Fish Oil)
- Vitamin D3
- Curcumin
- Green Tea Extract (Epigallocatechin Gallate (EGCG))
- Trans Resveratrol
- Quercetin
- Nettle (Urtica dioica)
- Pro-Resolving Mediators (PRMs): 18-HEPE (18-hydroxy eicosapentaenoic acid), 17-HDHA (17-hydroxy docosahexaenoic acid), 14-HDHA (14-hydroxy docosahexaenoic acid)

Antioxidants:
- Acerola Extract (Malpighia glabra)
- Grape Seed Extract (Vitis vinifera)
- Curcumin
- Garlic (Allium sativum)
- Ginkgo Extract (Ginkgo biloba)
- Quercetin
- Rutin
- Clove (Syzygium aromaticum)
- Allspice (Pimenta dioica)
- Sweet Basil (Ocimum basilicum)
- Sage (Salvia officinalis)
- Rosemary Extract (Rosmarinus officinalis)
- Lutein
- Lycopene
- Trans Resveratrol
- Vitamin A
- Vitamin E
- L-glutathione
- NAC (N-Acetyl-L-Cysteine)
- Broccoli Powder Extract
- Sulforaphane
- Olive Leaf Extract (Olea europaea)
- Bergamot
- Red Grape Powder
- Alpha Lipoic Acid
- Taurine
- MVM (Multi-vitamin/mineral)
- Glutathione (reduced)

Oxidized LDL (OxLDL)

Oxidized LDL is LDL cholesterol that has reacted with free radicals, becoming more atherogenic. High levels of oxidized LDL are associated with increased risk of atherosclerosis, coronary heart disease (CHD), and other cardiovascular events. This form of LDL is more readily taken up by macrophages, promoting plaque formation within the arteries, increasing risk of cardiovascular events independently of total cholesterol and LDL levels.

Normal Range	60 - 69 U/L

If HIGH or > 69 U/L:

High levels of oxidized LDL significantly increase the risk of plaque formation, vascular inflammation, and cardiovascular disease, including metabolic syndrome. This biomarker may predict a 4x higher risk of heart attack compared to other traditional risk factors alone.

Lifestyle Modifications:
- Quit Smoking: Seek support programs or medications if needed, as smoking elevates oxidized LDL.
- Dietary Adjustments: Increase intake of fruits, vegetables, and foods high in antioxidants while avoiding saturated and trans fats.

- Exercise: Engage in regular physical activity, as approved by your healthcare provider, to improve lipid profiles.

Anti-inflammatory Support:
- Phytocannabinoids
- Hemp Flower Extract
- Hemp Seed Oil
- Palmitoylethanolamide (PEA)
- Omega-3 Fatty Acids (Fish Oil)
- Vitamin D3
- Curcumin
- Green Tea Extract (Epigallocatechin Gallate (EGCG))
- Trans Resveratrol
- Quercetin
- Nettle (Urtica dioica)
- Pro-Resolving Mediators (PRMs): 18-HEPE (18-hydroxy eicosapentaenoic acid), 17-HDHA (17-hydroxy docosahexaenoic acid), 14-HDHA (14-hydroxy docosahexaenoic acid)

Antioxidants:
- Acerola Extract (Malpighia glabra)
- Grape Seed Extract (Vitis vinifera)
- Curcumin
- Garlic (Allium sativum)
- Ginkgo Extract (Ginkgo biloba)
- Quercetin
- Rutin
- Clove (Syzygium aromaticum)
- Allspice (Pimenta dioica)
- Sweet Basil (Ocimum basilicum)
- Sage (Salvia officinalis)
- Rosemary Extract (Rosmarinus officinalis)
- Lutein
- Lycopene
- Trans Resveratrol
- Vitamin A
- Vitamin E
- L-glutathione
- NAC (N-Acetyl-L-Cysteine)
- Broccoli Powder Extract
- Sulforaphane
- Olive Leaf Extract (Olea europaea)
- Bergamot
- Red Grape Powder
- Alpha Lipoic Acid
- Taurine
- MVM (Multi-vitamin/mineral)
- Glutathione (reduced)

Lipid Support (high):
- Red Yeast Rice (Monascus purpureus)
- Coenzyme Q10
- Sweet Orange (Citrus sinensis)
- Quercetin
- Gotu Kola (Centella asiatica)
- Horse Chestnut (Aesculus hippocastanum)
- Grape Seed Extract (Vitis vinifera)
- Vitamin C
- Plant Sterols/Stanols (Beta-Sitosterol, Campesterol, Campestanol, Sitostanol)
- Monostroma nitidum (seaweed) extract

Oxidized Phospholipids (OxPL-apoB)

OxPL-apoB measures oxidized phospholipids carried on the apoB protein, predominantly associated with lipoprotein(a) [Lp(a)]. Elevated OxPL-apoB is a marker of vascular inflammation and oxidative stress. High levels of OxPL-apoB are strongly associated with atherosclerosis and increase the risk for cardiovascular disease (CVD) events by two- to three-fold compared to individuals with lower levels.

| **Normal Range** | < 5.0 nmol/L |

INFLAMMATION PANEL

If **HIGH** or > 5.0 nmol/L:

 Elevated OxPL-apoB levels indicate increased vascular inflammation and oxidative stress, correlating with higher risk of cardiovascular events. Aggressive preventive and therapeutic measures are recommended to manage this risk.

 Lifestyle Modifications:
- Quit Smoking: Seek support programs or medications, as smoking elevates oxidative stress.
- Dietary Adjustments: Reduce intake of saturated fats and avoid trans fats. Increase antioxidant-rich fruits and vegetables.
- Exercise: Engage in physical activity as approved by a healthcare provider.

 Lipid Support (high):
- Red Yeast Rice (Monascus purpureus)
- Coenzyme Q10
- Sweet Orange (Citrus sinensis)
- Quercetin
- Gotu Kola (Centella asiatica)
- Horse Chestnut (Aesculus hippocastanum)
- Grape Seed Extract (Vitis vinifera)
- Vitamin C
- Plant Sterols/Stanols (Beta-Sitosterol, Campesterol, Campestanol, Sitostanol)
- Monostroma nitidum (seaweed) extract

Anti-inflammatory Support:
- Phytocannabinoids
- Hemp Flower Extract
- Hemp Seed Oil
- Palmitoylethanolamide (PEA)
- Omega-3 Fatty Acids (Fish Oil) docosahexaenoic acid), 14-HDHA (14-hydroxy docosahexaenoic acid)
- Vitamin D3
- Curcumin
- Green Tea Extract (Epigallocatechin Gallate (EGCG))
- Trans Resveratrol
- Quercetin
- Nettle (Urtica dioica)
- Pro-Resolving Mediators (PRMs): 18-HEPE (18-hydroxy eicosapentaenoic acid), 17-HDHA (17-hydroxy

Antioxidants:
- Acerola Extract (Malpighia glabra)
- Grape Seed Extract (Vitis vinifera)
- Curcumin
- Garlic (Allium sativum)
- Ginkgo Extract (Ginkgo biloba)
- Quercetin
- Rutin
- Clove (Syzygium aromaticum)
- Allspice (Pimenta dioica)
- Sweet Basil (Ocimum basilicum)
- Sage (Salvia officinalis)
- Rosemary Extract (Rosmarinus officinalis)
- Lutein
- Lycopene
- Trans Resveratrol
- Vitamin A
- Vitamin E
- L-glutathione
- NAC (N-Acetyl-L-Cysteine)
- Broccoli Powder Extract
- Sulforaphane
- Olive Leaf Extract (Olea europaea)
- Bergamot
- Red Grape Powder
- Alpha Lipoic Acid
- Taurine
- MVM (Multi-vitamin/mineral)
- Glutathione (reduced)

Erythrocyte Sedimentation Rate (ESR)

ESR measures the rate at which red blood cells settle in a tube over one hour. It is an indirect, non-specific marker of inflammation and is influenced by elevated fibrinogen and other plasma acute-phase proteins, which can cause red blood cells to clump and settle more rapidly. Though ESR lacks specificity, it can indicate the presence of inflammatory conditions.

MALE	
Normal Range	0.00–3.00 mg/L
Optimal Range	0.00–0.60 mg/L

FEMALE	
Normal Range	0.00 - 20.00 mm/hr
Optimal Range	0.00 - 10.00 mm/hr

If HIGH or > 0.60 mm/hr or >10.00 mm/hr:

An elevated ESR may be indicative of inflammation or chronic conditions. However, ESR is non-specific and can be affected by factors such as anemia, age, medications, or non-inflammatory conditions like pregnancy and menstruation.

Potential Causes:
- Inflammatory Conditions: Rheumatoid arthritis, inflammatory bowel disease, cardiovascular inflammation.
- Infections: Chronic infections such as periodontal disease, respiratory infections.
- Other Factors: Heart disease, kidney disease, certain cancers.

Lifestyle Modifications:
- Weight reduction, aerobic exercise, and smoking cessation to reduce overall inflammation.

Dietary Adjustments:
- Emphasize fruits, vegetables, legumes, soluble fiber, and omega-3 rich foods (e.g., cold-water fish).
- Limit intake of simple starches, sugars, trans fats, and alcohol.

Anti-inflammatory Support:
- Phytocannabinoids
- Hemp Flower Extract
- Hemp Seed Oil
- Palmitoylethanolamide (PEA)
- Omega-3 Fatty Acids (Fish Oil)
- Vitamin D3
- Curcumin
- Green Tea Extract (Epigallocatechin Gallate (EGCG))
- Trans Resveratrol
- Quercetin
- Nettle (Urtica dioica)
- Pro-Resolving Mediators (PRMs): 18-HEPE (18-hydroxy eicosapentaenoic acid), 17-HDHA (17-hydroxy docosahexaenoic acid), 14-HDHA (14-hydroxy docosahexaenoic acid)

Antioxidants:
- Acerola Extract (Malpighia glabra)
- Grape Seed Extract (Vitis vinifera)
- Curcumin
- Garlic (Allium sativum)
- Ginkgo Extract (Ginkgo biloba)
- Quercetin
- Rutin
- Clove (Syzygium aromaticum)
- Allspice (Pimenta dioica)
- Sweet Basil (Ocimum basilicum)
- Sage (Salvia officinalis)
- Rosemary Extract (Rosmarinus officinalis)
- Lutein

INFLAMMATION PANEL

- Lycopene
- Trans Resveratrol
- Vitamin A
- Vitamin E
- L-glutathione
- NAC (N-Acetyl-L-Cysteine)
- Broccoli Powder Extract
- Sulforaphane
- Olive Leaf Extract (Olea europaea)
- Bergamot
- Red Grape Powder
- Alpha Lipoic Acid
- Taurine
- MVM (Multi-vitamin/mineral)
- Glutathione (reduced)

Advanced Heart Markers

Includes more advanced cardiovascular disease risk marker than a Lipid Panel.

C-Reactive Protein (hs-CRP)

CRP is a protein that is produced in the liver in response to systemic inflammation and is an acute phase reactant. The "high sensitivity" CRP test is needed to detect very low levels of CRP that may be seen with vascular and/or systemic inflammation. Independent predictor of developing CVD events. Provides independent prognostic information after initiating protocol

MALE	
Normal Range	0 - 3.00 mg/L
Optimal Range	< 0.6 mg/L

FEMALE	
Normal Range	0 - 3.00 mg/L
Optimal Range	< 1.5 mg/L

If HIGH or > 0.6 mg/L or > 1.5mg/L:

Blood levels are usually low. If high with elevated lipids or suspected heart issues, order advanced cardiac markers.

hs-CRP may predict CVD events and provide independent prognostic information after support. High levels predict cardiovascular events and assess patient response to lifestyle changes and statins.

Consider hs-CRP levels >10 for inflammation due to infections, illnesses, or arthritis flare-ups. Avoid acute stress during measurement (preferably 2 weeks apart).

Statins and beta blockers decrease CoQ10, selenium, O3, carnitine, T3f, melatonin, electrolytes, minerals, and B9/B12. ACE inhibitors/blockers reduce zinc and sodium.

Rule out chronic inflammation, such as rheumatoid arthritis (RA) or infections like periodontitis, C. pneumonia, H. pylori, or CMV, which can increase cardiovascular inflammation and CAD risk. Note: Repeat the test after the transitory inflammation has subsided.

Lifestyle modifications include:
- Improving insulin sensitivity through weight reduction and aerobic exercise.
- Avoiding smoking.
- Following a diet rich in omega-3 fatty acids, choline, betaine, anti-inflammatory and mixed antioxidant agents.
- Insulin-sensitizing agents like chromium, alpha-lipoic acid, zinc, biotin, and magnesium.
- Low magnesium status is associated with higher CRP levels.

Pharmaceutical considerations include:
- Statins (used to reduce cardiovascular events regardless of their cholesterol-lowering effect);
- Always include CoQ10.
- Oral estrogens can increase hsCRP levels, while transdermal estrogen appears to have no effect.

Inflammation Support:
- Proteolytic enzyme blend
- Turmeric
- Boswellia
- Ginger, Quercetin, Rutin, Rosemary, Trans Resveratrol
- Curcumin (turmeric)
- Omega-3 Fatty Acids (fish oil)

Antioxidants:
- Acerola Extract (Malpighia glabra)
- Grape Seed Extract (Vitis vinifera)
- Curcumin
- Garlic (Allium sativum)
- Ginkgo Extract (Ginkgo biloba)
- Quercetin
- Rutin
- Clove (Syzygium aromaticum)
- Allspice (Pimenta dioica)
- Sweet Basil (Ocimum basilicum)
- Sage (Salvia officinalis)
- Rosemary Extract (Rosmarinus officinalis)
- Lutein
- Lycopene
- Trans Resveratrol
- Vitamin A
- Vitamin E
- L-glutathione
- NAC (N-Acetyl-L-Cysteine)
- Broccoli Powder Extract
- Sulforaphane
- Olive Leaf Extract (Olea europaea)
- Bergamot
- Red Grape Powder
- Alpha Lipoic Acid
- Taurine
- MVM (Multi-vitamin/mineral)
- Glutathione (reduced)

Lipid Support (high):
- Red Yeast Rice (Monascus purpureus)
- Coenzyme Q10
- Sweet Orange (Citrus sinensis)
- Quercetin
- Gotu Kola (Centella asiatica)
- Horse Chestnut (Aesculus hippocastanum)
- Grape Seed Extract (Vitis vinifera)
- Vitamin C
- Plant Sterols/Stanols (Beta-Sitosterol, Campesterol, Campestanol, Sitostanol)
- Monostroma nitidum (seaweed) extract

Small Dense LDL Cholesterol (sdLDL-C)

Small Dense LDL Cholesterol (sdLDL-C) - Small dense LDL particles are denser and more atherogenic compared to regular LDL particles. sdLDL-C measures the total amount of LDL-C in the small dense format. These particles are the culprits behind cardiovascular disease, increasing the risk by 2-3 times.

LDL-p, on the other hand, measures the number of LDL particles in the serum, while LDL-C measures the amount of cholesterol within the particles. Small-dense LDL is a more specific risk factor, enhancing the predictive power of cardiovascular disease in individuals.

Lipoproteins transport cholesterol throughout the body, but it's the actual lipoprotein particle, not the cholesterol within it, that penetrates the arterial wall and causes heart disease. Therefore, understanding the number of small LDL particles is crucial.

Non-Alcoholic Fatty Liver Disease (NAFLD) is closely linked to cardiovascular disease. High glucose and fructose levels in hepatocytes (liver cells) lead to increased oxidative stress, insulin resistance, hepatocyte injury, and ultimately, cell death. This process triggers an increase in liver enzymes, such as AST, ALT, and GGT.

These factors contribute significantly to the development of Cardiovascular Disease (CVD) and Coronary Artery Disease (CAD):
- Excessive consumption of vegetable oils and hydrogenated fats
- Excessive consumption of refined carbohydrates, including sugar and white flour
- Mineral deficiencies, particularly magnesium and iodine
- Deficiencies in vitamins C, E, D, and K2 due to Coronary Artery Disease
- Lack of antimicrobial fats obtained from the diet
- Inadequate protection against viruses and bacteria associated with the onset of pathogenic plaque leading to heart disease.

Normal Range	20 - 40 mg/dL
Optimal Range	20 - 40 mg/dL

If **HIGH** or **> 40 mg/dL**:

High levels of LDL cholesterol are associated with a two to three-fold increased risk of cardiovascular disease events. The size difference between LDL particles is crucial. Even if two individuals have the same LDL reading, such as 150 LDL, one may be at higher risk of coronary artery disease due to a higher particle number.

Small-Dense LDL is particularly harmful because smaller particles can more easily penetrate the arterial wall than larger ones. This is because their smaller size makes them more likely to enter the arterial endothelium, where they become oxidized and taken up by macrophage cells. These cells then transform into foam cells, which eventually stick together to form plaque within the arteries.

Evidence also suggests a link between small-dense LDL and vascular dementia.

Cardiovascular diseases and stroke collectively cause the deaths of one in every three women annually. This equates to approximately one woman losing life every 80 seconds. Cardiovascular disease is responsible for more women's deaths each year (around 400,000) than all types of cancer, respiratory illness, and diabetes combined.

A staggering 25% of all deaths occur due to cardiovascular disease, making it the leading cause of death for both men and women. Moreover, nearly two-thirds (64%) of women who die suddenly of coronary heart disease have had no prior symptoms.

Risk factors for cardiovascular disease include high blood pressure, high LDL cholesterol, smoking, diabetes, overweight and obesity (covered in FMA 5), poor diet, physical inactivity, and excessive alcohol consumption.

Lifestyle modifications, such as statins, niacin, fibrates, and omega-3 fatty acids, are essential for heart health. These changes help balance blood sugar levels and prevent diabetes and metabolic syndrome.

Key cardiovascular lifestyle changes that impact inflammation include:

- Non-inflammatory diet

- Proper sleep
- Movement
- Stress management
- Addressing nutritional deficiencies

Preventative measures include:
- Avoiding diabetes by balancing blood sugar levels
- Steering clear of canola oil or other polyunsaturated fatty acids (PUFAs)
- Eliminating or reducing sugars, as they can drive up triglycerides, lower the immune response, convert to fat in the body, elevate insulin, and tear up arteries leading to plaque formation
- Increasing healthy fats, including saturated fat
- Eliminating or limiting grains, or learning how to eat and prepare them correctly
- Eating cholesterol (e.g., eggs) Egg yolks, processed foods, and a Metabolic Reset & Weight Loss program can help improve cholesterol levels.
- Antioxidants and cholesterol antagonists can help reduce excess cholesterol in the bloodstream.
- Liver and adrenal health are also important for overall well-being.
- Managing stress can help improve adrenal health, which can impact blood sugar levels regardless of diet.
- Vitamin and mineral deficiencies should be addressed, and random vitamin and mineral supplements, including multivitamins, should be avoided.
- Smoking should be avoided, and getting out of the chair occasionally and considering getting a pet can also be beneficial.

Statins and beta blockers can have nutritional consequences, including decreased CoQ10, selenium, O3, carnitine, and T3f in statins, and melatonin in beta-blockers. Diuretics may reduce electrolytes and key minerals. Metformin reduces B9 and B12, while ACE inhibitors/blockers decrease zinc and sodium.

Arterosclerosis is a condition characterized by the buildup of plaque in the arteries. The endothelial glycocalyx (EG) is a thin, gel-like layer that coats the inside of the vascular endothelium, including every artery, vein, and capillary. EG plays a crucial role in maintaining arterial health by preventing cholesterol and other particles from adhering to or penetrating the endothelial wall.

Several factors contribute to the breakdown of the endothelial glycocalyx, including high blood glucose, oxidative stress, and inflammation. Pathologies associated with impaired endothelial glycocalyx (EG) include coronary heart disease, hyperglycemia, diabetes, renal diseases, lacunar stroke, and severe trauma.

Lipid Support (high):
- Red Yeast Rice (Monascus purpureus)
- Coenzyme Q10
- Sweet Orange (Citrus sinensis)
- Quercetin
- Gotu Kola (Centella asiatica)
- Horse Chestnut (Aesculus hippocastanum)
- Grape Seed Extract (Vitis vinifera)
- Vitamin C
- Plant Sterols/Stanols (Beta-Sitosterol, Campesterol, Campestanol, Sitostanol)
- Monostroma nitidum (seaweed) extract

Prescription: Statins, fibrates, anti-inflammatory support

Anti-inflammatory Support:
- Phytocannabinoids
- Hemp Flower Extract

- Hemp Seed Oil
- Palmitoylethanolamide (PEA)
- Omega-3 Fatty Acids (Fish Oil)
- docosahexaenoic acid), 14-HDHA (14-hydroxy docosahexaenoic acid)
- Vitamin D3
- Curcumin
- Green Tea Extract (Epigallocatechin Gallate (EGCG))
- Trans Resveratrol
- Quercetin
- Nettle (Urtica dioica)
- Pro-Resolving Mediators (PRMs): 18-HEPE (18-hydroxy eicosapentaenoic acid), 17-HDHA (17-hydroxy

Liver Support:
- Milk Thistle
- L-methionine
- Taurine
- Inositol
- Ox Bile
- Artichoke
- Beet Powder
- Vitamin A
- Vitamin B6
- Vitamin B12
- Plant protein powder with MVM (multi-vitamin/mineral)
- L-glutathione
- N-Acetyl-L-Cysteine (NAC)
- Quercetin
- Methylsulfonylmethane (MSM)
- Sodium Sulfate
- Green Tea Extract
- Reishi
- Cordyceps
- Chinese Skullcap
- Schisandra
- Burdock Extract
- Phosphatidylcholine

Thyroid Support:
- N-Acetyl-L-Tyrosine
- American Ginseng (Panax quinquefolius)
- Forskolin (Coleus forskohlii)
- Iodine
- Chromium
- Zinc
- Selenium
- Copper
- Manganese
- Vitamin A
- Vitamin B2
- Potassium Iodide
- Myo-Inositol

Fiber Support:
- Acacia gum
- Cellulose
- Guar gum
- Cranberry seed powder
- Carrot fiber
- Inulin
- Orange fiber
- Glucomannan
- Apple pectin
- Psyllium husk
- Flax seed
- Prune powder

LDL-p

LDL Particle Number (LDL-P): LDL-P measures the number of LDL particles in serum, unlike LDL-C, which measures cholesterol inside LDL particles. LDL-P is directly determined by nuclear magnetic resonance (NMR) spectroscopy and has been shown to better predict cardiovascular events than LDL-C concentrations, especially in patients with discordant LDL-P and LDL-C levels. NAFLD is associated with cardiovascular disease. High glucose/fructose intake increases fatty acids/adipose tissue in hepatocytes (liver cells), leading to oxidative stress, insulin resistance, hepatocyte injury, and cell death. This causes an increase in liver enzyme production, particularly AST, ALT, and GGT. REAL CONTRIBUTORS TO CVD/CAD: Excessive consumption of vegetable oils and hydrogenated fats, refined carbohydrates like

ADVANCED HEART MARKERS

sugar and white flour, mineral deficiencies (magnesium and iodine), vitamin deficiencies (C, E, D, K2 due to coronary artery disease), insufficient antimicrobial fats from the diet, and lack of protection against viruses and bacteria associated with pathogenic plaque leading to heart disease.

Normal Range	1200 - 1800 nmol/L
Optimal Range	<1100 nmol/L

If **HIGH** or **> 1800 nmol/L**:

 Smoking, diabetes, overweight and obesity (covered in FMA 5), poor diet, physical inactivity, and excessive alcohol use are all risk factors for health problems.

 Lifestyle modifications, such as adopting a reduced-calorie diet, losing excess weight, and exercising regularly, can alter LDL-P levels. Additionally, lipid-lowering drugs like statins and PCSK9-inhibitors can significantly reduce LDL-P levels.

For heart health, it's crucial to balance blood sugar levels and avoid developing diabetes or metabolic syndrome.

Statins and beta-blockers have nutritional consequences, including decreased CoQ10, selenium, O3, carnitine, T3f, melatonin, and potentially reduced electrolytes and key minerals. Metformin reduces B9 and B12, while ACE inhibitors/blockers decrease zinc and sodium.

Key cardiovascular lifestyle changes that impact inflammation include adopting a non-inflammatory diet, getting proper sleep, engaging in movement, managing stress, addressing nutritional deficiencies, and taking preventative measures.

Preventative measures include avoiding diabetes by balancing blood sugar levels, avoiding canola oil or other polyunsaturated fatty acids (PUFAs), eliminating or reducing sugars, as they can drive up triglycerides, lower the immune response, convert to fat in the body, elevate insulin levels, and tear up arteries leading to plaque formation.

To increase healthy fats, include saturated fats in the diet. Eliminate or limit grains or learn how to eat and prepare them correctly.

Additionally, consume cholesterol, such as found in eggs. Egg yolks, processed foods, and a Metabolic Reset & Weight Loss program can help improve cholesterol levels. Antioxidants and cholesterol antagonists can help reduce free radicals and excess cholesterol in the bloodstream. Liver and adrenal health are also crucial for overall well-being. Managing stress and addressing vitamin/mineral deficiencies are important. Smoking, sitting for long periods, and considering getting a pet can also contribute to better cholesterol levels. Statindecisionaid.mayoclinic.org is a helpful resource for medical professionals and patients who don't choose statins. Statins work by inhibiting HMG CoA reductase, effectively stopping the production of CoQ10, cholesterol, and lowering levels of vitamin D, estrogen, progesterone, testosterone, and cortisol.

 Lipid Support (high):
- Red Yeast Rice (Monascus purpureus)
- Coenzyme Q10
- Sweet Orange (Citrus sinensis)
- Quercetin
- Gotu Kola (Centella asiatica)
- Horse Chestnut (Aesculus hippocastanum)
- Grape Seed Extract (Vitis vinifera)
- Vitamin C
- Plant Sterols/Stanols (Beta-Sitosterol, Campesterol, Campestanol, Sitostanol)
- Monostroma nitidum (seaweed) extract

Prescription: Statins, fibrates, cholesterol absorption inhibitors (ezetimibe), bile acid sequestrants, anti-inflammatory support

Inflammation Support:
- Proteolytic enzyme blend
- Turmeric
- Boswellia
- Ginger, Quercetin, Rutin, Rosemary, Trans Resveratrol
- Curcumin (turmeric)
- Omega-3 Fatty Acids (fish oil)

Liver Support:
- Milk Thistle
- L-methionine
- Taurine
- Inositol
- Ox Bile
- Artichoke
- Beet Powder
- Vitamin A
- Vitamin B6
- Vitamin B12
- Plant protein powder with MVM (multi-vitamin/mineral)
- L-glutathione
- N-Acetyl-L-Cysteine (NAC)
- Quercetin
- Methylsulfonylmethane (MSM)
- Sodium Sulfate
- Green Tea Extract
- Reishi
- Cordyceps
- Chinese Skullcap
- Schisandra
- Burdock Extract
- Phosphatidylcholine

Thyroid Support:
- N-Acetyl-L-Tyrosine
- American Ginseng (Panax quinquefolius)
- Forskolin (Coleus forskohlii)
- Iodine
- Chromium
- Zinc
- Selenium
- Copper
- Manganese
- Vitamin A
- Vitamin B2
- Potassium Iodide
- Myo-Inositol

Fiber Support:
- Acacia gum
- Cellulose
- Guar gum
- Cranberry seed powder
- Carrot fiber
- Inulin
- Orange fiber
- Glucomannan
- Apple pectin
- Psyllium husk
- Flax seed
- Prune powder

HDL-p

Normal Range	34.9 umol/L
Optimal Range	34.9 umol/L

ADVANCED HEART MARKERS

If **LOW** or **< 34.9 umol/L:**

 Increase insulin sensitivity (refer to the section on Insulin Resistance & Dyslipidemia). Avoid a high-carbohydrate diet, as it reduces hepatic Apo-A1 production and decreases HDL-P. Consider niacin (refer to the section on LDL-C), fibrates (such as gemfibrozil), and/or thiazolidinediones (such as pioglitazone).

 Support immunity and inflammation for heart health. Balance blood sugar to prevent diabetes and metabolic syndrome.

Lifestyle Recommendations:
- Stay active to maintain ideal weight and body composition.
- Engage in a regular, balanced exercise program that includes a pedometer or Fitbit to track steps and ensure more movement.
- Incorporate high-intensity, short bursts (20-60 seconds) of activity throughout the day to boost growth hormone release.
- Aim for at least two sessions per week of resistance training that works all major muscle groups.
- Manage stress healthily by reducing or eliminating alcohol consumption and quitting smoking.
- Comprehensively assess your circulatory system with a test like an advanced lipid panel.
- Check thyroid, blood sugar, and hormonal levels.

Dietary Tips and Caveats:
- Limit starchy foods like potatoes, pasta, bread, crackers, and rice.
- Avoid simple sugars and sugary drinks and sodas.
- Incorporate heart-healthy, anti-inflammatory snacks like blueberries, pomegranate seeds, avocados, walnuts, and pistachios.
- Avoid hydrogenated vegetable oils, trans fats, and fried foods.
- Opt for coconut and avocado oils for cooking.
- Add olive oil to cooked foods and raw vegetables.
- Choose organic produce, organic, antibiotic-free, hormone-free, and grass-fed dairy and animal products.
- Consume freshly ground flax seeds or chia seeds to increase fiber intake.
- Eat the skin of fruits and vegetables.
- Consume adequate amounts of antioxidants and flavonoids, which can be obtained daily through 5-9 servings of organic vegetables and fruit.
- Eat garlic frequently.

 Lipid Support (high):
- Red Yeast Rice (Monascus purpureus)
- Coenzyme Q10
- Sweet Orange (Citrus sinensis)
- Quercetin
- Gotu Kola (Centella asiatica)
- Horse Chestnut (Aesculus hippocastanum)
- Grape Seed Extract (Vitis vinifera)
- Vitamin C
- Plant Sterols/Stanols (Beta-Sitosterol, Campesterol, Campestanol, Sitostanol)
- Monostroma nitidum (seaweed) extract

Prescription:
- Statins
- Fibrates
- Cholesterol absorption inhibitors (ezetimibe)
- Bile acid sequestrants

Anti-inflammatory Support:
- Phytocannabinoids
- Hemp Flower Extract
- Hemp Seed Oil
- Palmitoylethanolamide (PEA)
- Omega-3 Fatty Acids (Fish Oil)
- docosahexaenoic acid), 14-HDHA (14-hydroxy docosahexaenoic acid)
- Vitamin D3
- Curcumin
- Green Tea Extract (Epigallocatechin Gallate (EGCG))
- Trans Resveratrol
- Quercetin
- Nettle (Urtica dioica)
- Pro-Resolving Mediators (PRMs): 18-HEPE (18-hydroxy eicosapentaenoic acid), 17-HDHA (17-hydroxy

Liver Support:
- Milk Thistle
- L-methionine
- Taurine
- Inositol
- Ox Bile
- Artichoke
- Beet Powder
- Vitamin A
- Vitamin B6
- Vitamin B12
- Plant protein powder with MVM (multi-vitamin/mineral)
- L-glutathione
- N-Acetyl-L-Cysteine (NAC)
- Quercetin
- Methylsulfonylmethane (MSM)
- Sodium Sulfate
- Green Tea Extract
- Reishi
- Cordyceps
- Chinese Skullcap
- Schisandra
- Burdock Extract
- Phosphatidylcholine

Thyroid Support:
- N-Acetyl-L-Tyrosine
- American Ginseng (Panax quinquefolius)
- Forskolin (Coleus forskohlii)
- Iodine
- Chromium
- Zinc
- Selenium
- Copper
- Manganese
- Vitamin A
- Vitamin B2
- Potassium Iodide
- Myo-Inositol

Very low dose Iodine, for short and long-term use:
- Potassium iodide, selenium

Fiber Support:
- Acacia gum
- Cellulose
- Guar gum
- Cranberry seed powder
- Carrot fiber
- Inulin
- Orange fiber
- Glucomannan
- Apple pectin
- Psyllium husk
- Flax seed
- Prune powder

Lp(a)

Lipoprotein(a) (Lp(a)) is a plasma lipoprotein composed of two parts: a LDL-like particle and apolipoprotein (a) [apo(a)], a protein produced in the liver and attached to the apoB portion of the particle. Levels of Lp(a) are often influenced by genetic factors. Elevated levels are an independent risk factor for cardiovascular disease (CVD). Lp(a) predicts a 15-year risk of CVD outcomes and improves CVD risk prediction. It acts as a preferential lipoprotein carrier for oxidized phospholipids (OxPL-apoB), which are pro-atherogenic and pro-inflammatory biomarkers. These biomarkers adversely affect endothelial function, oxidative stress, and plaque stability.

Genetic factors play a crucial role in Lp(a) levels. The COMT gene, which encodes an enzyme involved in the metabolism of estrogen and catecholamines (neurotransmitters like epinephrine, norepinephrine, and dopamine), has an SNP that impairs its function and increases the risk of CVD. The MTHFR gene, which encodes a rate-limiting enzyme in the methyl cycle, a chemical process that regulates neurotransmitters, genetic function/repair, detoxification, and ATP production, has an SNP that alters DNA/RNA expression and can contribute to chronic diseases, including CVD.

Normal Range	30 - 50 mg/dL
Optimal Range	30 - 50 mg/dL

If **HIGH** or > 50 mg/dL:

Elevated levels of cholesterol are an independent risk factor for several cardiovascular diseases, including myocardial infarction, coronary artery disease, cerebrovascular disease, vein graft stenosis, and retinal artery occlusion. The risk is particularly high in young patients with premature atherosclerosis, particularly males below 55 and females below 65. The risk is further compounded by elevations in LDL-C, fibrinogen, or Lp-PLA2.

Although heredity plays a significant role, niacin (B3) can help lower LDL levels. For heart health, it's important to maintain a balanced blood sugar level and avoid developing diabetes or metabolic syndrome. Niacin, along with other supplements, can support heart health in the following ways:
- Niacin helps optimize LDL-C, sdLDL-C, and apoB levels.
- Aspirin reduces the risk of heart disease.
- Lifestyle support is important for heart health, including maintaining a healthy weight, eating a balanced diet, and exercising regularly.

Dietary changes can also help lower LDL levels. It's important to avoid trans fats, which increase Lp(a) levels. Instead, focus on eating antioxidant-rich fruits and vegetables, as Lp(a) promotes free radical production. Flaxseed is also a good source of antioxidants.

Supplemental support can also be helpful. Niacin can be taken in extended-release form (1-2 grams at bedtime) or as inositol hexaniacinate or nicotinate. L-carnitine (2 grams per day) can help lower free fatty acid inflow to the liver, which may reduce Lp(a) levels. N-acetylcysteine (about 1 gram per day) can also provide modest reductions in Lp(a) levels.

However, it's important to note that some medications may interact with these supplements. For example, estrogen replacement in women (and progestogens may mitigate the effect) and testosterone replacement in men with deficiency may be considered. Neomycin sulfate (2 grams per day) has been shown to have a greater effect when combined with niacin. Fibrates (which have variable effects) and statins (which are used to lower LDL-C) are also medications that may be considered for heart health.

Lipid Support (high):
- Red Yeast Rice (Monascus purpureus)
- Coenzyme Q10
- Sweet Orange (Citrus sinensis)
- Quercetin
- Gotu Kola (Centella asiatica)
- Horse Chestnut (Aesculus hippocastanum)
- Grape Seed Extract (Vitis vinifera)
- Vitamin C
- Plant Sterols/Stanols (Beta-Sitosterol, Campesterol, Campestanol, Sitostanol)

- Monostroma nitidum (seaweed) extract

Antioxidants:
- Acerola Extract (Malpighia glabra)
- Grape Seed Extract (Vitis vinifera)
- Curcumin
- Garlic (Allium sativum)
- Ginkgo Extract (Ginkgo biloba)
- Quercetin
- Rutin
- Clove (Syzygium aromaticum)
- Allspice (Pimenta dioica)
- Sweet Basil (Ocimum basilicum)
- Sage (Salvia officinalis)
- Rosemary Extract (Rosmarinus officinalis)
- Lutein
- Lycopene
- Trans Resveratrol
- Vitamin A
- Vitamin E
- L-glutathione
- NAC (N-Acetyl-L-Cysteine)
- Broccoli Powder Extract
- Sulforaphane
- Olive Leaf Extract (Olea europaea)
- Bergamot
- Red Grape Powder
- Alpha Lipoic Acid
- Taurine
- MVM (Multi-vitamin/mineral)
- Glutathione (reduced)

Anti-inflammatory Support:
- Phytocannabinoids
- Hemp Flower Extract
- Hemp Seed Oil
- Palmitoylethanolamide (PEA)
- Omega-3 Fatty Acids (Fish Oil) docosahexaenoic acid), 14-HDHA (14-hydroxy docosahexaenoic acid)
- Vitamin D3
- Curcumin
- Green Tea Extract (Epigallocatechin Gallate (EGCG))
- Trans Resveratrol
- Quercetin
- Nettle (Urtica dioica)
- Pro-Resolving Mediators (PRMs): 18-HEPE (18-hydroxy eicosapentaenoic acid), 17-HDHA (17-hydroxy

Liver Support:
- Milk Thistle
- L-methionine
- Taurine
- Inositol
- Ox Bile
- Artichoke
- Beet Powder
- Vitamin A
- Vitamin B6
- Vitamin B12
- Plant protein powder with MVM (multi-vitamin/mineral)
- L-glutathione
- N-Acetyl-L-Cysteine (NAC)
- Quercetin
- Methylsulfonylmethane (MSM)
- Sodium Sulfate
- Green Tea Extract
- Reishi
- Cordyceps
- Chinese Skullcap
- Schisandra
- Burdock Extract
- Phosphatidylcholine

ApoA-I

Oxidized LDL is LDL cholesterol that has reacted with free radicals, becoming more atherogenic. High levels of oxidized LDL are associated with increased risk of atherosclerosis, coronary heart disease (CHD), and other cardiovascular events. This form of LDL is more readily taken up by macrophages, promoting plaque formation within the arteries, increasing risk of cardiovascular events independently of total cholesterol and LDL levels.

MALE	
Normal Range	120 - 160 mg/dL
Optimal Range	75 - 160 mg/dL

FEMALE	
Normal Range	140 - 180 mg/dL
Optimal Range	80 - 175 mg/dL

If LOW or < 75 mg/dL or < 80 mg/dL:

 Low blood pressure is associated with a higher risk of cardiovascular disease (CVD). Cardiovascular diseases and stroke cause one in three women's deaths each year, resulting in approximately one woman's death every 80 seconds. Cardiovascular disease is the leading cause of death for both men and women, accounting for nearly 400,000 deaths annually, which is more than the combined number of deaths caused by all types of cancer, respiratory illness, and diabetes. Moreover, 25% of all deaths occur due to cardiovascular disease.

Almost two-thirds (64%) of women who die suddenly of coronary heart disease have had no previous symptoms. Several risk factors contribute to the development of CVD, including high blood pressure, high LDL cholesterol, smoking, diabetes, overweight and obesity (covered in FMA 5), poor diet, physical inactivity, excessive alcohol consumption, and nutritional consequences of statins and beta blockers.

Statins and beta blockers decrease CoQ10, selenium, O3, carnitine, and T3f, while beta-blockers decrease melatonin. Diuretics potentially reduce electrolytes and key minerals. Metformin reduces B9 (folate) and B12. ACE inhibitors/blockers decrease zinc and sodium.

Lifestyle modifications, including niacin and statins, support immunity and inflammation. For heart health, they help balance blood sugar and prevent diabetes or metabolic syndrome. Key cardiovascular lifestyle changes that impact inflammation include:
- Non-inflammatory diet
- Proper sleep
- Movement
- Stress management
- Addressing nutritional deficiencies

Preventative measures include:
- Avoiding diabetes by balancing blood sugar
- Steering clear of canola oil or other polyunsaturated fatty acids (PUFAs)
- Eliminating or reducing sugars, as they:
- Drive up triglyceride levels
- Lower the immune response
- Convert to fat in the body
- Elevate insulin levels
- Damage arteries, leading to plaque formation
- Increasing healthy fats, including saturated fat
- Eliminating or limiting grains, or learning how to eat and prepare them correctly
- Eating cholesterol (e.g., eggs) Egg yolks, processed foods, and a Metabolic Reset & Weight Loss program are all things to avoid.
- Antioxidants and free radicals should be consumed in moderation, as should cholesterol antagonists to reduce excess cholesterol in the bloodstream.
- Liver and adrenal health are crucial for overall well-being, so managing stress and addressing vitamin/mineral deficiencies are essential.

- Smoking should be avoided, and getting out of the chair occasionally and considering getting a pet are also beneficial.

Dietary Tips and Caveats:
- Limit starchy foods like potatoes, pasta, bread, crackers, and rice.
- Avoid simple sugars and sugary drinks and sodas.
- Incorporate heart-healthy, anti-inflammatory snacks like blueberries, pomegranate seeds, avocados, walnuts, and pistachios.
- Avoid hydrogenated vegetable oils, trans fats, and fried foods.
- Cook with coconut and avocado oils; add olive oil to cooked foods and raw vegetables.
- Choose organic produce, organic, antibiotic-free, hormone-free, grass-fed dairy, and animal products.
- Eat freshly ground flax seeds or chia seeds to increase fiber intake; eat the skin of fruits and vegetables.
- Consume adequate amounts of antioxidants and flavonoids, which can be obtained daily through 5-9 servings of organic vegetables/fruit.
- Eat garlic frequently.

Lipid Support (high):
- Red Yeast Rice (Monascus purpureus)
- Coenzyme Q10
- Sweet Orange (Citrus sinensis)
- Quercetin
- Gotu Kola (Centella asiatica)
- Horse Chestnut (Aesculus hippocastanum)
- Grape Seed Extract (Vitis vinifera)
- Vitamin C
- Plant Sterols/Stanols (Beta-Sitosterol, Campesterol, Campestanol, Sitostanol)
- Monostroma nitidum (seaweed) extract

Anti-inflammatory Support:
- Phytocannabinoids
- Hemp Flower Extract
- Hemp Seed Oil
- Palmitoylethanolamide (PEA)
- Omega-3 Fatty Acids (Fish Oil)
- docosahexaenoic acid), 14-HDHA (14-hydroxy docosahexaenoic acid)
- Vitamin D3
- Curcumin
- Green Tea Extract (Epigallocatechin Gallate (EGCG))
- Trans Resveratrol
- Quercetin
- Nettle (Urtica dioica)
- Pro-Resolving Mediators (PRMs): 18-HEPE (18-hydroxy eicosapentaenoic acid), 17-HDHA (17-hydroxy

Immune Support:
- Echinacea angustifolia
- Astragalus membranaceus
- Elderberry Extract (Sambucus nigra)
- Andrographis paniculate
- Green Tea Extract
- Arabinogalactan (larch tree)
- Lauric Acid
- Cordyceps mushroom
- Shiitake mushroom
- Maitake mushroom
- Reishi mushroom
- Beta 1,3 Glucans
- Vitamin A
- Vitamin D3
- Vitamin E
- Vitamin K2
- Wild cherry bark
- Ginger
- Lovage (Levisticum officinale)
- Wild Cherry Extract

If **HIGH** or **> 160 mg/dL** or **> 175 mg/dL:**

 High Apo A-1 is not a CVD risk factor, but rather it appears to be protective. Apo A-1 is the primary protein component associated with high-density lipoproteins (HDL). Apo A-1 also stabilizes prostacyclin (PGI2) thus giving it some potential for an anti-clotting effect. Protection from Alzheimer's disease by Apo A-1 may rely on a synergistic interaction with alpha-tocopherol. Apo A-1 may increase with the use of carbamazepine, phenobarbital, some statins and ethanol.

- Increased ApoA1 concentrations are more strongly associated with a reduction in risk of a first myocardial infarction than HDL-C concentrations.
- Increased ApoA1, but not HDL-C concentrations, are associated with reduced cardiovascular events among statin-treated patients, even when LDL-C <50 mg/dL.
- In statin-treated patients, patients whose ApoA1 increased while on treatment were at lower risk than those whose ApoA1 did not increase.

Apolipoprotein A levels may be high if you:
- Have high levels of apolipoprotein (familial hyperalphalipoproteinemia)
- Have a genetic disorder called familial cholesteryl ester transfer protein deficiency, or CETP
- Take medicines containing extra estrogens
- Take niacin or statins, a type of cholesterol-lowering medicine
- Take statins
- Lose weight

ApoB

Apolipoprotein B (apoB) is a structural protein found in low-density lipoproteins (LDL), very-low-density lipoproteins (VLDL), and intermediate-density lipoproteins (IDL). It plays a crucial role in the structure and function of these lipoproteins, which carry triglycerides (TGs) and other substances.

ApoB levels are used to assess the risk of cardiovascular disease. They provide a direct measure of the number of atherogenic lipoprotein particles in the bloodstream, which are particles that can contribute to plaque buildup in the arteries. ApoB is also a surrogate marker for LDL particle concentration or number, since LDL particles make up about 90% of the atherogenic lipoprotein particles.

In addition to apoB, other lipoproteins, such as chylomicrons, Lp(a), and VLDL, also contribute to cholesterol levels in the blood. However, apoB is particularly important in assessing cardiovascular risk, especially in individuals with diabetes and metabolic syndrome. These conditions often lead to the presence of small, dense LDL particles with relatively normal cholesterol levels but high apoB levels.

Normal Range	80 - 120 mg/dL
Optimal Range	< 100 mg/dL

If **LOW** or **< 80 mg/dL:**

 Apo B levels can be reduced by any condition that affects lipoprotein production or synthesis and packaging in the liver. Lower levels are often seen in secondary causes, including:
- Use of drugs such as estrogen (in post-menopausal women), lovastatin, simvastatin, niacin, and thyroxine
- Hyperthyroidism
- Malnutrition
- Reye syndrome
- Weight loss

- Severe illness
- Surgery
- Cirrhosis

 Identify the underlying cause. Reducing alcohol consumption might help increase ApoB levels by improving liver health.

 Liver Support:
- Milk Thistle
- L-methionine
- Taurine
- Inositol
- Ox Bile
- Artichoke
- Beet Powder
- Vitamin A
- Vitamin B6
- Vitamin B12
- Plant protein powder with MVM (multi-vitamin/mineral)
- L-glutathione
- N-Acetyl-L-Cysteine (NAC)
- Quercetin
- Methylsulfonylmethane (MSM)
- Sodium Sulfate
- Green Tea Extract
- Reishi
- Cordyceps
- Chinese Skullcap
- Schisandra
- Burdock Extract
- Phosphatidylcholine

If **HIGH** or > 120 mg/dL:

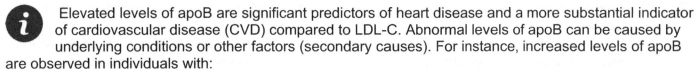 Elevated levels of apoB are significant predictors of heart disease and a more substantial indicator of cardiovascular disease (CVD) compared to LDL-C. Abnormal levels of apoB can be caused by underlying conditions or other factors (secondary causes). For instance, increased levels of apoB are observed in individuals with:
- Diabetes
- Use of drugs such as androgens, beta blockers, diuretics, and progestins (synthetic progesterones)
- Hypothyroidism
- Nephrotic syndrome (a kidney disease)
- Pregnancy (levels increase temporarily and decrease after delivery)

Elevated levels of apoB correspond to elevated levels of LDL-C and non-HDL-C and are associated with an increased risk of cardiovascular disease (CVD). Elevations may be attributed to a high-fat diet and/or reduced clearance of LDL from the blood. Certain genetic disorders are the direct (primary) cause of abnormal levels of apoB. For example, familial combined hyperlipidemia is an inherited disorder characterized by high blood levels of cholesterol and triglycerides. Abetalipoproteinemia, also known as Apolipoprotein B deficiency or Bassen-Kornzweig syndrome, is a rare genetic condition that can cause abnormally low levels of apoB. For more information about these disorders, refer to the Related Content section.

 Address nutritional deficiencies

Preventative measures include:
- Avoid diabetes by balancing your blood sugar
- Steer clear of CANOLA OIL or other PUFAs
- Eliminate or lessen sugars as they:
- Drive up your Triglycerides
- Lower your immune response
- Turns to fat in your body
- Elevates your insulin

ADVANCED HEART MARKERS

- Tears up your arteries leading to plaque formation
- Increase healthy fats including saturated fat
- Eliminate or limit grains, or know how to eat/prepare correctly
- Eat cholesterol (ex. Egg yolks)
- Avoid processed foods
- Consider doing a Metabolic Reset & Weight Loss program
- Consume Antioxidants and watch those free radicals
- Cholesterol Antagonists eat up the excess cholesterol in the bloodstream
- Be mindful of your Liver health, which is essential for good health
- Ensure good Adrenal health by managing your stress response which will drive up your blood sugar regardless of what you are eating
- Address vitamin/mineral deficiencies, and don't randomly take vitamins/minerals including a mult-ivitamin
- And of course - forget smoking, get out of the chair occasionally, and consider getting a pet

Statindecisionaid.mayoclinic.org is a helpful tool, particularly for documenting the standard of care for medical professionals and patients that do not elect a statin.

Statin's mechanism of action is to stop the HMG CoA reductase, thereby effectively turning off the production of CoQ10 and cholesterol, and lowering the levels of vitamin D, Estrogen, Progesterone, Testosterone and Cortisol.

Lipid Support (high):
- Red Yeast Rice (Monascus purpureus)
- Coenzyme Q10
- Sweet Orange (Citrus sinensis)
- Quercetin
- Gotu Kola (Centella asiatica)
- Horse Chestnut (Aesculus hippocastanum)
- Grape Seed Extract (Vitis vinifera)
- Vitamin C
- Plant Sterols/Stanols (Beta-Sitosterol, Campesterol, Campestanol, Sitostanol)
- Monostroma nitidum (seaweed) extract

Prescription: Statins, fibrates, cholesterol absorption inhibitors (ezetimibe), bile acid sequestrants, anti-inflammatory support.

Anti-inflammatory Support:
- Phytocannabinoids
- Hemp Flower Extract
- Hemp Seed Oil
- Palmitoylethanolamide (PEA)
- Omega-3 Fatty Acids (Fish Oil)
- docosahexaenoic acid), 14-HDHA (14-hydroxy docosahexaenoic acid)
- Vitamin D3
- Curcumin
- Green Tea Extract (Epigallocatechin Gallate (EGCG))
- Trans Resveratrol
- Quercetin
- Nettle (Urtica dioica)
- Pro-Resolving Mediators (PRMs): 18-HEPE (18-hydroxy eicosapentaenoic acid), 17-HDHA (17-hydroxy

Liver Support:
- Milk Thistle
- L-methionine
- Taurine
- Inositol
- Ox Bile
- Artichoke
- Beet Powder
- Vitamin A
- Vitamin B6
- Vitamin B12
- Plant protein powder with MVM (multi-vitamin/mineral)

- L-glutathione
- N-Acetyl-L-Cysteine (NAC)
- Quercetin
- Methylsulfonylmethane (MSM)
- Sodium Sulfate
- Green Tea Extract

Thyroid Support:
- N-Acetyl-L-Tyrosine
- American Ginseng (Panax quinquefolius)
- Forskolin (Coleus forskohlii)
- Iodine
- Chromium
- Zinc

Fiber Support:
- Acacia gum
- Cellulose
- Guar gum
- Cranberry seed powder
- Carrot fiber
- Inulin

- Reishi
- Cordyceps
- Chinese Skullcap
- Schisandra
- Burdock Extract
- Phosphatidylcholine

- Selenium
- Copper
- Manganese
- Vitamin A
- Vitamin B2
- Potassium Iodide
- Myo-Inositol

- Orange fiber
- Glucomannan
- Apple pectin
- Psyllium husk
- Flax seed
- Prune powder

Fatty Acids

This test measures the major fatty acids (FA) for the purposes of cardiovascular disease characterization and management

EPA (Eicosapentaenoic acid)

Eicosapentanoic acid (EPA), an omega-3 fatty acid, plays a crucial role in maintaining the health of cellular membranes, regulating lipid actions, and mitigating inflammatory responses within the body. EPA and DHA influence the production of inflammatory response mediators, favoring the synthesis of anti-inflammatory eicosanoids such as leukotrienes, prostaglandins, and thromboxanes. Additionally, EPA and DHA exhibit moderate to strong anti-depressant effects. Notably, EPA has been demonstrated to suppress the signaling of TNF-a in adipocytes. Furthermore, EPA enhances cerebral oxygenation and appears to exert beneficial effects on regulating leptin levels and increasing adiponectin. Moreover, EPA may stimulate adaptive immunity by enhancing B cell responsiveness.

Normal Range	0.16 - 1.45 %
Optimal Range	0.16 - 1.45 %

If **LOW** or < 0.16%:

Lower dietary intake of omega-3 fatty acids is the primary reason for the deficiency of EPA, or low levels of EPA. Certain genetic polymorphisms, such as reduced activity of the FADS1 and FADS2 genes, can lead to reduced conversion of ALA into EPA and DHA. EPA can be synthesized in the body from ALA and retroconverted from DHA. However, relying solely on ALA intake to provide adequate levels of EPA is not recommended due to poor or inefficient conversion from ALA to EPA. Lower levels of EPA or deficient intake of EPA have been associated with an increased risk of cardiovascular disease, arrhythmia, blood clots, heart attacks, stroke, elevated triglyceride levels, increased growth of atherosclerotic plaque, reduced vascular endothelial function, skin cancer, and increased inflammation. Lower levels of EPA are also linked to lower brain mass in older adults.

 Good sources of EPA include: fatty fish such as Pacific herring, salmon, oysters, tuna, and omega-3 enriched eggs.

Food sources of ALA, the essential fatty acid EPA precursor include: flaxseeds and flaxseed oil, chia seeds, walnuts, and canola oil.

Currently, no official dietary intake recommendations have been established. Several official health organizations have proposed a minimum dietary intake level of 500 mg/day of EPA+DHA. Because the efficiency of conversion of ALA to EPA is so low, supplementing EPA is generally recommended to meet therapeutic doses. High dose supplementation of omega-3 fatty acids (including EPA) has been shown to reduce the need for non-steroidal anti-inflammatory drugs (NSAIDS). Persons suffering from ulcerative colitis have been shown to need fewer corticosteroids when supplementing with high dose omega-3 fatty acids.

Adverse side effects observed with high dose omega-3 fatty acids from supplement form include gastrointestinal upset and loose stools.
Omega-3 supplements including EPA and DHA should be used with caution in persons with clotting disorders or on anti-clotting medication.

Nutritional support:
- Omega-3 Fatty Acids (fish oil)

If **HIGH** or > 1.45%:

 Currently, there are no official dietary intake recommendations for omega-3 fatty acids. However, several official health organizations have proposed a minimum daily intake of 500 mg of EPA and DHA. Since the body can only convert a small amount of ALA into EPA, supplementing with EPA is usually recommended to achieve therapeutic doses.

High-dose supplementation of omega-3 fatty acids, including EPA, has been shown to reduce the need for non-steroidal anti-inflammatory drugs (NSAIDs). Additionally, people with ulcerative colitis have been found to require fewer corticosteroids when supplementing with high-dose omega-3 fatty acids.

However, it's important to note that high doses of omega-3 fatty acids from supplements may cause gastrointestinal upset and loose stools as an adverse side effect. Therefore, omega-3 supplements, including EPA and DHA, should be used with caution in individuals with clotting disorders or those taking anti-clotting medication, as omega-3s may prolong clotting times.

Reduce any supplements that contain Omega 3 fatty acids. If appropriate, increase your intake of food sources of Omega 6 fatty acids, such as meat (pork, chicken, beef), fish (farmed salmon, flatfish, flounder, sardines), and dairy (cream cheese).

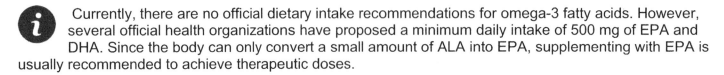

DPA (Docosapentanoic acid)

Docosapentanoic acid (DPA), a structurally similar omega-3 fatty acid to EPA, serves as an intermediary in the conversion of EPA to DHA. DPA plays a crucial role in supporting the production of healthy blood vessels and reducing the risk of clotting.

Normal Range	0.73% - 1.99%
Optimal Range	0.73% - 1.99%

If **LOW** or < 0.73%:

 Deficiency of DHA is typically due to low dietary intake of high DPA foods. Low levels of DPA are associated with increased risk of thrombosis and stroke death.

 Good sources of DPA include: fish oil, fatty fish such as salmon, and grass-fed beef. Adverse side effects observed with high dose omega-3 fatty acids from supplement form include gastrointestinal upset and loose stools.

 Nutritional support:
- Omega-3 Fatty Acids (fish oil)

If **HIGH** or > 1.99%:

 Adverse side effects observed with high doses of omega-3 fatty acids from supplement form include gastrointestinal upset and loose stools

Reduce any supplements that contain Omega 3 fatty acids. If appropriate, increase your intake of food sources of Omega 6 fatty acids, such as meat (pork, chicken, beef), fish (farmed salmon, flatfish, flounder, sardines), and dairy (cream cheese).

DHA (Docosahexanoic acid)

Docosahexanoic acid (DHA), an essential omega-3 fatty acid, can be synthesized from alpha linolenic acid (ALA) in the human body. However, this conversion is inefficient, and some individuals may not meet their physiological needs for DHA. Essential fatty acids, which are converted into omega-3 and omega-6 fatty acids in the body, play a crucial role in cell membrane structure and function. EPA and DHA influence the types of inflammatory response mediators, favoring less inflammatory eicosanoids like leukotrienes, prostaglandins, and thromboxanes. Additionally, EPA and DHA exhibit moderate to strong anti-depressant effects.

Specifically, DHA is a vital component of retinal and neuronal cell membranes, suggesting a potential role in neurological development, function, and visual function development. Furthermore, DHA, along with EPA, may help reduce lipids in individuals with Type 2 diabetes mellitus. The third trimester of pregnancy and the first three months of life after birth are the most critical periods for accumulating DHA in the infant's brain.

Normal Range	1.12 - 9.58 %
Optimal Range	1.12 - 9.58 %

If **LOW** or < 1.12%:

Low dietary intake of omega-3 fatty acids from fatty fish, fish oil, or krill oil is the primary reason for DHA deficiency. Only about 0-4% of dietary ALA is converted to DHA in men, while up to 9% of dietary ALA is converted to DHA in women due to estrogenic effects on fatty acid conversion. Certain genetic polymorphisms, such as reduced activity of the FADS1 and FADS2 genes, can lead to reduced conversion of ALA into EPA and DHA. Individuals with APOE4 genetic SNPs may experience lower serum levels of DHA due to increased oxidation of DHA in these individuals. In addition to assessing DHA status relative to the risk of Alzheimer's disease and dementia, it's important to consider the presence of APOE4 genetic SNPs. Fish oil supplementation has been shown to lower AA levels, likely through decreased activity of the delta-6-desaturase enzyme. Low DHA levels may be a risk factor for the development of neurological conditions like Alzheimer's disease and dementia. Depletion of DHA in the brain can lead to learning or cognitive deficits, increased aggression, and reduced vascular endothelial function. Lower levels of DHA or deficient intake of DHA have been associated with an increased risk of cardiovascular disease, including arrhythmia, blood clots, heart attacks, stroke, reduced vascular endothelial function, elevated triglyceride levels, skin cancer, and increased inflammation.

Good sources of DHA include fatty fish like Pacific herring, salmon, oysters, tuna, and omega-3 enriched eggs. Food sources of ALA, the essential fatty acid DHA precursor, include flaxseeds and flaxseed oil, chia seeds, walnuts, and canola oil. Since the human body is inefficient at converting ALA to DHA, it's generally recommended to obtain DHA from seafood sources or supplements. Similarly, since the body is inefficient at converting ALA to EPA, it's recommended to obtain EPA from seafood sources or supplements. AA can also be obtained directly from the diet and is found in egg yolks, bone marrow, and meats. However, there are currently no official dietary intake recommendations for AA. Several health organizations have proposed a minimum dietary intake level of 500 mg/day of EPA+DHA. Due to the low efficiency of ALA conversion to DHA, supplementing DHA is generally recommended to achieve therapeutic doses. The recommended minimum daily DHA supplementation for adults is 250 mg. Pregnant and lactating women are advised to consume at least 200 mg DHA daily. Diabetic individuals may benefit from supplementing

DHA (along with EPA) due to its triglyceride-lowering effects. High-dose supplementation of omega-3 fatty acids (including DHA) has been shown to reduce the need for non-steroidal anti-inflammatory drugs (NSAIDs). Individuals with ulcerative colitis have been found to require fewer corticosteroids when supplementing with high-dose omega-3 fatty acids. However, high-dose omega-3 fatty acid supplements from supplements may cause gastrointestinal upset and loose stools. Omega-3 supplements containing EPA and DHA should be used with caution in individuals with clotting disorders or those taking anti-clotting medication.

 Nutritional support:
- Omega-3 Fatty Acids (fish oil)

If **HIGH** or **> 9.58%**:

 Currently, there are no official dietary intake recommendations for omega-3 fatty acids. However, high-dose supplementation of omega-3s, particularly DHA, has been shown to reduce the need for non-steroidal anti-inflammatory drugs (NSAIDs). However, it's important to note that adverse side effects, such as gastrointestinal upset and loose stools, have been observed with high doses of omega-3 fatty acids obtained from supplements. Additionally, omega-3 supplements, including EPA and DHA, should be used with caution in individuals with clotting disorders or those taking anticlotting medication, as omega-3s may prolong clotting times.

 Reduce any supplements that contain Omega 3 fatty acids. If appropriate, increase your intake of food sources of Omega 6 fatty acids, such as meat (pork, chicken, beef), fish (farmed salmon, flatfish, flounder, sardines), and dairy (cream cheese).

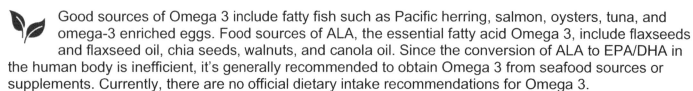

Total Omega-3

The total of EPA, DPA, and DHA.

Normal Range	1.89 - 12.82 %
Optimal Range	1.89 - 12.82 %

If **LOW** or **< 1.89%**:

 Low dietary intake of omega-3 fatty acids from fatty fish, fish oil, or krill oil is the primary reason for deficiency of Omega 3.

 Good sources of Omega 3 include fatty fish such as Pacific herring, salmon, oysters, tuna, and omega-3 enriched eggs. Food sources of ALA, the essential fatty acid Omega 3, include flaxseeds and flaxseed oil, chia seeds, walnuts, and canola oil. Since the conversion of ALA to EPA/DHA in the human body is inefficient, it's generally recommended to obtain Omega 3 from seafood sources or supplements. Currently, there are no official dietary intake recommendations for Omega 3.

 Nutritional support:
- Omega-3 Fatty Acids (fish oil)

If **HIGH** or **> 12.82%**:

FATTY ACIDS

 Supplementation with EPA+ DHA from fish oil capsules for approximately five months dose dependently increased the omega-3 index in 115 healthy young adults (ages 20-45 years), validating the use of the omega-3 index as a biomarker of EPA + DHA intake.

 Reduce any supplements that contain Omega 3 fatty acids. If appropriate, increase your intake of food sources of Omega 6 fatty acids, such as meat (pork, chicken, beef), fish (farmed salmon, flatfish, flounder, sardines), and dairy (cream cheese).

LA (Linolenic Acid)

Linolenic Acid is considered the "parent" omega-6 fatty acid. All other omega-6 fatty acids are synthesized from linolenic acid by desaturation and elongation reactions. Thus, linolenic acid must be consumed in the diet in order for all omega-6 fatty acids to be used and incorporated into the body's cells and cell membranes. LA stimulates cell division and repair.

Normal Range	1.36 - 8.62%
Optimal Range	1.36 - 8.62%

If LOW or < 1.36%:

 Given the significant amounts of vegetable oils in the typical Western diet, low levels of Linoleic Acid (LA) are usually only observed in a fat-free diet, a diet severely restricted in dietary fat, or in situations of fat malabsorption. Insufficient LA can lead to eczema-like skin manifestations and impaired wound healing. Conversely, excessive LA is typically associated with a high-fat diet, particularly one high in refined vegetable oils. High consumption of Linolenic Acid (LA) has been linked to pro-inflammatory conditions and various adverse health risks. There are also correlations with an increased risk of certain cancers, including breast, colon, and prostate, as excess amounts of this fatty acid can cause abnormal cell division.

 Linolenic acid, a crucial omega-3 fatty acid, is abundant in vegetable oils. Corn, soybean, sunflower, safflower, canola, and peanut oil are the primary sources of dietary linolenic acid. Other dietary sources include avocados, nuts, and seeds. Since linolenic acid is readily available in the Western diet, supplementation is usually unnecessary. However, reducing refined vegetable oil intake (corn, soy, peanut, canola, safflower oil) and replacing it with healthier alternatives like olive oil, coconut oil, avocado oil, or animal-based fats can effectively increase linoleic acid levels.

 Nutritional support:
- Omega-3 Fatty Acids (fish oil)

If HIGH or > 8.62%:

 Linoleic acid and omega-6 fatty acids are plentiful in the Western diet, so supplementation is typically unnecessary.

The best way to lower LA levels is to decrease the intake of refined vegetable oil (corn, soy, peanut, canola, safflower oil) and replace it with an alternative such as olive oil, coconut oil, avocado oil, or fat from animal sources.

 To reduce endogenous AA production, limit dietary intake of vegetable oils high in LA (corn, soy, canola, safflower oil).
Increase Omega 3 intake.

Cofactors for Delta-6-Desaturase and Delta-5-Desaturase enzymes: B2, B3, B6, Vitamin C, Zinc, Magnesium.
Cofactors for Elongase enzymes: B3, B5, B6, Biotin (B7), Vitamin C.

Essential Fatty Acid Support:
- Essential Fatty Acids with Vitamin D
- Omega-3 Fatty Acids with Probiotics
- Omega-3 Fatty Acids
- Essential Fatty Acids with PRMs

Nutritional Support:
- Magnesium Citrate
- Magnesium taurinate
- Magnesium glycinate
- Magnesium malate
- Zinc
- Vitamin B complex

- Riboflavin (Vitamin B2)
- Vitamin B3 / Niacin (as Nicotinic Acid)
- Vitamin B6
- Vitamin C
- MVM (Multi-vitamin/mineral)

Total Omega-6

Total of all Omega 6 fatty acids.

Normal Range	7.43% - 36.90%
Optimal Range	7.43% - 36.90%

If **LOW** or < 7.43%:

Given the significant amounts of vegetable oils in the typical Western diet, low levels of Linoleic Acid (LA) are usually only observed in a fat-free diet, a diet severely restricted in dietary fat, or in situations of fat malabsorption. Insufficient LA can lead to eczema-like skin manifestations and impaired wound healing. Conversely, excessive LA is typically associated with a high-fat diet, particularly one high in refined vegetable oils. High consumption of Linolenic Acid (LA) has been linked to pro-inflammatory conditions and various adverse health risks. There are also correlations with an increased risk of certain cancers, including breast, colon, and prostate, as excess amounts of this fatty acid can cause abnormal cell division.

Omega-6, a crucial fatty acid, is abundant in vegetable oils. Corn, soybean, sunflower, safflower, canola, and peanut oil are the primary sources of dietary omega-6. Other dietary sources include avocados, nuts, and seeds. Generally, supplementation of omega-6 fatty acids is unnecessary since they are readily available in the Western diet.

Nutritional support
- Borage oil (GLA - Gamma Linolenic Acid)

If **HIGH** or > 36.90%:

The majority of omega-6 fats in our diet originate from plant sources, including corn, soy, safflower, sunflower, and sesame oils. These foods contain linoleic acid (LA) and can be converted into arachidonic acid (AA) within the cell. Some animal sources, such as meat, milk, eggs, and shrimp, contain higher amounts of AA due to their higher consumption of omega-6-rich foods. Omega-6 and -3 fatty acids ultimately produce crucial signaling molecules called prostanoids and eicosanoids, which play a vital role in coordinating immunity, inflammation, and coagulation. Maintaining an appropriate ratio of omega-6s to omega-3s may be beneficial in reducing the risk of cardiovascular disease and depression. However, excessive intake of omega-6 can lead to increased inflammation and platelet aggregation, while omega-3s have the opposite effect, reducing inflammation and platelet aggregation.

Lower your intake of omega-6 fats by avoiding corn, soy, safflower, sunflower, and sesame oils. On the other hand, limit your consumption of foods high in omega-6 fatty acids, such as red meat, poultry, eggs, and nuts.

Nutritional support:
- Omega-3 Fatty Acids (fish oil)

Omega-3 Index

Normal Range	≥ 8.01 %
Optimal Range	8.00 - 12.65%

If **LOW** or **< 8.01%**:

The Omega-3 Index is a validated biomarker of tissue membrane omega−3 (n−3) polyunsaturated fatty acid (PUFA) status. The ratio is expressed as a percentage where the denominator is the sum off all fatty acids measured in the blood. Thus, a decrease in the ratio can be caused by a low intake of omega−3 fatty acids and incorporation of those fatty acids into cell membranes; or due to a proportionally high intake of other dietary fatty acids (saturated fatty acids, mono-unsaturated fatty acids and omega−6's poly unsaturated fatty acids) Low levels of omega-3 index are associated with increased risk for cardiac death.

If the omega-3 index is below 8.0%, it's recommended to increase dietary sources of EPA and DHA from both plant and animal sources. Since the omega-3 index is a relative ratio of omega-3 compared to all other fatty acids in the blood, it's also crucial to consider the intake of all other dietary fatty acids, including saturated fatty acids, mono-unsaturated fatty acids, and omega-6s. Currently, there are no official dietary intake recommendations for omega-3s. However, several official health organizations have proposed a minimum daily intake of 500 mg of EPA+DHA. Due to the low efficiency of converting ALA to DHA, supplementing DHA is generally recommended to achieve therapeutic doses. The recommended minimum daily DHA supplementation for adults is 250 mg. Pregnant and lactating women are advised to consume at least 200 mg of DHA daily. Diabetic individuals may benefit from supplementing DHA (along with EPA) due to its triglyceride-lowering effects. High-dose supplementation of omega-3 fatty acids (including DHA) has been shown to reduce the need for non-steroidal anti-inflammatory drugs (NSAIDs). Additionally, individuals with ulcerative colitis have been observed to require fewer corticosteroids when supplementing with high-dose omega-3 fatty acids. However, it's important to note that adverse side effects, such as gastrointestinal upset and loose stools, have been associated with high-dose omega-3 fatty acid supplements from supplements. Therefore, omega-3 supplements containing EPA and DHA should be used with caution in individuals with clotting disorders or those taking anti-clotting medication.

Nutritional support:
- Omega-3 Fatty Acids (fish oil)

If **HIGH** or **> 12.65%**:

 Supplementation with EPA+ DHA from fish oil capsules for approximately five months dosedependently increased the omega-3 index in 115 healthy young adults (ages 20-45 years), validating the use of the omega-3 index as a biomarker of EPA + DHA intake.

 Reduce any supplements that contain Omega 3 fatty acids. If appropriate, increase your intake of food sources of Omega 6 fatty acids, such as meat (pork, chicken, beef), fish (farmed salmon, flatfish, flounder, sardines), and dairy (cream cheese).

Sugar Panel

The sugar panel blood test is a comprehensive assessment of an individual's glucose metabolism and insulin sensitivity. This panel provides insights into how the body processes sugar (glucose) and the associated hormones. These markers are essential for understanding an individual's risk of metabolic conditions such as diabetes, insulin resistance, and obesity.

Glucose - Fasting

Blood sugar balance involves a complex interaction between the pancreas (insulin/glucagon), adrenal glands (cortisol), and liver (gluconeogenesis). Deviations in blood sugar levels can result from various factors such as impaired glycogen breakdown or storage, poor glucose absorption in the gastrointestinal tract, elevated hormone levels (e.g., cortisol, estrogen, insulin), and receptor insensitivity. Stable blood sugar levels are crucial for a healthy immune response.

Normal Range	65 - 99 mg/dL
Optimal Range	80 - 100 mg/dL

If **LOW** or **< 80 mg/dL:**

Low fasting glucose levels may indicate reactive hypoglycemia, impaired glycogen storage in the liver, excessive insulin, adrenal or thyroid hypofunction, or liver dysfunction.

Increase protein and fat intake.
Consider checking glucose handling capabilities at different intervals throughout the day.
Increase chromium intake to enhance insulin sensitivity.

Lifestyle Recommendations:
- Avoid stress and include relaxation techniques.
- Engage in balanced physical activity, incorporating high-intensity intervals and resistance training.
- Avoid stimulants (e.g., caffeine), alcohol, and smoking.
- Ensure adequate sleep and hydration.
- Use natural and organic personal care products.

Dietary Tips:
- Increase dietary fiber intake (50g/day recommended).
- Eat small, balanced meals with healthy fats (e.g., nuts, seeds, avocados).
- Avoid refined carbs; focus on lean protein and fiber-rich foods.
- Consume omega-3s, green leafy vegetables, and monounsaturated fats.

Glucose Metabolism Support:
- Magnesium
- Zinc
- Selenium
- Manganese
- Chromium
- Molybdenum
- Potassium Iodide
- Taurine
- Carnosine
- R-Lipoic Acid
- Vitamin A
- Vitamin D3
- Vitamin E
- Vitamin K1

- Benfotiamine (Fat-Soluble Vitamin B1)
- Vitamin B1
- Vitamin B2
- Vitamin B3
- Vitamin B5
- Vitamin B6
- Vitamin B7 (Biotin)
- Vitamin B9 (Folate)
- Vitamin B12
- Vitamin C
- Berberine
- Fenugreek
- Gymnema sylvestre
- Banaba (Lagerstroemia speciosa)
- Kudzu (Pueraria lobata)
- Cinnamon
- Inositol (as Myo and D-Chiro)
- Alpha Lipoic Acid
- MVM (Multi-vitamin/mineral)

Adrenal Support:
- gamma-Aminobutyric Acid (GABA)
- Eleutherococcus senticosus
- American Ginseng
- Ashwagandha
- Rhodiola
- Licorice
- Vitamin B2
- Vitamin B5
- Vitamin B6
- Vitamin C
- N-Acetyl-L-Tyrosine
- Phosphatidylserine
- Valerian
- Passion Flower
- Lemon Balm
- Chamomile
- L-theanine
- 5-HTP
- Melatonin
- Rhodiola rosea
- Pyrroloquinoline Quinone (PQQ)
- Taurine
- Vitamin B1
- Vitamin B12
- Magnesium Malate
- Magnesium Taurinate
- Magnesium Glycinate

If **HIGH** or > 100 mg/dL:

High fasting glucose may indicate insulin resistance, early-stage diabetes, or metabolic syndrome. It could also point to liver congestion, stress-related hormone insensitivity, or medication effects.

Consider assessing for insulin resistance, early diabetes, and liver health.
Regularly monitor fasting glucose and insulin levels.

Lifestyle Recommendations:
- Reduce stress and prioritize emotional well-being.
- Incorporate high-intensity interval training as part of a balanced exercise regimen.
- Ensure proper hydration and relaxation practices (e.g., meditation, yoga).

Dietary Tips:
- Start the day with a high-protein breakfast.
- Follow an anti-inflammatory diet rich in omega-3 fats.
- Focus on low-glycemic foods and high-fiber options (e.g., ground flax/chia seeds, legumes).
- Include antioxidant-rich herbs like turmeric, ginger, and rosemary.
- Avoid high-sugar foods, processed juices, and refined carbs.

SUGAR PANEL

Glucose - Non-Fasting

Blood sugar balance involves a complex interaction between the pancreas (insulin/glucagon), adrenal glands (cortisol), and liver (gluconeogenesis). Deviations in blood sugar levels can result from factors such as impaired glycogen breakdown or storage, poor glucose absorption, elevated hormone levels (e.g., cortisol, estrogen, insulin), and receptor insensitivity. Stable blood sugar levels are crucial for a healthy immune response.

Normal Range	65 - 125 mg/dL
Optimal Range	80 - 125 mg/dL

If LOW or < 80 mg/dL:

Low non-fasting glucose levels may indicate reactive hypoglycemia, impaired glycogen storage in the liver, excessive insulin, or adrenal or thyroid hypofunction.

Consider increasing protein and fat intake.
Monitor glucose handling at key intervals throughout the day.
Increase chromium intake to enhance insulin sensitivity.

Lifestyle Recommendations:
- Avoid stress and include relaxation techniques.
- Avoid alcohol, smoking, stimulants (e.g., caffeine).
- Engage in regular exercise, including high-intensity intervals and resistance training.
- Ensure adequate sleep, hydration, and use natural personal care products.

Dietary Tips:
- Increase dietary fiber intake (50g/day recommended) with adequate water.
- Eat small, balanced meals with healthy fats and proteins throughout the day.
- Avoid refined carbs; focus on lean protein and fiber-rich foods.
- Consume omega-3s, dark leafy greens, and monounsaturated fats.

Glucose Metabolism Support:
- Magnesium
- Zinc
- Selenium
- Manganese
- Chromium
- Molybdenum
- Potassium Iodide
- Taurine
- Carnosine
- R-Lipoic Acid
- Vitamin A
- Vitamin D3
- Vitamin E
- Vitamin K1
- Benfotiamine (Fat-Soluble Vitamin B1)
- Vitamin B1
- Vitamin B2
- Vitamin B3
- Vitamin B5
- Vitamin B6
- Vitamin B7 (Biotin)
- Vitamin B9 (Folate)
- Vitamin B12
- Vitamin C
- Berberine
- Fenugreek
- Gymnema sylvestre
- Banaba (Lagerstroemia speciosa)
- Kudzu (Pueraria lobata)
- Cinnamon
- Inositol (as Myo and D-Chiro)
- Alpha Lipoic Acid
- MVM (Multi-vitamin/mineral)

Adrenal Support:
- gamma-Aminobutyric Acid (GABA)
- Eleutherococcus senticosus
- American Ginseng
- Ashwagandha
- Rhodiola
- Licorice
- Vitamin B2
- Vitamin B5
- Vitamin B6
- Vitamin C
- N-Acetyl-L-Tyrosine
- Phosphatidylserine
- Valerian
- Passion Flower
- Lemon Balm
- Chamomile
- L-theanine
- 5-HTP
- Melatonin
- Rhodiola rosea
- Pyrroloquinoline Quinone (PQQ)
- Taurine
- Vitamin B1
- Vitamin B12
- Magnesium Malate
- Magnesium Taurinate
- Magnesium Glycinate

If **HIGH** or > 125 mg/dL:

High non-fasting glucose levels may indicate insulin resistance, early-stage diabetes, or metabolic syndrome. Liver congestion, B1 deficiency, and chronic stress should also be considered.

Assess for insulin resistance, early diabetes, and liver health.
Regularly monitor fasting glucose and insulin levels.

Lifestyle Recommendations:
- Reduce lifestyle stressors; engage in daily relaxation techniques (e.g., meditation, yoga).
- Avoid a sedentary lifestyle; incorporate high-intensity interval training as approved.
- Stay well-hydrated and establish an anti-inflammatory routine.

Dietary Tips:
- Start with a high-protein breakfast; eat every 4 hours.
- Follow an anti-inflammatory diet with omega-3 fats and low-glycemic foods.
- Consume antioxidant-rich herbs and spices, avoid high-glycemic snacks, and focus on low-glycemic vegetables and fruits.

Glucose Metabolism Support:
- Magnesium
- Zinc
- Selenium
- Manganese
- Chromium
- Molybdenum
- Potassium Iodide
- Taurine
- Carnosine
- R-Lipoic Acid
- Vitamin A
- Vitamin D3
- Vitamin E
- Vitamin K1
- Benfotiamine (Fat-Soluble Vitamin B1)
- Vitamin B1
- Vitamin B2
- Vitamin B3
- Vitamin B5
- Vitamin B6
- Vitamin B7 (Biotin)
- Vitamin B9 (Folate)
- Vitamin B12
- Vitamin C
- Berberine
- Fenugreek
- Gymnema sylvestre
- Banaba (Lagerstroemia speciosa)
- Kudzu (Pueraria lobata)
- Cinnamon
- Inositol (as Myo and D-Chiro)
- Alpha Lipoic Acid
- MVM (Multi-vitamin/mineral)

Anti-inflammatory Support:
- Phytocannabinoids
- Hemp Flower Extract
- Hemp Seed Oil
- Palmitoylethanolamide (PEA)
- Omega-3 Fatty Acids (Fish Oil)
- docosahexaenoic acid), 14-HDHA (14-hydroxy docosahexaenoic acid)
- Vitamin D3
- Curcumin
- Green Tea Extract (Epigallocatechin Gallate (EGCG))
- Trans Resveratrol
- Quercetin
- Nettle (Urtica dioica)
- Pro-Resolving Mediators (PRMs): 18-HEPE (18-hydroxy eicosapentaenoic acid), 17-HDHA (17-hydroxy

High Dose Probiotics:
- Multi-strain probiotic blend
- Saccharomyces boulardii
- Beta Glucans
- Lactobacillus plantarum strain L-137 (HK L-137)
- Xylooligosaccharide (XOS)

Antioxidant Support:
- Acerola Extract (Malpighia glabra)
- Grape Seed Extract (Vitis vinifera)
- Curcumin
- Garlic (Allium sativum)
- Ginkgo Extract (Ginkgo biloba)
- Quercetin
- Rutin
- Clove (Syzygium aromaticum)
- Allspice (Pimenta dioica)
- Sweet Basil (Ocimum basilicum)
- Sage (Salvia officinalis)
- Rosemary Extract (Rosmarinus officinalis)
- Lutein
- Lycopene
- Trans Resveratrol
- Vitamin A
- Vitamin E
- L-glutathione
- NAC (N-Acetyl-L-Cysteine)
- Broccoli Powder Extract
- Sulforaphane
- Olive Leaf Extract (Olea europaea)
- Bergamot
- Red Grape Powder
- Alpha Lipoic Acid
- Taurine
- MVM (Multi-vitamin/mineral)
- Glutathione (reduced)

Hemoglobin A1C

Hemoglobin A1C measures the glycosylation of red blood cells (RBCs) over the past 3-4 months, making it a key marker for diabetes risk. Hemoglobin A1C, or glycohemoglobin, forms when glucose binds with hemoglobin over an RBC's lifespan (approximately 120 days). High blood glucose (hyperglycemia) results in increased glycohemoglobin and elevated Hemoglobin A1C levels. Stable blood sugar is essential for a healthy immune response and maintaining immune function.

Normal Range	4.8 - 5.5%
Optimal Range	4.1 - 5.3%

If **LOW** or **< 4.1%:**

 Low Hemoglobin A1C may suggest hypoglycemia, liver storage dysfunction, or a high degree of insulin sensitivity.

Increase protein and fat intake.
Regularly monitor glucose handling at intervals throughout the day.
Consider Chromium GTF to enhance insulin action.

Lifestyle Recommendations:
- Avoid stress, incorporate relaxation, and avoid alcohol and stimulants (caffeine).
- Follow a balanced exercise program with high-intensity, short bursts.
- Stay hydrated, get adequate sleep, and avoid exposure to chemicals/toxins.

Dietary Tips:
- Increase fiber to slow carb absorption
- Eat small, balanced meals and snacks with healthy fats and proteins.
- Focus on omega-3 fatty acids, dark leafy greens, and monounsaturated fats like olive oil.

Glucose Metabolism Support:
- Magnesium
- Zinc
- Selenium
- Manganese
- Chromium
- Molybdenum
- Potassium Iodide
- Taurine
- Carnosine
- R-Lipoic Acid
- Vitamin A
- Vitamin D3
- Vitamin E
- Vitamin K1
- Benfotiamine (Fat-Soluble Vitamin B1)
- Vitamin B1
- Vitamin B2
- Vitamin B3
- Vitamin B5
- Vitamin B6
- Vitamin B7 (Biotin)
- Vitamin B9 (Folate)
- Vitamin B12
- Vitamin C
- Berberine
- Fenugreek
- Gymnema sylvestre
- Banaba (Lagerstroemia speciosa)
- Kudzu (Pueraria lobata)
- Cinnamon
- Inositol (as Myo and D-Chiro)
- Alpha Lipoic Acid
- MVM (Multi-vitamin/mineral)

Adrenal Support:
- gamma-Aminobutyric Acid (GABA)
- Eleutherococcus senticosus
- American Ginseng
- Ashwagandha
- Rhodiola
- Licorice
- Vitamin B2
- Vitamin B5
- Vitamin B6
- Vitamin C
- N-Acetyl-L-Tyrosine
- Phosphatidylserine
- Valerian
- Passion Flower
- Lemon Balm
- Chamomile
- L-theanine
- 5-HTP
- Melatonin
- Rhodiola rosea
- Pyrroloquinoline Quinone (PQQ)
- Taurine
- Vitamin B1
- Vitamin B12
- Magnesium Malate
- Magnesium Taurinate
- Magnesium Glycinate

If **HIGH** or **> 5.3%**:

SUGAR PANEL

 Elevated Hemoglobin A1C may indicate insulin resistance or diabetes. Elevated fasting insulin can signal insulin resistance years before A1C elevation.

 Consider insulin resistance or early diabetes as possible causes.
Regularly monitor fasting glucose and insulin levels.

Lifestyle Recommendations:
- Reduce stress, incorporate high-intensity interval training, and stay hydrated.
- Prioritize relaxation through meditation, yoga, or prayer.

Dietary Tips:
- Consume a high-protein breakfast, anti-inflammatory diet, and low-glycemic, high-fiber foods.
- Snack on healthy proteins/fats and avoid high-sugar snacks, beverages, and refined carbohydrates.

 Glucose Metabolism Support:
- Magnesium
- Zinc
- Selenium
- Manganese
- Chromium
- Molybdenum
- Potassium Iodide
- Taurine
- Carnosine
- R-Lipoic Acid
- Vitamin A
- Vitamin D3
- Vitamin E
- Vitamin K1
- Benfotiamine (Fat-Soluble Vitamin B1)
- Vitamin B1
- Vitamin B2
- Vitamin B3
- Vitamin B5
- Vitamin B6
- Vitamin B7 (Biotin)
- Vitamin B9 (Folate)
- Vitamin B12
- Vitamin C
- Berberine
- Fenugreek
- Gymnema sylvestre
- Banaba (Lagerstroemia speciosa)
- Kudzu (Pueraria lobata)
- Cinnamon
- Inositol (as Myo and D-Chiro)
- Alpha Lipoic Acid
- MVM (Multi-vitamin/mineral)

Anti-inflammatory Support:
- Phytocannabinoids
- Hemp Flower Extract
- Hemp Seed Oil
- Palmitoylethanolamide (PEA)
- Omega-3 Fatty Acids (Fish Oil)
- docosahexaenoic acid), 14-HDHA (14-hydroxy docosahexaenoic acid)
- Vitamin D3
- Curcumin
- Green Tea Extract (Epigallocatechin Gallate (EGCG))
- Trans Resveratrol
- Quercetin
- Nettle (Urtica dioica)
- Pro-Resolving Mediators (PRMs): 18-HEPE (18-hydroxy eicosapentaenoic acid), 17-HDHA (17-hydroxy

High Dose Probiotics:
- Multi-strain probiotic blend
- Saccharomyces boulardii
- Beta Glucans
- Lactobacillus plantarum strain L-137 (HK L-137)
- Xylooligosaccharide (XOS)

Antioxidant Support:
- Acerola Extract (Malpighia glabra)
- Grape Seed Extract (Vitis vinifera)

- Curcumin
- Garlic (Allium sativum)
- Ginkgo Extract (Ginkgo biloba)
- Quercetin
- Rutin
- Clove (Syzygium aromaticum)
- Allspice (Pimenta dioica)
- Sweet Basil (Ocimum basilicum)
- Sage (Salvia officinalis)
- Rosemary Extract (Rosmarinus officinalis)
- Lutein
- Lycopene
- Trans Resveratrol
- Vitamin A
- Vitamin E
- L-glutathione
- NAC (N-Acetyl-L-Cysteine)
- Broccoli Powder Extract
- Sulforaphane
- Olive Leaf Extract (Olea europaea)
- Bergamot
- Red Grape Powder
- Alpha Lipoic Acid
- Taurine
- MVM (Multi-vitamin/mineral)
- Glutathione (reduced)

Fasting Insulin

Insulin is a hormone that regulates blood glucose levels by transporting and storing glucose in cells. Elevated fasting insulin levels can indicate insulin resistance or poor blood glucose control, which may lead to Type 2 diabetes. Insulin resistance can develop long before blood glucose levels reflect an issue, making fasting insulin a valuable early indicator.

Normal Range	2.6 - 24.9 uIU/mL
Optimal Range	4.6 - 5.5 uIU/mL

If **LOW** or < 4.6 uIU/mL:

Low fasting insulin levels in non-diabetic individuals are generally not clinically significant. However, in patients with diabetes, low insulin may indicate Type 1 diabetes or late-stage Type 2 diabetes due to insufficient beta cell function. Low levels can also result from pancreatic issues, autoimmune destruction, or chronic pancreatitis.

Low insulin may indicate Type 1 diabetes if the patient requires insulin replacement for glucose processing. In such cases, insulin administration might be necessary. Elevated insulin-like growth factor (IGF) levels could be indicative of certain non-beta cell tumors.

Glucose Metabolism Support:
- Magnesium
- Zinc
- Selenium
- Manganese
- Chromium
- Molybdenum
- Potassium Iodide
- Taurine
- Carnosine
- R-Lipoic Acid
- Vitamin A
- Vitamin D3
- Vitamin E
- Vitamin K1
- Benfotiamine (Fat-Soluble Vitamin B1)
- Vitamin B1
- Vitamin B2
- Vitamin B3
- Vitamin B5
- Vitamin B6
- Vitamin B7 (Biotin)
- Vitamin B9 (Folate)
- Vitamin B12
- Vitamin C
- Berberine
- Fenugreek
- Gymnema sylvestre
- Banaba (Lagerstroemia speciosa)

- Kudzu (Pueraria lobata)
- Cinnamon
- Inositol (as Myo and D-Chiro)

Adrenal Support:
- gamma-Aminobutyric Acid (GABA)
- Eleutherococcus senticosus
- American Ginseng
- Ashwagandha
- Rhodiola
- Licorice
- Vitamin B2
- Vitamin B5
- Vitamin B6
- Vitamin C
- N-Acetyl-L-Tyrosine
- Phosphatidylserine
- Valerian
- Passion Flower
- Alpha Lipoic Acid
- MVM (Multi-vitamin/mineral)
- Lemon Balm
- Chamomile
- L-theanine
- 5-HTP
- Melatonin
- Rhodiola rosea
- Pyrroloquinoline Quinone (PQQ)
- Taurine
- Vitamin B1
- Vitamin B12
- Magnesium Malate
- Magnesium Taurinate
- Magnesium Glycinate

If **HIGH** or > 5.5 uIU/mL:

 Elevated fasting insulin levels may indicate early insulin resistance, obesity, steroid use, or endocrine disorders such as Cushing syndrome and acromegaly. High insulin levels can also result from insulin-secreting tumors or excessive administration of insulin or insulin secretagogues. Elevated levels of insulin in the context of normal or high blood glucose could suggest insulin resistance, a precursor to Type 2 diabetes and metabolic syndrome.

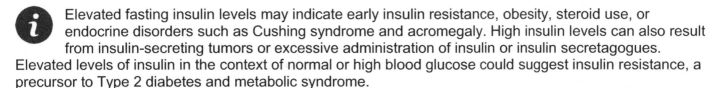 High fasting insulin levels, often associated with insulin resistance, indicate an increased risk for Type 2 diabetes, hypertension, and cardiovascular disease. Conditions like Type 2 diabetes and insulinoma (insulin-secreting tumors) also feature high insulin levels.

Lifestyle Recommendations:
- Diet: Implement a blood sugar-balancing diet, such as keto or low-carb, high-fat (LCHF).
- Exercise: Regular physical activity can improve insulin sensitivity.
- Sleep & Stress Management: Adequate sleep and stress reduction techniques support balanced insulin levels.

 Glucose Metabolism Support:
- Magnesium
- Zinc
- Selenium
- Manganese
- Chromium
- Molybdenum
- Potassium Iodide
- Taurine
- Carnosine
- R-Lipoic Acid
- Vitamin A
- Vitamin D3
- Vitamin E
- Vitamin K1
- Benfotiamine (Fat-Soluble Vitamin B1)
- Vitamin B1
- Vitamin B2
- Vitamin B3
- Vitamin B5
- Vitamin B6
- Vitamin B7 (Biotin)
- Vitamin B9 (Folate)
- Vitamin B12
- Vitamin C
- Berberine
- Fenugreek
- Gymnema sylvestre
- Banaba (Lagerstroemia speciosa)

- Kudzu (Pueraria lobata)
- Cinnamon
- Inositol (as Myo and D-Chiro)
- Alpha Lipoic Acid
- MVM (Multi-vitamin/mineral)

Anti-inflammatory Support:
- Phytocannabinoids
- Hemp Flower Extract
- Hemp Seed Oil
- Palmitoylethanolamide (PEA)
- Omega-3 Fatty Acids (Fish Oil)
- docosahexaenoic acid), 14-HDHA (14-hydroxy docosahexaenoic acid)
- Vitamin D3
- Curcumin
- Green Tea Extract (Epigallocatechin Gallate (EGCG))
- Trans Resveratrol
- Quercetin
- Nettle (Urtica dioica)
- Pro-Resolving Mediators (PRMs): 18-HEPE (18-hydroxy eicosapentaenoic acid), 17-HDHA (17-hydroxy

High Dose Probiotics:
- Multi-strain probiotic blend
- Saccharomyces boulardii
- Beta Glucans
- Lactobacillus plantarum strain L-137 (HK L-137)
- Xylooligosaccharide (XOS)

Antioxidant Support:
- Acerola Extract (Malpighia glabra)
- Grape Seed Extract (Vitis vinifera)
- Curcumin
- Garlic (Allium sativum)
- Ginkgo Extract (Ginkgo biloba)
- Quercetin
- Rutin
- Clove (Syzygium aromaticum)
- Allspice (Pimenta dioica)
- Sweet Basil (Ocimum basilicum)
- Sage (Salvia officinalis)
- Rosemary Extract (Rosmarinus officinalis)
- Lutein
- Lycopene
- Trans Resveratrol
- Vitamin A
- Vitamin E
- L-glutathione
- NAC (N-Acetyl-L-Cysteine)
- Broccoli Powder Extract
- Sulforaphane
- Olive Leaf Extract (Olea europaea)
- Bergamot
- Red Grape Powder
- Alpha Lipoic Acid
- Taurine
- MVM (Multi-vitamin/mineral)
- Glutathione (reduced)

C-Peptide

C-Peptide, or Connecting Peptide, is produced by β-cells of the pancreas alongside insulin. It provides an accurate measure of insulin production, particularly helpful in patients receiving insulin medication. Since C-peptide remains in the body longer than insulin, it is often a better indicator of insulin levels. This test is useful to show how much insulin the body produces naturally.

Normal Range	1.1 - 4.4 ng/mL
Optimal Range	1.1 - 4.4 ng/mL

If **LOW** or **< 1.1 ng/mL:**

SUGAR PANEL

 Low C-peptide levels may indicate insulin deficiency, which could be associated with Type 1 diabetes, Addison's disease, or liver disease. It could also suggest that diabetes treatment isn't effectively managing blood sugar levels.

 Decreased C-peptide levels may result from conditions such as starvation, hypoglycemia, Addison's disease, or post-pancreatectomy.
Insulin medication may be necessary for diabetic patients with low levels.

Lifestyle Recommendations:
- Patients should refrain from biotin supplementation (if over 5 mg/day) at least 3 days before testing as it may interfere with results.

 Glucose Metabolism Support:
- Magnesium
- Zinc
- Selenium
- Manganese
- Chromium
- Molybdenum
- Potassium Iodide
- Taurine
- Carnosine
- R-Lipoic Acid
- Vitamin A
- Vitamin D3
- Vitamin E
- Vitamin K1
- Benfotiamine (Fat-Soluble Vitamin B1)
- Vitamin B1
- Vitamin B2
- Vitamin B3
- Vitamin B5
- Vitamin B6
- Vitamin B7 (Biotin)
- Vitamin B9 (Folate)
- Vitamin B12
- Vitamin C
- Berberine
- Fenugreek
- Gymnema sylvestre
- Banaba (Lagerstroemia speciosa)
- Kudzu (Pueraria lobata)
- Cinnamon
- Inositol (as Myo and D-Chiro)
- Alpha Lipoic Acid
- MVM (Multi-vitamin/mineral)

Adrenal Support:
- gamma-Aminobutyric Acid (GABA)
- Eleutherococcus senticosus
- American Ginseng
- Ashwagandha
- Rhodiola
- Licorice
- Vitamin B2
- Vitamin B5
- Vitamin B6
- Vitamin C
- N-Acetyl-L-Tyrosine
- Phosphatidylserine
- Valerian
- Passion Flower
- Lemon Balm
- Chamomile
- L-theanine
- 5-HTP
- Melatonin
- Rhodiola rosea
- Pyrroloquinoline Quinone (PQQ)
- Taurine
- Vitamin B1
- Vitamin B12
- Magnesium Malate
- Magnesium Taurinate
- Magnesium Glycinate

If **HIGH** or > 4.4 ng/mL:

 High C-peptide levels may indicate Type 2 diabetes, insulin resistance, obesity, or Cushing's syndrome. Elevated levels may also suggest a pancreatic tumor.

Elevated C-peptide is associated with hyperinsulinemia, insulin resistance, and renal insufficiency.

Lifestyle Recommendations:
- Adopt lifestyle modifications, exercise, and stress management.
- Follow a blood sugar balancing diet, such as keto or low-carb, high-fat (LCHF) diets.

 Glucose Metabolism Support:
- Magnesium
- Zinc
- Selenium
- Manganese
- Chromium
- Molybdenum
- Potassium Iodide
- Taurine
- Carnosine
- R-Lipoic Acid
- Vitamin A
- Vitamin D3
- Vitamin E
- Vitamin K1
- Benfotiamine (Fat-Soluble Vitamin B1)
- Vitamin B1
- Vitamin B2
- Vitamin B3
- Vitamin B5
- Vitamin B6
- Vitamin B7 (Biotin)
- Vitamin B9 (Folate)
- Vitamin B12
- Vitamin C
- Berberine
- Fenugreek
- Gymnema sylvestre
- Banaba (Lagerstroemia speciosa)
- Kudzu (Pueraria lobata)
- Cinnamon
- Inositol (as Myo and D-Chiro)
- Alpha Lipoic Acid
- MVM (Multi-vitamin/mineral)

Anti-inflammatory Support:
- Phytocannabinoids
- Hemp Flower Extract
- Hemp Seed Oil
- Palmitoylethanolamide (PEA)
- Omega-3 Fatty Acids (Fish Oil)
- docosahexaenoic acid), 14-HDHA (14-hydroxy docosahexaenoic acid)
- Vitamin D3
- Curcumin
- Green Tea Extract (Epigallocatechin Gallate (EGCG))
- Trans Resveratrol
- Quercetin
- Nettle (Urtica dioica)
- Pro-Resolving Mediators (PRMs): 18-HEPE (18-hydroxy eicosapentaenoic acid), 17-HDHA (17-hydroxy

High Dose Probiotics:
- Multi-strain probiotic blend
- Saccharomyces boulardii
- Beta Glucans
- Lactobacillus plantarum strain L-137 (HK L-137)
- Xylooligosaccharide (XOS)

Antioxidant Support:
- Acerola Extract (Malpighia glabra)
- Grape Seed Extract (Vitis vinifera)
- Curcumin
- Garlic (Allium sativum)
- Ginkgo Extract (Ginkgo biloba)
- Quercetin
- Rutin
- Clove (Syzygium aromaticum)
- Allspice (Pimenta dioica)
- Sweet Basil (Ocimum basilicum)
- Sage (Salvia officinalis)
- Rosemary Extract (Rosmarinus officinalis)
- Lutein
- Lycopene
- Trans Resveratrol
- Vitamin A
- Vitamin E
- L-glutathione
- NAC (N-Acetyl-L-Cysteine)
- Broccoli Powder Extract
- Sulforaphane

SUGAR PANEL

- Olive Leaf Extract (Olea europaea)
- Bergamot
- Red Grape Powder
- Alpha Lipoic Acid
- Taurine
- MVM (Multi-vitamin/mineral)
- Glutathione (reduced)

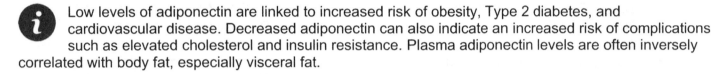

Adiponectin

Normal Range	2.5 - 12.3 µg/mL
Optimal Range	2.5 - 12.3 µg/mL

If LOW or < 2.5 µg/mL:

Low levels of adiponectin are linked to increased risk of obesity, Type 2 diabetes, and cardiovascular disease. Decreased adiponectin can also indicate an increased risk of complications such as elevated cholesterol and insulin resistance. Plasma adiponectin levels are often inversely correlated with body fat, especially visceral fat.

Low adiponectin is associated with insulin resistance, Type 2 diabetes, and could contribute to obesity-related conditions.
It may play a role in atherogenesis, endothelial function, and vascular remodeling.

Lifestyle Recommendations:
- Incorporate weight loss, physical exercise, and a healthy diet to increase adiponectin.
- Avoid smoking and practice stress management for improved insulin sensitivity.

Glucose Metabolism Support:
- Magnesium
- Zinc
- Selenium
- Manganese
- Chromium
- Molybdenum
- Potassium Iodide
- Taurine
- Carnosine
- R-Lipoic Acid
- Vitamin A
- Vitamin D3
- Vitamin E
- Vitamin K1
- Benfotiamine (Fat-Soluble Vitamin B1)
- Vitamin B1
- Vitamin B2
- Vitamin B3
- Vitamin B5
- Vitamin B6
- Vitamin B7 (Biotin)
- Vitamin B9 (Folate)
- Vitamin B12
- Vitamin C
- Berberine
- Fenugreek
- Gymnema sylvestre
- Banaba (Lagerstroemia speciosa)
- Kudzu (Pueraria lobata)
- Cinnamon
- Inositol (as Myo and D-Chiro)
- Alpha Lipoic Acid
- MVM (Multi-vitamin/mineral)

Anti-inflammatory Support:
- Phytocannabinoids
- Hemp Flower Extract
- Hemp Seed Oil
- Palmitoylethanolamide (PEA)
- Omega-3 Fatty Acids (Fish Oil)
- docosahexaenoic acid), 14-HDHA (14-hydroxy docosahexaenoic acid)
- Vitamin D3
- Curcumin

- Green Tea Extract (Epigallocatechin Gallate (EGCG))
- Trans Resveratrol
- Quercetin

High Dose Probiotics:
- Multi-strain probiotic blend
- Saccharomyces boulardii
- Beta Glucans

Antioxidant Support:
- Acerola Extract (Malpighia glabra)
- Grape Seed Extract (Vitis vinifera)
- Curcumin
- Garlic (Allium sativum)
- Ginkgo Extract (Ginkgo biloba)
- Quercetin
- Rutin
- Clove (Syzygium aromaticum)
- Allspice (Pimenta dioica)
- Sweet Basil (Ocimum basilicum)
- Sage (Salvia officinalis)
- Rosemary Extract (Rosmarinus officinalis)
- Lutein
- Lycopene
- Nettle (Urtica dioica)
- Pro-Resolving Mediators (PRMs): 18-HEPE (18-hydroxy eicosapentaenoic acid), 17-HDHA (17-hydroxy
- Lactobacillus plantarum strain L-137 (HK L-137)
- Xylooligosaccharide (XOS)
- Trans Resveratrol
- Vitamin A
- Vitamin E
- L-glutathione
- NAC (N-Acetyl-L-Cysteine)
- Broccoli Powder Extract
- Sulforaphane
- Olive Leaf Extract (Olea europaea)
- Bergamot
- Red Grape Powder
- Alpha Lipoic Acid
- Taurine
- MVM (Multi-vitamin/mineral)
- Glutathione (reduced)

If **HIGH** or > 12.3 μg/mL:

High adiponectin levels are generally associated with a lower risk of heart disease and certain cancers, but may predict rheumatoid arthritis development in obese individuals.

Elevated adiponectin levels can reduce risk for heart disease and certain cancers, such as prostate cancer.
High adiponectin levels may indicate reduced inflammation and potentially support cardiovascular health.

Lifestyle Recommendations:
- Implement a heart-healthy lifestyle with an anti-inflammatory diet, proper sleep, regular exercise, and stress management.
- Limit sugar, processed foods, and refined carbohydrates, and incorporate healthy fats.

Anti-inflammatory Support:
- Phytocannabinoids
- Hemp Flower Extract
- Hemp Seed Oil
- Palmitoylethanolamide (PEA)
- Omega-3 Fatty Acids (Fish Oil)
- Vitamin D3
- Curcumin
- Green Tea Extract (Epigallocatechin Gallate (EGCG))
- Trans Resveratrol
- Quercetin
- Nettle (Urtica dioica)
- Pro-Resolving Mediators (PRMs): 18-HEPE (18-hydroxy eicosapentaenoic acid), 17-HDHA (17-hydroxy docosahexaenoic acid), 14-HDHA (14-hydroxy docosahexaenoic acid)

Antioxidant Support:
- Acerola Extract (Malpighia glabra)
- Grape Seed Extract (Vitis vinifera)
- Curcumin
- Garlic (Allium sativum)
- Ginkgo Extract (Ginkgo biloba)
- Quercetin
- Rutin
- Clove (Syzygium aromaticum)
- Allspice (Pimenta dioica)
- Sweet Basil (Ocimum basilicum)
- Sage (Salvia officinalis)
- Rosemary Extract (Rosmarinus officinalis)
- Lutein
- Lycopene
- Trans Resveratrol
- Vitamin A
- Vitamin E
- L-glutathione
- NAC (N-Acetyl-L-Cysteine)
- Broccoli Powder Extract
- Sulforaphane
- Olive Leaf Extract (Olea europaea)
- Bergamot
- Red Grape Powder
- Alpha Lipoic Acid
- Taurine
- MVM (Multi-vitamin/mineral)
- Glutathione (reduced)

Lipid Support (high):
- Red Yeast Rice (Monascus purpureus)
- Coenzyme Q10
- Sweet Orange (Citrus sinensis)
- Quercetin
- Gotu Kola (Centella asiatica)
- Horse Chestnut (Aesculus hippocastanum)
- Grape Seed Extract (Vitis vinifera)
- Vitamin C
- Plant Sterols/Stanols (Beta-Sitosterol, Campesterol, Campestanol, Sitostanol)
- Monostroma nitidum (seaweed) extract

Homeostasis Model of Insulin Resistance (HOMA-IR)

HOMA-IR is a standard measure for assessing insulin resistance using fasting insulin and glucose levels. This test helps evaluate insulin sensitivity and potential risks of impaired glucose tolerance and diabetes. The model is a convenient alternative to the more resource-intensive "clamp" method. It provides an estimate of insulin resistance that can assist in clinical decision-making for metabolic health.

Homeostasis Model of Insulin Resistance (HOMA-IR) is calculated by multiplying fasting insulin (uU/ml) by fasting glucose (mg/dL) and then dividing the result by 401.85.

Normal Range	0.4 - 2.4
Optimal Range	< 2.0

If HIGH or > 2.0 md/dL:

A HOMA-IR result > 3.0 indicates the presence of insulin resistance and a heightened risk for conditions like coronary heart disease, stroke, peripheral vascular disease, Type 2 diabetes, hypertension, and hyperlipidemia.

Insulin resistance increases risks of cardiovascular diseases and metabolic disorders. Management focuses on improving insulin sensitivity and reducing inflammation.

Lifestyle Recommendations:
- Reduce stress: Set boundaries for emotional health.
- Increase physical activity: Incorporate high-intensity interval training (HIIT) with approval, alongside aerobic and resistance exercises.
- Stay hydrated: Drink plenty of filtered water daily.
- Practice relaxation: Use meditation, yoga, or biofeedback.

Dietary Tips:
- High protein breakfast: Eat within 2 hours of waking to stabilize blood glucose.
- Anti-inflammatory diet: Incorporate omega-3-rich foods, nuts, seeds, and fatty fish.
- Low glycemic foods: Focus on fiber-rich vegetables and low-sugar fruits (e.g., berries, apples, plums).
- Avoid high-sugar foods: Limit sodas, processed fruit juices, and refined carbs.
- Balanced meals: Include snacks with healthy fats and proteins; avoid starchy, high-glycemic foods.

Glucose Metabolism Support:
- Magnesium
- Zinc
- Selenium
- Manganese
- Chromium
- Molybdenum
- Potassium Iodide
- Taurine
- Carnosine
- R-Lipoic Acid
- Vitamin A
- Vitamin D3
- Vitamin E
- Vitamin K1
- Benfotiamine (Fat-Soluble Vitamin B1)
- Vitamin B1
- Vitamin B2
- Vitamin B3
- Vitamin B5
- Vitamin B6
- Vitamin B7 (Biotin)
- Vitamin B9 (Folate)
- Vitamin B12
- Vitamin C
- Berberine
- Fenugreek
- Gymnema sylvestre
- Banaba (Lagerstroemia speciosa)
- Kudzu (Pueraria lobata)
- Cinnamon
- Inositol (as Myo and D-Chiro)
- Alpha Lipoic Acid
- MVM (Multi-vitamin/mineral)

Anti-inflammatory Support:
- Phytocannabinoids
- Hemp Flower Extract
- Hemp Seed Oil
- Palmitoylethanolamide (PEA)
- Omega-3 Fatty Acids (Fish Oil)
- docosahexaenoic acid), 14-HDHA (14-hydroxy docosahexaenoic acid)
- Vitamin D3
- Curcumin
- Green Tea Extract (Epigallocatechin Gallate (EGCG))
- Trans Resveratrol
- Quercetin
- Nettle (Urtica dioica)
- Pro-Resolving Mediators (PRMs): 18-HEPE (18-hydroxy eicosapentaenoic acid), 17-HDHA (17-hydroxy

High Dose Probiotics:
- Multi-strain probiotic blend
- Saccharomyces boulardii
- Beta Glucans
- Lactobacillus plantarum strain L-137 (HK L-137)
- Xylooligosaccharide (XOS)

Antioxidant Support:
- Acerola Extract (Malpighia glabra)
- Grape Seed Extract (Vitis vinifera)

- Curcumin
- Garlic (Allium sativum)
- Ginkgo Extract (Ginkgo biloba)
- Quercetin
- Rutin
- Clove (Syzygium aromaticum)
- Allspice (Pimenta dioica)
- Sweet Basil (Ocimum basilicum)
- Sage (Salvia officinalis)
- Rosemary Extract (Rosmarinus officinalis)
- Lutein
- Lycopene
- Trans Resveratrol
- Vitamin A
- Vitamin E
- L-glutathione
- NAC (N-Acetyl-L-Cysteine)
- Broccoli Powder Extract
- Sulforaphane
- Olive Leaf Extract (Olea europaea)
- Bergamot
- Red Grape Powder
- Alpha Lipoic Acid
- Taurine
- MVM (Multi-vitamin/mineral)
- Glutathione (reduced)

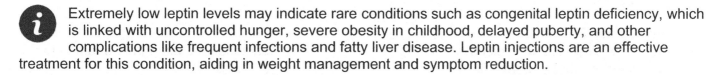

Leptin

Leptin is a hormone produced by fat cells that regulates appetite and energy balance. It signals the brain to stop eating once fat stores are sufficient. Blood levels of leptin generally correlate with body fat levels. High leptin levels typically reduce appetite and increase energy expenditure, while low leptin levels may lead to increased appetite. Issues such as leptin resistance—where the brain doesn't respond to leptin signals—are associated with obesity and its complications, including diabetes and cardiovascular diseases.

Normal Range	0.3 - 13.4 ng/mL
Optimal Range	4.1 - 5.3 ng/mL

If **LOW** or < 4.1 ng/mL:

 Extremely low leptin levels may indicate rare conditions such as congenital leptin deficiency, which is linked with uncontrolled hunger, severe obesity in childhood, delayed puberty, and other complications like frequent infections and fatty liver disease. Leptin injections are an effective treatment for this condition, aiding in weight management and symptom reduction.

 A deficiency in leptin can lead to issues like hypogonadism, growth hormone deficiency, and thyroid dysfunction due to the hormone's influence on the hypothalamic-pituitary axis.

If **HIGH** or > 5.3 ng/mL:

 Elevated leptin levels are common in obesity due to leptin resistance, where the brain does not respond to leptin's satiety signal, causing overeating. This condition is similar to insulin resistance in diabetes, where excess insulin does not lower blood glucose effectively.

 Factors such as inflammation, elevated triglycerides, and a diet high in processed foods contribute to leptin resistance. Managing leptin resistance may help reduce obesity-related risks.

Lifestyle Recommendations:
- Exercise: Regular physical activity can improve leptin sensitivity.
- Diet: Include more proteins, soluble fibers, and reduce processed carbohydrates and high-fat foods to lower inflammation and improve satiety.
- Sleep: Ensure adequate sleep to regulate leptin levels.

- Weight management: Work toward achieving a healthy weight to reduce leptin resistance.

Glucose Metabolism Support:
- Magnesium
- Zinc
- Selenium
- Manganese
- Chromium
- Molybdenum
- Potassium Iodide
- Taurine
- Carnosine
- R-Lipoic Acid
- Vitamin A
- Vitamin D3
- Vitamin E
- Vitamin K1
- Benfotiamine (Fat-Soluble Vitamin B1)
- Vitamin B1
- Vitamin B2
- Vitamin B3
- Vitamin B5
- Vitamin B6
- Vitamin B7 (Biotin)
- Vitamin B9 (Folate)
- Vitamin B12
- Vitamin C
- Berberine
- Fenugreek
- Gymnema sylvestre
- Banaba (Lagerstroemia speciosa)
- Kudzu (Pueraria lobata)
- Cinnamon
- Inositol (as Myo and D-Chiro)
- Alpha Lipoic Acid
- MVM (Multi-vitamin/mineral)

Anti-inflammatory Support:
- Phytocannabinoids
- Hemp Flower Extract
- Hemp Seed Oil
- Palmitoylethanolamide (PEA)
- Omega-3 Fatty Acids (Fish Oil)
- docosahexaenoic acid), 14-HDHA (14-hydroxy docosahexaenoic acid)
- Vitamin D3
- Curcumin
- Green Tea Extract (Epigallocatechin Gallate (EGCG))
- Trans Resveratrol
- Quercetin
- Nettle (Urtica dioica)
- Pro-Resolving Mediators (PRMs): 18-HEPE (18-hydroxy eicosapentaenoic acid), 17-HDHA (17-hydroxy

High Dose Probiotics:
- Multi-strain probiotic blend
- Saccharomyces boulardii
- Beta Glucans
- Lactobacillus plantarum strain L-137 (HK L-137)
- Xylooligosaccharide (XOS)

Antioxidant Support:
- Acerola Extract (Malpighia glabra)
- Grape Seed Extract (Vitis vinifera)
- Curcumin
- Garlic (Allium sativum)
- Ginkgo Extract (Ginkgo biloba)
- Quercetin
- Rutin
- Clove (Syzygium aromaticum)
- Allspice (Pimenta dioica)
- Sweet Basil (Ocimum basilicum)
- Sage (Salvia officinalis)
- Rosemary Extract (Rosmarinus officinalis)
- Lutein
- Lycopene
- Trans Resveratrol
- Vitamin A
- Vitamin E
- L-glutathione
- NAC (N-Acetyl-L-Cysteine)
- Broccoli Powder Extract
- Sulforaphane
- Olive Leaf Extract (Olea europaea)
- Bergamot
- Red Grape Powder
- Alpha Lipoic Acid
- Taurine
- MVM (Multi-vitamin/mineral)
- Glutathione (reduced)

Thyroid

The evaluation of thyroid gland function and the diagnosis and monitoring of thyroid disorders can be facilitated through a thyroid panel, which utilizes a blood sample.

TSH (Thyroid Stimulating Hormone)

TSH is a hormone produced by the anterior pituitary gland that stimulates thyroid hormone production. TSH levels are regulated by the hypothalamus, which releases thyrotropin-releasing hormone (TRH) to maintain a balanced thyroid function cascade. When thyroid hormones decrease, TSH increases, and vice versa. This test screens for thyroid function but can sometimes be insufficient alone due to variations in individual metabolism and influences on TSH levels. Cholesterol often inversely correlates with thyroid function, and liver health is crucial for proper thyroid activity.

Normal Range	0.45 - 4.5 uIU/mL
Optimal Range	1.0 - 2.0 uIU/mL

If **LOW** or < 1.0 uIU/mL:

Low TSH may indicate overactive thyroid function (primary hyperthyroidism) or other conditions affecting thyroid activity, potentially due to medication, high cortisol, or heavy metal toxicity.

Low TSH can signal excessive T4 or iodine, hyperthyroidism, or HPA axis issues. Possible conditions include secondary/tertiary hypothyroidism, hyperthyroidism (e.g., Grave's disease), Cushing's, pregnancy, high testosterone, or thyroid nodules.

Dietary and Lifestyle Recommendations:
- Avoid gluten, caffeine, and consider a Paleo or anti-inflammatory diet.
- Address HPA axis function, ensure sleep hygiene, and consider mitochondrial health and thyroid antibody testing.
- Consider addressing leaky gut if autoimmune.

Thyroid Support:
- N-Acetyl-L-Tyrosine
- American Ginseng (Panax quinquefolius)
- Forskolin (Coleus forskohlii)
- Iodine
- Chromium
- Zinc
- Selenium
- Copper
- Manganese
- Vitamin A
- Vitamin B2
- Potassium Iodide
- Myo-Inositol

Herbal Support: Bugleweed herb, Lemon Balm, Motherwort, gamma-Aminobutyric acid (GABA)
- **Immune & Gut Support:** N-Acetyl-L-Cysteine, Milk Thistle, Reishi, Cordyceps, Chinese Skullcap, Schisandra, Burdock Extract, Full spectrum mushroom blend: Reishi Blend, Chaga (Inonotus obliquus), Lion's Mane (Hericium erinaceus), Cordyceps Blend, Maitake (Grifola frondosa), Shiitake (Lentinula edodes), Agaricus (Agaricus blazel), Turkey Tail (Trametes versiocolor), Multi-strain probiotic blend

Energy Support:

- L-Carnitine
- Acetyl-L-Carnitine

Nutritional Support:
- Vitamin A
- Borage oil (GLA - Gamma Linolenic Acid)
- Vitamin D3
- Vitamin K2
- Omega-3 Fatty Acids (fish oil)

If HIGH or > 2.0 uIU/mL:

Elevated TSH often indicates underactive thyroid (primary hypothyroidism) and can be associated with issues like high reverse T3, cortisol dysregulation, estrogen excess, and pregnancy.

High TSH may reflect hypothyroidism, Hashimoto's thyroiditis, iodine deficiency, or factors affecting thyroid hormone uptake and conversion. Conditions like fatty liver, low T3 uptake, mercury exposure, and extreme stress may elevate TSH levels.

Dietary and Lifestyle Recommendations:
- Avoid gluten and caffeine, consider Paleo or anti-inflammatory diets.
- Support HPA axis, sleep, heavy metal detox, and consider thyroid antibody testing.
- Address gut health, zinc, magnesium, and essential vitamins (A, B, C, D) intake.

Thyroid Support:
- N-Acetyl-L-Tyrosine
- American Ginseng (Panax quinquefolius)
- Forskolin (Coleus forskohlii)
- Iodine
- Chromium
- Zinc
- Selenium
- Copper
- Manganese
- Vitamin A
- Vitamin B2
- Potassium Iodide
- Myo-Inositol

Adrenal Support:
- gamma-Aminobutyric Acid (GABA)
- Eleutherococcus senticosus
- American Ginseng
- Ashwagandha
- Rhodiola
- Licorice
- Vitamin B2
- Vitamin B5
- Vitamin B6
- Vitamin C
- N-Acetyl-L-Tyrosine
- Phosphatidylserine
- Valerian
- Passion Flower
- Lemon Balm
- Chamomile
- L-theanine
- 5-HTP
- Melatonin
- Rhodiola rosea
- Pyrroloquinoline Quinone (PQQ)
- Taurine
- Vitamin B1
- Vitamin B12
- Magnesium Malate
- Magnesium Taurinate
- Magnesium Glycinate

- **Immune & Gut Support:** N-Acetyl-L-Cysteine, Milk Thistle, Reishi, Cordyceps, Chinese Skullcap, Schisandra, Burdock Extract, Full spectrum mushroom blend: Reishi Blend, Chaga (Inonotus obliquus), Lion's Mane (Hericium erinaceus), Cordyceps Blend, Maitake (Grifola frondosa), Shiitake (Lentinula edodes), Agaricus (Agaricus blazel), Turkey Tail (Trametes versiocolor), Multi-strain probiotic blend

Nutritional Support:
- Vitamin A
- Borage oil (GLA - Gamma Linolenic Acid)
- Vitamin D3
- Vitamin K2
- Omega-3 Fatty Acids (fish oil)
- Magnesium Citrate
- Vitamin C

Thyroxine (T4), Total

Total T4 measures both bound and free thyroxine in the blood. Estrogen dominance can lead to high total T4 levels without high free T4, potentially misinterpreted as hyperthyroidism. T4 affects TSH, reducing it when T4 is high. Abnormal T4 levels should be assessed alongside TSH and checked for potential issues like mineral deficiencies or liver conversion problems. A well-functioning thyroid supports liver cell stimulation, aiding cholesterol and bile production. Insufficient thyroid hormone can cause systemic cellular decline.

Normal Range	4.5 - 12 ug/dL
Optimal Range	7.5 - 8.1 ug/dL

If LOW or < 7.5 ug/dL:

Low T4 levels suggest hypothyroid conditions or adrenal fatigue, potentially leading to reduced cellular function. Assess liver health, as T4 supports cholesterol synthesis and bile production.

Low total T4 can indicate thyroid gland failure, lack of anterior pituitary stimulation, or adrenal fatigue.

Dietary and Lifestyle Recommendations:
- Eliminate gluten and caffeine, and consider a Paleo or anti-inflammatory diet.
- Focus on HPA axis health, check for leaky gut (especially if autoimmune), ensure adequate sleep, and address any heavy metal burdens.

Thyroid Support:
- N-Acetyl-L-Tyrosine
- American Ginseng (Panax quinquefolius)
- Forskolin (Coleus forskohlii)
- Iodine
- Chromium
- Zinc
- Selenium
- Copper
- Manganese
- Vitamin A
- Vitamin B2
- Potassium Iodide
- Myo-Inositol

Glandular Thyroid Cytotrophin Support (thyroxine free):
- Thyroid Glandular
- Hypothalamus Glandular
- Iodine
- Zinc
- Selenium
- Copper
- Manganese
- N-Acetyl L-Tyrosine

- Thyroid Cytotrophin

Adrenal Support:
- gamma-Aminobutyric Acid (GABA)
- Eleutherococcus senticosus
- American Ginseng
- Ashwagandha
- Rhodiola
- Licorice
- Vitamin B2
- Vitamin B5
- Vitamin B6
- Vitamin C
- N-Acetyl-L-Tyrosine
- Phosphatidylserine
- Valerian
- Passion Flower
- Lemon Balm
- Chamomile
- L-theanine
- 5-HTP
- Melatonin
- Rhodiola rosea
- Pyrroloquinoline Quinone (PQQ)
- Taurine
- Vitamin B1
- Vitamin B12
- Magnesium Malate
- Magnesium Taurinate
- Magnesium Glycinate

- **Immune & Gut Support:** N-Acetyl-L-Cysteine, Milk Thistle, Reishi, Cordyceps, Chinese Skullcap, Schisandra, Burdock Extract, Full spectrum mushroom blend: Reishi Blend, Chaga (Inonotus obliquus), Lion's Mane (Hericium erinaceus), Cordyceps Blend, Maitake (Grifola frondosa), Shiitake (Lentinula edodes), Agaricus (Agaricus blazel), Turkey Tail (Trametes versiocolor), Multi-strain probiotic blend

Nutritional Support:
- Vitamin A
- Borage oil (GLA - Gamma Linolenic Acid)
- Vitamin D3
- Vitamin K2
- Omega-3 Fatty Acids (fish oil)
- Magnesium Citrate
- Vitamin C

If HIGH or > 8.1 ug/dL:

Elevated T4 may indicate an overactive thyroid, requiring monitoring, especially in cases of medication use, pregnancy, or thyroid disorders.

High T4 may signal hyperthyroidism, thyroiditis, or excess thyroid medication. Certain medications can reduce TBG, falsely elevating T4.

Dietary and Lifestyle Recommendations:
- Avoid gluten and caffeine; consider an anti-inflammatory or Paleo diet.
- Focus on HPA axis health, check for leaky gut (especially if autoimmune), ensure sleep hygiene, and monitor for heavy metal accumulation.
- Regularly monitor thyroid antibody levels.

Thyroid Support:
- N-Acetyl-L-Tyrosine
- American Ginseng (Panax quinquefolius)
- Forskolin (Coleus forskohlii)
- Iodine
- Chromium
- Zinc
- Selenium
- Copper
- Manganese

- Vitamin A
- Vitamin B2
- Potassium Iodide
- Myo-Inositol

- **Herbal Support:** Bugleweed herb, Lemon Balm, Motherwort, gamma-Aminobutyric acid (GABA)
- **Immune & Gut Support:** N-Acetyl-L-Cysteine, Milk Thistle, Reishi, Cordyceps, Chinese Skullcap, Schisandra, Burdock Extract, Full spectrum mushroom blend: Reishi Blend, Chaga (Inonotus obliquus), Lion's Mane (Hericium erinaceus), Cordyceps Blend, Maitake (Grifola frondosa), Shiitake (Lentinula edodes), Agaricus (Agaricus blazel), Turkey Tail (Trametes versiocolor), Multi-strain probiotic blend

Energy Support:
- L-Carnitine
- Acetyl-L-Carnitine

Nutritional Support:
- Vitamin A
- Borage oil (GLA - Gamma Linolenic Acid)
- Vitamin D3
- Vitamin K2
- Omega-3 Fatty Acids (fish oil)

T3 (Triiodothyronine), Total

Total T3 measures both the protein-bound (inactive) and free T3 in the blood. Estrogen dominance can cause high total T3 even if free T3 is low. T3 levels are affected by cortisol, which inhibits T4-to-T3 conversion by deactivating 5'-deiodinase. T4 is converted to T3 in the liver, but liver dysfunction can reduce this conversion. Gut bacteria also aid T3 metabolism, so dysbiosis or infections can impair T3 production.

Normal Range	71.0 - 180.0 ng/dL
Optimal Range	90.0 - 168.0 ng/dL

If LOW or < 90.0 ng/dL:

Low T3 levels may lead to fatigue, poor metabolism, and hypothyroid symptoms due to decreased thyroid hormone activity.

Low T3 levels could indicate thyroid gland failure, liver congestion impacting T4-to-T3 conversion, anterior pituitary dysfunction, adrenal fatigue, or high reverse T3 due to toxic metals.

Dietary and Lifestyle Recommendations:
- Avoid gluten and caffeine, and consider a Paleo or anti-inflammatory diet.
- Address liver function, blood sugar, HPA axis health, leaky gut, and monitor for heavy metal exposure.
- Ensure sufficient sleep and mitochondrial health, and check thyroid antibody levels.

Thyroid Support:
- N-Acetyl-L-Tyrosine
- American Ginseng (Panax quinquefolius)
- Forskolin (Coleus forskohlii)
- Iodine
- Chromium
- Zinc
- Selenium
- Copper

- Manganese
- Vitamin A
- Vitamin B2

Adrenal Support:
- gamma-Aminobutyric Acid (GABA)
- Eleutherococcus senticosus
- American Ginseng
- Ashwagandha
- Rhodiola
- Licorice
- Vitamin B2
- Vitamin B5
- Vitamin B6
- Vitamin C
- N-Acetyl-L-Tyrosine
- Phosphatidylserine
- Valerian
- Passion Flower

Liver Support:
- Milk Thistle
- L-methionine
- Taurine
- Inositol
- Ox Bile
- Artichoke
- Beet Powder
- Vitamin A
- Vitamin B6
- Vitamin B12
- Plant protein powder with MVM (multi-vitamin/mineral)

Gut & Glucose Support:
- Multi-strain Probiotic Blend
- Magnesium
- Zinc
- Selenium
- Manganese
- Chromium
- Molybdenum
- Potassium Iodide
- Taurine
- Carnosine
- R-Lipoic Acid
- Vitamin A
- Vitamin D3

Nutritional Support:
- Vitamin A
- Borage oil (GLA - Gamma Linolenic Acid)

- Potassium Iodide
- Myo-Inositol

- Lemon Balm
- Chamomile
- L-theanine
- 5-HTP
- Melatonin
- Rhodiola rosea
- Pyrroloquinoline Quinone (PQQ)
- Taurine
- Vitamin B1
- Vitamin B12
- Magnesium Malate
- Magnesium Taurinate
- Magnesium Glycinate

- L-glutathione
- N-Acetyl-L-Cysteine (NAC)
- Quercetin
- Methylsulfonylmethane (MSM)
- Sodium Sulfate
- Green Tea Extract
- Reishi
- Cordyceps
- Chinese Skullcap
- Schisandra
- Burdock Extract
- Phosphatidylcholine

- Vitamin E
- Vitamin K1
- Benfotiamine (Fat Soluble Vitamin B1)
- Vitamin B1
- Vitamin B2
- Vitamin B3
- Vitamin B5
- Vitamin B6
- Vitamin B7 (Biotin)
- Vitamin B9 (Folate)
- Vitamin B12
- Vitamin C

- Vitamin D3
- Vitamin K2
- Omega-3 Fatty Acids (fish oil)
- Magnesium Citrate
- Vitamin C

If **HIGH** or > 168.0 ng/dL:

Elevated T3 levels may cause symptoms of hyperthyroidism, such as increased heart rate, anxiety, and heat intolerance. If symptoms persist, consider referral to a healthcare provider for potential treatment.

High T3 may result from excessive T4 or iodine intake, thyroid hormone medication, or pregnancy. It is important to monitor as high T3 can lead to hyperthyroid symptoms.

Dietary and Lifestyle Recommendations:
- Remove gluten and caffeine; consider Paleo or anti-inflammatory diet.
- Address HPA axis health, check for leaky gut (especially if autoimmune), ensure sleep hygiene, and monitor for heavy metals.
- Regularly check thyroid antibodies and monitor T3 levels to ensure levels remain stable..

Thyroid Support:
- N-Acetyl-L-Tyrosine
- American Ginseng (Panax quinquefolius)
- Forskolin (Coleus forskohlii)
- Iodine
- Chromium
- Zinc
- Selenium
- Copper
- Manganese
- Vitamin A
- Vitamin B2
- Potassium Iodide
- Myo-Inositol

Adrenal Support:
- gamma-Aminobutyric Acid (GABA)
- Eleutherococcus senticosus
- American Ginseng
- Ashwagandha
- Rhodiola
- Licorice
- Vitamin B2
- Vitamin B5
- Vitamin B6
- Vitamin C
- N-Acetyl-L-Tyrosine
- Phosphatidylserine
- Valerian
- Passion Flower
- Lemon Balm
- Chamomile
- L-theanine
- 5-HTP
- Melatonin
- Rhodiola rosea
- Pyrroloquinoline Quinone (PQQ)
- Taurine
- Vitamin B1
- Vitamin B12
- Magnesium Malate
- Magnesium Taurinate
- Magnesium Glycinate

Immune Support:
- Echinacea angustifolia
- Astragalus membranaceus
- Elderberry Extract (Sambucus nigra)
- Andrographis paniculate
- Green Tea Extract
- Arabinogalactan (larch tree)

- Lauric Acid
- Cordyceps mushroom
- Shiitake mushroom
- Maitake mushroom
- Reishi mushroom
- Beta 1,3 Glucans
- Vitamin A
- Vitamin D3
- Vitamin E
- Vitamin K2
- Wild cherry bark
- Ginger
- Lovage (Levisticum officinale)
- Wild Cherry Extract

Energy & Gut Support:
- L-Carnitine
- Acetyl-L-Carnitine
- Multi-strain probiotic blend

Nutritional Support:
- Vitamin A
- Borage oil (GLA - Gamma Linolenic Acid)
- Vitamin D3
- Vitamin K2
- Omega-3 Fatty Acids (fish oil)

T4, Free (Direct)

Free T4 is the biologically active form of thyroxine in the blood, which is not bound to proteins and is available for conversion to T3 or reverse T3. The level of free T4 provides insight into thyroid function, liver health, and potential thyroid disorders.

Normal Range	0.82 - 1.77 ng/dL
Optimal Range	1.0 - 1.5 ng/dL

If LOW or < 1.0 ng/dL:

Lower-than-optimal levels of free T4 may lead to symptoms of hypothyroidism, such as fatigue, weight gain, and cold intolerance.

Low free T4 may indicate thyroid gland dysfunction, lack of pituitary stimulation, adrenal fatigue, or liver dysfunction affecting T4 conversion.

Dietary and Lifestyle Recommendations:
- Remove gluten and caffeine; consider a Paleo or anti-inflammatory diet.
- Support liver health, balance blood sugar, strengthen the HPA axis, improve sleep hygiene, and address potential heavy metal toxicity.
- Assess and monitor thyroid antibodies, especially if autoimmune thyroid conditions are suspected.

Thyroid Support:
- N-Acetyl-L-Tyrosine
- American Ginseng (Panax quinquefolius)
- Forskolin (Coleus forskohlii)
- Iodine
- Chromium
- Zinc
- Selenium
- Copper
- Manganese

- Vitamin A
- Vitamin B2
- Potassium Iodide
- Myo-Inositol

Adrenal Support:
- gamma-Aminobutyric Acid (GABA)
- Eleutherococcus senticosus
- American Ginseng
- Ashwagandha
- Rhodiola
- Licorice
- Vitamin B2
- Vitamin B5
- Vitamin B6
- Vitamin C
- N-Acetyl-L-Tyrosine
- Phosphatidylserine
- Valerian
- Passion Flower
- Lemon Balm
- Chamomile
- L-theanine
- 5-HTP
- Melatonin
- Rhodiola rosea
- Pyrroloquinoline Quinone (PQQ)
- Taurine
- Vitamin B1
- Vitamin B12
- Magnesium Malate
- Magnesium Taurinate
- Magnesium Glycinate

Liver Support:
- Milk Thistle
- L-methionine
- Taurine
- Inositol
- Ox Bile
- Artichoke
- Beet Powder
- Vitamin A
- Vitamin B6
- Vitamin B12
- Plant protein powder with MVM (multi-vitamin/mineral)
- L-glutathione
- N-Acetyl-L-Cysteine (NAC)
- Quercetin
- Methylsulfonylmethane (MSM)
- Sodium Sulfate
- Green Tea Extract
- Reishi
- Cordyceps
- Chinese Skullcap
- Schisandra
- Burdock Extract
- Phosphatidylcholine

Immune Support:
- Echinacea angustifolia
- Astragalus membranaceus
- Elderberry Extract (Sambucus nigra)
- Andrographis paniculate
- Green Tea Extract
- Arabinogalactan (larch tree)
- Lauric Acid
- Cordyceps mushroom
- Shiitake mushroom
- Maitake mushroom
- Reishi mushroom
- Beta 1,3 Glucans
- Vitamin A
- Vitamin D3
- Vitamin E
- Vitamin K2
- Wild cherry bark
- Ginger
- Lovage (Levisticum officinale)
- Wild Cherry Extract

Gut & Glucose Support:
- Multi-strain Probiotic Blend
- Magnesium
- Zinc
- Selenium
- Manganese
- Chromium
- Molybdenum
- Potassium Iodide
- Taurine
- Carnosine

- R-Lipoic Acid
- Vitamin A
- Vitamin D3
- Vitamin E
- Vitamin K1
- Benfotiamine (Fat Soluble Vitamin B1)
- Vitamin B1
- Vitamin B2
- Vitamin B3
- Vitamin B5
- Vitamin B6
- Vitamin B7 (Biotin)
- Vitamin B9 (Folate)
- Vitamin B12
- Vitamin C

Nutritional Support:
- Vitamin A
- Borage oil (GLA - Gamma Linolenic Acid)
- Vitamin D3
- Vitamin K2
- Omega-3 Fatty Acids (fish oil)
- Magnesium Citrate
- Vitamin C

If **HIGH** or **> 1.5 ng/dL:**

Elevated free T4 may lead to hyperthyroid symptoms, including anxiety, weight loss, increased heart rate, and heat intolerance. Ongoing monitoring and possibly referral for further evaluation are advised if symptoms persist.

High levels of free T4 could be due to excess T4 or iodine intake, thyroid hormone medication, or conditions like hyperthyroidism and thyroiditis. It is essential to monitor closely, as high free T4 can cause hyperthyroid symptoms.

Dietary and Lifestyle Recommendations:
- Avoid gluten and caffeine; consider Paleo or anti-inflammatory diet.
- Address HPA axis health, assess for leaky gut, improve sleep hygiene, and monitor heavy metal levels.
- Monitor thyroid antibody levels to confirm or rule out autoimmune thyroid conditions.

Thyroid Support:
- N-Acetyl-L-Tyrosine
- American Ginseng (Panax quinquefolius)
- Forskolin (Coleus forskohlii)
- Iodine
- Chromium
- Zinc
- Selenium
- Copper
- Manganese
- Vitamin A
- Vitamin B2
- Potassium Iodide
- Myo-Inositol

Adrenal Support:
- gamma-Aminobutyric Acid (GABA)
- Eleutherococcus senticosus
- American Ginseng
- Ashwagandha
- Rhodiola
- Licorice
- Vitamin B2
- Vitamin B5
- Vitamin B6
- Vitamin C
- N-Acetyl-L-Tyrosine
- Phosphatidylserine
- Valerian
- Passion Flower
- Lemon Balm
- Chamomile
- L-theanine
- 5-HTP

- Melatonin
- Rhodiola rosea
- Pyrroloquinoline Quinone (PQQ)
- Taurine
- Vitamin B1
- Vitamin B12
- Magnesium Malate
- Magnesium Taurinate
- Magnesium Glycinate

Immune Support:
- Echinacea angustifolia
- Astragalus membranaceus
- Elderberry Extract (Sambucus nigra)
- Andrographis paniculate
- Green Tea Extract
- Arabinogalactan (larch tree)
- Lauric Acid
- Cordyceps mushroom
- Shiitake mushroom
- Maitake mushroom
- Reishi mushroom
- Beta 1,3 Glucans
- Vitamin A
- Vitamin D3
- Vitamin E
- Vitamin K2
- Wild cherry bark
- Ginger
- Lovage (Levisticum officinale)
- Wild Cherry Extract

Energy & Gut Support:
- L-Carnitine
- Acetyl-L-Carnitine
- Multi-strain probiotic blend

Nutritional Support:
- Vitamin A
- Borage oil (GLA - Gamma Linolenic Acid)
- Vitamin D3
- Vitamin K2
- Omega-3 Fatty Acids (fish oil)

T3, Free, Serum

Free T3 reflects the biologically active form of T3 that supports energy production (ATP). Stable blood sugar is essential for optimal immune function, as imbalances can lead to immune dysfunction. Factors like estrogen dominance and cortisol elevation can affect free T3 levels, while liver and gut health are also critical for T4-to-T3 conversion.

Normal Range	2.0 - 4.4 pg/mL
Optimal Range	3.0 - 3.25 pg/mL

If **LOW** or < 3.0 pg/mL:

Low free T3 can lead to symptoms of hypothyroidism such as low energy, cold sensitivity, and weight gain.

Low free T3 can be due to issues with liver conversion, adrenal fatigue, heavy metal burden, or poor T3 receptor activity. Optimal free T3 levels are critical as free T3 is more biologically active than free T4.

Dietary and Lifestyle Recommendations:
- Remove gluten and caffeine; consider a Paleo or anti-inflammatory diet.
- Address liver health, balance blood sugar, support the HPA axis, improve sleep hygiene, and check for heavy metal toxicity.
- Regularly monitor thyroid antibody levels, especially if autoimmune issues are suspected.

Thyroid Support:
- N-Acetyl-L-Tyrosine
- American Ginseng (Panax quinquefolius)
- Forskolin (Coleus forskohlii)
- Iodine
- Chromium
- Zinc
- Selenium
- Copper
- Manganese
- Vitamin A
- Vitamin B2
- Potassium Iodide
- Myo-Inositol

Adrenal Support:
- gamma-Aminobutyric Acid (GABA)
- Eleutherococcus senticosus
- American Ginseng
- Ashwagandha
- Rhodiola
- Licorice
- Vitamin B2
- Vitamin B5
- Vitamin B6
- Vitamin C
- N-Acetyl-L-Tyrosine
- Phosphatidylserine
- Valerian
- Passion Flower
- Lemon Balm
- Chamomile
- L-theanine
- 5-HTP
- Melatonin
- Rhodiola rosea
- Pyrroloquinoline Quinone (PQQ)
- Taurine
- Vitamin B1
- Vitamin B12
- Magnesium Malate
- Magnesium Taurinate
- Magnesium Glycinate

Liver Support:
- Milk Thistle
- L-methionine
- Taurine
- Inositol
- Ox Bile
- Artichoke
- Beet Powder
- Vitamin A
- Vitamin B6
- Vitamin B12
- Plant protein powder with MVM (multi-vitamin/mineral)
- L-glutathione
- N-Acetyl-L-Cysteine (NAC)
- Quercetin
- Methylsulfonylmethane (MSM)
- Sodium Sulfate
- Green Tea Extract
- Reishi
- Cordyceps
- Chinese Skullcap
- Schisandra
- Burdock Extract
- Phosphatidylcholine

Immune Support:
- Echinacea angustifolia
- Astragalus membranaceus
- Elderberry Extract (Sambucus nigra)
- Andrographis paniculate
- Green Tea Extract
- Arabinogalactan (larch tree)
- Lauric Acid
- Cordyceps mushroom
- Shiitake mushroom
- Maitake mushroom

- Reishi mushroom
- Beta 1,3 Glucans
- Vitamin A
- Vitamin D3
- Vitamin E

Gut & Glucose Support:
- Multi-strain Probiotic Blend
- Magnesium
- Zinc
- Selenium
- Manganese
- Chromium
- Molybdenum
- Potassium Iodide
- Taurine
- Carnosine
- R-Lipoic Acid
- Vitamin A
- Vitamin D3

Nutritional Support:
- Vitamin A
- Borage oil (GLA - Gamma Linolenic Acid)
- Vitamin D3
- Vitamin K2
- Omega-3 Fatty Acids (fish oil)
- Magnesium Citrate
- Vitamin C

- Vitamin K2
- Wild cherry bark
- Ginger
- Lovage (Levisticum officinale)
- Wild Cherry Extract

- Vitamin E
- Vitamin K1
- Benfotiamine (Fat Soluble Vitamin B1)
- Vitamin B1
- Vitamin B2
- Vitamin B3
- Vitamin B5
- Vitamin B6
- Vitamin B7 (Biotin)
- Vitamin B9 (Folate)
- Vitamin B12
- Vitamin C

If **HIGH** or > 3.25 pg/mL:

High free T3 can result in hyperthyroid-like symptoms, such as increased heart rate, heat intolerance, and nervousness. Monitoring with a primary care provider is advised to avoid prolonged hyperthyroid states.

Elevated free T3 may be due to excessive T4 or iodine intake, thyroid hormone therapy, or hyperthyroidism. Careful monitoring is essential as hyperthyroid states can cause symptoms like restlessness, palpitations, and unintended weight loss.

Dietary and Lifestyle Recommendations:
- Avoid gluten and caffeine; consider a Paleo or anti-inflammatory diet.
- Support liver health, address HPA axis function, and improve gut health to manage T4-to-T3 conversion.
- Consider testing thyroid antibodies to rule out autoimmune thyroid conditions.

Thyroid Support:
- N-Acetyl-L-Tyrosine
- American Ginseng (Panax quinquefolius)
- Forskolin (Coleus forskohlii)
- Iodine
- Chromium

- Zinc
- Selenium
- Copper
- Manganese
- Vitamin A
- Vitamin B2

- Potassium Iodide

Adrenal Support:
- gamma-Aminobutyric Acid (GABA)
- Eleutherococcus senticosus
- American Ginseng
- Ashwagandha
- Rhodiola
- Licorice
- Vitamin B2
- Vitamin B5
- Vitamin B6
- Vitamin C
- N-Acetyl-L-Tyrosine
- Phosphatidylserine
- Valerian
- Passion Flower
- Myo-Inositol
- Lemon Balm
- Chamomile
- L-theanine
- 5-HTP
- Melatonin
- Rhodiola rosea
- Pyrroloquinoline Quinone (PQQ)
- Taurine
- Vitamin B1
- Vitamin B12
- Magnesium Malate
- Magnesium Taurinate
- Magnesium Glycinate

Immune Support:
- Echinacea angustifolia
- Astragalus membranaceus
- Elderberry Extract (Sambucus nigra)
- Andrographis paniculate
- Green Tea Extract
- Arabinogalactan (larch tree)
- Lauric Acid
- Cordyceps mushroom
- Shiitake mushroom
- Maitake mushroom
- Reishi mushroom
- Beta 1,3 Glucans
- Vitamin A
- Vitamin D3
- Vitamin E
- Vitamin K2
- Wild cherry bark
- Ginger
- Lovage (Levisticum officinale)
- Wild Cherry Extract

Energy & Gut Support:
- L-Carnitine
- Acetyl-L-Carnitine
- Multi-strain probiotic blend

Nutritional Support:
- Vitamin A
- Borage oil (GLA - Gamma Linolenic Acid)
- Vitamin D3
- Vitamin K2
- Omega-3 Fatty Acids (fish oil)

TPO Thyroid Peroxidase

A normal TPO test result is negative. Elevated TPO antibodies are typically associated with autoimmune thyroid diseases, such as Hashimoto's and Graves' disease, as well as other autoimmune conditions. TPO antibodies may also be influenced by microbiome dysregulation, including the presence of gram-negative bacteria that produce lipopolysaccharide (LPS), an inflammatory mediator that can interfere with thyroid function. Gluten intolerance and blood sugar imbalances are also known contributors to inflammatory and autoimmune conditions.

Normal Range	0 - 34 IU/mL
Optimal Range	0 IU/mL

If POSITIVE or > 34.0 IU/mL:

Elevated TPO antibodies are often associated with autoimmune conditions. However, a negative TPO result does not completely rule out autoimmunity, as some individuals with autoimmune thyroiditis do not produce detectable antibodies at all times. Additionally, TPO antibodies may appear in other autoimmune conditions, such as rheumatoid arthritis, lupus, and Type 1 diabetes.

Elevated TPO antibodies may indicate autoimmune thyroiditis. Testing for Thyroid Stimulating Immunoglobulin (TsIg) can help differentiate Graves' disease from Hashimoto's if other thyroid markers are inconclusive. Symptoms like goiter (thyroid enlargement) are common in both Hashimoto's and Graves' disease, while exophthalmos (protruding eyes) is more specific to Graves' disease.

Dietary and Lifestyle Recommendations:
- Dietary: Consider eliminating gluten and caffeine, and explore a Paleo, anti-inflammatory, or autoimmune diet.
- Lifestyle: Focus on sleep hygiene, HPA axis support, and liver health. Maintain stable blood sugar levels to support immune function and thyroid health.
- Gut Health: Address gut dysbiosis and monitor for gram-negative bacteria that produce LPS. Improve intestinal barrier function to reduce autoimmune triggers.

Thyroid Support:
- N-Acetyl-L-Tyrosine
- American Ginseng (Panax quinquefolius)
- Forskolin (Coleus forskohlii)
- Iodine
- Chromium
- Zinc
- Selenium
- Copper
- Manganese
- Vitamin A
- Vitamin B2
- Potassium Iodide
- Myo-Inositol

Immune Support (if autoimmune):
- Cordyceps
- N-Acetyl-L-Cysteine (NAC)
- Milk Thistle
- Reishi
- Chinese Skullcap
- Schisandra
- Burdock Extract
- Full Spectrum Mushroom Blend:
- Reishi Blend
- Chaga (Inonotus obliquus)
- Lion's Mane (Hericium erinaceus)
- Cordyceps Blend
- Maitake (Grifola frondosa)
- Shiitake (Lentinula edodes)
- Agaricus (Agaricus blazei)
- Turkey Tail (Trametes versicolor)

Adrenal Support:

- gamma-Aminobutyric Acid (GABA)
- Eleutherococcus senticosus
- American Ginseng
- Ashwagandha
- Rhodiola
- Licorice
- Vitamin B2
- Vitamin B5
- Vitamin B6
- Vitamin C
- N-Acetyl-L-Tyrosine
- Phosphatidylserine
- Valerian
- Passion Flower
- Lemon Balm
- Chamomile
- L-theanine
- 5-HTP
- Melatonin
- Rhodiola rosea
- Pyrroloquinoline Quinone (PQQ)
- Taurine
- Vitamin B1
- Vitamin B12
- Magnesium Malate
- Magnesium Taurinate
- Magnesium Glycinate

Energy Support:
- L-Carnitine
- Acetyl-L-Carnitine

Gut Support:
- Multi-strain probiotic blend

Nutritional Support:
- Vitamin A
- Borage oil (GLA - Gamma Linolenic Acid)
- Vitamin D3
- Vitamin K2
- Omega-3 Fatty Acids (fish oil)

TGAb Thyroglobulin Antibody

A normal TGAb (Thyroglobulin Antibody) test result is negative. Elevated TGAb (also known as Anti-Tg or ATA) can be indicative of autoimmune thyroid conditions, such as Hashimoto's thyroiditis or Graves' disease. Dysbiosis in the microbiome, especially from gram-negative bacteria releasing lipopolysaccharides (LPS), can influence thyroid function, particularly TSH and T4 levels. Gluten intolerance and blood sugar imbalances may also contribute to autoimmune activity, impacting immune coordination and response.

Normal Range	0 - 15 IU/mL
Optimal Range	0 IU/mL

If POSITIVE or > 0 IU/mL:

Elevated TGAb levels are often seen in autoimmune thyroid conditions. Further testing, such as Thyroid Stimulating Immunoglobulin (TsIg), may help distinguish between Hashimoto's and Graves' disease. Physical indicators of these conditions include goiter (common in Hashimoto's and Graves') and exophthalmos (enlarged/protruding eyes, specific to Graves').

Although elevated TGAb suggests autoimmune activity, it is possible to have autoimmune thyroiditis without detectable antibodies, so a negative test does not exclude autoimmunity. Elevated thyroid antibodies may also appear in other autoimmune diseases, including Type 1 diabetes, rheumatoid arthritis, lupus, and Sjogren's. As autoimmune thyroid tests are not fully reliable, a thorough clinical history and assessment of symptoms remain essential.

Dietary and Lifestyle Recommendations:
- Dietary: Consider gluten and caffeine elimination. Adopt an anti-inflammatory, Paleo, or autoimmune protocol.
- Lifestyle: Prioritize liver health, stress management, and intestinal barrier function to reduce LPS endotoxin and systemic inflammation. Investigate gut health, focusing on gut dysbiosis and addressing allergens or mast cell activation, as these can exacerbate autoimmune responses.

Thyroid Support:
- N-Acetyl-L-Tyrosine
- American Ginseng (Panax quinquefolius)
- Forskolin (Coleus forskohlii)
- Iodine
- Chromium
- Zinc
- Selenium
- Copper
- Manganese
- Vitamin A
- Vitamin B2
- Potassium Iodide
- Myo-Inositol

Immune Support (if autoimmune):
- Cordyceps
- N-Acetyl-L-Cysteine (NAC)
- Milk Thistle
- Reishi
- Chinese Skullcap
- Schisandra
- Burdock Extract
- Full Spectrum Mushroom Blend:
- Reishi Blend
- Chaga (Inonotus obliquus)
- Lion's Mane (Hericium erinaceus)
- Cordyceps Blend
- Maitake (Grifola frondosa)
- Shiitake (Lentinula edodes)
- Agaricus (Agaricus blazei)
- Turkey Tail (Trametes versicolor)

Adrenal Support:
- gamma-Aminobutyric Acid (GABA)
- Eleutherococcus senticosus
- American Ginseng
- Ashwagandha
- Rhodiola
- Licorice
- Vitamin B2
- Vitamin B5
- Vitamin B6
- Vitamin C
- N-Acetyl-L-Tyrosine
- Phosphatidylserine
- Valerian
- Passion Flower
- Lemon Balm
- Chamomile
- L-theanine
- 5-HTP
- Melatonin
- Rhodiola rosea
- Pyrroloquinoline Quinone (PQQ)
- Taurine
- Vitamin B1
- Vitamin B12
- Magnesium Malate
- Magnesium Taurinate
- Magnesium Glycinate

THYROID

Energy Support:
- L-Carnitine
- Acetyl-L-Carnitine

Gut Support:
- Multi-strain probiotic blend

Nutritional Support:
- Vitamin A
- Borage oil (GLA - Gamma Linolenic Acid)
- Vitamin D3
- Vitamin K2
- Omega-3 Fatty Acids (fish oil)

T3 Uptake

T3 Uptake measures the availability of binding sites on proteins for T3, which indicates the amount of unsaturated thyroid-binding globulin (TBG) available. A lower T3 Uptake indicates more binding sites, while a higher T3 Uptake indicates fewer binding sites. This marker does not measure actual T3 levels, but rather assesses the thyroid's protein binding capacity. Testosterone may lower binding sites (raising T3 Uptake), while estrogen dominance increases binding sites (lowering T3 Uptake).

Normal Range	24-39%
Optimal Range	30-35%

If **LOW** or **< 30%**:

Low T3 Uptake often results from an excess of binding sites, potentially due to elevated T4, high estrogen levels, or iodine deficiency. Low uptake could indicate underlying hyperthyroidism, the use of estrogen or anti-ovulatory drugs, or thyroid gland hypofunction.

Dietary and Lifestyle Recommendations:
- Dietary: Consider a gluten-free, caffeine-free, Paleo, or anti-inflammatory diet. Address gut health and liver function, which are essential for proper thyroid function.
- Lifestyle: Focus on HPA axis balance, sleep hygiene, and mitochondrial health.
- Monitor: Regularly check thyroid antibody levels and work with a healthcare provider to manage any hyperthyroid symptoms if present.

Thyroid Support:
- N-Acetyl-L-Tyrosine
- American Ginseng (Panax quinquefolius)
- Forskolin (Coleus forskohlii)
- Iodine
- Chromium
- Zinc
- Selenium
- Copper
- Manganese
- Vitamin A
- Vitamin B2
- Potassium Iodide
- Myo-Inositol

Adrenal Support:
- gamma-Aminobutyric Acid (GABA)
- Eleutherococcus senticosus
- American Ginseng
- Ashwagandha
- Rhodiola
- Licorice

- Vitamin B2
- Vitamin B5
- Vitamin B6
- Vitamin C
- N-Acetyl-L-Tyrosine
- Phosphatidylserine
- Valerian
- Passion Flower
- Lemon Balm
- Chamomile
- L-theanine

- 5-HTP
- Melatonin
- Rhodiola rosea
- Pyrroloquinoline Quinone (PQQ)
- Taurine
- Vitamin B1
- Vitamin B12
- Magnesium Malate
- Magnesium Taurinate
- Magnesium Glycinate

Immune Support (if autoimmune):
- Cordyceps
- N-Acetyl-L-Cysteine (NAC)
- Milk Thistle
- Reishi
- Chinese Skullcap
- Schisandra
- Burdock Extract
- Full Spectrum Mushroom Blend:
- Reishi Blend
- Chaga (Inonotus obliquus)
- Lion's Mane (Hericium erinaceus)
- Cordyceps Blend
- Maitake (Grifola frondosa)
- Shiitake (Lentinula edodes)
- Agaricus (Agaricus blazei)
- Turkey Tail (Trametes versicolor)

Energy Support:
- L-Carnitine
- Acetyl-L-Carnitine

Nutritional Support:
- Vitamin A
- Borage oil (GLA - Gamma Linolenic Acid)
- Vitamin D3
- Vitamin K2
- Omega-3 Fatty Acids (fish oil)

If **HIGH** or > 35%:

High T3 Uptake may result from reduced binding sites, which could indicate increased metabolic activity or sensitivity to catecholamines. Elevated T3 Uptake might relate to hypothyroidism, renal dysfunction, or protein malnutrition.

Dietary and Lifestyle Recommendations:
- Dietary: A nutrient-dense, thyroid-supportive diet with B vitamins and trace minerals can aid metabolic and thyroid function.
- Lifestyle: Support liver health, which can impact thyroid binding sites, and manage estrogen and testosterone levels as these affect binding capacity.

Thyroid Support:
- N-Acetyl-L-Tyrosine
- American Ginseng (Panax quinquefolius)
- Forskolin (Coleus forskohlii)
- Iodine
- Chromium
- Zinc
- Selenium
- Copper
- Manganese
- Vitamin A
- Vitamin B2
- Potassium Iodide
- Myo-Inositol

Anti-inflammatory/Liver Support:
- Vitamin C
- Sodium Bicarbonate
- Potassium Bicarbonate
- Guduchi (Tinospora cordifolia)
- Nettle
- Quercetin

Gland Support:
- Broccoli Powder Extract
- Vitex agnus castus (Chasteberry)
- Black Cohosh
- Calcium D-Glucarate (CDG)
- Diindolylmethane (DIM)
- Green Tea Extract
- Mustard Powder (Sinapis alba)
- Trans Resveratrol
- Chrysin
- Magnesium Malate
- Vitamin B6
- Vitamin B9 (Folate)
- Vitamin B12

Reverse T3

Reverse T3 (rT3) is an inactive form of T3 that serves as a regulatory "brake" during periods of stress, fasting, and trauma, slowing down the thyroid's activity. Elevated cortisol can increase Reverse T3 and reduce the ability of T3 to bind to receptors, preventing its entry into cells. Typically, a 10:1 ratio of Free T3 (FT3) to Reverse T3 is ideal, though some clinical situations may show deviations. High rT3 may indicate reduced T4 levels or the body's response to stress, inflammation, or other metabolic disturbances.

Normal Range	9.2 - 24.1 ng/dL
Optimal Range	14.9 - 24.1 ng/dL

If LOW or < 14.9 ng/dL:

Low Reverse T3 may indicate lower T4 levels. Though not clinically significant in all cases, low rT3 can signal reduced T4 conversion to rT3 and may warrant a review of T4 status. Evaluate the balance of Free T3 (FT3) and T4 for optimal thyroid performance.

Dietary and Lifestyle Recommendations:
- Dietary: Gluten-free, caffeine-free, Paleo, or anti-inflammatory diets can support thyroid and overall health. Address liver health, blood sugar control, HPA axis, sleep quality, and heavy metal detoxification.
- Lifestyle: Regularly assess thyroid antibody levels and incorporate liver-supportive practices if needed.

Thyroid Support:
- N-Acetyl-L-Tyrosine
- American Ginseng (Panax quinquefolius)
- Forskolin (Coleus forskohlii)
- Iodine
- Chromium
- Zinc
- Selenium
- Copper
- Manganese
- Vitamin A
- Vitamin B2
- Potassium Iodide
- Myo-Inositol

Adrenal Support:
- gamma-Aminobutyric Acid (GABA)
- Eleutherococcus senticosus
- American Ginseng
- Ashwagandha
- Rhodiola
- Licorice
- Vitamin B2
- Vitamin B5
- Vitamin B6
- Vitamin C
- N-Acetyl-L-Tyrosine
- Phosphatidylserine
- Valerian
- Passion Flower
- Lemon Balm
- Chamomile
- L-theanine
- 5-HTP
- Melatonin
- Rhodiola rosea
- Pyrroloquinoline Quinone (PQQ)
- Taurine
- Vitamin B1
- Vitamin B12
- Magnesium Malate
- Magnesium Taurinate
- Magnesium Glycinate

Liver Support:
- Milk Thistle
- L-methionine
- Taurine
- Inositol
- Ox Bile
- Artichoke
- Beet Powder
- Vitamin A
- Vitamin B6
- Vitamin B12
- Plant protein powder with MVM (multi-vitamin/mineral)
- L-glutathione
- N-Acetyl-L-Cysteine (NAC)
- Quercetin
- Methylsulfonylmethane (MSM)
- Sodium Sulfate
- Green Tea Extract
- Reishi
- Cordyceps
- Chinese Skullcap
- Schisandra
- Burdock Extract
- Phosphatidylcholine

Immune & Gut Support:
- Serum-Derived Bovine Immunoglobulin Concentrate
- Immunoglobulin G
- N-Acetyl-D-Glucosamine
- Colostrum
- Protein Powder
- Mixed Amino Acids
- Zinc L-Carnosine
- L-Glutamine
- Citrus Pectin
- Deglycyrrhizinated Licorice Extract (DGL)
- Aloe Vera
- Slippery Elm
- Mucin
- Chamomile Extract
- Marshmallow
- Okra
- Cat's Claw
- Methylsulfonylmethane (MSM)
- Quercetin
- Prune Powder
- Aloe Vera Leaf Gel Extract
- Apple Pectin

- Iron

Nutritional Support:
- Vitamin A
- Borage oil (GLA - Gamma Linolenic Acid)
- Vitamin D3
- Vitamin K2
- Omega-3 Fatty Acids (fish oil)
- Magnesium Citrate
- Vitamin C

- Glucosamine HCl

If **HIGH** or > 24.1 ng/dL:

Elevated Reverse T3 levels may indicate conditions like hypothyroidism or "non-thyroidal illness syndrome" (also called low T3 syndrome) driven by stress, trauma, or other physiological strain. Elevated cortisol, low selenium, zinc, B12, or iron deficiency, and factors such as inflammation and toxins may drive up Reverse T3. Monitor the 10:1 ratio of FT3 to rT3 for further assessment.

Dietary and Lifestyle Recommendations:
- Dietary: Consider a gluten-free, anti-inflammatory, or Paleo diet, and support thyroid and liver function by balancing blood sugar and reducing inflammation.
- Lifestyle: Address chronic stress, which may exacerbate rT3 levels; ensure adequate sleep and address heavy metal detoxification as needed.

Thyroid Support:
- N-Acetyl-L-Tyrosine
- American Ginseng (Panax quinquefolius)
- Forskolin (Coleus forskohlii)
- Iodine
- Chromium
- Zinc
- Selenium
- Copper
- Manganese
- Vitamin A
- Vitamin B2
- Potassium Iodide
- Myo-Inositol

Adrenal and Liver Support:
- Eleurococcus senticosus, American Ginseng, Ashwagandha, Rhodiola, Licorice, Vitamins B2, B5, B6, C, N-Acetyl L-Tyrosine, Ashwagandha, plant protein powder with MVM (multi-vitamin / mineral), L-methionine, L-glutathione, N-Acetyl-L-Cysteine (NAC), Milk Thistle, quercetin, Taurine, Inositol, Methylsulfonylmethane (MSM), Sodium Sulfate, Green Tea Extract

Immune & Gut Support:
- Serum-Derived Bovine Immunoglobulin Concentrate
- Immunoglobulin G
- N-Acetyl-D-Glucosamine
- Colostrum
- Protein Powder
- Mixed Amino Acids
- Zinc L-Carnosine
- L-Glutamine
- Citrus Pectin
- Deglycyrrhizinated Licorice Extract (DGL)
- Aloe Vera
- Slippery Elm
- Mucin
- Chamomile Extract
- Marshmallow
- Okra
- Cat's Claw
- Methylsulfonylmethane (MSM)
- Quercetin
- Prune Powder
- Aloe Vera Leaf Gel Extract
- Apple Pectin
- Iron
- Glucosamine HCl

Nutritional Support:
- Vitamin A
- Borage oil (GLA - Gamma Linolenic Acid)
- Vitamin D3
- Vitamin K2
- Omega-3 Fatty Acids (fish oil)
- Magnesium Citrate
- Vitamin C

Free Thyroxine Index (FTI or T7)

The Free Thyroxine Index (FTI or T7) assesses the amount of free or unbound T4 activity in the blood by using total T4 (TT4) and T3 uptake. This index indicates the balance of T4 and binding proteins in circulation, where low TT4 should correspond with high T3 uptake, and high TT4 with low T3 uptake. The calculation is typically: T7 = (T4 x T3-Uptake) / 100

Normal Range	1.2 - 4.9 ng/dL
Optimal Range	1.2 - 4.9 ng/dL

If LOW or < 1.2 ng/dL:

A low Free Thyroxine Index can indicate potential hypothyroidism, as it reflects reduced free T4 activity. Supporting adrenal and thyroid health, gut health, and overall immunity may help improve T4 availability.

Dietary and Lifestyle Recommendations:
- Dietary: Consider gluten-free, caffeine-free, Paleo, or anti-inflammatory diets to support thyroid health.
- Lifestyle: Focus on liver health, stable blood sugar, HPA axis support, and proper sleep and detoxification routines. Regularly monitor thyroid antibody levels to assess immune status.

Thyroid Support:
- N-Acetyl-L-Tyrosine
- American Ginseng (Panax quinquefolius)
- Forskolin (Coleus forskohlii)
- Iodine
- Chromium
- Zinc
- Selenium
- Copper
- Manganese
- Vitamin A
- Vitamin B2
- Potassium Iodide
- Myo-Inositol

Adrenal Support:
- gamma-Aminobutyric Acid (GABA)
- Eleutherococcus senticosus
- American Ginseng
- Ashwagandha
- Rhodiola
- Licorice
- Vitamin B2
- Vitamin B5
- Vitamin B6
- Vitamin C
- N-Acetyl-L-Tyrosine
- Phosphatidylserine
- Valerian
- Passion Flower
- Lemon Balm
- Chamomile
- L-theanine
- 5-HTP

- Melatonin
- Rhodiola rosea
- Pyrroloquinoline Quinone (PQQ)
- Taurine
- Vitamin B1

Immune & Gut Support:
- Serum-Derived Bovine Immunoglobulin Concentrate
- Immunoglobulin G
- N-Acetyl-D-Glucosamine
- Colostrum
- Protein Powder
- Mixed Amino Acids
- Zinc L-Carnosine
- L-Glutamine
- Citrus Pectin
- Deglycyrrhizinated Licorice Extract (DGL)
- Aloe Vera

- Vitamin B12
- Magnesium Malate
- Magnesium Taurinate
- Magnesium Glycinate

- Slippery Elm
- Mucin
- Chamomile Extract
- Marshmallow
- Okra
- Cat's Claw
- Methylsulfonylmethane (MSM)
- Quercetin
- Prune Powder
- Aloe Vera Leaf Gel Extract
- Apple Pectin
- Iron
- Glucosamine HCl

Nutritional Support:
- Vitamin A
- Borage oil (GLA - Gamma Linolenic Acid)
- Vitamin D3
- Vitamin K2
- Omega-3 Fatty Acids (fish oil)
- Magnesium Citrate
- Vitamin C

If **HIGH** or > 4.9 ng/dL:

A high Free Thyroxine Index may suggest hyperthyroidism, often requiring additional monitoring. Excessive T4, iodine intake, or thyroid medication could elevate this index.

Dietary and Lifestyle Recommendations:
- Dietary: Avoid gluten and caffeine, and consider Paleo or anti-inflammatory diets. Address thyroid antibody levels, gut health, and heavy metal detoxification.
- Lifestyle: Emphasize stress management, sleep quality, and liver health to support overall thyroid function.

Thyroid Support:
- N-Acetyl-L-Tyrosine
- American Ginseng (Panax quinquefolius)
- Forskolin (Coleus forskohlii)
- Iodine
- Chromium
- Zinc

- Selenium
- Copper
- Manganese
- Vitamin A
- Vitamin B2
- Potassium Iodide
- Myo-Inositol

Herbal Thyroid Support:
- Bugleweed herb
- Lemon Balm

- Motherwort

Adrenal Support:
- gamma-Aminobutyric Acid (GABA)
- Eleutherococcus senticosus
- American Ginseng
- Ashwagandha
- Rhodiola
- Licorice
- Vitamin B2
- Vitamin B5
- Vitamin B6
- Vitamin C
- N-Acetyl-L-Tyrosine
- Phosphatidylserine
- Valerian
- Passion Flower
- Lemon Balm
- Chamomile
- L-theanine
- 5-HTP
- Melatonin
- Rhodiola rosea
- Pyrroloquinoline Quinone (PQQ)
- Taurine
- Vitamin B1
- Vitamin B12
- Magnesium Malate
- Magnesium Taurinate
- Magnesium Glycinate

Immune & Gut Support:
- Serum-Derived Bovine Immunoglobulin Concentrate
- Immunoglobulin G
- N-Acetyl-D-Glucosamine
- Colostrum
- Protein Powder
- Mixed Amino Acids
- Zinc L-Carnosine
- L-Glutamine
- Citrus Pectin
- Deglycyrrhizinated Licorice Extract (DGL)
- Aloe Vera
- Slippery Elm
- Mucin
- Chamomile Extract
- Marshmallow
- Okra
- Cat's Claw
- Methylsulfonylmethane (MSM)
- Quercetin
- Prune Powder
- Aloe Vera Leaf Gel Extract
- Apple Pectin
- Iron
- Glucosamine HCl

Energy Support:
- L-Carnitine
- Acetyl-L-Carnitine

Nutritional Support:
- Vitamin A
- Borage oil (GLA - Gamma Linolenic Acid)
- Vitamin D3
- Vitamin K2
- Omega-3 Fatty Acids (fish oil)

Thyroxine Binding Globulin (TBG)

Thyroxine Binding Globulin (TBG) is used to assess whether changes in thyroid hormone levels (Total T3 or Total T4) are due to alterations in free T4/T3 levels or bound TBG. Additionally, it helps identify hyper- or hypothyroidism and assess organ function, especially in the liver, ovaries, and kidneys.

Normal Range	14 - 30 mcg/mL
Optimal Range	14 - 28 mcg/mL

If **LOW** or < 14 mcg/mL:

Low TBG can indicate hypoproteinemia, renal protein loss, or liver dysfunction. It may also be associated with low estrogen levels, ovarian hypofunction, or high-dose aspirin use. Support for thyroid, kidney, digestive, and liver function may be beneficial.

Focus on thyroid, digestive, kidney, and liver health, and investigate estrogen levels if they are suspected to be low.

Thyroid Support:
- N-Acetyl-L-Tyrosine
- American Ginseng (Panax quinquefolius)
- Forskolin (Coleus forskohlii)
- Iodine
- Chromium
- Zinc
- Selenium
- Copper
- Manganese
- Vitamin A
- Vitamin B2
- Potassium Iodide
- Myo-Inositol

Digestive Support:
- Digestive enzymes
- Betaine HCl
- Ox Bile
- L-taurine
- Gentian extract
- Dandelion extract
- Fennel
- Amylase
- Protease SP
- Protease
- Diastase
- Lactase
- Glucoamylase
- Alpha-galactosidase
- Beta-glucanase
- Acid protease
- Phytase
- Cellulase
- Hemicellulase
- Invertase
- Lipase
- Bromelain
- Papain
- Pepsin
- Triphala (Emblica officinalis, Terminalia bellirica, Terminalia chebula)
- Magnesium Hydroxide
- Mastic Gum
- DGL (Deglycyrrhizinated Licorice)
- Methylmethionine Sulfonium Chloride (MMSC)
- Zinc L-Carnosine
- Vitamin C
- Berberine
- Ginger
- Bismuth

Kidney Support:
- Champignon (Agaricus bisporus)
- Cordyceps (Cordyceps sinensis)
- Poria (Poria cocos)
- American Ginseng (Panax quinquefolius)
- Astragalus (Astragalus membranaceus)

Liver Support:
- Milk Thistle
- L-methionine
- Taurine
- Inositol
- Ox Bile
- Artichoke
- Beet Powder
- Vitamin A
- Vitamin B6
- Vitamin B12

- Plant protein powder with MVM (multi-vitamin/mineral)
- L-glutathione
- N-Acetyl-L-Cysteine (NAC)
- Quercetin
- Methylsulfonylmethane (MSM)
- Sodium Sulfate
- Green Tea Extract
- Reishi
- Cordyceps
- Chinese Skullcap
- Schisandra
- Burdock Extract
- Phosphatidylcholine

If **HIGH** or > 28 mcg/mL:

 Elevated TBG may be linked to hypothyroidism, pregnancy, liver dysfunction, estrogen therapy, or oral contraceptive use. Additionally, ovarian hyperfunction or other hormone imbalances may contribute to increased TBG.

 Address thyroid and adrenal health, monitor sex hormones (especially estrogen), and consider liver support.

Thyroid Support:
- N-Acetyl-L-Tyrosine
- American Ginseng (Panax quinquefolius)
- Forskolin (Coleus forskohlii)
- Iodine
- Chromium
- Zinc
- Selenium
- Copper
- Manganese
- Vitamin A
- Vitamin B2
- Potassium Iodide
- Myo-Inositol

Glandular Thyroid Cytotrophin Support (thyroxine free):
- Thyroid Glandular
- Hypothalamus Glandular
- Iodine
- Zinc
- Selenium
- Copper
- Manganese
- N-Acetyl L-Tyrosine
- Thyroid Cytotrophin

Adrenal Support:
- gamma-Aminobutyric Acid (GABA)
- Eleutherococcus senticosus
- American Ginseng
- Ashwagandha
- Rhodiola
- Licorice
- Vitamin B2
- Vitamin B5
- Vitamin B6
- Vitamin C
- N-Acetyl-L-Tyrosine
- Phosphatidylserine
- Valerian
- Passion Flower
- Lemon Balm
- Chamomile
- L-theanine
- 5-HTP
- Melatonin
- Rhodiola rosea
- Pyrroloquinoline Quinone (PQQ)
- Taurine
- Vitamin B1
- Vitamin B12
- Magnesium Malate
- Magnesium Taurinate
- Magnesium Glycinate

Hormone Metabolism Support:
- CDG (Calcium-D-Glucarate)
- Diindolylmethane (DIM)
- Broccoli Powder Extract
- Vitex agnus castus (Chasteberry)
- Black Cohosh
- Green Tea Extract

- Mustard Powder (Sinapis alba)
- Trans Resveratrol
- Chrysin
- Magnesium Malate
- Vitamin B6
- Vitamin B9 (Folate)
- Vitamin B12
- Sulforaphane

Nutrient

Blood

Vitamins

Minerals

Antioxidants

Vibrant Micronutrient

Get LabDx Online Here:

Vitamins

A vitamin panel helps assess a person's nutritional status and identify any deficiencies or excesses in specific vitamins.

Vitamin A (Retinol)

Vitamin A (Retinol) is essential for vision, immune function, cell growth, and skin health. Its blood test measures the levels of retinol, the active form of Vitamin A. Deficiency can lead to night blindness, skin issues, and impaired immune function. Vitamin A encompasses a group of fat-soluble vitamins (retinol, retinal, retinoic acid, and provitamin A carotenoids, especially beta-carotene) and plays a role in:
- Growth and development
- Immune system function
- Vision health
- Gene transcription, haematopoiesis, and antioxidant activity

Daily Recommended Intake:
- Women: 700 mcg RAE/day (about 2500 IU from animal sources)
- Men: 900 mcg RAE/day (about 3000 IU from animal sources)
- Upper Intake Level (UL): 3,000 mcg RAE/day to prevent toxicity.

Normal Range	42.0 - 153.7 mcg/dL
Optimal Range	42.0 - 153.7 mcg/dL

If **LOW** or **< 42.0 mcg/dL:**

Low Vitamin A levels can be caused by dietary deficiency, liver or gallbladder disorders, digestive issues, or a low-fat diet (Vitamin A requires fat for absorption). Deficiency can result in night blindness, dry skin, impaired immunity, growth retardation, and infection risk. Chronic alcoholism, zinc deficiency, and hypothyroidism are also risk factors.

Include Vitamin A-rich foods such as liver, cod liver oil, fortified milk, eggs, sweet potato, carrots, and leafy greens.

Nutritional Support:
- Vitamin A

If **HIGH** or **> 153.7 mcg/dL:**

High Vitamin A levels may indicate excessive intake from supplements, overconsumption of animal liver (especially from big game), or certain acne medications containing retinoids. Toxicity may lead to symptoms such as abdominal pain, nausea, dizziness, bone pain, poor appetite, and potential birth defects.

Remove or reduce supplements and foods providing excessive Vitamin A to prevent toxicity.

High Vitamin A intake should be closely monitored, especially during pregnancy, due to the risk of birth defects.

Vitamin B1 (Thiamin)

Vitamin B1 (Thiamin) is essential for energy conversion, nervous system health, and muscle function. It acts as a coenzyme in carbohydrate and amino acid metabolism and aids in producing hydrochloric acid for digestion. Vitamin B1 is closely tied to energy, cholesterol, and neurotransmitter production.

- **RDA:** 1.0 mg/day for females, 1.2 mg/day for males, and 1.4 mg/day during pregnancy/lactation.
- **Therapeutic Intake:** Commonly 25-100 mg/day, with no established upper limit for toxicity.

Normal Range	2.2 - 107.3 nmol/L
Optimal Range	2.2 - 107.3 nmol/L

If LOW or < 2.2 nmol/L:

Low levels of Vitamin B1 can result in fatigue, neuropathy, irritability, depression, and potentially serious conditions like beriberi. Severe deficiency, especially with alcohol abuse, can lead to neurological and cardiovascular symptoms.

Risk Factors for Deficiency:
Poor diet, chronic alcohol use, gastric bypass surgery, diabetes, heavy intake of tea/coffee (contains thiaminase which depletes thiamine), and consuming raw freshwater fish/shellfish (thiaminase content).

Include thiamin-rich foods such as pork, organ meats, legumes, sweet potatoes, brown rice, brewer's yeast, sunflower seeds, and enriched grains.

Nutritional Support:
- Borage oil (GLA - Gamma Linolenic Acid)

If HIGH or > 107.3 nmol/L:

High Vitamin B1 levels are rare but may result from excessive supplement intake or overconsumption of B1-rich foods. While toxicity is uncommon, excessive thiamin intake should be minimized if not medically indicated.

Remove supplements or foods providing high amounts of Vitamin B1.

Vitamin B2 (Riboflavin)

Vitamin B2 (Riboflavin) plays an essential role in energy production, cell function, and supporting antioxidant defenses. It forms coenzymes that aid in oxidation-reduction reactions, important for metabolism and detoxification. Riboflavin also supports nitric oxide production, which benefits cardiovascular health and enhances glutathione activity for antioxidant defense.

- **RDA**: 1.7 mg/day
- **Therapeutic Intake**: 25-50 mg/day (no established upper limit due to low toxicity risk)

Normal Range	9.9 - 261.7 nmol/L
Optimal Range	9.9 - 261.7 nmol/L

If **LOW** or **< 9.9 nmol/L:**

Low levels of riboflavin can cause symptoms such as fatigue, skin issues (red, cracking skin around lips and mouth), and sensitivity to touch, heat, or pain. Riboflavin deficiency may be exacerbated by excessive alcohol intake, and the elderly may have increased riboflavin requirements.

Symptoms of Deficiency:
- Cracked, red lips and mouth corners
- Red, scaly skin (especially around nostrils, ears, and eyelids)
- Increased sensitivity in hands and feet

Foods high in riboflavin include organ meats, dairy products, eggs, leafy greens (e.g., spinach), and enriched grains.

Nutritional Support:
- Borage oil (GLA - Gamma Linolenic Acid)

If **HIGH** or **> 261.7 nmol/L:**

Elevated riboflavin levels have no known toxicity or adverse effects. High levels may result from supplementation or riboflavin-rich foods.

No action is typically required, but high levels of riboflavin do not pose toxicity concerns.

Vitamin B3 (Niacin)

Vitamin B3 (Niacin) is essential for energy metabolism, cell function, and maintaining healthy skin, and plays a critical role in over 200 enzyme reactions, including fatty acid synthesis, DNA repair, and lowering cholesterol. It is especially important for mental, gut, and skin health, and for healthy aging and DNA repair. Niacin can be depleted by factors like stress, injury, certain medications, and dietary deficiencies.

- **RDA:** 20 mg/day
- **UL:** 35 mg/day, though doses up to 6g per day are sometimes used under supervision for lipid management

Normal Range	2.6 - 76.8 ng/mL
Optimal Range	2.6 - 76.8 ng/mL

If LOW or < 2.6 ng/mL:

Niacin deficiency can lead to pellagra, characterized by dermatitis, diarrhea, and dementia, as well as fatigue, circulatory issues, and digestive disturbances. A deficiency may be linked to dietary insufficiency, digestive disorders, or conditions affecting tryptophan metabolism.

Symptoms of Deficiency:
- Pigmented skin rash (especially on sun-exposed areas)
- Red, swollen tongue
- Fatigue, memory loss, and, in severe cases, hallucinations

Rich food sources include pork, peanuts, tofu, eggs, and enriched grains. Niacin is synthesized from tryptophan, so adequate intake of iron, B6, and riboflavin, which are required for niacin synthesis, is also essential.

Nutritional Support:
- Borage oil (GLA - Gamma Linolenic Acid)
- Vitamin B3 / Niacin (as Nicotinic Acid)

If HIGH or > 76.8 ng/mL:

High levels of niacin may cause adverse effects such as skin flushing, gastrointestinal discomfort, low blood pressure, and, in rare cases, liver toxicity. Monitoring liver function is recommended with high-dose supplementation.

Limit niacin intake: Consider reducing supplemental or food sources to avoid excessive intake. Symptoms to monitor: Look for signs of overdose such as nausea, headache, dizziness, or gastrointestinal upset.

Vitamin B5 (Pantothenic Acid)

Vitamin B5, or Pantothenic Acid, is essential for energy metabolism and synthesizing various compounds, including coenzyme A (CoA), which is necessary for fatty acid metabolism. It supports the synthesis and breakdown of proteins, carbohydrates, and fats. Pantothenic acid is widely available in foods, and gut bacteria can produce some, although not enough to meet daily needs.

- **AI (Adequate Intake):** 5 mg/day for adults, 6 mg/day during pregnancy, 7 mg/day during lactation
- **Food Sources:** Beef, pork, chicken, fish, egg yolks, whole grains, legumes, lentils

Normal Range	2.0 - 4.4 pg/mL
Optimal Range	3.0 - 3.25 pg/mL

If LOW or < 3.0 pg/mL:

Although B5 deficiency is rare, low levels may lead to fatigue, neurological symptoms, and mood changes. High levels of dietary biotin or biotin supplementation can compete with B5 for intestinal absorption, potentially contributing to deficiency.

Symptoms of Deficiency:
- Fatigue, loss of enthusiasm
- Mood changes, numbness, or tingling in hands and feet
- Gastrointestinal issues: nausea, cramps, and vomiting
- Increased heart rate with minor exertion

- **Increase Dietary Sources:** Include B5-rich foods such as beef, pork, chicken, fish, eggs, whole grains, and legumes.
- **Supplemental Support:** Consider adding Borage oil (GLA - Gamma Linolenic Acid) to address low levels if dietary intake is insufficient.

If HIGH or > 3.25 pg/mL:

Vitamin B5 has no known toxicity. However, high doses can interfere with the absorption of biotin and lipoic acid. If taking B5 at high doses, consider supplementing with 100-300 mcg of biotin and 100 mg of R-lipoic acid at least 3 hours apart from the nearest dose of B5 to avoid interference.

- **Monitor Intake:** Remove any excessive B5 supplements or foods contributing to high levels.
- **Ensure Nutritional Balance:** If high doses are necessary, pair with biotin and lipoic acid supplements as suggested above to prevent absorption issues.

Vitamin B6 (Pyridoxine)

Vitamin B6 (Pyridoxine) is essential for brain development, neurotransmitter production, immune function, and energy metabolism. It supports the breakdown of amino acids, hemoglobin production, and the synthesis of serotonin and dopamine. It also plays a role in managing blood sugar and reducing homocysteine levels, which are associated with cardiovascular health.

- **RDA:** 2 mg/day
- **UL:** 100 mg/day (doses >1000 mg/day over extended periods may cause neuropathy)

Normal Range	0.7 - 447.6 ng/mL
Optimal Range	0.7 - 447.6 ng/mL

If LOW or < 0.7 ng/mL:

B6 deficiency may cause anemia, immune dysfunction, mood changes, and skin disorders. It can arise from malabsorption, chronic illnesses, and certain medications (e.g., oral contraceptives, NSAIDs). Low B6 levels can also lead to elevated homocysteine, which increases cardiovascular risk.

Symptoms of Deficiency:
- Depression, confusion, irritability
- Inflamed tongue, sores at the corners of the mouth
- PMS symptoms, morning sickness, and increased inflammation

Foods rich in B6 include poultry, fish, beef liver, and plant-based sources such as legumes, whole grains, and nuts. Animal sources tend to be better absorbed than plant sources.

Nutritional Support:
- Borage oil (GLA - Gamma Linolenic Acid)
- Vitamin B-6

If **HIGH** or **> 447.6 ng/mL:**

High B6 levels can result from excessive supplementation and may lead to adverse effects such as neuropathy or sensory nerve damage with prolonged use. The body uses B6 for many enzymatic processes, including those essential for neurotransmitter synthesis and protein metabolism.

- **Reduce intake:** Discontinue or reduce supplements or foods high in vitamin B6.
- **Monitor for symptoms:** Be aware of signs such as tingling or numbness in hands and feet, which may indicate nerve damage.

Vitamin B9 (Folate)

Vitamin B9, also known as folate (naturally occurring in foods) or folic acid (synthetic/supplemental form), is vital for cell division, DNA synthesis, and red blood cell production. Folate plays a critical role in methylation reactions with vitamin B12, which supports mental health, DNA synthesis, and homocysteine reduction.

- **Functions:** Folate supports DNA synthesis, cell growth, and proper methylation, which is crucial for mood stability, energy production, immune health, and pregnancy.
- **RDA:** 400 mcg/day for adults, 600 mcg/day during pregnancy.
- **Supplementation:** Common therapeutic doses range from 400 to 1000 mcg/day, with caution to avoid masking B12 deficiency.

Methylation status (related to MTHFR mutations) may influence folate needs; methylated forms like methyl-tetrahydrofolate may be necessary for optimal absorption and function.

Normal Range	1.5 - 20.6 ng/mL
Optimal Range	1.5 - 20.6 ng/mL

If **LOW** or **< 1.5 ng/mL:**

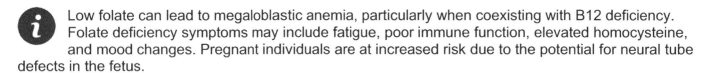
Low folate can lead to megaloblastic anemia, particularly when coexisting with B12 deficiency. Folate deficiency symptoms may include fatigue, poor immune function, elevated homocysteine, and mood changes. Pregnant individuals are at increased risk due to the potential for neural tube defects in the fetus.

- **Risk Factors:** Poor diet, alcohol dependence, malabsorption disorders, MTHFR mutation, and use of certain medications (e.g., anticonvulsants, antacids, methotrexate).
- **Anemia:** Folate deficiency can contribute to megaloblastic anemia, especially in combination with B12 deficiency.
- **Mood and Cognitive Issues:** Folate is involved in mental health via methylation; low levels can exacerbate anxiety, depression, and cognitive issues.
- **Pregnancy Risks:** Folate deficiency during pregnancy is linked to neural tube defects.

- **Dietary Sources:** Increase intake of green leafy vegetables, legumes (e.g., black-eyed peas, lentils), brewer's yeast, and enriched grains.
- **Check MTHFR Status:** For individuals with the MTHFR mutation, consider methylated folate forms to ensure effective absorption and function.

Nutritional Support:
- Borage oil (GLA - Gamma Linolenic Acid)
- Vitamins B9 (folate), B12

If **HIGH** or > 20.6 ng/mL:

It is extremely rare to reach a toxic level when eating folate from food sources. However, an upper limit for folic acid is set at 1,000 mcg daily because studies have shown that taking higher amounts can mask a vitamin B12 deficiency.

High levels may mean either an excess intake or possibly a B12 deficiency

Vitamin B12 (Cobalamin)

Vitamin B12 (Cobalamin) is essential for nerve function, DNA synthesis, and red blood cell production. It plays a critical role in methylation, neurological health, and homocysteine metabolism. B12 requires intrinsic factor, a glycoprotein in the stomach, for absorption. Risk factors for B12 deficiency include age, certain medications (such as PPIs), and specific genetic factors (e.g., MTHFR SNPs).

- **RDA:** 6 mcg/day
- **Therapeutic Range:** Common doses are 1000-5000 mcg in cases of deficiency. B12 is safe in high doses with no established toxicity.

Normal Range	232 - 1245 ng/L
Optimal Range	232 - 1245 ng/L

If **LOW** or < 232 ng/L:

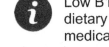
Low B12 levels may lead to anemia, neurological issues, and fatigue. Causes include insufficient dietary intake (especially in vegans), malabsorption due to gastrointestinal conditions, and medication effects. Pernicious anemia, celiac disease, and chronic alcohol use can also impair B12 absorption.

Symptoms of Deficiency:
- Fatigue, weakness
- Cognitive decline, dementia
- Numbness or tingling in the hands and feet
- Anemia (megaloblastic anemia, pernicious anemia)

Foods rich in B12 include fish, meat, eggs, and dairy. B12 is not naturally found in plant foods, so those on a vegan diet should consider supplementation or fortified foods.

Nutritional Support:
- Borage oil (GLA - Gamma Linolenic Acid)
- Vitamin B12
- Vitamins B9 (folate), B12

VITAMINS

If HIGH or > 1245 ng/L:

Elevated B12 may occur due to liver diseases (e.g., cirrhosis or hepatitis) or myeloproliferative disorders. However, these conditions are not typically diagnosed based on B12 levels alone.

- **Rule Out Contributing Conditions:** If high B12 persists, consider evaluating liver function and blood markers for possible myeloproliferative conditions.
- **Monitor Levels:** Continue to check B12 levels if there are any concerning symptoms, but no toxicity is associated with high B12 levels from dietary or supplemental intake.

Vitamin C (Ascorbic Acid)

Vitamin C (Ascorbic Acid) is a powerful antioxidant that plays a significant role in immune function, wound healing, and collagen synthesis. It supports the regeneration of vitamin E, reduces oxidative stress, and promotes healthy skin, gums, and blood vessels. Vitamin C is also crucial for carnitine synthesis, aiding in the breakdown of fats for energy.

- **RDA:** 75 mg/day for women, 90 mg/day for men, and 120 mg/day during pregnancy and lactation.
- **Food Sources:** Oysters, tropical fruits (e.g., guava, papaya, oranges), leafy greens (e.g., kale, spinach), cruciferous vegetables (e.g., broccoli, cauliflower), berries, and bell peppers.

Normal Range	0.4 - 2.2 mg/dL
Optimal Range	0.4 - 2.2 mg/dL

If LOW or < 0.4 mg/dL:

Vitamin C deficiency can result in symptoms such as fatigue, weakened immunity, slow wound healing, bleeding gums, and joint pain. Severe deficiency, known as scurvy, is rare but possible in cases of prolonged low intake.

Symptoms of Deficiency:
- Fatigue, easy bruising
- Prolonged wound healing
- Bleeding gums and joint pain
- Symptoms of scurvy in severe cases (e.g., swollen gums, skin issues)

Consume more vitamin C-rich foods like citrus fruits, leafy greens, cruciferous vegetables, and berries.

Consider adding Vitamin C.

If HIGH or > 2.2 mg/dL:

High levels of vitamin C generally pose no toxicity; however, excessive intake may cause digestive issues like loose stools in some individuals. Those with conditions such as glucose-6-phosphate dehydrogenase deficiency, hemochromatosis, or a history of kidney stones should be cautious with high doses.

VITAMINS

- **Reduce Supplement Intake:** Discontinue or reduce supplements or foods that contribute excessive amounts of vitamin C.
- **Monitor Symptoms:** Watch for signs of gastrointestinal discomfort or symptoms related to high intake, especially if taking doses over 1-2 grams.

Vitamin D3

Vitamin D3 (Cholecalciferol) is crucial for maintaining bone health and regulating calcium and phosphorus levels. It also plays a role in immune function, mood regulation, and gene expression. Vitamin D is synthesized in the skin through sunlight exposure, but adequate levels are often challenging to achieve without supplementation. Low levels are associated with conditions such as osteoporosis, rickets, and other health complications. Excessive supplementation, however, can lead to toxicity and hypercalcemia.

- **Forms:** Vitamin D3 (cholecalciferol) and D2 (ergocalciferol)
- **RDA:** Typically insufficient for therapeutic needs; common doses range from 1,000 to 10,000 IU/day.
- **Toxicity:** Rare but can occur with doses exceeding 50,000 IU/day.
- **Supplementation Note:** Vitamin K2 is often recommended alongside vitamin D3 to help balance calcium levels in the body.
- **Food Sources:** Fatty fish, fortified dairy, egg yolks, and mushrooms exposed to sunlight.

Normal Range	1.3 - 9.5 ng/mL
Optimal Range	1.3 - 9.5 ng/mL

If **LOW** or < 1.3 ng/mL:

Low vitamin D levels can contribute to weakened bones, immune dysfunction, and an increased risk of several chronic conditions such as osteoporosis, cardiovascular disease, and mood disorders. Deficiency is common, especially in those with limited sun exposure, darker skin, or malabsorption issues.

Symptoms of Deficiency:
- Fatigue, mood disturbances
- Bone pain and muscle weakness
- Increased susceptibility to infections

- **Increase Sun Exposure:** Safe, limited sun exposure may help increase vitamin D levels.
- **Increase Dietary Sources:** Include more vitamin D-rich foods like fortified milk, fatty fish, egg yolks, and mushrooms.

Consider Vitamin D3, K2 to achieve optimal levels. Supplementing with vitamin K2 is also recommended to help regulate calcium levels when taking high doses of vitamin D.

If **HIGH** or > 9.5 ng/mL:

Excessive vitamin D can lead to toxicity, a condition typically caused by high-dose supplementation rather than diet or sun exposure. High vitamin D levels can lead to hypercalcemia, causing symptoms like nausea, vomiting, loss of appetite, and potential long-term organ damage.

- **Discontinue or Reduce Supplements:** Remove or reduce high-dose vitamin D supplements or any food sources contributing to excessive intake.
- **Monitor Symptoms:** Watch for signs of hypercalcemia and consult a healthcare provider if symptoms occur.

Vitamin D, 25-OH

Vitamin D, 25-OH, also known as calcidiol, is the storage form of vitamin D and is commonly measured to assess overall vitamin D status. It reflects both vitamin D2 and D3 levels and is a precursor to the active form, 1,25-OHD3. This marker helps evaluate bone health, calcium and phosphorus metabolism, and general immune function. It is particularly useful in identifying deficiency or toxicity, as well as potential underlying health conditions.

- **Forms:** Vitamin D2 (ergocalciferol) and D3 (cholecalciferol)
- **RDA:** Traditional recommendation of 400 IU/day is considered insufficient for optimal levels; typical therapeutic doses range from 1,000–10,000 IU/day.
- **Toxicity:** Rare, but possible with doses above 50,000 IU/day. Intake of less than 10,000 IU/day is unlikely to cause toxicity.
- **Food Sources:** Fortified milk, egg yolks, fatty fish, liver, and sunlight exposure.
- **Supplementation:** Vitamin D supplementation is usually necessary due to challenges in obtaining adequate levels from diet and sunlight alone, especially in higher-risk groups (e.g., individuals with darker skin, those in northern latitudes, and people with limited sun exposure). Vitamin K2 is often recommended alongside vitamin D to help regulate calcium.

Normal Range	≥ 30 ng/mL
Optimal Range	≥ 30 ng/mL

If LOW or < 30 ng/mL:

Low levels of vitamin D are associated with increased risks of conditions such as cardiovascular disease, diabetes, osteoporosis, and weakened immune function. Vitamin D deficiency is particularly common in individuals with limited sun exposure, those living in northern latitudes, people with darker skin, and those with malabsorption issues.

Conditions associated with low vitamin D levels include:
- Bone and joint issues (e.g., osteoporosis, osteomalacia)
- Immune system dysregulation (e.g., increased susceptibility to colds, flus)
- Mood disorders and cognitive impairments
- Increased risks of chronic illnesses such as heart disease and diabetes

- **Increase Sun Exposure:** Safe exposure to sunlight may aid in natural vitamin D production.
- **Include Dietary Sources:** Fortified dairy, fatty fish, and egg yolks can help boost vitamin D intake.
- **Monitor Levels:** Routine monitoring is recommended to assess response to supplementation and maintain optimal levels.

Vitamin D3, K2 to help raise serum levels. Consult with a healthcare provider for an optimal target.

Vitamin E

Vitamin E (alpha-tocopherol) is a key antioxidant that helps protect cells from oxidative damage. It supports immune function, reduces blood clotting risk, and is important for nerve and muscle health. As a fat-soluble vitamin, vitamin E reduces reactive oxygen species (ROS) from fat oxidation, regulates cell signaling, and aids in immune responses.

- **RDA:** 15 mg/day
- **UL:** 1,000 mg/day (to prevent interference with vitamin K pathways)
- **Supplemental Forms:** Only alpha-tocopherol reverses deficiency symptoms, with a-Lipoic acid as an essential co-factor.
- **Food Sources:** Found in seeds, nuts, oils, leafy greens, and fortified foods.

Normal Range	7.1 - 43.1 mg/L
Optimal Range	7.1 - 43.1 mg/L

If LOW or < 7.1 mg/L:

Low vitamin E levels can lead to neurological and muscle-related symptoms, including peripheral neuropathy, muscle weakness, and impaired immune function. Vitamin E deficiency is typically associated with absorption disorders or low dietary intake and is rare in healthy individuals.

Associated Conditions:
- Potential Health Risks: Neuropathy, ataxia, muscle weakness, increased risk of cardiovascular disease (CVD), retinopathy, and oxidative stress-related conditions.
- Conditions Leading to Deficiency: Malabsorption syndromes (e.g., Crohn's disease, cystic fibrosis), liver disease, smoking, or low-fat diets.

- **Increase Dietary Sources:** Foods rich in vitamin E include sunflower seeds, nuts, avocado, spinach, and olive oil.
- **Assess Malabsorption:** If deficiency persists, further tests may be needed to evaluate digestive health or absorption capacity.

- Vitamin E tocotrienols

If HIGH or > 43.1 mg/L

High levels of vitamin E, often from supplementation rather than dietary sources, can increase bleeding risks, especially for patients on anticoagulation therapy. Elevated vitamin E levels may also interact with various medications.

- **Reduce Supplementation:** Discontinue or reduce supplemental vitamin E if excessive intake is identified.
- **Monitor for Symptoms:** Watch for symptoms of toxicity, including nausea, fatigue, blurred vision, and bleeding risk in those on blood-thinning medications.
- **Consult Healthcare Provider:** Adjust dosage under medical supervision, especially if high vitamin E supplementation is used.

Vitamin K1

Vitamin K1, also known as phylloquinone, is a fat-soluble vitamin crucial for blood clotting and bone health. It assists with clotting factor production, calcium regulation, and converting glucose to glycogen in the liver. As a member of the vitamin K group, which includes K1 and K2, vitamin K1 is found mainly in leafy green vegetables.

- **AI:** 90 µg/day for women and 120 µg/day for men
- **Primary Sources:** Dark leafy greens (e.g., kale, spinach), cruciferous vegetables, and some plant oils.
- **Clinical Uses:** Important for those on anticoagulants (e.g., warfarin) or with conditions affecting clotting, bone health, or calcium metabolism.

Note: Individuals taking vitamin K2 supplements or with certain absorption disorders may have altered or undetectable vitamin K1 levels.

Normal Range	0.2 - 13.3 ng/mL
Optimal Range	0.2 - 13.3 ng/mL

If LOW or < 0.2 ng/mL:

Low vitamin K1 levels can lead to bleeding disorders due to insufficient blood clotting. Symptoms may include easy bruising, excessive bleeding, and in severe cases, menorrhagia or capillary rupture. Low vitamin K1 levels may stem from insufficient dietary intake, fat malabsorption, or extended antibiotic use, which reduces vitamin K synthesis by gut bacteria.

- **Risk Factors:** Conditions causing fat malabsorption (e.g., Crohn's disease, cystic fibrosis), chronic kidney disease, liver or biliary disorders, and use of anticoagulants or certain antibiotics.
- **Genetic Risks:** Individuals with the ApoE4 genotype may have an increased risk of vitamin K deficiency.

- **Risk Factors:** Conditions causing fat malabsorption (e.g., Crohn's disease, cystic fibrosis), chronic kidney disease, liver or biliary disorders, and use of anticoagulants or certain antibiotics.
- **Genetic Risks:** Individuals with the ApoE4 genotype may have an increased risk of vitamin K deficiency.

Vitamins K1, K2, Trans-Geranylgeraniol

If HIGH or > 13.3 ng/mL:

High levels of vitamin K are typically not associated with health risks in individuals not on blood-thinning medications. Vitamin K does not increase clotting in excess; however, those on anticoagulant therapy (such as warfarin) must manage their vitamin K intake to prevent interference with medication efficacy.

- **Adjust Supplementation:** Consider reducing dietary or supplemental vitamin K intake, especially if taking anticoagulants.
- **Monitor:** Discuss any changes in vitamin K levels with a healthcare provider, particularly if taking blood-thinning medications.

Vitamin K2

Vitamin K2, a fat-soluble vitamin, is primarily involved in calcium metabolism, bone health, and cardiovascular health. It helps prevent arterial calcification by activating matrix GLA protein (MGP), which inhibits calcium buildup in blood vessels. Vitamin K2 comes in several forms, called menaquinones (MK), with MK-4 and MK-7 being the most common.

- **Sources:** Found in animal-based foods (butter, egg yolks) and fermented foods (e.g., natto, kefir). The body can also convert K1 from plant foods to K2.
- **Function:** Essential for calcium regulation, supports heart health, bone density, and helps shuttle calcium into bones, reducing risk of heart disease and kidney stones.
- **Recommended Intake:** Daily therapeutic dose of 360-500 mcg is commonly suggested.

Note: Vitamin K1 levels may not be reliable when taking K2 supplements due to potential interferences.

Normal Range	≥ 0.08 ng/mL
Optimal Range	≥ 0.08 ng/mL

If LOW or < 0.08 ng/mL:

Low vitamin K2 can increase the risk of cardiovascular diseases, osteoporosis, and uncontrolled bleeding. Since vitamin K2 assists with calcium homeostasis, low K2 may cause unregulated calcium release from bones, especially if vitamin D3 supplementation is being used without K2.

- **Risk Factors:** Blood-thinning medications, antibiotic use, insufficient dietary intake, high doses of vitamins A or E, or malabsorption conditions (e.g., cystic fibrosis, liver disorders).
- **Increased Risk:** Heart disease, stroke, and arterial calcification due to calcium deposits in blood vessels.
- **Bone Health:** Chronic low vitamin K2 can be linked to osteoporosis.

- **Dietary Focus:** Increase consumption of vitamin K2-rich foods, such as natto, liver, egg yolk, and fermented cheeses.
- **Vitamin D Co-Supplementation:** If taking vitamin D3, ensure adequate K2 intake to aid in proper calcium balance and prevent potential calcium buildup in soft tissues.

Vitamins K1, K2, Trans-Geranylgeraniol

Minerals

A mineral panel helps assess a person's nutritional status and identify any deficiencies or excesses in specific minerals.

Calcium

Calcium, a crucial mineral, plays a vital role in maintaining strong bones and teeth, facilitating muscle contraction, nerve transmission, cellular metabolism, and aiding in blood clotting. The recommended daily intake (RDI) for adults aged 19 to 50 is 1000 mg. However, adolescents require a higher intake of 1300 mg/day due to their growing bone mass. For individuals aged nine to 18, the RDI is further increased to 1300 mg/day. For those aged 51 and above, the RDI is reduced to 1200 mg/day.

The upper limit (UL) for calcium intake is set at 2,500 milligrams to prevent mineral imbalances caused by excessive calcium consumption. This mineral interferes with the absorption of iron, magnesium, zinc, and other essential nutrients.

Several forms of calcium supplementation are available, including calcium carbonate, calcium citrate, calcium citrate malate, calcium gluconate, and calcium lactate. Calcium citrate is particularly preferred for individuals with hypo- or achlorhydria (low or insufficient stomach acid). To optimize calcium absorption, it is advisable to limit each dose to no more than 500 mg.

Concurrent adequate vitamin D supplementation is essential when taking calcium supplements. Vitamin D deficiency impairs cellular calcium absorption, potentially leading to atopic calcium deposits in epidermal tissue. Iron supplementation may also interfere with calcium absorption, so it is recommended to take iron supplements at least two hours apart from meals containing calcium-rich foods.

Calcium is essential for the proper functioning of bones, the heart, nerves, muscles, and blood clotting. As the most abundant mineral element in the body, calcium is primarily found in bones. However, serum and red blood cell calcium levels do not accurately reflect bone mineral content or dietary adequacy. While most of the body's calcium is stored in bones, a significant portion circulates in the blood. Approximately 40% of the calcium in blood is bound to proteins, primarily albumin. This protein-bound calcium serves as a reserve source for cells but lacks active physiological functions.

Normal Range	8.9 - 10.6 mg/dL
Optimal Range	8.9 - 10.6 mg/dL

If **LOW** or < 8.9 mg/dL:

A deficiency of calcium can lead to osteoporosis. Some research suggests that low calcium intake may increase the risk of high blood pressure, colon cancer, and preeclampsia (high blood pressure and excess protein in the urine of a woman more than 20 weeks pregnant). However, calcium stores in the blood remain relatively stable, while calcium stores in other parts of the body may become depleted under certain conditions, such as increased demand.

Low dietary calcium intake during periods of growth or stress can result in reduced calcium stores. It's important to consider vitamin D and magnesium levels alongside calcium status. Iron supplementation can interfere with calcium absorption, so it's recommended to take iron supplements at least 2 hours apart from a meal containing calcium-rich foods. Hypocalcemia, or low calcium levels, typically occurs when too much calcium is lost in urine or when not enough calcium is transferred from bones to the blood. Several factors can contribute to hypocalcemia, including:

- Hypoparathyroidism
- Pseudohypoparathyroidism
- Absence of parathyroid glands at birth
- Hypomagnesemia
- Vitamin D deficiency
- Kidney dysfunction
- Inadequate calcium intake
- Disorders that decrease calcium absorption

 Good sources of calcium are: dairy foods, salmon, turnip greens, Chinese cabbage, kale, bok choy and broccoli. Sardines and other canned fish with bones are additional sources. Some foods such as orange juice and bread are fortified with calcium. Chinese cabbage, kale and turnip greens contain absorbable calcium. Spinach and some other vegetables contain calcium that is poorly absorbed.

Support: Calcium supplements, given by mouth, are often all that is needed to support hypocalcemia. If a cause is identified, supporting the disorder causing hypocalcemia or changing drugs may restore the calcium level. Sometimes vitamin D

Nutritional support
- Calcium malate, Vitamin D3
- Trans-Geranylgeraniol, calcium, magnesium, zinc, copper, manganese, boron, Vitamins D3, E, K1, K2, Vitamin C
- Vitamins A, D, E, K
- Vitamins K1, K2, Trans-Geranylgeraniol

If **HIGH** or > 10.6 mg/dL:

Symptoms and conditions associated with excess calcium include calcification of soft tissues (including the heart and arteries), parathyroid disorders, and kidney stones. Causes of excess calcium in the blood include low levels of parathyroid hormone (PTH), high or excessive intake of vitamin D2 or D3 supplements (unlikely with D2), hyperparathyroidism, reduced conversion of 25-hydroxyvitamin D (25-OHD) to 1,25-dihydroxyvitamin D (1,25-OHD) in the kidneys, renal failure, and parathyroid cancer.

Caution with calcium supplements: Calcium supplements may cause an excess of calcium in the blood if one has parathyroid dysfunction or renal failure. It is not recommended to take calcium supplements if these conditions exist, unless under the direction of a doctor. Calcium supplementation should almost always be accompanied by supplementation of vitamin D and possibly vitamin K2 to ensure calcium is assimilated into bone and not ectopically deposited into soft tissue.

Hypercalcemia is a condition in which the calcium level in the blood is above normal. Too much calcium in the blood can weaken bones, create kidney stones, and interfere with how the heart and brain function. Symptoms include excessive thirst and frequent urination (kidneys have to work harder to filter calcium), upset stomach, nausea, vomiting, and constipation, bone pain, muscle weakness, and depression (due to calcium leaching from bones), confusion, lethargy, and fatigue (calcium can interfere with brain functions), palpitations, fainting, and cardiac arrhythmia (severe hypercalcemia can disrupt heart functions in severe cases).

Causes include overactive parathyroid glands (hyperparathyroidism), cancer (lung, breast, blood can increase risk), tuberculosis or sarcoidosis can increase serum vitamin D levels and trigger the GI tract to absorb more calcium, genetic disorders (check for familial hypocalciuric hypercalcemia), excessive sitting or lying down, severe dehydration, certain drugs, excessive amounts of calcium or vitamin D supplements.

 Support depends on the cause.

 Support depends on the cause.

Manganese

Manganese plays a crucial role in numerous enzyme-mediated chemical reactions, particularly those involving enzymes in antioxidant actions within mitochondria and enzymes responsible for cartilage synthesis in the skin and bones. Additionally, manganese activates enzymes involved in the metabolism of carbohydrates, amino acids, and cholesterol. Furthermore, enzymes that incorporate manganese convert the neuro-excitatory glutamate into glutamine.

Iron supplementation can potentially reduce the absorption of dietary manganese. Iron stores (ferritin levels) tend to be higher in men than in women, which can lead to a reduction in intestinal manganese absorption. Magnesium supplementation has also been demonstrated to decrease manganese levels through reduced intestinal absorption or increased urinary excretion.

The Adequate Intake (AI) for manganese is set at 1.8 mg per day, while the Upper Limit (UL) is 11 mg per day. Generally, supplementation of manganese is not necessary and may even lead to toxicity.

Normal Range	≤ 2.2 ng/mL
Optimal Range	≤ 2.2 ng/mL

If **HIGH** or **> 2.2 ng/mL:**

Toxicity is also uncommon and is most frequently the result of exposure to airborne manganese dust. Symptoms of toxicity include multiple neurological problems that resemble Parkinson's disease In children, exposure to elevated levels of manganese in drinking water has been associated with increased rates of attention deficit hyperactivity disorder, cognitive decline, and behavioral problems. Individuals with liver failure are at risk for manganese toxicity-associated neurological symptoms.

Tea and coffee are significant sources of manganese in the American diet. Additional sources are nuts, whole grains, legumes and some fruits and vegetables, such as leafy greens. Tea and coffee are signikcant sources of manganese in the American diet. Additional sources are nuts, whole grains, legumes and some fruits and vegetables, such as leafy greens.

Zinc

Zinc is essential for normal growth and sexual maturation. It plays a crucial role in the immune system and is involved in the proper functioning of at least 300 enzymes. Zinc is vital for the structure of proteins and cell membranes. Additionally, it regulates gene function, influences cell signaling, hormone release, and nerve signaling.

The recommended daily allowance (RDA) for zinc is 8 milligrams (mg) per day for women and 11 mg per day for men. The upper limit (UL) for zinc is 40 mg per day. Long-term supplementation of zinc at levels exceeding 60 mg per day can interfere with copper absorption.

Zinc lozenges are commonly used to shorten the duration of the common cold. Zinc is available in various forms, including zinc acetate, zinc gluconate, zinc picolinate, zinc sulfate, and zinc carnosine. Zinc carnosine has been used in combination therapies to support the health of the epithelial linings of both the stomach and intestines during times of physiological stress, such as stomach ulcers and impaired intestinal barrier function.

However, consuming large doses of zinc or taking it for prolonged periods without addressing a zinc deficiency can lead to toxicity. Single doses of 200-450 mg of zinc may cause vomiting and gastrointestinal distress.

Normal Range	0.7 - 1.6 mcg/mL
Optimal Range	0.7 - 1.6 mcg/mL

If LOW or < 0.7 mcg/mL:

Insufficient dietary intake, particularly in populations that heavily rely on cereal grains for caloric intake, is a concern due to the high levels of phytic acid that impairs zinc absorption. While higher doses of supplementary zinc can impair copper uptake, copper intake does not affect zinc absorption except when zinc status is already marginally deficient. Supplementation of elemental iron may decrease zinc absorption. Therefore, pregnant women and individuals with anemia who are supplementing iron may need to take supplemental zinc separately from iron supplements.

Zinc deficiency can lead to delayed growth and sexual development, decreased immune function, altered sense of taste, hair loss, pregnancy complications, and gastrointestinal distress. Loss of zinc from cell membranes impairs their function and increases the susceptibility of the membrane to oxidative damage. Loss of zinc through malabsorption increases susceptibility to infections due to depressed immune function. Increased urination in individuals with diabetes mellitus may lead to marginal zinc deficiency.

Individuals who may be at higher risk of zinc deficiency include pregnant and lactating women, patients receiving total parenteral nutrition (TPN), malnourished individuals, individuals with eating disorders such as anorexia nervosa, individuals with impaired intestinal absorption and/or persistent diarrhea like celiac disease, Crohn's disease, and ulcerative colitis, alcoholics, and individuals with liver disease. Additionally, individuals over 65 years of age and strict vegetarians may also be at risk.

Subnormal levels are associated with alcoholic cirrhosis, cystic fibrosis, myocardial infarction, acute and chronic infections. Oysters, beef and clams are rich sources of absorbable zinc. Whole grains also contain zinc, but it is less available for absorption due to high phytic acid content of grains.

Nutritional support - Zinc

If HIGH or > 1.6 mcg/mL:

Zinc can be toxic when consumed in large doses, or when taken for prolonged periods of time in the absence of a zinc deficiency.

High levels may be due to industrial exposure or over supplementation Look to copper levels - can be deficient when zinc is elevated and vice versa Zinc supplements can cause copper deficiency. Avoid zinc supplements over 50 mg/d unless you have a strong reason to use higher doses, and if supplementing with zinc use a zinc-to-copper ratio between 2:1 and 15:1.

Copper

Copper plays a vital role in various bodily functions. It aids in the transportation of iron, supports energy production within cells, facilitates methylation and gene transcription that influences cellular detoxification mechanisms, contributes to neurotransmitter generation, supports the myelin sheath around nerves, and aids in connective tissue development. Copper is essential for redox reactions and possesses potent antioxidant properties. Additionally, it supports melanin production in the cells of hair, skin, and nails.

Most serum copper is bound to ceruloplasmin, and elevated levels may indicate increased inflammation and oxidative stress rather than specific excess copper in the blood. The Recommended Dietary Allowance (RDA) for copper in adults is 900 μg/day, while the Upper Limit (UL) is 10 mg/day, which has been shown not to cause liver damage in healthy individuals. Copper supplementation of 2 mg/day is usually sufficient to correct copper deficiencies.

Copper is commonly available in supplemental forms such as cupric oxide, copper gluconate, copper sulfate, and copper amino acid chelates. Some research suggests that elevated blood levels of free unbound copper, which depletes zinc levels, may be associated with the onset of Alzheimer's disease. Therefore, copper supplementation in this population is not recommended if zinc deficiency is suspected.

Copper is involved in enzymes, which are proteins that facilitate biochemical reactions in every cell. It plays a crucial role in iron absorption, storage, and metabolism. The symptoms of copper deficiency are similar to iron deficiency anemia. (The liver produces a special protein called ceruloplasmin to transport copper and assist in converting iron into a form usable by other tissues.) Copper is utilized by most cells as a component of enzymes involved in energy production, protecting cells from free radical damage, strengthening connective tissue, and supporting brain neurotransmitter function.

Normal Range	0.7 - 1.8 mcg/mL
Optimal Range	0.7 - 1.8 mcg/mL

If LOW or < 0.7 mcg/mL:

Copper deficiencies or excesses are uncommon in healthy individuals. However, copper deficiency can occur in specific populations, including infants or children fed exclusively cow's milk formula, premature infants, infants or children with persistent diarrhea, individuals with malabsorption syndromes like celiac disease, bowel resections, Crohn's disease, and ulcerative colitis, individuals with cystic fibrosis, and individuals with prolonged high supplemental zinc intake. To assess the possibility of copper deficiency, consider testing for celiac disease or neurological indicators of demyelination. Copper deficiency can also develop due to prolonged supplemental zinc intake exceeding 60mg/day. Since copper is essential for iron metabolism and red blood cell formation and function, anemia can be a clinical sign of copper deficiency as iron accumulates in the liver without sufficient copper for transport. Copper depletion is rare but can be observed in Wilson's disease, where dietary copper intake has no impact on copper status. Severe copper deficiency may also lead to cardiovascular abnormalities and cardiomyopathy. However, some epidemiological studies suggest a possible association between elevated copper levels and increased atherosclerosis. Copper deficiency can also result in low neutrophil counts, anemias that don't respond to iron supplementation, and impaired growth, neurological problems, and skin pigmentation in children.

Rich sources of copper include liver, shellfish, cashews, hazelnuts, almonds, peanut butter, lentils, mushrooms, and sunflower seeds. Copper supplementation of 2 mg/day is usually sufficient to correct deficiencies of copper. Some research suggests elevated blood levels of free unbound copper, which depletes zinc levels, may have an association with the onset of Alzheimer's disease, and supplementation of copper in this population is not recommended if zinc deficiency is suspected.

Nutritional support - Copper

If **HIGH** or > 1.8 mcg/mL:

 Most serum copper is found in ceruloplasmin and elevated levels may be an indicator of increase inflammation and oxidative stress, rather than specifically excess copper in the blood.

 Address inflammation and oxidative stress. Look to zinc levels - can be deficient when copper is elevated and vice versa

Chromium

Chromium, an essential nutrient found in trace amounts in humans, plays a crucial role as a cofactor for chromodulin, a peptide that enhances the effectiveness of insulin on target tissues. This interaction aids in regulating blood sugar and lipid metabolism. The recommended daily intake of chromium varies depending on sex: 35 µg/day for men and 25 µg/day for women. However, increased needs may arise during pregnancy and lactation.

While supplemental chromium is generally not necessary as dietary consumption typically meets physiological requirements, it's important to note that its effectiveness is poorly studied, and insufficient evidence exists to provide specific recommendations. Nevertheless, chromium picolinate is a commonly used form in the treatment of insulin resistance and diabetes.

Normal Range	≤ 0.3 ng/mL
Optimal Range	≤ 0.3 ng/mL

If **LOW**:

 Dietary deficiency of chromium is believed to be widespread in the United States. Chromium deficiency may increase the likelihood of insulin resistance, metabolic syndrome, coronary artery disease, PCOS, dyslipidemia

 Food sources of chromium: Brewer's yeast (especially yeast grown in soil high in chromium) Whole grain bread and cereals Molasses Spices Some bran cereals Organ meats Mushrooms Oatmeal Prunes Nuts Asparagus

If **HIGH** or > 0.3 ng/mL:

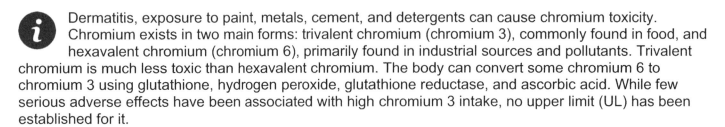 Dermatitis, exposure to paint, metals, cement, and detergents can cause chromium toxicity. Chromium exists in two main forms: trivalent chromium (chromium 3), commonly found in food, and hexavalent chromium (chromium 6), primarily found in industrial sources and pollutants. Trivalent chromium is much less toxic than hexavalent chromium. The body can convert some chromium 6 to chromium 3 using glutathione, hydrogen peroxide, glutathione reductase, and ascorbic acid. While few serious adverse effects have been associated with high chromium 3 intake, no upper limit (UL) has been established for it.

Overexposure to chromium 6 can occur among welders and other workers in the metallurgical industry, individuals using chromium-containing paints and primers, those with metallic surgical implants, and those who ingest chromium salts. Chromium toxicity can result from oral, inhaled, or dermal absorption. Depending on the route of exposure, it can lead to nausea, vomiting, diarrhea, muscle cramps, skin lesions, sinus, nasal, and lung cancer, renal failure, liver damage, circulatory collapse, coma, and death.

Balance gut microflora, phytates

Iron

Normal Range	35 - 150 mcg/dL
Optimal Range	35 - 150 mcg/dL

If LOW or < 35.0 mcg/dL:

Iron is lost from the body through various means, including urination, defecation, sweating, and exfoliation of old skin cells. Bleeding further contributes to iron loss, explaining why women have a higher iron demand than men. When iron stores are low, normal hemoglobin production slows down, reducing oxygen transport and causing symptoms like fatigue, dizziness, lowered immunity, and reduced athletic performance. Since our bodies can't produce iron, we must ensure sufficient iron intake through our diet. Mild iron deficiency can be prevented or corrected by consuming iron-rich foods and cooking in iron skillets. Iron is essential for most plants and animals, so a diverse range of foods provide iron. Heme-iron, which is most easily absorbed and not inhibited by medications or other components, is found in good sources like red meat and poultry. Non-heme iron, found in lentils, beans, leafy greens, pistachios, tofu, fortified bread, and fortified breakfast cereals, is also available but has reduced bioavailability.

Iron absorption and processing vary among foods; heme iron from meat is more easily absorbed than non-heme iron from grains and vegetables. However, heme iron from red meat may increase the risk of colorectal cancer. Minerals and chemicals in one food can inhibit iron absorption from another. For instance, oxalates and phytic acid form insoluble complexes that bind iron in the gut, preventing absorption. Since iron from plant sources is less easily absorbed than heme-bound iron from animal sources, vegetarians and vegans should consume slightly more iron daily than those who eat meat, fish, or poultry. Legumes and dark green leafy vegetables like broccoli, kale, and oriental greens are excellent iron sources for vegetarians and vegans. However, spinach and Swiss chard contain oxalates that bind iron, making it almost entirely unavailable for absorption. Consuming iron from non-heme sources with foods containing heme-bound iron or vitamin C enhances absorption.

Consuming iron-rich foods will support optimal iron levels. Consuming both heme iron food categories and non-heme sources of iron will provide various options to support the various physiological processes that require this mineral. When optimizing iron levels, an additional avenue is to consider foods high in Vitamin C. Heme Iron Sources: Oysters Mussels Duck Bison Duck Egg Beef Sardines, canned Crab Lamb Shrimp Non-Heme Iron Sources: Spinach Artichokes Soybeans Canned stewed tomatoes Lentils Asparagus, raw Beets, cooked Sesame seeds Cashews

 Nutritional support - Iron (Ferrous Bisglycinate Chelate)

If HIGH or > 150.0 mcg/dL:

Iron levels are typically evaluated in conjunction with other iron tests or a full anemia panel. High levels of serum iron can occur as the result of multiple blood transfusions, excessive iron supplementation or injections, lead poisoning, liver or kidney disease. Elevated iron levels can also be due to the genetic disease hemochomatosis—when too much iron accumulates in the body and can damage organs. High iron levels from dietary or supplementation are more likely in men, and women after menopause because they do not lose iron in blood. High levels of iron in the serum are associated with too much iron, vitamin B6 or vitamin B12. Some specific causes of high iron might be: - anemia where the blood cells rupture, called hemolytic anemia - iron overdose, where you have consumed more iron than what your body requires and can successfully deal with - an overload of iron, where your body is not eliminating iron as it should - liver health issues such as hemosiderosis, hemochromatosis, liver failure or hepatitis - too many blood transfusions - lead poisoning - use of birth control pills

Increased levels may be seen in alcohol abuse, acute hepatitis, and infections. In severe cases of hemochromatosis, periodic removal of a prescribed amount of blood, also known as therapeutic phlebotomy, may be necessary.

Magnesium

Normal Range	1.6 - 2.6 mg/dL
Optimal Range	1.6 - 2.6 mg/dL

If LOW or < 1.6 mg/dL:

 Alcohol consumption leads to increased urine excretion. Prolonged use of diuretics further exacerbates this effect. Excessive sweating, particularly during prolonged endurance exercise, and hyperparathyroidism, chronic renal failure, malabsorbent conditions such as celiac disease, Crohn's disease, and partial bowel resection, diabetes (30% of which show signs of depletion), and aging are all risk factors for magnesium depletion. Intestinal absorption of magnesium declines with age, and high doses of zinc supplements in supplemental form can interfere with its absorption. Primary magnesium deficiency is rare, and deficiency is usually secondary to another condition.

Signs and symptoms of magnesium deficiency include weakness, heart irregularities, muscle cramps and twitches, insomnia, mental confusion, fatigue, irritability, and impaired Vitamin D and calcium absorption, increasing the risk of bone mineral density disorders. Magnesium depletion is commonly associated with various disease states, including both type 1 and type 2 diabetes, hypertension, endothelial dysfunction, asthma, and migraine headaches.

 Magnesium is part of chlorophyll so leafy greens are rich in magnesium. Best food sources include: oats, brown rice, spinach, swiss chard, almonds, cashews, hazelnuts, potatoes, bananas, milk, raisins, halibut, avocado, black strap molasses, and chocolate.

 Nutritional support: Magnesium Citrate

If HIGH or > 2.6 mg/dL:

Severe toxicity may cause confusion, loss of kidney function, difficulty breathing and cardiac arrest individuals with kidney disease are at higher risk for magnesium toxicity. The use of supraphysiological doses of magnesium can be used therapeutically.

Magnesium, when consumed in excess from food, doesn't pose a health risk to healthy individuals since the kidneys efficiently eliminate any excess through urine. However, high doses of magnesium from dietary supplements or medications can lead to diarrhea, nausea, and abdominal cramping. Magnesium salts, particularly magnesium carbonate, chloride, gluconate, and oxide, are the most common forms that cause diarrhea. The laxative effects of magnesium salts are attributed to the osmotic activity of unabsorbed salts in the intestine and colon, as well as the stimulation of gastric motility.

It's important to note that the Upper Limit (UL) for magnesium only applies to supplemental magnesium intake. The ULs are as follows:
- 1-3 years: 65 mg per day
- 4-8 years: 110 mg per day
- 9-18 years and adults: 350 mg per day

Very large doses of magnesium-containing laxatives and antacids (typically exceeding 5,000 mg per day) have been associated with magnesium toxicity, which can be fatal in severe cases. Symptoms of magnesium toxicity may include hypotension, nausea, vomiting, facial flushing, urine retention, ileus, depression, and lethargy. As the condition progresses, it can lead to muscle weakness, difficulty breathing, extreme hypotension, irregular heartbeat, and cardiac arrest. The risk of magnesium toxicity increases with impaired renal function or kidney failure, as the kidneys' ability to eliminate excess magnesium is compromised.

Copper to Zinc Ratio

Copper and zinc, being antagonists, compete for binding sites and work against each other. An imbalance in their ratio can lead to health problems, including impaired insulin balance and other hormone imbalances. Part of the normal immune response depletes infected tissues of zinc to starve pathogens and moves it to other locations to support the immune response. Copper also assists in the immune response by regulating macrophage (white blood cell, especially in response to infection) pathways. Many of these changes are not related to nutritional or supplemental intake of the metals. A balanced copper to zinc ratio plays a crucial role in maintaining the immune system, aiding in disease resistance, and potentially indicating oxidative stress.

Normal Range	0.7 - 1.0 ratio
Optimal Range	0.7 - 1.0 ratio

If LOW or < 0.7 RATIO:

Zinc supplements can cause copper deficiency. Avoid zinc supplements over 50 mg/d unless you have a strong reason to use higher doses, and if supplementing with zinc use a zinc-to-copper ratio between 2:1 and 15:1. High blood levels of copper have been seen in Wilson's disease and in the elderly. Autistic children have been shown to have high serum copper-zinc ratio and low ceruloplasmin. Copper dysregulation is present in some neurodegenerative conditions such as amyotrophic lateral sclerosis (ALS), Parkinson's disease, Down's syndrome, and idiopathic seizure disorder.

Rich sources of copper include liver, shellfish, cashews, hazelnuts, almonds, peanut butter, lentils, mushrooms, and sunflower seeds. Copper supplementation of 2 mg/day is usually sufficient to correct deficiencies of copper. Some research suggests elevated blood levels of free unbound copper, which depletes zinc levels, may have an association with the onset of Alzheimer's disease, and supplementation of copper in this population is not recommended if zinc deficiency is suspected.

Nutritional support - Copper

If HIGH or > 1.0 RATIO:

Imbalanced copper/zinc ratio can be implicated in oxidative stress, poor mood and brain health and poor sleep. Excess zinc intake can result in a copper deficiency when intake of copper is insufficient.

Evaluate the use of copper cookware or water lines. Other potential serum imbalances include low serum albumin, high CRP, high ESR, and high IL-6. In the elderly, ratios above 2.0 appear to correlate with an increased inflammatory response.

 Nutritional support: Zinc

Antioxidants

Antioxidants are molecules that play a crucial role in protecting cells from damage caused by oxidative stress, which is a natural process associated with the production of harmful molecules called free radicals. An imbalance between free radicals and antioxidants can lead to various health issues, including chronic diseases and aging-related conditions.

Coenzyme Q10

Coenzyme Q10 (CoQ10): CoQ10, also known as ubiquinone, is a fat-soluble antioxidant that is vital for cellular energy production in the form of ATP (adenosine triphosphate). It is present in the mitochondria, the energy-producing organelles of cells. CoQ10 not only contributes to energy production but also acts as an antioxidant, protecting cell membranes from damage caused by free radicals. Measurement of CoQ10 levels can provide insights into mitochondrial health and overall energy metabolism. CoQ10 is a fat-soluble compound primarily synthesized by the body and also consumed in the diet. It is found in virtually all cell membranes and participates in the mitochondria to convert carbohydrates and fatty acids into ATP. CoQ10 also supports cell signaling, gene expression, stimulation of cell growth, inhibition of apoptosis, control of thiol groups, formation of hydrogen peroxide, and control of membrane channels

Normal Range	0.59 - 2.07 mcg/mL
Optimal Range	0.59 - 2.07 mcg/mL

If LOW or < 0.59 mcg/mL:

CoQ10 is most commonly depleted through use of cholesterol-lowering medication, such as statins. Other causes of CoQ10 deficiency include genetic mutations that limit biosynthesis, unknown reasons in the aging process, cancer, and smoking. Signs of CoQ10 deficiency include muscle weakness and fatigue, high blood pressure, and slowed thinking; more extreme symptoms of CoQ10 deficiency include chest pain, heart failure, and seizures.

CoQ10, a nutrient found in various foods, is considered a poor source. However, organ meats from red meat sources are richer in CoQ10. Nuts are considered a moderate source but require excessive consumption to meet the daily requirement. Currently, there are no established Recommended Dietary Allowances (RDAs), Adequate Intakes (AIs), or Upper Limits (ULs) for CoQ10.

CoQ10 exists in two forms: ubiquinone and ubiquinol. Ubiquinol is considered the active form, but the body utilizes both forms as needed. Typically, doses of 100-200 mg/day are required to restore minimum CoQ10 levels while taking statin drugs. Intestinal absorption of CoQ10 is limited but can be optimized by consuming it with a meal containing fat.

While high-dose CoQ10 supplementation generally does not cause adverse symptoms, it is not typically recommended for pregnant or lactating women due to the lack of controlled studies.

Nutritional support
- Coenzyme Q10 (Ubiquinone)

ANTIOXIDANTS

If HIGH or > 2.07 mcg/mL:

 Abnormally high levels of coenzyme Q10 are only practically possible through the use of supplements. It is unclear whether moderately excessive amounts of coenzyme Q10 are harmful to humans. While it is fat soluble, CoQ10 does not accumulate after supplementation has stopped.

There is currently no established RDA, AI, or UL for CoQ10.

There have been no reports of significant adverse side effects of oral coenzyme Q10 supplementation at doses as high as 3,000 mg/day for up to eight months, 1,200 mg/day for up to 16 months), and 600 mg/day for up to 30 months.

According to the observed safe level (OSL) risk assessment method, evidence of safety is strong with doses up to 1,200 mg/day of coenzyme Q10.

Because reliable data on lactating women are unavailable, supplementation should be avoided during breastfeeding.

Stop or reduce Coenzyme Q10 supplementation

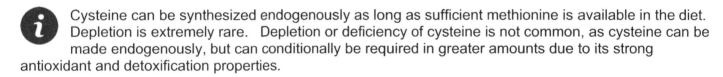

Cysteine

Cysteine is an amino acid that plays a crucial role in the synthesis of glutathione, another potent antioxidant. It also has direct antioxidant properties. Cysteine is important for maintaining the balance of antioxidants in the body, as it serves as a precursor for glutathione production. Cysteine has antioxidant properties itself, but is also a precursor molecule to glutathione production, the master antioxidant. Cysteine is also an important source of sulfide for iron-sulfide metabolism. Cysteine will bind metals easily to its thiol group, such as iron, nickel, copper, zinc, and heavy metals such as mercury and lead, which may confer some chelation benefits. Cysteine counteracts acetaldehyde effects from consumption of alcohol and can reduce hangovers.

Normal Range	11.0 - 36.1 nmol/mL
Optimal Range	11.0 - 36.1 nmol/mL

If LOW or < 11.0 nmol/mL:

 Cysteine can be synthesized endogenously as long as sufficient methionine is available in the diet. Depletion is extremely rare. Depletion or deficiency of cysteine is not common, as cysteine can be made endogenously, but can conditionally be required in greater amounts due to its strong antioxidant and detoxification properties.

Dietary sources of cysteine include: meat, poultry, eggs, dairy, red peppers, garlic, onions, broccoli, Brussels sprouts, oats, granola, wheat germ, and lentils. There is currently no established RDA, AI, or UL for cysteine. Cysteine is typically purchased in supplement form as N-acetyl-cysteine (NAC). Cysteine can be purchased as L-cysteine in powder form. For general antioxidant support, doses start at 500mg/day and can increase depending upon direction from medical provider. AVOID: D-cysteine or D-cystine, which are toxic

Nutritional support:
- S-Acetyl Glutathione
- N-Acetyl-L-Cysteine (NAC)
- Vitamin B6 (P5P)

If **HIGH** or > 36.1 nmol/mL:

There is currently no established RDA, AI, or UL for cysteine.

Excess supplementation:
- Cysteine is typically purchased in supplement form as N-acetyl cysteine (NAC).
- For general antioxidant support, doses start at 500 mg/day and can increase depending upon direction from the medical provider.
- AVOID: D-cysteine or D-cystine, which are toxic.
- A diet high in cysteine-rich proteins can elevate cysteine levels. As with all sulfur-containing amino acids, the enzyme sulfite oxidase catabolizes the amino acid into sulfite for excretion.

An important cofactor for this enzyme is molybdenum. With that, insufficient molybdenum can contribute to elevated cysteine.

Homocysteine is pulled into the transsulfuration pathway via the enzyme cystathionine-beta-synthase (CBS) to become cysteine, with cystathionine formation as an intermediate step. Cysteine levels may be elevated due to a CBS SNP which results in an upregulation of the enzyme and more cystathionine and cysteine production.

Zinc is an important cofactor downstream from cysteine in transsulfuration. Because of this, cysteine elevations can also be seen in zinc insufficiency.

Vitamin B12 may also be a cofactor in the peripheral utilization of cysteine; therefore functional deficiencies of vitamin B12 can contribute to higher levels.

Stop or reduce cysteine / NAC supplementation
Consider co-factors for trans-sulfuration: molybdenum, zinc, magnesium, manganese, B12, B-Complex

Nutritional support:
- Molybdenum
- Zinc
- Multi-mineral
- Vitamin B12
- Vitamin B9 (folate)
- Vitamin B complex

Glutathione

Glutathione is often referred to as the "master antioxidant" due to its widespread presence in cells and its ability to neutralize a variety of free radicals and toxins. It plays a significant role in detoxification processes and helps protect cells from oxidative damage. Measuring glutathione levels can provide information about the body's ability to counteract oxidative stress and maintain cellular health. Glutathione is the master intracellular antioxidant. Glutathione is the main non-enzymatic antioxidant in intestinal epithelium. The only cells in the body that have been found to be able to absorb intact GSH are hepatocytes, intestinal mucosal cells, and retinal cells. GSH can also conjugate target compounds for removal through hepatic/renal excretion or through removal into the intestinal lumen and through fecal elimination. Alpha-lipoic acid appears to support the transport of cystine (two bonded cysteine molecules) between cells for uptake to generate glutathione, and therefore, may increase glutathione synthesis provided that cysteine levels are adequate.

Normal Range	0.5 - 1.9 nmol/mL
Optimal Range	0.5 - 1.9 nmol/mL

If LOW or < 0.5 nmol/mL:

Glutathione levels deplete naturally during aging, however, this could be related to decreased protein intake in aging individuals. Pro-inflammatory states and elevated oxidative stress will drain GSH stores and require a conditionally greater intake of either high cysteine foods or NAC as a supplement to increase endogenous GSH production. Conversion of depleted glutathione back to its active state is achieved through an NADPH-dependent enzyme, so it stands to reason that low levels of NAD (or niacin, nicotinic acid) could further limit this conversion back to active GSH forms. Consider mutations in GSHPx gene to determine if deficiency or depletion is genetically influenced. Symptoms of glutathione depletion or deficiency include: fatigue, increased oxidative stress, inflammation, cancer, and infections.

Dietary glutathione consumption does not correlate with systemic levels of glutathione, but sources of glutathione are fruits and vegetables such as: asparagus, avocado, spinach, broccoli, cantaloupe, tomato, carrot, grapefruit, orange, zucchini, strawberry, watermelon, papaya, red bell pepper, peaches, lemons, mangoes, cauliflower, and cabbage. There currently is no RDA, AI, or UL established for glutathione intake. Glutathione cannot enter cells intact, and must be synthesized inside the cell in order to be effective, therefore, supplementation usually has negligible benefit. Supplementing the building blocks such as N-acetyl-cysteine, glutamic acid and glycine, of which NAC is the only one that may be necessary to supplement, may increase cellular production of glutathione. Direct glutathione supplementation has only been shown to benefit slowing the breakdown of nitric oxide in the bloodstream.

Nutritional support:
- S-Acetyl Glutathione
- N-Acetyl-L-Cysteine (NAC)
- Vitamin B6 (P5P)

If HIGH or > 1.9 nmol/mL:

There currently is no RDA, AI, or UL established for glutathione intake.

Excess supplementation:
- High-dose supplementation is sometimes used for various purposes, including skin lightening and antioxidant support.
- Glutathione cannot enter cells intact and must be synthesized inside the cell to be effective. Therefore, supplementation usually has negligible benefit.
- Supplementing the building blocks such as NAC, glutamic acid, and glycine may increase cellular production of glutathione; however, NAC may be most impactful as the amino acid cysteine is known to be rate-limiting for the synthesis of glutathione.
- Direct glutathione supplementation has only been shown to benefit slowing the breakdown of nitric oxide in the bloodstream.

Stop or reduce glutathione supplementation
Consider support cellular production of glutathione with precursors and co-factors if appropriate (i.e. supplementary glutathione is high but you suspect antioxidant status overall is still poor)

Nutritional support:
- NAC (N-Acetyl-L-Cysteine)
- Glycine
- Molybdenum
- Vitamin B complex

Selenium

Selenium is a trace element that is an essential component of various antioxidant enzymes, including glutathione peroxidases. These enzymes play a crucial role in neutralizing hydrogen peroxide and lipid peroxides, which are harmful byproducts of oxidative reactions. Adequate selenium levels are important for the proper function of these antioxidant enzymes. Selenium is an essential trace element required for immune function and for the synthesis of thyroid hormones, through its actions in selenoproteins such as iodothyronine deiodinase, and the direct conversion of thyroxine (T4) to triiodothyronine (T3). Additionally, this mineral assists enzymes in protecting cell membranes from damage and selenium is a critical component of antioxidant reactions, by supporting the production of selenoproteins, such as glutathione peroxidase. Selenium helps to regenerate vitamin C and vitamin E from their oxidized forms, supporting antioxidant action of these vitamins.

Normal Range	168.0 - 276.3 ng/mL
Optimal Range	168.0 - 276.3 ng/mL

If **LOW** or < 168.0 ng/ml:

Individuals at risk for low levels of selenium or selenium depletion are patients who have had bariatric surgery, celiac patients, and Crohn's disease patients. Selenium deficiency is very rare in developed countries. Low selenium intake may decrease an individual's ability to fight viral infections. Some research also links low intakes to some cancers. Toxicity causes brittle hair and nails and is most likely to occur with supplements. Selenium deficiency may not always produce overt symptoms of disease, but may manifest as increased oxidative stress in deficient individuals, due to decreased action of glutathione peroxidase, decreased antioxidant regeneration, decreased conversion of thyroid hormones, and reduced methionine metabolism. Severe selenium deficiency can result in Keshan disease, in which the heart becomes enlarged alongside cardiac insufficiency. Selenium supplementation prevents further progression of the condition, but does not reverse damage that has already occurred.

Food sources of selenium include: Brazil nuts, tuna, cod, turkey, chicken breast, beef roast, sunflower seeds, and ground beef. Organ meats, seafood, other meats, and whole grains are additional sources. Depending upon the soil in which they are grown, Brazil nuts are one of the richest sources of selenium. The RDA for selenium is 55 µg/day. The UL for selenium is 400 µg/day, including food sources. Protein-based food sources of selenium appear to be the most effective at increasing circulating levels of glutathione peroxidase. Selenium supplementation in individuals with autoimmune thyroiditis has been shown to reduce circulating autoantibody levels. Selenium supplementation has been found to reduce viral load progression in individuals with HIV. Selenium supplementation in persons with sepsis and septic shock has been shown to reduce mortality. Selenium comes in the following supplemental forms: sodium, selenite, sodium selenate, selenomethionine. Selenomethionine has been shown to increase blood levels of selenium more effectively than the inorganic forms of selenium (selenite and selenate). Sodium selenate is absorbed to a lesser extent than sodium selenite, but sodium selenate is retained in greater amounts. Selenium supplements are not recommended for individuals with or at risk for diabetes mellitus.

Nutritional support
- Selenium

If **HIGH** or > 276.3 ng/mL:

Excess levels can lead to selenium poisoning or toxicity, and this can potentially be fatal or lead to heart attack and respiratory (lung) For most people, selenium requirements can be met through food sources. Symptoms of selenium toxicity include nausea; vomiting; nail discoloration, brittleness, and loss; hair loss; fatigue; irritability; and foul breath odor (often described as "garlic breath").

Vibrant Micronutrient

The Micronutrients Panel from Vibrant America is the only test that provides a comprehensive extracellular and intracellular assessment of the levels of the most important vitamins, minerals, antioxidants, fatty acids, and amino acids.

Micronutrient 'Dial Charts' categorize micronutrients based on body system, structure, and function. Each 'Dial Chart' is scored on a scale of 0-100, indicating risk. Green (86 or above) indicates optimal levels, yellow (40-85) indicates moderate risk, and red (<40) indicates high risk. The Dial Chart Summary Scores assign different weights to each micronutrient based on its clinical importance and significance in each category. Consequently, not all micronutrients are scored or weighted equally. For instance, EPA will have a higher weightage in the Cardiovascular Health Dial Chart compared to vitamin E, while zinc will have a lower weightage compared to vitamin D or vitamin K2 in the Bone Joint & Muscle Health Dial Chart.

Lymphocyte Count (Cellular)

Lymphocytes, a type of white blood cell, play a crucial role in the immune system, helping the body fight diseases and infections. They are primarily found in lymph organs and blood, where they function as phagocytes, engulfing and eliminating bacteria, fungi, and viruses.

Lymphocytes comprise three main types: T cells, B cells, and natural killer cells. Together, they constitute the primary component of the adaptive immune response, accounting for approximately 20-40% of total white blood cells.

Lymphocytes identify foreign objects, such as bacteria and viruses, and generate a specific response tailored to eliminate the invader. They have a lifespan of 13-20 days before being destroyed by the lymph system. The number of WBCs is regulated by the endocrine system, which can be elevated during stress and impaired by elevated blood sugar levels.

In addition to their role in the adaptive immune response, lymphocytes also possess the ability to remember antigens, which are foreign substances that trigger the immune system. After encountering an antigen, some lymphocytes differentiate into memory cells, enabling the body to mount a more potent response upon subsequent encounters with the same antigen. When memory lymphocytes encounter an antigen for a second time, they swiftly and precisely respond to it. This is the reason why vaccines can prevent specific diseases. Lymphocytes continuously monitor the body's environment, identifying potential foreign antigens ranging from the common cold to malignant tumors. They interact with other cells, including phagocytes (monocytes, macrophages, histiocytes, and similar cells) and more specialized cells called dendritic cells.

Optimal Range	1.32 - 3.57 (x 10^3/µL)

If LOW or < 1.32 x 10^3/µL:

- Chronic viral or bacterial infection
- Bone marrow insufficiency, Free radical activity/oxidative stress. Low levels can be seen in autoimmune disorders, bone marrow damage, and immune deficiency.

Immune Support:
- Echinacea angustifolia
- Astragalus membranaceus
- Elderberry Extract (Sambucus nigra)
- Andrographis paniculate
- Lovage (Levisticum officinale)
- Green Tea Extract
- Arabinogalactan (larch tree)
- Lauric Acid
- Ginger
- Wild Cherry Extract
- Wild cherry bark
- Cordyceps mushroom
- Shiitake mushroom
- Maitake mushroom
- Reishi mushroom
- Beta 1,3 Glucans
- Zinc
- Vitamin C
- Vitamin D3
- Vitamin K2
- L-Glutamine
- Zinc Carnosine
- Slippery Elm
- Aloe Vera Leaf Gel Extract
- Apple Pectin
- Deglycyrrhizinated Licorice (DGL)
- Marshmallow
- Chamomile
- MSM (methylsulfonylmethane)
- Mucin
- Okra
- Prune
- Iron
- Glucosamine HCl
- Cat's Claw

If **HIGH** or > 3.57 (x 10^3/μL):

- Actue viral or bacterial infection, Parasites, Inflammation
- Compromised detox pathways, Overall toxicity.
- High levels of lymphocytes may be seen in acute viral infections and certain bacterial infections.

Support immune & build up natural defense mech.   Anti-inflammatories Gut healing and anti-parasites if necessary

Immune Support:
- Echinacea angustifolia
- Astragalus membranaceus
- Elderberry Extract (Sambucus nigra)
- Andrographis paniculate
- Lovage (Levisticum officinale)
- Green Tea Extract
- Arabinogalactan (larch tree)
- Lauric Acid
- Ginger
- Wild Cherry Extract
- Wild cherry bark
- Cordyceps mushroom
- Shiitake mushroom
- Maitake mushroom
- Reishi mushroom
- Beta 1,3 Glucans
- Zinc
- Vitamin C
- Vitamin D3
- Vitamin K2
- L-Glutamine
- Zinc Carnosine
- Slippery Elm
- Aloe Vera Leaf Gel Extract
- Apple Pectin
- Deglycyrrhizinated Licorice (DGL)
- Marshmallow
- Chamomile
- MSM (methylsulfonylmethane)
- Mucin
- Okra
- Prune
- Iron
- Glucosamine HCl
- Cat's Claw

Neutrophil Count (Cellular)

Measures the number of neutrophils which are the most abundant white blood cell in healthy adults and are the body's main defense against bacterial, viral and fungal infections. 60-70% of WBC are Neutros, 8 day life span, first resp to infection, react to inflammation digest bacteria.

Neutrophils are the most common type of white blood cell in your body. Neutrophils grow in your bone's soft tissue (bone marrow) and migrate through your circulation system in your blood and tissues. Neutrophils are phagocytic, meaning that they engulf and destroy things like bacteria and viruses at the site of an injury. Like all other white blood cells, they also play a part in our body's inflammatory response to things like allergens.

Neutrophils are clear in color. Neutrophils have a spherical shape when at rest but change shape to fight infection.

| Optimal Range | 1.78 - 5.38 (x 10^3/µL) |

If LOW or < 1.78 x 10^3/µL:

- Chronic viral or bacterial infection, Pancreatic insuff (WBC "rescue" as digest enzyme
- Bone marrow insufficiency, B12, B6 and folic acid anemia's, Nutrient def, Intestinal parasites (chronic).

Support immune, Protocol for incl B9/B12.

Immune Support:
- Echinacea angustifolia
- Astragalus membranaceus
- Elderberry Extract (Sambucus nigra)
- Andrographis paniculate
- Lovage (Levisticum officinale)
- Green Tea Extract
- Arabinogalactan (larch tree)
- Lauric Acid
- Ginger
- Wild Cherry Extract
- Wild cherry bark
- Cordyceps mushroom
- Shiitake mushroom
- Maitake mushroom
- Reishi mushroom
- Beta 1,3 Glucans
- Zinc
- Vitamin C
- Vitamin D3
- Vitamin K2
- L-Glutamine
- Zinc Carnosine
- Slippery Elm
- Aloe Vera Leaf Gel Extract
- Apple Pectin
- Deglycyrrhizinated Licorice (DGL)
- Marshmallow
- Chamomile
- MSM (methylsulfonylmethane)
- Mucin
- Okra
- Prune
- Iron
- Glucosamine HCl
- Cat's Claw

If HIGH or > 5.38 x 10^3/µL:

- Acute viral or bacterial infections, Inflammation, Leaky gut
- Emotional/physical stress, Intestinal parasites.

High levels of neutrophils can be caused by acute bacterial, viral or fungal infections, inflammatory diseases, physiological stress, rigorous exercise, smoking, and chronic leukemia.

- Vit C, PMGs, adrenals, bacterial response, enzyme clean up support.
- Inflamm protocols.
- Leaky gut (food sensit)

Immune Support:
- Echinacea angustifolia
- Astragalus membranaceus
- Elderberry Extract (Sambucus nigra)
- Andrographis paniculate
- Lovage (Levisticum officinale)
- Green Tea Extract
- Arabinogalactan (larch tree)
- Lauric Acid
- Ginger
- Wild Cherry Extract
- Wild cherry bark
- Cordyceps mushroom
- Shiitake mushroom
- Maitake mushroom
- Reishi mushroom
- Beta 1,3 Glucans
- Zinc
- Vitamin C
- Vitamin D3
- Vitamin K2
- L-Glutamine
- Zinc Carnosine
- Slippery Elm
- Aloe Vera Leaf Gel Extract
- Apple Pectin
- Deglycyrrhizinated Licorice (DGL)
- Marshmallow
- Chamomile
- MSM (methylsulfonylmethane)
- Mucin
- Okra
- Prune
- Iron
- Glucosamine HCl
- Cat's Claw

WBC (Cellular)

A WBC count, a blood test, measures the number of white blood cells (WBCs) in your blood. These cells, also known as leukocytes, play a crucial role in fighting infections. There are five primary types of WBCs:

- Neutrophils: The most abundant WBCs, neutrophils are produced by the bone marrow and are essential for combating a wide range of inflammatory and infectious diseases.
- Lymphocytes: Lymphocytes, including B-cells and T-cells, primarily reside in the lymph system and actively fight bacteria and other pathogens circulating in the blood.
- Monocytes: Monocytes collaborate with neutrophils to combat infections and illnesses while simultaneously eliminating damaged or dead cells.
- Eosinophils: Eosinophils are activated WBCs triggered by allergies and certain types of infections.
- Basophils: Basophils are involved in the early detection of infections, wound repair, and allergic reactions.

An elevated WBC count could indicate inflammation, infection, a medical reaction, or another underlying health condition. Conversely, a low WBC count may elevate your susceptibility to infections. Medications, viral infections, or bone marrow diseases can also cause a decrease in WBC count.

| Optimal Range | 4.23 - 9.07 (x $10^3/\mu L$) |

If LOW or < 4.23 x 10^3/µL:

- Chronic viral or bacterial infection, Pancreatic insuff (WBC "rescue" as digest enzyme)
- Bone marrow insufficiency, B12, B6 and folic acid anemia's, Nutrient def, Intestinal parasites (chronic).

Immunological suppl, support adrenal syst, FYS. Foods - carrots, red, yellow, organce and dark leafy greens, garlic, kale, almonds, chicken.

Immune Support:
- Echinacea angustifolia
- Astragalus membranaceus
- Elderberry Extract (Sambucus nigra)
- Andrographis paniculate
- Lovage (Levisticum officinale)
- Green Tea Extract
- Arabinogalactan (larch tree)
- Lauric Acid
- Ginger
- Wild Cherry Extract
- Wild cherry bark
- Cordyceps mushroom
- Shiitake mushroom
- Maitake mushroom
- Reishi mushroom
- Beta 1,3 Glucans
- Zinc
- Vitamin C
- Vitamin D3
- Vitamin K2
- L-Glutamine
- Zinc Carnosine
- Slippery Elm
- Aloe Vera Leaf Gel Extract
- Apple Pectin
- Deglycyrrhizinated Licorice (DGL)
- Marshmallow
- Chamomile
- MSM (methylsulfonylmethane)
- Mucin
- Okra
- Prune
- Iron
- Glucosamine HCl
- Cat's Claw

If HIGH or > 9.07 x 10^3/µL:

- Acute viral or bacterial infection, Stress, Diet high in refined foods
- Intestinal parasites, Neoplasms.

Immunological suppl, support adrenal syst.

Immune Support:
- Echinacea angustifolia
- Astragalus membranaceus
- Elderberry Extract (Sambucus nigra)
- Andrographis paniculate
- Lovage (Levisticum officinale)
- Green Tea Extract
- Arabinogalactan (larch tree)
- Lauric Acid
- Ginger
- Wild Cherry Extract
- Wild cherry bark
- Cordyceps mushroom
- Shiitake mushroom
- Maitake mushroom
- Reishi mushroom
- Beta 1,3 Glucans
- Zinc
- Vitamin C
- Vitamin D3
- Vitamin K2
- L-Glutamine
- Zinc Carnosine
- Slippery Elm
- Aloe Vera Leaf Gel Extract
- Apple Pectin
- Deglycyrrhizinated Licorice (DGL)
- Marshmallow
- Chamomile
- MSM (methylsulfonylmethane)
- Mucin

- Okra
- Prune
- Iron
- Glucosamine HCl
- Cat's Claw

AA (Arachidonic acid) (Cellular)

Arachidonic Acid (AA) is an essential polyunsaturated fatty Acid (PUFA). It is a precursor in the biosynthesis of important molecules like prostaglandins, thromboxanes, and leukotrienes. It is also an integral constituent of the cell membrane, providing it with fluidity and flexibility.

Thus, it is important for the function of most cells, especially in the nervous system, skeletal muscles, and immune system. Metabolites obtained from the oxidation of arachidonic acid contribute to inflammation and wound healing processes.

| Optimal Range | 5.50 - 19.01% |

If LOW or < 5.50%:

How it gets depleted A low AA level with a high or normal LA level likely indicates a delta-6-desaturase deficiency. Activity of this enzyme can be impaired with increased age, alcohol use, certain genetic defects or nutrient deficiency or excess.

Fish oil supplementation has been shown to lower AA, likely through decreasing activity of the delta-6-desaturase enzyme.

Malabsorption disorders: Essential fatty acid deficiency has been found to occur in patients with chronic fat malabsorption and in patients with cystic fibrosis.

Clinical Manifestations of Depletion Low levels of AA are somewhat rare but can lead to an impairment to cell membrane functions of the central nervous system. Children with attention deficient or hyperactivity disorders have been shown to have low levels. Low levels could also lead to an inappropriate or insufficient immune response or delayed wound healing.

Food Sources of AA can be synthesized endogenously within the body from the parent compound Linolenic Acid. The rate of conversion is largely influenced by the activity of the delta-6-desaturase enzyme.

Food sources of AA include:
- Meat (pork, chicken, beef)
- Fish (farmed salmon, flatfish, flounder, sardines)
- Dairy (cream cheese)

Supplement Options: It is uncommon to require supplementation with AA. If levels are deficient, consider checking linolenic acid levels and factors that could affect the activity of the delta-6-desaturase enzyme.

Cofactors for Delta-6-Desaturase and Delta-5-Desaturase enzymes involved in converting Linoleic Acid (LA) include: B2, B3, B6, Vitamin C, Zinc, Magnesium

Additionally, fish oil supplementation or increasing the intake of EPA fatty acids in the diet can also lower AA levels.

Nutritional support:
- Magnesium Citrate
- Magnesium taurinate, Magnesium glycinate, Magnesium malate
- Zinc
- Vitamin B complex
- Riboflavin (Vitamin B2)
- Vitamin B3 / Niacin (as Nicotinic Acid)
- Vitamin B6
- Vitamin C
- MVM (Multi-vitamin/mineral)

If **HIGH** or **> 19.01%:**

Arachidonic acid can have two origins: the diet or endogenous synthesis from a precursor, particularly linoleic acid, which is consumed in fairly high amounts in most diets. The rate of conversion is largely dependent on the activity of the delta-6-desaturase.

Excessive Intake: Dietary sources of preformed arachidonic acid are eggs and meat; fish also contain arachidonic acid. In western cultures, high levels of AA tend to be more problematic (than low levels) as they are associated with many proinflammatory conditions including heart disease, diabetes, arthritis and other autoimmune conditions. High levels of AA stimulate the production of proinflammatory cytokines.

To reduce endogenous AA production, reduce dietary intake of vegetables oils high in LA (corn, soy, canola, safflower oil). Increase intake of Omega 3 sources

Essential Fatty Acid Support:
- Essential Fatty Acids with Vitamin D
- Omega-3 Fatty Acids with Probiotics
- Omega-3 Fatty Acids
- Essential Fatty Acids with PRMs

Nutritional Support:
- Magnesium Citrate
- Magnesium taurinate
- Magnesium glycinate
- Magnesium malate
- Zinc
- Vitamin B complex
- Riboflavin (Vitamin B2)
- Vitamin B3 / Niacin (as Nicotinic Acid)
- Vitamin B6
- Vitamin C
- MVM (Multi-vitamin/mineral)

AA/EPA Ratio (Cellular)

Eicosapentaenoic acid (EPA) is a key antiinflammatory/ anti-aggregatory long-chain polyunsaturated omega-3 fatty acid. Conversely, the omega-6 fatty acid arachidonic acid (AA) is a precursor to several proinflammatory/ pro-aggregatory mediators.

EPA acts competitively with AA for the key cyclooxygenase and lipoxygenase enzymes to form less inflammatory products.

Optimal Range	2.5 - 10.9

If **LOW** or < 2.5:

 A low AA:EPA ratio reflects a low AA relative to EPA, which might shift the balance towards an overly anti-inflammatory /anti-aggregatory state, which may not be beneficial as inflammation is a natural and necessary part of the immune response, and platelet aggregation is a natural and necessary part of blood clotting and wound healing.

Additionally, as AA is a crucial component of cell membranes, a low AA:EPA ratio may negatively impact cellular membrane integrity, permeability, and function.

Furthermore, as AA is important to brain development and cognitive function, a low AA:EPA ratio may negatively impact neurological and cognitive function.

 Food Sources of AA can be synthesized endogenously within the body from the parent compound Linolenic Acid. The rate of conversion is largely influenced by the activity of the delta-6-desaturase enzyme.

Food sources of AA include:
- Meat (pork, chicken, beef)
- Fish (farmed salmon, flatfish, flounder, sardines)
- Dairy (cream cheese)

Supplement Options: It is uncommon to require supplementation with AA. If levels are deficient, consider checking linolenic acid levels and factors that could affect the activity of the delta-6-desaturase enzyme.

Cofactors for Delta-6-Desaturase and Delta-5-Desaturase enzymes involved in converting Linoleic Acid (LA) include: B2, B3, B6, Vitamin C, Zinc, Magnesium

Additionally, fish oil supplementation or increasing the intake of EPA fatty acids in the diet can also lower AA levels.

Nutritional Support:
- Magnesium Citrate
- Magnesium taurinate
- Magnesium glycinate
- Magnesium malate
- Zinc
- Vitamin B complex
- Riboflavin (Vitamin B2)
- Vitamin B3 / Niacin (as Nicotinic Acid)
- Vitamin B6
- Vitamin C
- MVM (Multi-vitamin/mineral)

If **HIGH** or > 10.9:

 A high AA:EPA ratio corresponds with higher levels of inflammation. Epidemiological studies have shown that a higher AA:EPA ratio is associated with an increased risk of coronary artery disease, acute coronary syndrome, myocardial infarction, stroke, chronic heart failure, peripheral artery disease, and vascular disease.

Decreasing the AA:EPA ratio through treatment with purified EPA has been shown in clinical studies to be effective in primary and secondary prevention of coronary artery disease and reduces the risk of cardiovascular events following percutaneous coronary intervention. The AA:EPA ratio is a valuable predictor of cardiovascular risk.

To reduce endogenous AA production, reduce dietary intake of vegetables oils high in LA (corn, soy, canola, safflower oil). Increase intake of Omega 3 sources

Essential Fatty Acid Support:
- Essential Fatty Acids with Vitamin D
- Omega-3 Fatty Acids with Probiotics
- Omega-3 Fatty Acids
- Essential Fatty Acids with PRMs

Nutritional Support:
- Magnesium Citrate
- Magnesium taurinate
- Magnesium glycinate
- Magnesium malate
- Zinc
- Vitamin B complex
- Riboflavin (Vitamin B2)
- Vitamin B3 / Niacin (as Nicotinic Acid)
- Vitamin B6
- Vitamin C
- MVM (Multi-vitamin/mineral)

DHA (Cellular)

Docosahexaenoic acid (DHA) is an omega-3 fatty acid that can be synthesized from alpha-linolenic acid (ALA) in the human body. Still, conversion is inefficient and may not meet physiological needs for some. Essential fatty acids, which are converted to omega-3 and omega-6 fatty acids in the body, play a critical role in cell membrane structure and function.

Eicosapentaenoic acid (EPA) and DHA influence the types of inflammatory response mediators in favor of less inflammatory eicosanoids such as leukotrienes, prostaglandins, and thromboxanes. EPA and DHA are also noted for moderate to strong anti-depressant effects.

Specific to DHA, it makes up an important component of retinal and neuronal cell membranes and, therefore, may playa role in neurological development and function, as well as visual function development. DHA, along with EPA, may help to lower lipids in individuals with Type 2 diabetes mellitus.

The third trimester of pregnancy and the first three months of life after birth are the most critical times for the accumulation of DHA in the infant brain.

Optimal Range	2.42 - 10.52%

If **LOW** or < 2.42%:

Inadequate intake of omega-3 fatty acids, primarily from fatty fish, fish oil, or krill oil, is the primary cause of DHA deficiency. Only about 0-4% of dietary ALA is converted to DHA in men, while up to 9% of dietary ALA is converted to DHA in women due to estrogenic effects on fatty acid conversion. Malabsorption disorders, such as chronic fat malabsorption and cystic fibrosis, have also been associated with essential fatty acid deficiency. Genetic factors play a role in DHA deficiency. Specific genetic polymorphisms, like reduced activity of the FADS1 and FADS2 genes, can lead to reduced conversion of ALA into EPA and DHA. Individuals with APOE4 genetic SNPs may experience lower serum levels of DHA due to increased DHA oxidation. In addition to assessing DHA status in relation to Alzheimer's disease and dementia risk, consider evaluating for the presence of APOE4 genetic SNPs.

Alphalinolenic acid (ALA), the precursor to EPA and DHA, is abundant in chia and flax seeds. Other food sources include Atlantic salmon, herring, sardines, mackerel, trout, and oysters.

B2, B3, B6, Vitamin C, Zinc, and Magnesium are cofactors for Delta-6-Desaturase and Delta-5-Desaturase enzymes, which convert ALA to EPA and DHA.

B3, B5, B6, Biotin (B7), and Vitamin C are cofactors for Elongase enzymes, which further convert ALA to EPA and DHA.

Essential Fatty Acid Support:
- Essential Fatty Acids with Vitamin D
- Omega-3 Fatty Acids with Probiotics
- Omega-3 Fatty Acids
- Essential Fatty Acids with PRMs

Nutritional Support:
- Magnesium Citrate
- Magnesium taurinate
- Magnesium glycinate
- Magnesium malate
- Zinc
- Vitamin B complex
- Riboflavin (Vitamin B2)
- Vitamin B3 / Niacin (as Nicotinic Acid)
- Vitamin B6
- Vitamin C
- MVM (Multi-vitamin/mineral)

If **HIGH** or **> 10.52%**:

Currently, there are no official dietary intake recommendations for omega-3 fatty acids. However, high-dose supplementation of omega-3s, particularly DHA, has been shown to reduce the need for non-steroidal anti-inflammatory drugs (NSAIDs). However, it's important to note that adverse side effects, such as gastrointestinal upset and loose stools, have been observed with high doses of omega-3 fatty acids obtained from supplements. Therefore, omega-3 supplements, including EPA and DHA, should be used with caution in individuals with clotting disorders or those taking anticlotting medication, as omega-3s may prolong clotting times.

Reduce any supplements that contain Omega 3 fatty acids. If appropriate, increase your intake of food sources of Omega 6 fatty acids:
- Meat (pork, chicken, beef)
- Fish (farmed salmon, flatfish, flounder, sardines)
- Dairy (cream cheese)

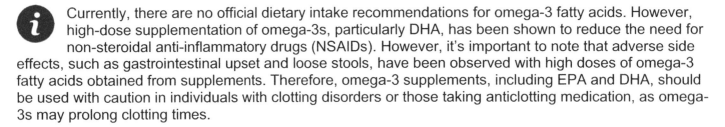

DPA (Cellular)

Docosapentaenoic acid (DPA) is an omega-3 fatty acid that is structurally similar EPA. DPA is an intermediary omega-3 fatty acid between the conversion of EPA and DHA.

DPA supports the production of healthy blood vessels and reduces clotting.

Optimal Range	0.45 - 1.80%

If **LOW** or **< 0.45%**:

Inadequate intake of DHA is usually caused by a low dietary intake of high-DHA foods. Malabsorption disorders, such as chronic fat malabsorption and cystic fibrosis, have also been associated with essential fatty acid deficiency.

- Food Sources: Salmon, Atlantic Mackerel, Pompano, Herring, Rainbow trout, Sablefish, Whitefish, Bluefin tuna, Grass-fed beef, Lamb.
- Cofactors for Delta-6-Desaturase and Delta-5-Desaturase enzymes: Vitamin C, Zinc, Magnesium.
- Cofactors for Elongase enzymes: Vitamin C, Biotin (B7), B3, B5, B6.

Essential Fatty Acid Support:
- Essential Fatty Acids with Vitamin D
- Omega-3 Fatty Acids with Probiotics
- Omega-3 Fatty Acids
- Essential Fatty Acids with PRMs

Nutritional Support:
- Magnesium Citrate
- Magnesium taurinate
- Magnesium glycinate
- Magnesium malate
- Zinc
- Vitamin B complex
- Riboflavin (Vitamin B2)
- Vitamin B3 / Niacin (as Nicotinic Acid)
- Vitamin B6
- Vitamin C
- MVM (Multi-vitamin/mineral)

If **HIGH** or **> 1.80%**:

Adverse side effects observed with high doses of omega-3 fatty acids from supplement form include gastrointestinal upset and loose stools

Reduce any supplements that contain Omega 3 fatty acids. If appropriate, increase your intake of food sources of Omega 6 fatty acids:
- Meat (pork, chicken, beef)
- Fish (farmed salmon, flatfish, flounder, sardines)
- Dairy (cream cheese)

EPA (Cellular)

Eicosapentaenoic acid (EPA), an omega-3 fatty acid, plays a crucial role in maintaining the health of cellular membranes, regulating lipid actions, and mitigating inflammatory responses within the body. EPA, along with docosahexaenoic acid (DHA), influences the production of inflammatory response mediators, favoring the synthesis of anti-inflammatory eicosanoids such as leukotrienes, prostaglandins, and thromboxanes. Notably, EPA and DHA exhibit moderate to strong anti-depressant effects. EPA stands out for its ability to suppress the signaling of TNF-a in adipocytes, while it also enhances cerebral oxygenation. Additionally, EPA appears to exert beneficial effects on regulating leptin levels and increasing adiponectin. Furthermore, EPA may stimulate adaptive immunity by enhancing B cell responsiveness.

Optimal Range	0.15 - 2.26%

If **LOW** or **< 0.15%**:

Inadequate intake of omega-3 fatty acids is the primary reason for deficiency of EPA, or low levels of EPA.

- Malabsorption disorders: Essential fatty acid deficiency has been found in patients with chronic fat malabsorption and cystic fibrosis.
- Genetics: Certain genetic polymorphisms, such as reduced activity of the FADS1 and FADS2 genes, may lead to reduced conversion of ALA into EPA and DHA.

 Alphalinolenic acid (ALA), the precursor to EPA and DHA, is abundant in chia and flax seeds. Other food sources include Atlantic salmon, herring, sardines, mackerel, trout, and oysters.

B2, B3, B6, Vitamin C, Zinc, and Magnesium are cofactors for Delta-6-Desaturase and Delta-5-Desaturase enzymes, which convert ALA to EPA and DHA.

B3, B5, B6, Biotin (B7), and Vitamin C are cofactors for Elongase enzymes, which further convert ALA to EPA and DHA.

Essential Fatty Acid Support:
- Essential Fatty Acids with Vitamin D
- Omega-3 Fatty Acids with Probiotics
- Omega-3 Fatty Acids
- Essential Fatty Acids with PRMs

Nutritional Support:
- Magnesium Citrate
- Magnesium taurinate
- Magnesium glycinate
- Magnesium malate
- Zinc
- Vitamin B complex
- Riboflavin (Vitamin B2)
- Vitamin B3 / Niacin (as Nicotinic Acid)
- Vitamin B6
- Vitamin C
- MVM (Multi-vitamin/mineral)

If **HIGH** or > 2.26%:

Currently, there are no official dietary intake recommendations for omega-3 fatty acids. However, several health organizations have proposed a minimum daily intake of 500 mg of EPA and DHA. Since the body can only convert a small amount of ALA into EPA, supplementing with EPA is usually recommended to achieve therapeutic doses.

High-dose supplementation of omega-3 fatty acids, including EPA, has been shown to reduce the need for non-steroidal anti-inflammatory drugs (NSAIDs). Additionally, people with ulcerative colitis have been found to require fewer corticosteroids when supplementing with high-dose omega-3 fatty acids.

However, it's important to note that high doses of omega-3 fatty acids from supplements can cause gastrointestinal upset and loose stools. Therefore, omega-3 supplements, including EPA and DHA, should be used with caution in individuals with clotting disorders or those taking anti-clotting medication, as omega-3s may prolong clotting times.

 Reduce any supplements that contain Omega 3 fatty acids. If appropriate, increase your intake of food sources of Omega 6 fatty acids:
- Meat (pork, chicken, beef)
- Fish (farmed salmon, flatfish, flounder, sardines)
- Dairy (cream cheese)

LA (Linoleic acid) (Cellular)

Linoleic Acid (LA) is considered the "parent" omega-6 fatty acid. All other omega-6 fatty acids are synthesized from linoleic acid by desaturation and elongation reactions. Thus, LA must be consumed in the diet for all omega- 6 fatty acids to be used and incorporated into the body's cells and cell membranes.

LA stimulates cell division and repair.

Optimal Range	3.22 - 10.49%

If LOW or < 3.22%:

- Inadequate intake: Given the large quantities of vegetable oils in the typical Western diet, depletion or low levels of LA are usually only seen on a fat-free diet, a diet very restricted in dietary fat, or in situations of fat malabsorption.
- Malabsorption disorders: Essential fatty acid deficiency has been found to occur in patients with chronic fat malabsorption and in patients with cystic fibrosis.

Food sources include vegetable oils (corn, soybean, sunflower, safflower, canola, peanut), avocado, walnuts, and seeds.

Essential Fatty Acid Support:
- Borage oil (GLA - Gamma Linolenic Acid)
- Mixed fatty acids (Omega 3, 6, 7, 9)

If HIGH or > 10.49%

Linoleic acid and omega-6 fatty acids are plentiful in the Western diet, so supplementation is typically unnecessary.

The best way to lower LA levels is to decrease the intake of refined vegetable oil (corn, soy, peanut, canola, safflower oil) and replace it with an alternative such as olive oil, coconut oil, avocado oil, or fat from animal sources.

To reduce endogenous AA production, reduce your intake of vegetables oils high in LA (corn, soy, canola, safflower oil). Instead, increase your intake of Omega 3 sources. Additionally, you need cofactors for the conversion of Linoleic acid (LA) to AA:
- B2, B3, B6, Vitamin C, Zinc, Magnesium for Delta-6-Desaturase and Delta-5-Desaturase enzymes.
- B3, B5, B6, Biotin (B7), Vitamin C for Elongase enzymes.

Essential Fatty Acid Support:
- Essential Fatty Acids with Vitamin D
- Omega-3 Fatty Acids with Probiotics
- Omega-3 Fatty Acids
- Essential Fatty Acids with PRMs

Nutritional Support:
- Magnesium Citrate
- Magnesium taurinate
- Magnesium glycinate
- Magnesium malate
- Zinc
- Vitamin B complex

- Riboflavin (Vitamin B2)
- Vitamin B3 / Niacin (as Nicotinic Acid)
- Vitamin B6
- Vitamin C
- MVM (Multi-vitamin/mineral)

Omega-3 Index (Cellular)

Omega-3 Index is the sum of EPA % and DHA % as measured in whole blood, and derived by validated calculations to yield the equivalent sum of EPA % and DHA % in red blood cell membranes. Please note this value is a percentage, with the denominator being the sum of all Fatty Acids measured in the blood and thus the index can vary based on fatty acid composition of the diet.

The omega-3 index is the amount of EPA plus DHA in red blood cell membranes expressed as the percent of total red blood cell membrane fatty acids.

Please note this value is a percentage, with the denominator being the sum of all fatty acids measured in the red blood cells; thus, the index can vary based on the fatty acid composition of the diet.

Optimal Range	8.00 - 12.65%

If **LOW** or < 8.00%:

How it gets depleted The Omega-3 Index is a validated biomarker of tissue membrane omega-3 (n-3) polyunsaturated fatty acid (PUFA) status. It's expressed as a percentage, where the denominator is the sum of all fatty acids measured in the blood. A decrease in the ratio can be caused by low omega-3 fatty acid intake and their incorporation into cell membranes, or by a proportionally high intake of other dietary fatty acids, including saturated, mono-unsaturated, and omega-6 polyunsaturated fatty acids.

Clinical Manifestations of Depletion Low levels of the Omega-3 Index are associated with an increased risk of cardiac death. The EPA + DHA content of red blood cell membranes is similar to that of cardiac muscle cells. Several observational studies have shown that a lower Omega-3 Index is linked to an increased risk of coronary heart disease mortality. Therefore, it's proposed that the Omega-3 Index be used as a biomarker for cardiovascular disease risk, with suggested cutoffs as follows: high risk, <4%; intermediate risk, 4%-8%; and low risk, >8%.

Food Sources: If the omega-3 index is below 8.0%, it's recommended to increase dietary sources of omega-3s (EPA and DHA) from both plant and animal sources. Since the omega-3 index is a relative ratio of omega-3 compared to all other fatty acids in the blood, it's also crucial to consider the intake of all other dietary fatty acids, including saturated fatty acids, mono-unsaturated fatty acids, and omega-6 polyunsaturated fatty acids.

Omega-3 Sources:
- Salmon
- Atlantic Mackerel
- Pompano
- Herring
- Rainbow trout
- Sablefish
- Whitefish
- Bluefin tuna
- Grass-fed beef
- Lamb

Supplement Options: Currently, there are no official dietary intake recommendations for omega-3s. However, several official health organizations have proposed a minimum daily intake of 500 mg of EPA+DHA. Since the conversion of ALA to DHA is relatively low, supplementing DHA is generally recommended to achieve therapeutic doses. The recommended minimum daily intake of DHA supplementation for adults is 250 mg. Pregnant and lactating women are advised to consume at least 200 mg of DHA daily. Diabetic individuals may benefit from supplementing DHA (along with EPA) due to its potential triglyceride-lowering effects.

High-dose supplementation of omega-3 fatty acids, including DHA, has been shown to reduce the need for non-steroidal anti-inflammatory drugs (NSAIDs). Additionally, individuals with ulcerative colitis have been observed to require fewer corticosteroids when supplementing with high-dose omega-3 fatty acids.

However, it's important to note that high-dose omega-3 fatty acid supplements from supplements may cause gastrointestinal upset and loose stools as adverse side effects. Therefore, omega-3 supplements, including EPA and DHA, should be used with caution in individuals with clotting disorders or those taking anti-clotting medication.

Essential Fatty Acid Support:
- Essential Fatty Acids with Vitamin D
- Omega-3 Fatty Acids with Probiotics
- Omega-3 Fatty Acids
- Essential Fatty Acids with PRMs

Nutritional Support:
- Magnesium Citrate
- Magnesium taurinate
- Magnesium glycinate
- Magnesium malate
- Zinc
- Vitamin B complex
- Riboflavin (Vitamin B2)
- Vitamin B3 / Niacin (as Nicotinic Acid)
- Vitamin B6
- Vitamin C
- MVM (Multi-vitamin/mineral)

If **HIGH** or **> 12.65%**:

Supplementation with EPA+ DHA from fish oil capsules for approximately five months dosedependently increased the omega-3 index in 115 healthy young adults (ages 20-45 years), validating the use of the omega-3 index as a biomarker of EPA + DHA intake.

Reduce any supplements that contain Omega 3 fatty acids. If appropriate, increase your intake of food sources of Omega 6 fatty acids:
- Meat (pork, chicken, beef)
- Fish (farmed salmon, flatfish, flounder, sardines)
- Dairy (cream cheese)

Total Omega-3 (Cellular)

The Total Omega-3 test, a crucial component of Vibrant America's Micronutrient panel, provides a comprehensive assessment of omega-3 fatty acids in red blood cells (RBCs). These fatty acids are essential for various bodily functions, including cardiovascular health, brain function, and anti-inflammatory processes.

The test measures the total amount of omega-3 fatty acids, including EPA (Eicosapentaenoic Acid), DHA (Docosahexaenoic Acid), and DPA (Docosapentaenoic Acid), rather than transient serum levels. Adequate omega-3 levels are associated with a reduced risk of heart disease, improved cognitive function, and lower inflammation.

The RBC measurement is particularly valuable for individuals with dietary restrictions, cardiovascular risks, or cognitive concerns. Vibrant America's Micronutrient panel, including the Total Omega-3 test, is indispensable for healthcare providers in developing targeted nutritional interventions.

This test is particularly relevant for individuals seeking to optimize their omega-3 intake through diet or supplementation, especially in populations with limited fish consumption or those following plant-based diets. It plays a critical role in preventive healthcare, aiding in the early detection and management of conditions related to omega-3 deficiencies, thereby contributing to overall health and well-being.

| Optimal Range | 3.25 - 13.99% |

If LOW or < 3.25%:

How it gets depleted The Omega-3 Index is a validated biomarker of tissue membrane omega-3 (n-3) polyunsaturated fatty acid (PUFA) status. It's expressed as a percentage, where the denominator is the sum of all fatty acids measured in the blood. A decrease in the ratio can be caused by low omega-3 fatty acid intake and their incorporation into cell membranes, or by a proportionally high intake of other dietary fatty acids, including saturated, mono-unsaturated, and omega-6 polyunsaturated fatty acids.

Clinical Manifestations of Depletion Low levels of the Omega-3 Index are associated with an increased risk of cardiac death. The EPA + DHA content of red blood cell membranes is similar to that of cardiac muscle cells. Several observational studies have shown that a lower Omega-3 Index is linked to an increased risk of coronary heart disease mortality. Therefore, it's proposed that the Omega-3 Index be used as a biomarker for cardiovascular disease risk, with suggested cutoffs as follows: high risk, <4%; intermediate risk, 4%-8%; and low risk, >8%.

Food Sources: If the total omega-3 content is less than 3.25%, it's recommended to increase dietary sources of EPA and DHA from both plant and animal sources. Since the omega-3 index compares omega-3 to all other fatty acids in the blood, it's also important to consider the intake of other dietary fatty acids, including saturated, mono-unsaturated, and omega-6 polyunsaturated fatty acids.

Salmon, Atlantic Mackerel, Pompano, Herring, Rainbow trout, Sablefish, Whitefish, Bluefin tuna, Grass-fed beef, and Lamb are all excellent sources of omega-3 fatty acids.

Supplement Options: Currently, there are no official dietary intake recommendations for omega-3 fatty acids. However, several health organizations have proposed a minimum daily intake of 500 mg of EPA+DHA. Since the body's conversion of ALA to DHA is relatively low, supplementing DHA is generally recommended to achieve therapeutic doses. The recommended minimum daily intake of DHA supplementation for adults is 250 mg. Pregnant and lactating women are advised to consume at least 200 mg of DHA daily. Diabetic individuals may benefit from supplementing DHA (along with EPA) due to its potential triglyceride-lowering effects.

High-dose supplementation of omega-3 fatty acids, including DHA, has been shown to reduce the need for non-steroidal anti-inflammatory drugs (NSAIDs). Additionally, individuals with ulcerative colitis have been observed to require fewer corticosteroids when supplementing with high-dose omega-3 fatty acids.

However, it's important to use omega-3 supplements, including EPA and DHA, with caution in individuals with clotting disorders or those taking anti-clotting medication.

Adverse side effects associated with high-dose omega-3 fatty acid supplements from supplements include gastrointestinal upset and loose stools.

Essential Fatty Acid Support:
- Essential Fatty Acids with Vitamin D
- Omega-3 Fatty Acids with Probiotics
- Omega-3 Fatty Acids
- Essential Fatty Acids with PRMs

Nutritional Support:
- Magnesium Citrate
- Magnesium taurinate
- Magnesium glycinate
- Magnesium malate
- Zinc
- Vitamin B complex
- Riboflavin (Vitamin B2)
- Vitamin B3 / Niacin (as Nicotinic Acid)
- Vitamin B6
- Vitamin C
- MVM (Multi-vitamin/mineral)

If **HIGH** or **> 13.99%:**

Supplementation with EPA+ DHA from fish oil capsules for approximately five months dosedependently increased the omega-3 index in 115 healthy young adults (ages 20-45 years), validating the use of the omega-3 index as a biomarker of EPA + DHA intake.

Reduce any supplements that contain Omega 3 fatty acids. If appropriate, increase your intake of food sources of Omega 6 fatty acids:
- Meat (pork, chicken, beef)
- Fish (farmed salmon, flatfish, flounder, sardines)
- Dairy (cream cheese)

Total Omega-6 (Cellular)

The Total Omega-6 test, a crucial component of Vibrant America's Micronutrient panel, delves into the comprehensive analysis of total omega-6 fatty acids present in red blood cells (RBCs). These essential fatty acids, including linoleic acid (LA) and arachidonic acid (AA), play pivotal roles in cellular health, inflammation regulation, and various bodily functions. By measuring omega-6 levels in RBCs, this test offers a more precise and long-term assessment of the body's fatty acid profile, unlike transient serum levels that only reflect short-term fluctuations. This analysis is vital for identifying imbalances between omega-6 and omega-3 fatty acids, which are key to managing inflammatory conditions, cardiovascular health, and overall well-being. Individuals following diets high in processed foods or vegetable oils, which can lead to an excess of omega-6 fatty acids, find this test particularly beneficial. Healthcare providers use this test to tailor dietary recommendations and supplement strategies, aiming to achieve a balanced omega-6 to omega-3 ratio. Vibrant America's Micronutrient panel, including the Total Omega-6 test, plays a significant role in preventive healthcare, aiding in the early detection and management of conditions related to omega-6 excess or deficiency. Accurate monitoring of omega-6 levels contributes to personalized healthcare approaches, promoting long-term health and well-being.

Optimal Range	11.03 - 34.96%

If **LOW** or **< 11.03%:**

- Inadequate intake: Given the large quantities of vegetable oils in the typical Western diet, depletion or low levels of Omega 6 fatty acids are usually only seen on a fat-free diet, a diet very restricted in dietary fat, or in situations of fat malabsorption.

- Malabsorption disorders: Essential fatty acid deficiency has been found to occur in patients with chronic fat malabsorption and in patients with cystic fibrosis.

Food sources include vegetable oils (corn, soybean, sunflower, safflower, canola, peanut), avocado, walnuts, and seeds.

Essential Fatty Acid Support
- Borage oil (GLA - Gamma Linolenic Acid)
- Mixed fatty acids (Omega 3, 6, 7, 9)

If **HIGH** or **> 34.96%**:

If the results fall within the upper range of the reference ranges, it suggests a higher-than-average concentration of omega-6 fatty acids in red blood cells. While omega-6 fatty acids are essential for health, playing roles in brain function, growth, and development, an excess can have implications:

- Inflammatory Response: Omega-6 fatty acids can be precursors to inflammatory molecules. High levels may predispose to or exacerbate inflammatory conditions like arthritis, cardiovascular diseases, and certain autoimmune disorders.
- Omega-6/Omega-3 Ratio Imbalance: A high omega-6 level indicates an imbalance in the omega-6 to omega-3 ratio. Ideally, this ratio should be balanced, as excessive omega-6 can negate the anti-inflammatory effects of omega-3 fatty acids.
- Dietary Factors: Elevated omega-6 levels often reflect a diet high in certain vegetable oils (such as corn, soybean, and sunflower oils) and processed foods, which are rich in omega-6 fatty acids.

- Dietary Modifications: Reducing the intake of foods high in omega-6 fatty acids and increasing omega-3-rich foods (like fish, flaxseeds, and walnuts) can help restore a healthier balance.
- Supplementation: In some cases, supplementing with omega-3 fatty acids may be recommended to counterbalance the high omega-6 levels.
- Lifestyle Changes: Regular exercise and maintaining a healthy weight can positively influence the body's inflammatory status and overall health.
- Regular Monitoring: Follow-up testing can be valuable in monitoring the effectiveness of these interventions and ensuring that fatty acid levels are moving toward a more balanced range.

Essential Fatty Acid Support:
- Essential Fatty Acids with Vitamin D
- Omega-3 Fatty Acids with Probiotics
- Omega-3 Fatty Acids
- Essential Fatty Acids with PRMs

Nutritional Support:
- Magnesium Citrate
- Magnesium taurinate
- Magnesium glycinate
- Magnesium malate
- Zinc
- Vitamin B complex
- Riboflavin (Vitamin B2)
- Vitamin B3 / Niacin (as Nicotinic Acid)
- Vitamin B6
- Vitamin C
- MVM (Multi-vitamin/mineral)

Arginine (Serum)

L-Arginine, a conditionally essential amino acid found in the diet, is primarily used by athletes as a dietary supplement. It plays a crucial role in producing nitric oxide through the nitric oxide synthase enzymes. Arginine aids in healing injuries, supports kidney function by aiding waste removal, and enhances immune system function.

During periods of illness and chronic conditions such as hypertension and type II diabetes, arginine becomes particularly important. These conditions often lead to an increase in arginase, an enzyme that degrades L-arginine, resulting in a temporary deficiency. This deficiency precedes a rise in blood pressure in these states and can be partially alleviated by increasing L-arginine intake or resolving the underlying illness or disease.

Arginine has numerous functions in the body, including:
- Ammonia disposal in the urea cycle
- Immune function
- Stimulation of insulin release
- Muscle metabolism (creatine/creatinine precursor)
- Nitric oxide (NO) formation
- Glutamic acid and proline formation
- Glucose/glycogen conversion
- Stimulation of the release of growth hormone, vasopressin, and prolactin
- Wound healing

Given its role as a precursor for nitric oxide synthesis, arginine is often therapeutically used in cardiovascular disease to achieve its vasodilatory effects.

Optimal Range	81.6 - 249.0 nmol/mL

If LOW or < 81.6 nmol/mL:

HoWith depletion, arginine becomes crucial during illness and chronic conditions like hypertension and type II diabetes. These states often lead to an increase in arginase, the enzyme that degrades L-arginine, causing a temporary deficiency. This deficiency precedes a rise in blood pressure and can be partially alleviated by increasing L-arginine intake or resolving the underlying illness or disease.

Nutrient Interaction: Low arginine may indicate excessive lysine or histidine supplementation, competing for absorption or consumption of lysine-rich foods like meat and dairy products. Additionally, low arginine is associated with elevated ammonia levels.

Increased Utilization: During illness and chronic conditions, arginine becomes essential. These states often lead to an increase in arginase, resulting in a temporary arginine deficiency. This deficiency precedes a rise in blood pressure and can be partially remedied by increasing L-arginine intake or resolving the underlying illness or disease.

Clinical Manifestations of Depletion: Arginine plays a vital role in the formation of creatine, a crucial nutrient that can induce mental retardation in deficiency. It also contributes to the production of agmatine, a signaling molecule in the body. Arginine serves as an intermediate in both the urea cycle (with L-ornithine, L-citrulline, and arginosuccinate) and the nitric oxide cycle (with ornithine and arginosuccinate). Through ornithine, arginine produces polyamine structures that regulate cellular function. In some individuals with viral infections like shingles, arginine supplementation may exacerbate symptoms, necessitating consultation with a healthcare provider.

Dietary arginine constitutes 40-60% of serum arginine. Food sources include red meat, poultry, fish, dairy, soy, quinoa, buckwheat, nuts, seeds, and beans. Supplement options include taking arginine up to three times daily, with a combined dose of 15-18g. L-citrulline supplementation is more effective at maintaining elevated arginine levels for extended periods. However, consuming more than 10g of arginine at once can lead to gastrointestinal distress and diarrhea.

 Amino Acid Support:
- Amino Acid Blend
- Vitamin B6
- Mixed Branch Chain Amino Acids (BCAAs)
- L-Arginine
- Taurine
- L-Tyrosine
- L-Lysine
- L-Methionine
- L-Citrulline
- Creatine
- Magnesium
- L-Glutathione
- Grape Extract (Vitis vinifera)
- Apple Extract (Malus pumila)
- Vitamin B5
- Vitamin B9 (Folate)
- Vitamin C

If HIGH or > 249.0 nmol/mL:

Excessive supplementation of arginine can lead to gastrointestinal distress, diarrhea, and potentially trigger cold sores or genital herpes in individuals with a history of these conditions. Additionally, it's not recommended for people who have recently had a heart attack due to concerns about increased risk of death.

A diet high in arginine or exogenous supplementation with arginine or citrulline can elevate arginine levels. Furthermore, manganese (Mn) insufficiency can also elevate arginine levels since Mn is a necessary cofactor in the conversion of arginine to ornithine (and urea) in the urea cycle. Lastly, some literature suggests that vitamin B_6 supplementation can alter plasma amino acids, resulting in increased arginine levels.

- Reduce any supplements providing L-arginine
- Consider manganese
- Consider if B6 supplementation is high

 Nutritional Support:
- Manganese (from Manganese Bisglycinate)
- Mixed greens powder from fruits and vegetables
- Mixed reds powder from fruits and vegetables
- Multi-vitamin/mineral (MVM) powdered formula

Asparagine (Serum)

Asparagine, a non-essential amino acid that the body can synthesize, plays a crucial role in brain development and function. It's found in various fruits and vegetables, including asparagus, hence its name. Other dietary sources include meat, potatoes, eggs, nuts, and dairy.

Asparagine can also be synthesized from aspartic acid and glutamine using the enzyme asparagine synthetase. Additionally, it can be formed from glutamine and aspartate. Beyond its role in protein synthesis, asparagine is essential for DNA and RNA synthesis, as well as the removal of cellular waste product ammonia.

Asparagine serves three primary functions:
- Incorporation into amino acid sequences of proteins.
- Storage as a precursor for the synthesis of DNA, RNA, and ATP.
- Providing amino groups for the production of other essential amino acids through transaminases.

In proteins, asparagine acts as an attachment site for carbohydrates, facilitating the assembly of collagen, enzymes, and cell-cell recognition. Moreover, asparagine can be readily converted into aspartate, allowing for its on-demand availability for various cellular functions. Aspartate contributes carbon skeletons to the Citric Acid Cycle, enhancing cellular energy production. It also plays a role in the urea cycle, effectively eliminating excess ammonia.

The conversion of asparagine to aspartate involves the transfer of the extra amino group from asparagine to another keto acid, resulting in the formation of a dispensable amino acid. This process enables asparagine to serve as a precursor for the production of numerous amino acids on demand to meet the cell's requirements.

Asparagine offers several health benefits, including maintaining a balance within the central nervous system, protecting the liver, and combating fatigue.

| Optimal Range | 39.2 - 89.8 nmol/mL |

If LOW or < 39.2 nmol/mL:

How it gets depleted: Asparagine deficiency is not likely due to its endogenous synthesis and ubiquitous presence in both plant and animal foods.

Lower levels of asparagine can reflect functional need for magnesium in the conversion from aspartic acid.

Clinical manifestations of depletion: There are no known deficiency symptoms of asparagine that have been well reported or well studied, but possible symptoms of asparagine depletion could include fatigue or cognitive decline in adults.

Food Sources: Red meat, poultry, fish, dairy, soy, quinoa, buckwheat, nuts, seeds, and beans are all good sources of asparagine. On the other hand, most fruits and vegetables are low in asparagine.

Supplement Options: There is currently no established Recommended Daily Allowance (RDA), Adequate Intake (AI), or Upper Limit (UL) for asparagine. Asparagine is rarely supplemented directly because the body produces it endogenously. However, it could be indirectly supplemented through glutamine.

Amino Acid Support:
- Amino Acid Blend
- Vitamin B6
- Mixed Branch Chain Amino Acids (BCAAs)
- L-Arginine
- Taurine
- L-Tyrosine
- L-Lysine
- L-Methionine
- L-Citrulline
- Creatine
- Magnesium
- L-Glutathione
- Grape Extract (Vitis vinifera)
- Apple Extract (Malus pumila)
- Vitamin B5
- Vitamin B9 (Folate)
- Vitamin C

Nutritional Support:
- Magnesium Citrate
- Magnesium Taurinate
- Magnesium Glycinate
- Magnesium Malate
- Multi-vitamin/mineral (iron/copper-free)

If **HIGH** or > 89.8 nmol/mL:

Higher levels of asparagine can indicate problems with purine (therefore protein) synthesis.

Consider reducing supplements that contain L-glutamine and reducing your food sources. Here are some food sources to consider:
- Red meat
- Poultry
- Fish
- Dairy
- Soy
- Quinoa
- Buckwheat
- Nuts
- Seeds
- Beans

Foods low in asparagine include most fruits and vegetables.

Asparagine (Cellular)

Asparagine, a non-essential amino acid that the body can synthesize, plays a crucial role in brain development and function. It's found in various fruits and vegetables, including asparagus, hence its name. Other dietary sources include meat, potatoes, eggs, nuts, and dairy.

Asparagine can also be synthesized from aspartic acid and glutamine using the enzyme asparagine synthetase. Additionally, it can be formed from glutamine and aspartate. Beyond its role in protein synthesis, asparagine is essential for DNA and RNA synthesis, as well as the removal of cellular waste product ammonia.

Asparagine serves three primary functions:
- Incorporation into amino acid sequences of proteins.
- Storage as a precursor for the synthesis of DNA, RNA, and ATP.
- Providing amino groups for the production of other essential amino acids through transaminases.

In proteins, asparagine acts as an attachment site for carbohydrates, facilitating the assembly of collagen, enzymes, and cell-cell recognition. Moreover, asparagine can be readily converted into aspartate, allowing for its on-demand availability for various cellular functions. Aspartate contributes carbon skeletons to the Citric Acid Cycle, enhancing cellular energy production. It also plays a role in the urea cycle, effectively eliminating excess ammonia.

The conversion of asparagine to aspartate involves the transfer of the extra amino group from asparagine to another keto acid, resulting in the formation of a dispensable amino acid. This process enables asparagine to serve as a precursor for the production of numerous amino acids on demand to meet the cell's requirements.

Asparagine offers several health benefits, including maintaining a balance within the central nervous system, protecting the liver, and combating fatigue.

Optimal Range	0.5 - 2.8 ng/MM WBC

If **LOW** or < 0.5 ng/MM WBC:

How it gets depleted: Asparagine deficiency is not likely due to its endogenous synthesis and ubiquitous presence in both plant and animal foods.

Lower levels of asparagine can reflect functional need for magnesium in the conversion from aspartic acid.

Clinical manifestations of depletion: There are no known deficiency symptoms of asparagine that have been well reported or well studied, but possible symptoms of asparagine depletion could include fatigue or cognitive decline in adults.

Food Sources: Red meat, poultry, fish, dairy, soy, quinoa, buckwheat, nuts, seeds, and beans are all good sources of asparagine. On the other hand, most fruits and vegetables are low in asparagine.

Supplement Options: There is currently no established Recommended Daily Allowance (RDA), Adequate Intake (AI), or Upper Limit (UL) for asparagine. Asparagine is rarely supplemented directly because the body produces it endogenously. However, it could be indirectly supplemented through glutamine.

Amino Acid Support:
- Amino Acid Blend
- Vitamin B6
- Mixed Branch Chain Amino Acids (BCAAs)
- L-Arginine
- Taurine
- L-Tyrosine
- L-Lysine
- L-Methionine
- L-Citrulline
- Creatine
- Magnesium
- L-Glutathione
- Grape Extract (Vitis vinifera)
- Apple Extract (Malus pumila)
- Vitamin B5
- Vitamin B9 (Folate)
- Vitamin C

Nutritional Support:
- Magnesium Citrate
- Magnesium Taurinate
- Magnesium Glycinate
- Magnesium Malate
- Multi-vitamin/mineral (iron/copper-free)

If **HIGH** or > 2.8 ng/MM WBC:

Higher levels of asparagine can indicate problems with purine (therefore protein) synthesis.

Consider reducing supplements that contain L-glutamine and reducing your food sources. Here are some food sources to consider:
- Red meat
- Poultry
- Fish
- Dairy
- Soy
- Quinoa
- Buckwheat
- Nuts
- Seeds
- Beans

Foods low in asparagine include most fruits and vegetables.

Citrulline (Serum)

Citrulline, an intermediate amino acid in the urea cycle, can be produced through two mechanisms: directly from arginine, which releases nitric oxide (involved in the nitric oxide cycle), or indirectly from arginine's conversion into ornithine (part of the urea cycle, which sequesters ammonia). Citrulline, derived from watermelon (Citrullus vulgaris), where it was initially isolated and identified, is easily absorbed by the gut and bypasses the liver, making it an effective way to replenish arginine levels. Other food sources of citrulline include muskmelons, bitter melons, squashes, gourds, cucumbers, and pumpkins.

Enterocytes, located in the small intestine, can also synthesize citrulline from arginine and glutamine. This citrulline can then be metabolized by the kidneys and converted back into arginine. Consequently, citrulline has been proposed as a marker of enterocyte mass in conditions characterized by villous atrophy.

Given its role in nitric oxide production for vasodilation and muscle protein synthesis, citrulline is sometimes administered therapeutically to deliver arginine to endothelial and immune cells. Additionally, it is supplemented in sarcopenia to stimulate protein synthesis in skeletal muscle through the rapamycin (mTOR) pathway.

Citrulline supplementation has been investigated in various conditions, including erectile dysfunction, sickle cell anemia, short bowel syndrome, hyperlipidemia, cancer chemotherapy, urea cycle disorders, Alzheimer's disease, multi-infarct dementia, and as an immunomodulator.

Optimal Range	18.7 - 47.5 nmol/mL

If LOW or < 18.7 nmol/mL:

 Low arginine intake can occur due to several factors. Firstly, the majority of L-citrulline either passes through the bloodstream passively or is transported to the kidneys for conversion into arginine. Secondly, citrulline can be produced from arginine through two mechanisms: either directly by arginine releasing a nitric oxide molecule (which is involved in the nitric oxide cycle) or indirectly by arginine converting into ornithine (which is involved in the urea cycle), thereby sequestering ammonia. Thirdly, low citrulline levels may be secondary to a relatively low protein diet and/or intestinal malabsorption. Additionally, since citrulline can be formed from glutamine, glutamine depletion has been associated with low citrulline levels in plasma.

 Food sources include red meat, poultry, fish, dairy, soy, quinoa, buckwheat, nuts, seeds, and beans. Consider supplementing with L-arginine.

Amino Acid Support:
- Amino Acid Blend
- Vitamin B6
- Mixed Branch Chain Amino Acids (BCAAs)
- L-Arginine
- Taurine
- L-Tyrosine
- L-Lysine
- L-Methionine
- L-Citrulline
- Creatine
- Magnesium
- L-Glutathione
- Grape Extract (Vitis vinifera)
- Apple Extract (Malus pumila)
- Vitamin B5
- Vitamin B9 (Folate)
- Vitamin C

If **HIGH** or > 47.5 nmol/mL:

 High plasma or urinary citrulline levels can indicate a functional enzyme block in the urea cycle, leading to an ammonia buildup. Genetics play a crucial role in this condition.

- Citrullinemia type I (CTLN1) is a rare autosomal recessive genetic disorder caused by a deficiency of argininosuccinate synthase, an enzyme that converts citrulline and aspartate into argininosuccinate. Complete defects in this enzyme result in extremely elevated levels of citrulline.
- Citrullinemia type II (CTLN2) occurs in adults and is characterized by recurrent hyperammonemia and neuropsychiatric symptoms due to impairment of the argininosuccinate synthase 1 step of the urea cycle.

To manage this condition, low-protein diets are recommended to minimize ammonia production. Arginine, on the other hand, helps remove ammonia from the blood.

- Supplement magnesium and aspartic acid add to drive the cycle. Lower protein intake is suggested in ammonia toxicities.
- Consider genetic testing
- Administration of thiamine (vitamin B_1) has been found to lower elevated citrulline, as well as other amino acids, in thiamine deficiency.

Nutritional support
- Magnesium Citrate
- Magnesium Taurinate
- Magnesium Glycinate
- Magnesium Malate
- Multi-vitamin/mineral (iron/copper-free)

Glutamine (Serum)

Glutamine, a conditionally essential amino acid, is primarily required during times of disease or muscle wasting, such as HIV/AIDS, cancer, or severe infections. In the intestinal lining, it serves as the preferred fuel source for intestinal epithelial cells and the primary energy source for leukocytes (immune cells). Beyond its role in energy production, glutamine plays several crucial functions:
- Transporting nitrogen between cells
- Acting as a precursor to glutathione production
- Serving as a precursor to nucleotides (essential for DNA and RNA synthesis)
- Participating in gluconeogenesis when carbohydrate intake is insufficient
- Mitigating the rapid rise in blood glucose levels after consuming carbohydrate-rich meals
- Regulating intestinal tight junctions

Optimal Range	1.4 - 7.0 ng/MM WBC

If **LOW** or < 1.4 ng/MM WBC:

 Glutamine depletion or deficiency is uncommon because the body can produce it endogenously and it's abundant in the food supply from both plant and animal sources.

Health conditions: Some studies indicate that intestinal permeability may increase when intestinal epithelial cells lack sufficient glutamine, as well as insufficient availability for leukocyte function.

Glutamine is known to be depleted in certain types of physiological stress, such as burns, major trauma, and cancers that consume available intracellular glutamine stores more rapidly than skeletal muscle can generate it, leading to increased muscle wasting.

Exercise: During physical activity, serum glutamine is consumed for extended endurance events (2+ hours); some evidence suggests that chronic endurance exercise reduces glutamine levels, which may affect immune cell function and proliferation.

Food sources include red meat, poultry, fish, dairy, soy, quinoa, buckwheat, nuts, seeds, and beans. Glutamine consumption often leads to an increase in serum insulin levels due to its conversion into glucose, which may affect individuals with insulin resistance. Additionally, glutamine supplementation has been shown to potentially enhance mental focus and concentration, while also reducing cravings for sugar and alcohol.

Amino Acid Support:
- Amino Acid Blend
- Vitamin B6
- Mixed Branch Chain Amino Acids (BCAAs)
- L-Arginine
- Taurine
- L-Tyrosine
- L-Lysine
- L-Methionine
- L-Citrulline
- Creatine
- Magnesium
- L-Glutathione
- Grape Extract (Vitis vinifera)
- Apple Extract (Malus pumila)
- Vitamin B5
- Vitamin B9 (Folate)
- Vitamin C

If **HIGH** or **> 7.0 ng/MM WBC**:

There is currently no established RDA, AI, or UL for glutamine.

Glutamine is typically sold as L-glutamine, and doses have been studied in humans ranging from 500 mg/day to 50 g/day. Higher doses (>10 g/day) are commonly used in the treatment of intestinal barrier permeability.

In some individuals, glutamine is converted more efficiently to glutamate, which can lead to a neuron-excitatory state, increased anxiety, tension headaches/migraines, and even tachycardia. If any of these symptoms occur after consuming glutamine, supplementation should be discontinued. If glutamate appears to be an issue, consider supporting these co-factors:
- Magnesium and manganese are required for the conversion of glutamate to glutamine.
- Magnesium is also required for the conversion of glutamine to glutamate.
- Zinc and Vitamin B6 are required for the conversion of glutamate to GABA.

Nutritional support:
- Magnesium Citrate
- Magnesium Taurinate
- Magnesium Glycinate
- Zinc
- Manganese
- Vitamin B6
- Vitamin B Complex
- Liposomal Vitamin B Complex
- Multivitamin and Mineral (iron/copper-free)

Isoleucine (Serum)

Isoleucine, an essential amino acid that must be obtained through diet, is one of the three branched-chain amino acids (BCAAs), alongside leucine and valine. It plays a crucial role in hemoglobin formation, regulating blood sugar and energy levels. Isoleucine is particularly concentrated in muscle tissues in humans.

Isoleucine is a common component of proteins, peptides, and hormones. Leucine, on the other hand, is catabolized during exercise in skeletal muscle to provide carbon for energy production. Compared to the other two BCAAs, isoleucine has an intermediate ability to induce muscle protein synthesis. While it is stronger than valine but weaker than leucine, it can significantly increase glucose uptake and utilization during exercise.

Unlike other amino acids, BCAAs are not precursors for bile acids or neurotransmitters. However, they are involved in controlling mechanisms for neurotransmitters, muscle development and repair, and blood sugar regulation. Isoleucine is also involved in carbohydrate and fat metabolism.

Optimal Range	25.5 - 158.9 nmol/mL

If LOW or < 25.5 nmol/mL:

Inadequate Intake: A diet lacking sufficient protein or deficient in sources of BCAAs (e.g., meat, dairy, eggs, legumes, and certain grains) can lead to deficiencies in isoleucine, leucine, and valine. Low levels of essential BCAA may indicate a poor-quality diet or maldigestion due to deficient digestive peptidase activity or pancreatic dysfunction. Supplementation with zinc, vitamin B_3, and vitamin B_6 has improved outcomes in various conditions associated with low BCAA levels.

Vegetarian and Vegan Diets: Individuals following strict vegetarian or vegan diets may have a higher risk of BCAA deficiency since plant-based diets generally provide lower amounts of BCAAs.

Medical Conditions:
- Malnutrition: General malnutrition or starvation can result in BCAA deficiencies along with other nutrient deficiencies.
- Malabsorption Disorders: Gastrointestinal conditions like celiac disease or Crohn's disease can hinder the absorption of amino acids, potentially leading to BCAA deficiencies.
- Conditions that increase protein requirements, such as growth, pregnancy, or certain medical conditions, can lead to an increased demand for BCAAs. In such cases, a diet that doesn't meet these increased requirements can result in deficiency.
- Medications like valproic acid (used for epilepsy and mood disorders) can interfere with BCAA metabolism and lead to deficiency.

Food Sources: Red meat, poultry, fish, dairy, soy, quinoa, buckwheat, nuts, seeds, and beans are all excellent sources of protein. Supplement options include branched-chain amino acids, especially leucine, which are crucial for muscle health. However, if you consume a well-balanced diet that includes a variety of protein-rich foods, supplementation may not be necessary. Zinc, B3 (niacin), and B6 are also important nutrients that can be obtained from food sources.

Amino Acid Support:
- Amino Acid Blend
- Vitamin B6
- Mixed Branch Chain Amino Acids (BCAAs)
- L-Arginine
- Taurine
- L-Tyrosine
- L-Lysine

- L-Methionine
- L-Citrulline
- Creatine
- Magnesium
- L-Glutathione
- Grape Extract (Vitis vinifera)
- Apple Extract (Malus pumila)
- Vitamin B5
- Vitamin B9 (Folate)
- Vitamin C

Nutritional Support:
- Zinc (as Zinc Picolinate)
- Niacin (as Nicotinic Acid)
- Vitamin B6 (as Pyridoxine HCl)
- B vitamins (including B1, B2, B3, B5, B6, B12)
- Folate (as L-methylfolate)
- Biotin
- Vitamin C
- Magnesium (as Magnesium Taurinate, Magnesium Glycinate, Magnesium Malate)

If **HIGH** or **> 158.9 nmol/mL:**

High-protein diets, especially those rich in animal sources, often lead to excessive supplementation of branched-chain amino acids (BCAAs), which are commonly used by athletes and bodybuilders. During the breakdown of BCAAs, branched-chain aminotransferase and the branched-chain alpha ketoacid dehydrogenase complex (BCKDC) require several cofactors, including vitamin B6, vitamin B1, and lipoic acid. Therefore, the functional need for these cofactors may contribute to elevated levels of BCAAs.

Additionally, liver dysfunction has been associated with elevated BCAA levels. Non-alcoholic fatty liver diseases (NAFLD), cirrhosis, and hepatocellular carcinoma (HCC) have all been linked to increased BCAA concentrations.

Furthermore, genetics play a role in the development of elevated BCAA levels. Maple Syrup Urine Disease (MSUD) is a rare inherited disorder that affects the body's ability to metabolize BCAAs. As a result, individuals with MSUD accumulate isoleucine, leucine, and valine in their blood and tissues, which can potentially lead to neurological problems and other health issues.

Reduce dietary and supplement sources of co-factors, including vitamins B6, B1, B2, B3, B5, biotin (B7), magnesium, and lipoic acid. Conduct additional investigations, such as liver function tests and genetic testing.

Nutritional support
- Magnesium Citrate
- Magnesium Taurinate
- Magnesium Glycinate
- Vitamin B1 (Thiamine)
- Vitamin B2 (Riboflavin)
- Vitamin B3 (Niacin)
- Vitamin B5 (Pantothenic Acid)
- Vitamin B6
- Vitamin B7 (Biotin)
- Vitamin B Complex
- Alpha Lipoic Acid
- Multivitamin and Mineral (iron/copper-free)

Leucine (Serum)

Leucine is one of nine essential amino acids (it must be obtained via diet) and one of three branchedchain amino acids (alongside isoleucine and valine). Leucine is important for protein synthesis and many metabolic functions. It contributes to regulating blood sugar levels, growing and repairing muscle and bone tissue, producing growth hormones, and healing wounds. Leucine also prevents the breakdown of muscle proteins after trauma or severe stress and may be beneficial for individuals with phenylketonuria.

BCAAs are used for the synthesis of enzymes, transport proteins, and structural components of cells. Unlike other amino acids, BCAAs do not serve as precursors for bile acids or neurotransmitters, but are involved in control mechanisms for neurotransmitters, muscle development and repair, and blood-sugar regulation.

| Optimal Range | 101.2 - 249.3 nmol/mL |

If LOW or < 101.2 nmol/mL:

Leucine, an essential amino acid, is abundant in various foods and is rarely deficient. However, inadequate intake can occur when a diet lacks sufficient protein or is deficient in sources of BCAAs, such as meat, dairy, eggs, legumes, and certain grains. This can lead to deficiencies in isoleucine, leucine, and valine. Low levels of essential BCAA may indicate a poor-quality diet or maldigestion due to deficient digestive peptidase activity or pancreatic dysfunction.

Supplementation with zinc, vitamin B_3, and vitamin B_6 has shown promising results in various conditions associated with low BCAA levels.

Individuals following strict vegetarian or vegan diets may be at higher risk of BCAA deficiency due to the generally lower BCAAs found in plant-based diets.

Several medical conditions can also contribute to BCAA deficiencies. These include:
- Malnutrition: General malnutrition or starvation can result in BCAA deficiencies along with other nutrient deficiencies.
- Malabsorption Disorders: Gastrointestinal conditions like celiac disease or Crohn's disease can hinder the absorption of amino acids, potentially leading to BCAA deficiencies.
- Conditions that increase protein requirements, such as growth, pregnancy, or certain medical conditions, can lead to an increased demand for BCAAs. In such cases, a diet that fails to meet these increased requirements can result in deficiency.
- Medications like valproic acid (used for epilepsy and mood disorders) can interfere with BCAA metabolism and lead to deficiency.

Clinical manifestations of BCAA depletion include:
- Leucine supplementation alone can exacerbate pellagra and cause psychosis in pellagra patients by increasing niacin excretion in the urine.
- Leucine may lower brain serotonin and dopamine levels.

Leucine, one of the essential amino acids, is more concentrated in certain foods compared to others. For instance, a cup of milk contains approximately 800 mg of leucine, while it only has 500 mg of isoleucine and valine. On the other hand, a cup of wheat germ provides about 1.6 grams of leucine, along with 1 gram of isoleucine and valine. Interestingly, the ratio of leucine to other branched-chain amino acids (BCAAs) is balanced in eggs and cheese. Each egg and an ounce of most cheeses contain approximately 400 mg of leucine, along with 400 mg of valine and isoleucine. Notably, pork has the highest ratio of leucine to other BCAA, with leucine comprising 7 to 8 grams, while the other BCAA together account for only 3-4 grams.

Food sources that are rich in leucine include red meat, poultry, fish, dairy, soy, quinoa, buckwheat, nuts, seeds, and beans.

Regarding supplement options, branched-chain amino acids (BCAAs), particularly leucine, are among the most essential amino acids for maintaining muscle health. However, supplementation is generally not necessary if a well-balanced diet that includes a variety of protein sources is sufficient. Additionally, zinc and B3 (niacin) are other nutrients that play important roles in overall health and well-being.

Amino Acid Support:
- Amino Acid Blend
- Vitamin B6
- Mixed Branch Chain Amino Acids (BCAAs)
- L-Arginine
- Taurine
- L-Tyrosine
- L-Lysine
- L-Methionine
- L-Citrulline
- Creatine
- Magnesium
- L-Glutathione
- Grape Extract (Vitis vinifera)
- Apple Extract (Malus pumila)
- Vitamin B5
- Vitamin B9 (Folate)
- Vitamin C

Nutritional Support:
- Zinc (as Zinc Picolinate)
- Niacin (as Nicotinic Acid)
- Vitamin B6 (as Pyridoxine HCl)
- B vitamins (including B1, B2, B3, B5, B6, B12)
- Folate (as L-methylfolate)
- Biotin
- Vitamin C
- Magnesium (as Magnesium Taurinate, Magnesium Glycinate, Magnesium Malate)

If **HIGH** or **> 249.3 nmol/mL:**

High-protein diets, especially those rich in animal sources, often lead to excessive supplementation of branched-chain amino acids (BCAAs), which are commonly used by athletes and bodybuilders. During the breakdown of BCAAs, branched-chain aminotransferase and the branched-chain alpha ketoacid dehydrogenase complex (BCKDC) require several cofactors, including vitamin B6, vitamin B1, and lipoic acid. Therefore, the functional need for these cofactors may contribute to elevated levels of BCAAs.

Additionally, liver dysfunction has been associated with elevated BCAA levels. Non-alcoholic fatty liver diseases (NAFLD), cirrhosis, and hepatocellular carcinoma (HCC) have all been linked to increased BCAA concentrations.

Furthermore, genetics play a role in the development of elevated BCAA levels. Maple Syrup Urine Disease (MSUD) is a rare inherited disorder that affects the body's ability to metabolize BCAAs. As a result, individuals with MSUD accumulate isoleucine, leucine, and valine in their blood and tissues, which can potentially lead to neurological problems and other health issues.

Reduce dietary and supplement sources of co-factors, including vitamins B6, B1, B2, B3, B5, biotin (B7), magnesium, and lipoic acid. Conduct additional investigations, such as liver function tests and genetic testing.

Nutritional support
- Magnesium Citrate
- Magnesium Taurinate
- Magnesium Glycinate
- Vitamin B1 (Thiamine)
- Vitamin B2 (Riboflavin)
- Vitamin B3 (Niacin)
- Vitamin B5 (Pantothenic Acid)
- Vitamin B6
- Vitamin B7 (Biotin)
- Vitamin B Complex
- Alpha Lipoic Acid
- Multivitamin and Mineral (iron/copper-free)

Serine (Serum)

Serine is a non-essential amino acid (it can be synthesized in the body to some extent). It can be synthesized endogenously from dietary glycine, which is not considered an essential amino acid. D-serine is a neuromodulator produced in the glial cells of the brain and modulates the functions of neurons. Serine can be considered a nootropic nutrient. Serine enhances the binding of other compounds at NMDA (N-methyl-Daspartate) receptors. Serine can be used as an energy source. Formed from threonine and phosphoserine (requiring B6, manganese, and magnesium), serine is necessary for the biosynthesis of acetylcholine, a neurotransmitter used in memory function. Serine is a nonessential amino acid used in protein biosynthesis and can be derived from four possible sources: dietary intake, degradation of protein and phospholipids, biosynthesis from glycolysis intermediate 3-phosphoglycerate, or from glycine. Serine is found in soybeans, nuts, eggs, lentils, shellfish, and meats.

Optimal Range	1.8 - 19.8 ng/MM WBC

If LOW or < 1.8 ng/MM WBC:

Inadequate Dietary Intake:
A diet lacking sufficient protein or primarily plant-based, such as vegetarian and vegan diets, may increase the risk of serine deficiency. Serine can be synthesized endogenously from dietary glycine, which is not considered an essential amino acid. However, serine deficiency would be rare, and supra-physiological doses may be necessary to confer benefits over standard dietary intake.

It does not appear that depletion of serine is common, but side effects of low levels of serine in the brain appear to be correlated with a higher risk for addiction behaviors and some neurodegenerative conditions. Low serine may be due to decreased intake, gastrointestinal malabsorption, or maldigestion. One pathway of serine biosynthesis requires the vitamin B6-dependent enzyme phosphoserine aminotransferase. Therefore, a functional need for vitamin B6 may contribute to low serine levels. Given its association with the folate cycle, plasma serine levels may be low or high with homocysteinemia and methylation defects. Supplementation with vitamin B6, B12, folate, or betaine (trimethylglycine [TMG]) can result in normalized homocysteine levels as well as serine levels.

Foods high in serine include fish, meat, dairy, sugar cane, soybeans, spinach, kale, cauliflower, cabbage, pumpkin, banana, kiwi, cucumber, and beans.

Currently, there is no established Recommended Dietary Allowance (RDA), Adequate Intake (AI), or Upper Limit (UL) for serine supplementation or intake.

Serine can be supplemented to reduce symptoms of cognitive decline and reduce symptoms of cocaine dependence and schizophrenia.

Phosphatidylserine is a common supplemental phospholipid that contains serine. Doses of 30mg/kg of bodyweight are commonly used in patients with cognitive decline.

Food sources include red meat, poultry, fish, dairy, soy, quinoa, buckwheat, nuts, seeds, and beans. Co-factors include B6, B12, folate, or betaine (trimethylglycine [TMG]), and manganese. Low serine levels can disrupt methionine metabolism and impair acetylcholine synthesis. If simultaneous high threonine or phosphoserine (from other tests), then a need for vitamin B6, folate, and manganese is indicated. Low serine may lead to memory problems and depression. Additional investigations include genetic testing (methylation /folate pathways), homocysteine, and folate, B12 status.

Nutritional support:
- B Vitamins (B1, B2, B3, B5, B6, B7, B9, B12)
- Magnesium Taurinate
- Magnesium Glycinate
- Magnesium Malate
- Manganese Bisglycinate
- Folate
- Vitamin B6
- Vitamin B12
- Iron-free Multivitamin
- Magnesium

If **HIGH** or **> 19.8 ng/MM WBC:**

High dietary intake of serine-rich foods or supplementation may lead to elevated levels. When accompanied by low threonine, high serine levels indicate glucogenic compensation and catabolism. To address this, supplement threonine and BCAAs. Serine's association with the folate cycle means plasma serine levels can be low or high with homocysteinemia and methylation defects. Supplementing with vitamin B6, B12, folate, or betaine (trimethylglycine [TMG]) can normalize homocysteine and serine levels. However, there is currently no established Recommended Dietary Allowance (RDA), Acceptable Daily Intake (ADI), or Upper Limit (UL) for serine supplementation or intake. Excessive supplementation can be beneficial in reducing symptoms of cognitive decline, cocaine dependence, and schizophrenia. Phosphatidylserine, a common supplemental phospholipid containing serine, is commonly used in cognitive decline patients. Doses of 30 mg/kg of body weight are commonly used. Deficiencies in nutrients required for serine metabolism, such as vitamin B6 or B1, can lead to elevated serine levels, as well as other amino acids.

Reduce dietary and supplement sources of co-factors, including vitamins B6, B1, B12, folate, or betaine (trimethylglycine [TMG]). Additional investigations include genetic testing (methylation /folate pathways), homocysteine levels, and folate and B12 status.

Nutritional support:
- B Vitamins (B1, B2, B3, B5, B6, B7, B9, B12)
- Magnesium Taurinate
- Magnesium Glycinate
- Magnesium Malate
- Manganese Bisglycinate
- Folate
- Vitamin B6
- Vitamin B12
- Iron-free Multivitamin
- Magnesium

Valine (Serum)

Essential amino acid (must be obtained via diet). Valine is a branched-chain essential amino acid that has stimulant activity. It promotes muscle growth and tissue repair. It is a precursor in the penicillin biosynthetic pathway. Valine maintains mental vigor, muscle coordination, and emotional calm as a glycogenic amino acid.

BCAAs are used for the synthesis of enzymes, transport proteins, and structural components of cells. Unlike other amino acids, BCAAs do not serve as precursors for bile acids or neurotransmitters, but are involved in control mechanisms for neurotransmitters, muscle development and repair, and blood-sugar regulation.

| Optimal Range | 155.9 - 368.0 nmol/mL |

If LOW or < 155.9 nmol/mL:

Inadequate Intake: A diet lacking sufficient protein or deficient in sources of BCAAs (e.g., meat, dairy, eggs, legumes, and certain grains) can lead to deficiencies in isoleucine, leucine, and valine. Low levels of essential BCAA may indicate a poor-quality diet or maldigestion due to deficient digestive peptidase activity or pancreatic dysfunction. Supplementation with zinc, vitamin B_3, and vitamin B_6 has improved outcomes in various conditions associated with low BCAA levels.

Vegetarian and Vegan Diets: Individuals following strict vegetarian or vegan diets may have a higher risk of BCAA deficiency since plant-based diets generally provide lower amounts of BCAAs.

Medical Conditions:
- Malnutrition: General malnutrition or starvation can result in BCAA deficiencies along with other nutrient deficiencies.
- Malabsorption Disorders: Gastrointestinal conditions like celiac disease or Crohn's disease can hinder the absorption of amino acids, potentially leading to BCAA deficiencies.
- Conditions that increase protein requirements, such as growth, pregnancy, or certain medical conditions, can lead to an increased demand for BCAAs. In such cases, a diet that doesn't meet these increased requirements can result in deficiency.
- Medications like valproic acid (used for epilepsy and mood disorders) can interfere with BCAA metabolism and lead to deficiency.

Food Sources: Red meat, poultry, fish, dairy, soy, quinoa, buckwheat, nuts, seeds, and beans are all excellent sources of protein. Supplement options include branched-chain amino acids, especially leucine, which are crucial for muscle health. However, if you consume a well-balanced diet that includes a variety of protein-rich foods, supplementation may not be necessary. Zinc, B3 (niacin), and B6 are also important nutrients that can be obtained from food sources.

Amino Acid Support:
- Amino Acid Blend
- Vitamin B6
- Mixed Branch Chain Amino Acids (BCAAs)
- L-Arginine
- Taurine
- L-Tyrosine
- L-Lysine
- L-Methionine
- L-Citrulline
- Creatine
- Magnesium
- L-Glutathione
- Grape Extract (Vitis vinifera)
- Apple Extract (Malus pumila)
- Vitamin B5
- Vitamin B9 (Folate)
- Vitamin C

Nutritional Support:
- Zinc (as Zinc Picolinate)
- Niacin (as Nicotinic Acid)
- Vitamin B6 (as Pyridoxine HCl)
- B vitamins (including B1, B2, B3, B5, B6, B12)
- Folate (as L-methylfolate)
- Biotin
- Vitamin C

- Magnesium (as Magnesium Taurinate, Magnesium Glycinate, Magnesium Malate)

If **HIGH** or **> 368.0 nmol/mL:**

High-protein diets, especially those rich in animal sources, often lead to excessive supplementation of branched-chain amino acids (BCAAs), which are commonly used by athletes and bodybuilders. During the breakdown of BCAAs, branched-chain aminotransferase and the branched-chain alpha ketoacid dehydrogenase complex (BCKDC) require several cofactors, including vitamin B6, vitamin B1, and lipoic acid. Therefore, the functional need for these cofactors may contribute to elevated levels of BCAAs.

Additionally, liver dysfunction has been associated with elevated BCAA levels. Non-alcoholic fatty liver diseases (NAFLD), cirrhosis, and hepatocellular carcinoma (HCC) have all been linked to increased BCAA concentrations.

Furthermore, genetics play a role in the development of elevated BCAA levels. Maple Syrup Urine Disease (MSUD) is a rare inherited disorder that affects the body's ability to metabolize BCAAs. As a result, individuals with MSUD accumulate isoleucine, leucine, and valine in their blood and tissues, which can potentially lead to neurological problems and other health issues.

Reduce dietary and supplement sources of co-factors, including vitamins B6, B1, B2, B3, B5, biotin (B7), magnesium, and lipoic acid. Conduct additional investigations, such as liver function tests and genetic testing.

Nutritional support
- Magnesium Citrate
- Magnesium Taurinate
- Magnesium Glycinate
- Vitamin B1 (Thiamine)
- Vitamin B2 (Riboflavin)
- Vitamin B3 (Niacin)
- Vitamin B5 (Pantothenic Acid)
- Vitamin B6
- Vitamin B7 (Biotin)
- Vitamin B Complex
- Alpha Lipoic Acid
- Multivitamin and Mineral (iron/copper-free)

Calcium (Serum)

Calcium is a mineral that is a major component of bones and teeth, is required for muscle contraction, nerve transmission, cellular metabolism, and aids in blood clotting.

| Optimal Range | 8.9 - 10.6 mg/dL |

If **LOW** or **< 8.9 mg/dL:**

Calcium stores in the blood remain metabolically stable, but calcium stores elsewhere in the body may become depleted, conditionally, due to increased demand. Low dietary calcium intake during growth or stress can lead to low calcium stores. It's important to evaluate vitamin D and magnesium levels alongside calcium status.

Iron supplementation can interfere with calcium absorption, so it's recommended to take iron supplements at least 2 hours apart from a meal containing calcium-rich foods.

Conditions that can cause calcium depletion include:

- Metabolic alkalosis: This condition can lead to decreased serum ionized calcium due to calcium-binding albumin being more readily released during alkalotic states.
- Chronic diseases: Hypoparathyroidism, chronic kidney disease, liver disease, and vitamin D deficiency can all contribute to calcium depletion.
- Acute illnesses: Sepsis, pancreatitis (due to fat saponification), and acute kidney injury can also result in hypocalcemia.
- Severe hypomagnesemia can sometimes cause hypocalcemia, as is sometimes seen in proton pump inhibitor (PPI) therapy. PPI therapy also reduces stomach acidity, which can decrease calcium absorption through the intestinal tract.

Calcium deficiency can lead to osteoporosis. Some research suggests a link between low calcium intake and an increased risk of high blood pressure, colon cancer, and preeclampsia (high blood pressure and excess protein in the urine of a woman more than 20 weeks pregnant).

Calcium interacts with various drugs, including:
- Calcium supplementation along with thiazide diuretics can increase the risk of hypercalcemia.
- High-dose calcium supplementation can increase the risk of abnormal heart rhythms if taken with digitalis (digoxin).
- Calcium may decrease the absorption of tetracycline, quinolone class of antibiotics, bisphosphonates, and levothyroxine.
- H2 blockers and proton pump inhibitors can decrease calcium absorption.
- Long-term use of corticosteroids, antiepileptics, aminoglycosides, cisplatin, and bisphosphonates can also lead to calcium depletion.

Acute hypocalcemia is common among patients receiving large transfusions, such as during treatment of traumatic hemorrhage, due to citrate and chelation products. Trauma patients receiving blood transfusions should be closely monitored to avoid severe hypocalcemic events.

Good sources of calcium include dairy products like whole milk, plain yogurt, and part-skim mozzarella cheese; fortified soy milk; salmon; turnip greens; Chinese cabbage, kale, bok choy, and broccoli; and sardines and other canned fish with bones. Some foods, such as orange juice and bread, are also fortified with calcium. However, Chinese cabbage, kale, and turnip greens contain absorbable calcium, while spinach and some other vegetables contain calcium that is poorly absorbed.

For adults aged 19 to 50, the Adequate Intake (AI) for calcium is 1000 mg per day. Since calcium is crucial for preventing bone disease later in life, the AI is higher for adolescents aged 9 to 18, at 1300 mg per day. For individuals aged 51 and older, the AI is 1200 mg per day.

The Upper Limit (UL) for calcium is 2,500 milligrams per day. Excess calcium intake can lead to mineral imbalances because it interferes with the absorption of iron, magnesium, zinc, and other minerals.

Calcium supplements are available in various forms, including calcium carbonate, calcium citrate, calcium citrate malate, calcium gluconate, and calcium lactate. Calcium citrate is the preferred form of calcium for individuals with hypo- or achlorhydria (low or insufficient stomach acid).

To maximize the absorption of calcium supplements, it's recommended to limit doses to no more than 500 mg per dose. Additionally, calcium supplementation should be accompanied by adequate vitamin D supplementation, as insufficient vitamin D levels impair cellular calcium absorption, which can lead to atopic calcium deposits in epidermal tissue.

It's also important to note that iron supplementation may interfere with calcium absorption. Therefore, it's recommended to take iron supplements at least 2 hours apart from a meal containing calcium-rich foods.

Nutritional support:
- Calcium malate
- Vitamin D
- Zinc
- Magnesium
- Manganese
- Copper
- Potassium
- Vitamin C
- Vitamin K
- Boron
- Iodine
- Vitamin B6
- Vitamin B12
- Folate
- Biotin
- Chromium
- Selenium
- Sodium
- Iron
- Omega-3 fatty acids
- Vitamin A
- Vitamin E

If **HIGH** or > 10.6 mg/dL:

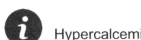

Hypercalcemia, a condition characterized by elevated calcium levels in the blood, has not been linked to excessive calcium intake from natural food sources. Instead, it arises from various factors, including:

- Calcification of soft tissues: This occurs when calcium deposits in tissues like the heart and arteries.
- Parathyroid disorders: These conditions involve the malfunction of the parathyroid glands, which regulate calcium levels in the body.
- Kidney stones: These hardened deposits of calcium and other minerals in the kidneys can cause pain and discomfort.

Causes of excess calcium in the blood include:
- Low levels of PTH: Parathyroid hormone (PTH) plays a crucial role in calcium regulation. Low PTH levels can lead to hypercalcemia.
- Malignancy and primary hyperparathyroidism: These conditions are the most common causes of elevated calcium concentrations in the blood.
- High or excessive intake of vitamin D2 or D3 supplements: While vitamin D2 is less likely to cause hypercalcemia, excessive vitamin D intake can lead to this condition.
- Vitamin D toxicity: This condition can occur when vitamin D levels become too high, causing symptoms such as nausea, vomiting, and abdominal pain. It can also lead to bone loss, kidney stones, and calcification of organs like the heart and kidneys if left untreated for an extended period.
- Over-the-counter calcium supplements combined with antacids: Certain individuals, such as postmenopausal women, pregnant women, transplant recipients, patients with bulimia, and those on dialysis, are at risk of hypercalcemia from these supplements when combined with antacids.
- Reduced conversion of 25-OHD to 1,25-OHD in the kidneys: This condition occurs when the kidneys are unable to convert vitamin D into its active form, leading to elevated calcium levels.
- Renal failure: Kidney failure can also cause hypercalcemia by impairing calcium regulation.
- Parathyroid cancer: This type of cancer can disrupt the parathyroid glands' ability to produce PTH, leading to hypercalcemia.

Considerations for Support:
- Evaluate if diet or supplements are affecting calcium levels and reduce them as necessary.
- Assess parathyroid and renal function.

Caution with Excess Calcium Supplements:
- Calcium supplements may cause excessive calcium in the blood if there's parathyroid dysfunction or renal failure.

- It's not recommended to take calcium supplements unless under medical supervision.
- Calcium supplementation should always be accompanied by Vitamin D and possibly Vitamin K2 to ensure calcium is absorbed into bones and not deposited in soft tissues.

Additional Investigations:
- Vitamin D levels
- Parathyroid hormone
- Kidney function

Calcium (Cellular)

Calcium is a mineral that is a major component of bones and teeth, is required for muscle contraction, nerve transmission, cellular metabolism, and aids in blood clotting.

Optimal Range	15 - 120 ng/MM WBC

If LOW or < 15 ng/MM WBC:

Calcium stores in the blood remain metabolically stable, but calcium stores elsewhere in the body may become depleted, conditionally, due to increased demand. Low dietary calcium intake during growth or stress can lead to low calcium stores. It's important to evaluate vitamin D and magnesium levels alongside calcium status.

Iron supplementation can interfere with calcium absorption, so it's recommended to take iron supplements at least 2 hours apart from a meal containing calcium-rich foods.

Conditions that can cause calcium depletion include:
- Metabolic alkalosis: This condition can lead to decreased serum ionized calcium due to calcium-binding albumin being more readily released during alkalotic states.
- Chronic diseases: Hypoparathyroidism, chronic kidney disease, liver disease, and vitamin D deficiency can all contribute to calcium depletion.
- Acute illnesses: Sepsis, pancreatitis (due to fat saponification), and acute kidney injury can also result in hypocalcemia.
- Severe hypomagnesemia can sometimes cause hypocalcemia, as is sometimes seen in proton pump inhibitor (PPI) therapy. PPI therapy also reduces stomach acidity, which can decrease calcium absorption through the intestinal tract.

Calcium deficiency can lead to osteoporosis. Some research suggests a link between low calcium intake and an increased risk of high blood pressure, colon cancer, and preeclampsia (high blood pressure and excess protein in the urine of a woman more than 20 weeks pregnant).

Calcium interacts with various drugs, including:
- Calcium supplementation along with thiazide diuretics can increase the risk of hypercalcemia.
- High-dose calcium supplementation can increase the risk of abnormal heart rhythms if taken with digitalis (digoxin).
- Calcium may decrease the absorption of tetracycline, quinolone class of antibiotics, bisphosphonates, and levothyroxine.
- H2 blockers and proton pump inhibitors can decrease calcium absorption.
- Long-term use of corticosteroids, antiepileptics, aminoglycosides, cisplatin, and bisphosphonates can also lead to calcium depletion.

Acute hypocalcemia is common among patients receiving large transfusions, such as during treatment of traumatic hemorrhage, due to citrate and chelation products. Trauma patients receiving blood transfusions should be closely monitored to avoid severe hypocalcemic events.

Good sources of calcium include dairy products like whole milk, plain yogurt, and part-skim mozzarella cheese; fortified soy milk; salmon; turnip greens; Chinese cabbage, kale, bok choy, and broccoli; and sardines and other canned fish with bones. Some foods, such as orange juice and bread, are also fortified with calcium. However, Chinese cabbage, kale, and turnip greens contain absorbable calcium, while spinach and some other vegetables contain calcium that is poorly absorbed.

For adults aged 19 to 50, the Adequate Intake (AI) for calcium is 1000 mg per day. Since calcium is crucial for preventing bone disease later in life, the AI is higher for adolescents aged 9 to 18, at 1300 mg per day. For individuals aged 51 and older, the AI is 1200 mg per day.

The Upper Limit (UL) for calcium is 2,500 milligrams per day. Excess calcium intake can lead to mineral imbalances because it interferes with the absorption of iron, magnesium, zinc, and other minerals.

Calcium supplements are available in various forms, including calcium carbonate, calcium citrate, calcium citrate malate, calcium gluconate, and calcium lactate. Calcium citrate is the preferred form of calcium for individuals with hypo- or achlorhydria (low or insufficient stomach acid).

To maximize the absorption of calcium supplements, it's recommended to limit doses to no more than 500 mg per dose. Additionally, calcium supplementation should be accompanied by adequate vitamin D supplementation, as insufficient vitamin D levels impair cellular calcium absorption, which can lead to atopic calcium deposits in epidermal tissue.

It's also important to note that iron supplementation may interfere with calcium absorption. Therefore, it's recommended to take iron supplements at least 2 hours apart from a meal containing calcium-rich foods.

Nutritional support:
- Calcium malate
- Vitamin D
- Zinc
- Magnesium
- Manganese
- Copper
- Potassium
- Vitamin C
- Vitamin K
- Boron
- Iodine
- Vitamin B6
- Vitamin B12
- Folate
- Biotin
- Chromium
- Selenium
- Sodium
- Iron
- Omega-3 fatty acids
- Vitamin A
- Vitamin E

If **HIGH** or **> 120 ng/MM WBC:**

Hypercalcemia, a condition characterized by elevated calcium levels in the blood, has not been linked to excessive calcium intake from natural food sources. Instead, it arises from various factors, including:
- Calcification of soft tissues: This occurs when calcium deposits in tissues like the heart and arteries.
- Parathyroid disorders: These conditions involve the malfunction of the parathyroid glands, which regulate calcium levels in the body.
- Kidney stones: These hardened deposits of calcium and other minerals in the kidneys can cause pain and discomfort.

Causes of excess calcium in the blood include:
- Low levels of PTH: Parathyroid hormone (PTH) plays a crucial role in calcium regulation. Low PTH levels can lead to hypercalcemia.
- Malignancy and primary hyperparathyroidism: These conditions are the most common causes of elevated calcium concentrations in the blood.
- High or excessive intake of vitamin D2 or D3 supplements: While vitamin D2 is less likely to cause hypercalcemia, excessive vitamin D intake can lead to this condition.
- Vitamin D toxicity: This condition can occur when vitamin D levels become too high, causing symptoms such as nausea, vomiting, and abdominal pain. It can also lead to bone loss, kidney stones, and calcification of organs like the heart and kidneys if left untreated for an extended period.
- Over-the-counter calcium supplements combined with antacids: Certain individuals, such as postmenopausal women, pregnant women, transplant recipients, patients with bulimia, and those on dialysis, are at risk of hypercalcemia from these supplements when combined with antacids.
- Reduced conversion of 25-OHD to 1,25-OHD in the kidneys: This condition occurs when the kidneys are unable to convert vitamin D into its active form, leading to elevated calcium levels.
- Renal failure: Kidney failure can also cause hypercalcemia by impairing calcium regulation.
- Parathyroid cancer: This type of cancer can disrupt the parathyroid glands' ability to produce PTH, leading to hypercalcemia.

Considerations for Support:
- Evaluate if diet or supplements are affecting calcium levels and reduce them as necessary.
- Assess parathyroid and renal function.

Caution with Excess Calcium Supplements:
- Calcium supplements may cause excessive calcium in the blood if there's parathyroid dysfunction or renal failure.
- It's not recommended to take calcium supplements unless under medical supervision.
- Calcium supplementation should always be accompanied by Vitamin D and possibly Vitamin K2 to ensure calcium is absorbed into bones and not deposited in soft tissues.

Additional Investigations:
- Vitamin D levels
- Parathyroid hormone
- Kidney function

Chromium (Serum)

Chromium, an essential nutrient found in trace amounts in humans, plays a crucial role as a cofactor for chromodulin. This peptide enhances the effectiveness of insulin on target tissues, thereby aiding in the regulation of blood sugar and lipid metabolism. Chromium exists in two primary states: trivalent chromium (chromium 3), commonly found in foods, and hexavalent chromium (chromium 6), primarily found in industrial sources and pollutants. While chromium 3 is significantly less toxic than chromium 6, the body can convert some chromium 6 to chromium 3 using glutathione, hydrogen peroxide, glutathione reductase, and ascorbic acid. Notably, few serious adverse effects have been associated with high intakes of chromium 3, hence the absence of an established upper limit (UL) for chromium 3. However, overexposure to chromium 6 can occur among welders and individuals in the metallurgical industry, as well as those who use chromium-containing paints and primers, individuals with metallic surgical implants, and those who consume chromium salts. Chromium toxicity can manifest through oral, inhaled, or dermal absorption.

Depending on the route of exposure, chromium toxicity can lead to various symptoms, including nausea, vomiting, diarrhea, muscle cramps, skin lesions, sinus, nasal, and lung cancer, renal failure, liver damage, circulatory collapse, coma, and even death.

Optimal Range	0.1 - 0.7 ng/mL

If LOW or < 0.1 ng/mL:

 How it gets depleted: Deficiency is rare, but it can occur in patients receiving IV parenteral nutrition without supplemental chromium or individuals who engage in regular endurance exercise. Clinical manifestations of depletion include the development of diabetes and metabolic syndrome. Even mild chromium deficiencies can disrupt blood sugar metabolism and contribute to symptoms like anxiety and fatigue.

DIET/MEDICATION INTERACTIONS: The interactions between chromium and drugs in humans are still poorly understood.

 Food sources include grape juice, ham, English muffin, brewer's yeast, orange juice, and beef.

Nutritional support:
- Chromium
- Manganese
- Zinc
- Vanadium
- Taurine
- Vitamin D3
- Magnesium
- Potassium
- Calcium
- Sodium
- Vitamin B1
- Vitamin B2
- Vitamin B3
- Vitamin B5
- Vitamin B6
- Vitamin B7 (Biotin)
- Vitamin B9 (Folate)
- Vitamin B12
- Vitamin A
- Vitamin C
- Vitamin E
- Vitamin K
- Copper
- Iodine
- Selenium
- Iron
- Omega-3 fatty acids
- L-Carnitine
- Acetyl-L-Carnitine
- Coenzyme Q10
- L-glutathione
- L-Glutamine
- N-Acetyl-L-Cysteine (NAC)
- Curcumin
- Chromium Picolinate

If HIGH or > 0.7 ng/mL:

Supplemental chromium is generally not necessary as dietary intake easily meets physiological requirements. However, excessive supplementation has been studied. Many studies have shown the safety of daily doses of up to 1,000 mcg of chromium for several months. Most concerns about the long-term safety of trivalent chromium supplementation stem from studies in cell culture, suggesting that trivalent chromium, particularly in the form of chromium picolinate, may increase DNA damage. A study of 10 women taking 400 mcg/day of chromium as chromium picolinate found no evidence of increased oxidative damage to DNA as measured by antibodies to an oxidized DNA base. Nevertheless, there have been a few isolated reports of severe adverse reactions to chromium picolinate. For instance, kidney failure was reported five months after a six-week course of 600 mcg/day of chromium in the form of chromium picolinate. In contrast, kidney failure and impaired liver function were reported after the use of 1,200 to 2,400 mcg/day of chromium in the form of chromium picolinate over four to five months.

Consider if diet or supplements are impacting calcium levels and reduce as necessary

Copper (Serum)

Copper plays a vital role in various bodily functions. It aids in the transport of iron, supports energy production within cells, and facilitates methylation and gene transcription, which are crucial for cellular detoxification mechanisms and neurotransmitter generation. Copper also contributes to the development of the myelin sheath around nerves and supports the formation of connective tissue. Additionally, it is essential for redox reactions and acts as a potent antioxidant. Furthermore, copper supports melanin production in hair, skin, and nail cells. The human body requires approximately 50 to 80 milligrams of copper to function optimally. Copper is absorbed into the bloodstream from ingested food. Once in the blood, it attaches to a protein called ceruloplasmin, which serves as a transporter, carrying copper throughout the body. Any copper remaining in the blood that is not bound to ceruloplasmin is referred to as free copper. Excessive free copper in the blood can be hazardous. It begins to migrate out of the bloodstream and into the tissues of the brain, eyes, and kidneys. As the copper accumulates, it damages the cells surrounding it, leading to a decline in the functioning of these organs.

Optimal Range	0.6 - 1.8 mcg/mL

If LOW or < 0.6 mcg/mL:

Deficiencies or excesses of copper are uncommon in healthy individuals. However, copper deficiency can occur in specific populations, including infants or children fed exclusively cow's milk formula, premature infants, infants or children with persistent diarrhea, individuals with malabsorption syndromes such as celiac disease, bowel resections, Crohn's disease, and ulcerative colitis, individuals with cystic fibrosis, and individuals with prolonged high supplemental zinc intake. To assess the possibility of copper deficiency, consider testing for celiac disease or neurological indications of demyelination. Additionally, excessive use of denture cream containing zinc can lead to hypocupremia. Furthermore, copper may become deficient or depleted in the presence of supplemental zinc intake exceeding 60 mg/day for extended periods.

MEDICATION INTERACTIONS: The interaction of copper with other medications is relatively unknown.

 Food Sources:
- Beef
- liver
- Oysters
- Baking chocolate
- Potatoes
- Shiitake mushrooms
- Cashew nuts
- Dungeness crab
- Sunflower seed kernels
- Turkey giblets
- Dark chocolate (70-85% cocoa)
- Tofu

Support Considerations:
- Assess if your diet or supplement sources of zinc are high, as these can interfere with copper absorption.

Additional Investigations:
- Ceruloplasmin levels
- Zinc levels
- Celiac disease or inflammatory bowel disease (IBD)
- Genetic testing for Menke's disease

Nutritional support includes:
- Copper (Glycinate)
- Multi-mineral
- Multi-vitamin/mineral
- Magnesium taurinate
- Magnesium glycinate
- Magnesium malate

If **HIGH** or **> 1.8 mcg/mL:**

Most serum copper is found in ceruloplasmin. Elevated levels may indicate increased inflammation and oxidative stress rather than excess copper in the blood. Copper supplementation of 2 mg/day is usually sufficient to correct copper deficiencies. The UL for copper is 10 mg/day, which has been shown not to cause liver damage in healthy individuals. Some research suggests that elevated blood levels of free unbound copper, which depletes zinc levels, may be associated with the onset of Alzheimer's disease. Therefore, copper supplementation in this population is not recommended if zinc deficiency is suspected. Elevated copper levels have also been linked to Wilson's disease, a rare, autosomal recessive disorder caused by abnormal copper accumulation in the body, particularly affecting the brain, liver, and cornea.

Considerations for Support:
- Evaluate if dietary changes or supplements are affecting copper levels and make adjustments as needed.
- If Wilson's disease is a possibility, consider referring the patient to a specialist for further evaluation.

Additional Investigations:
- Ceruloplasmin levels
- Liver panel
- Inflammation markers (hsCRP, ESR)
- Zinc levels
- Genetic testing for Wilson's disease

Nutritional support
- Zinc
- Magnesium Taurinate
- Magnesium Glycinate
- Magnesium Malate

Copper (Cellular)

Copper plays a vital role in various bodily functions. It aids in the transport of iron, supports energy production within cells, and facilitates methylation and gene transcription, which are crucial for cellular detoxification mechanisms and neurotransmitter generation. Copper also contributes to the development of the myelin sheath around nerves and supports the formation of connective tissue. Additionally, it is essential for redox reactions and acts as a potent antioxidant. Furthermore, copper supports melanin production in hair, skin, and nail cells. The human body requires approximately 50 to 80 milligrams of copper to function optimally. Copper is absorbed into the bloodstream from ingested food. Once in the blood, it attaches to a protein called ceruloplasmin, which serves as a transporter, carrying copper throughout the body. Any copper remaining in the blood that is not bound to ceruloplasmin is referred to as free copper. Excessive free copper in the blood can be hazardous. It begins to migrate out of the bloodstream and into the tissues of the brain, eyes, and kidneys. As the copper accumulates, it damages the cells surrounding it, leading to a decline in the functioning of these organs.

Optimal Range	2.0 - 15.0 ng/MM WBC

If **LOW** or **< 2.0 ng/MM WBC**:

Deficiencies or excesses of copper are uncommon in healthy individuals. However, copper deficiency can occur in specific populations, including infants or children fed exclusively cow's milk formula, premature infants, infants or children with persistent diarrhea, individuals with malabsorption syndromes such as celiac disease, bowel resections, Crohn's disease, and ulcerative colitis, individuals with cystic fibrosis, and individuals with prolonged high supplemental zinc intake. To assess the possibility of copper deficiency, consider testing for celiac disease or neurological indications of demyelination. Additionally, excessive use of denture cream containing zinc can lead to hypocupremia. Furthermore, copper may become deficient or depleted in the presence of supplemental zinc intake exceeding 60 mg/day for extended periods.

MEDICATION INTERACTIONS: The interaction of copper with other medications is relatively unknown.

Food Sources:
- Beef liver
- Oysters
- Baking chocolate
- Potatoes
- Shiitake mushrooms
- Cashew nuts
- Dungeness crab
- Sunflower seed kernels
- Turkey giblets
- Dark chocolate (70-85% cocoa)
- Tofu

Support Considerations:
- Assess if your diet or supplement sources of zinc are high, as these can interfere with copper absorption.

Additional Investigations:
- Ceruloplasmin levels
- Zinc levels
- Celiac disease or inflammatory bowel disease (IBD)

- Genetic testing for Menke's disease

Nutritional support includes:
- Copper (Glycinate)
- Multi-mineral
- Multi-vitamin/mineral
- Magnesium taurinate
- Magnesium glycinate
- Magnesium malate

If **HIGH** or **> 15 ng/MM WBC:**

Most serum copper is found in ceruloplasmin. Elevated levels may indicate increased inflammation and oxidative stress rather than excess copper in the blood. Copper supplementation of 2 mg/day is usually sufficient to correct copper deficiencies. The UL for copper is 10 mg/day, which has been shown not to cause liver damage in healthy individuals. Some research suggests that elevated blood levels of free unbound copper, which depletes zinc levels, may be associated with the onset of Alzheimer's disease. Therefore, copper supplementation in this population is not recommended if zinc deficiency is suspected. Elevated copper levels have also been linked to Wilson's disease, a rare, autosomal recessive disorder caused by abnormal copper accumulation in the body, particularly affecting the brain, liver, and cornea.

Considerations for Support:
- Evaluate if dietary changes or supplements are affecting copper levels and make adjustments as needed.
- If Wilson's disease is a possibility, consider referring the patient to a specialist for further evaluation.

Additional Investigations:
- Ceruloplasmin levels
- Liver panel
- Inflammation markers (hsCRP, ESR)
- Zinc levels
- Genetic testing for Wilson's disease

Nutritional support
- Zinc
- Magnesium Taurinate
- Magnesium Glycinate
- Magnesium Malate

Copper to Zinc Ratio (Serum)

The copper-to-zinc ratio, a crucial indicator of overall health, quantifies the relative proportion of copper to zinc in the body. Both copper and zinc, essential trace minerals, play vital roles in various physiological processes. An optimal balance between these minerals is essential for immune system efficiency, antioxidant defense, and neurological function. Imbalances in this ratio, whether excessive copper or deficient zinc, can lead to various health concerns.

Physiological and hormonal factors, including estrogen, progesterone, and testosterone, influence the minerals zinc and copper. Zinc is crucial for progesterone and testosterone production, while copper is affected by estrogen. Additionally, zinc and copper are associated with the antioxidant activity of superoxide dismutase (SOD). Their balance reflects the activity of zinc and copper-activated SOD.

Physiological conditions such as pregnancy, growth, and development, as well as virus and bacterial infections, can also affect the Zn/Cu ratio.

Optimal Range	0.9 - 2.6

If LOW or < 0.9:

A low ratio indicates higher levels of zinc compared to copper. A lower copper-to-zinc ratio may suggest copper deficiency (or zinc toxicity), which can affect red blood cell formation and iron metabolism. A decreased copper-to-zinc ratio imbalance can have various consequences:
- Copper Deficiency: Although less common than zinc deficiency, copper deficiency can occur and may lead to symptoms like anemia, a lower white blood cell count (increasing susceptibility to infections), neuropathy, and weakened bones.
- Neurological Implications: While an elevated ratio has been associated with neurodegenerative diseases, a decreased ratio due to excessive zinc supplementation can impair neurologic function, as both copper and zinc play crucial roles in the central nervous system.
- Cardiovascular Issues: Copper is essential for cardiovascular health. Copper deficiency can lead to irregular heartbeats and other cardiovascular complications.
- Collagen Synthesis: Copper plays a role in collagen synthesis. A deficiency can impact skin health, wound healing, and the structural integrity of tissues.
- Compromised Immune Function: Although zinc is essential for the immune system, copper also plays a role. A decreased copper-to-zinc ratio, implying copper deficiency, can hinder the immune response.
- Potential Over-supplementation: A decreased copper-to-zinc ratio could indicate excessive zinc supplementation, which can lead to copper deficiency if not balanced. High zinc intake can act as a copper antagonist, reducing its absorption and utilization in the body.
- Gastrointestinal Problems: Excessive zinc intake, leading to a lowered copper-to-zinc ratio, can result in gastrointestinal disturbances, including nausea, vomiting, loss of appetite, stomach cramps, diarrhea, and headaches.

Food Sources of Copper:
- Beef liver
- Oysters
- Baking chocolate
- Potatoes
- Shiitake mushrooms
- Cashew nuts
- Dungeness crab
- Sunflower seed kernels
- Turkey giblets
- Dark chocolate (70-85% cocoa)
- Tofu

Considerations:
- If your diet or supplement sources of zinc are high, they can reduce copper absorption.
- Additional investigations may include ceruloplasmin, zinc, celiac disease, or inflammatory bowel disease (IBD), as well as genetic testing for Menke's disease.

Nutritional support includes:
- Copper (Glycinate)
- Multi-mineral

- Multi-vitamin/mineral
- Magnesium taurinate
- Magnesium glycinate
- Magnesium malate

If **HIGH** or > 2.6:

 A high copper-to-zinc ratio indicates higher copper levels compared to zinc. Systemic inflammation can elevate this ratio. For instance, a high copper-to-zinc ratio has been associated with neurodegenerative diseases, increased oxidative stress, and certain cardiovascular conditions. Elevated copper levels in the body suggest an imbalance between copper and zinc. This imbalance can lead to various health implications, including:

- Neurological Issues: High copper levels relative to zinc can be linked to neurodegenerative diseases. Copper can produce oxidative stress, which, when unopposed by zinc's antioxidant effects, can cause neuronal damage.
- Mood and Behavior Disturbances: Elevated copper-to-zinc ratios have been implicated in some mood disorders, such as depression, anxiety, and even ADHD. Copper influences neurotransmitter levels, and its imbalance with zinc can affect mood and cognition.
- Immune Function: An imbalanced copper-to-zinc ratio can impact immune system function. Zinc is crucial for various immune functions, including T-cell activity. A skewed ratio may potentially decrease immune system efficiency.
- Cardiovascular Concerns: High copper levels relative to zinc have been associated with certain cardiovascular diseases. The oxidative stress induced by copper may contribute to these conditions.
- Estrogen Dominance: Copper levels can rise with increased estrogen in the body. This can be observed in conditions like polycystic ovary syndrome (PCOS) or during specific menstrual cycle phases. Elevated copper can thus indicate hormonal imbalances in certain cases.
- Oxidative Stress and Inflammation: Copper can induce oxidative stress, which, when not counteracted by zinc's antioxidant properties, can lead to cellular damage and inflammation. This increased risk of chronic diseases is a potential consequence of this imbalance.

 Food Sources of Zinc: Oysters, Beef, Blue Crab, Fortified Breakfast Cereal, Pumpkin Seeds

Considerations:
- Assess if diet or supplements are affecting copper levels and adjust as necessary.
- Consult a healthcare professional if Wilson's disease is a possibility.

Addressing this imbalance often involves reducing copper intake and increasing zinc, along with other supportive measures. Here are some general strategies to consider:

Adjust Diet:
- Reduce Copper Intake: Limit foods high in copper, such as shellfish, organ meats, nuts, seeds, chocolate, and some grains.
- Increase Zinc Intake: Consume foods rich in zinc like beef, poultry, oysters, beans, nuts, and whole grains.

Supplementation:
- Zinc Supplementation: Zinc can act as a copper antagonist, helping to balance the ratio. A healthcare professional can guide appropriate dosages.
- Molybdenum: This trace mineral supports the body's copper processing and elimination.

Enhance Detoxification:
- Drink Plenty of Water: This aids in the removal of excess copper from the body.

- Sauna and Sweating: Some believe sweating can help expel excess copper, although more research is needed in this area.

Be cautious of copper plumbing and cookware, as they can be sources of copper exposure. If you're concerned about copper exposure, consider the following steps:
- Have your water tested or use a filter: Copper can be found in drinking water from copper pipes.
- Be aware of other sources of copper exposure: Some intrauterine devices (IUDs) and dental materials can also contain copper.
- Support liver function: The liver plays a crucial role in metabolizing and excreting copper. Consuming liver-supportive foods and herbs, such as milk thistle, can be beneficial.
- Evaluate supplements and medications: Ensure that multivitamins or other supplements you're taking don't contain excessive copper. Some medications can also influence copper metabolism, so it's essential to consult with a healthcare provider.
- Monitor and test regularly: Regularly test your copper-to-zinc ratio to monitor your progress and adjust your strategies as needed.
- Seek professional guidance: It's crucial to consult with a healthcare professional, such as a nutritionist or naturopath, who can provide tailored advice based on your individual needs and circumstances.

Additionally, consider the following tests:
- ceruloplasmin
- liver panel
- inflammation markers (hsCRP, ESR)
- zinc
- genetic testing (Wilson's disease)

Nutritional support
- Zinc
- Magnesium Taurinate
- Magnesium Glycinate
- Magnesium Malate

Iron (Serum)

Iron is essential for producing red blood cells (hematopoiesis) and is a component of hemoglobin, the pigment that gives red blood cells their characteristic red color. Hemoglobin binds to oxygen and facilitates its transport from the lungs to all cells in the body through the arteries. Once oxygen is delivered, the iron (part of hemoglobin) binds to carbon dioxide, which is then transported back to the lungs for exhalation. Iron also plays a role in converting blood sugar into energy.

Additionally, the production of enzymes, which are crucial for producing new cells, amino acids, hormones, and neurotransmitters, depends on iron. This aspect becomes particularly important during recovery from illnesses or strenuous exercise. Furthermore, the immune system relies on iron for its efficient functioning. Sufficient iron levels are essential for physical and mental growth, especially during childhood and pregnancy, when the developing fetus solely depends on its mother's iron supply.

| Optimal Range | 59.0 - 158.0 ug/dL |

If LOW or < 59.0 ug/dL:

Inadequate iron intake can lead to iron deficiency, which can cause various symptoms. Iron is essential for producing hemoglobin, a protein in red blood cells that carries oxygen throughout the body. When iron stores are low, hemoglobin production slows down, reducing oxygen transport and causing fatigue, dizziness, lowered immunity, and reduced athletic performance.

Since our bodies can't produce iron, it's crucial to consume sufficient amounts through diet. Iron is lost from the body through various processes, including urination, defecation, sweating, and exfoliation of old skin cells. Bleeding further contributes to iron loss, explaining why women have a higher iron demand than men.

To prevent or correct iron deficiency, it's important to eat iron-rich foods and cook in iron skillets. Iron is found in various foods, including heme-iron sources like red meat and poultry, which are easily absorbed, and non-heme sources like lentils, beans, leafy vegetables, pistachios, tofu, fortified bread, and fortified breakfast cereals.

However, iron from different foods is absorbed and processed differently by the body. Heme iron from meat is more easily absorbed than non-heme iron from grains and vegetables. Additionally, heme iron from red meat may increase the risk of colorectal cancer. Minerals and chemicals in one food type can also inhibit the absorption of iron from another food consumed simultaneously. For instance, oxalates and phytic acid form insoluble complexes that bind iron in the gut, preventing its absorption. Iron from plant sources, such as legumes and dark-green leafy vegetables like broccoli, kale, and oriental greens, is less easily absorbed than heme-bound iron from animal sources. Therefore, vegetarians and vegans should consume slightly more iron daily than meat-eaters, fish-eaters, and poultry-eaters. However, spinach and Swiss chard contain oxalates that bind iron, making it almost entirely unavailable for absorption.

To enhance iron absorption from nonheme sources, it's best to consume them with foods containing heme-bound iron or vitamin C. Iron deficiency can manifest even before iron deficiency anemia develops. Iron deficiency symptoms aren't exclusive to anemia; they arise because iron is essential for many enzymes to function normally. Consequently, a wide range of symptoms may eventually emerge, either as secondary effects of anemia or as primary results of iron deficiency.

Common iron deficiency symptoms include fatigue, dizziness, pale skin, hair loss, twitches, irritability, weakness, pica, brittle or grooved nails, and nausea.

Common forms of iron in supplements include ferrous and ferric iron salts, such as ferrous sulfate, ferrous gluconate, ferric citrate, and ferric sulfate. Ferrous iron in dietary supplements is more bioavailable than ferric iron. However, high doses of supplemental iron (45 mg or more daily) may cause gastrointestinal side effects like nausea and constipation.

Other forms of supplemental iron, such as heme iron polypeptides, carbonyl iron, iron amino-acid chelates, and polysaccharide-iron complexes, may have fewer gastrointestinal side effects than ferrous or ferric salts.

Many medicinal herbs can boost iron levels in individuals with iron deficiency. These herbs can be easily assimilated into the bloodstream by making a hot water infusion (tea). Iron-enhancing herbs include yellow dock, red raspberry leaf, gentian, yellow root, turmeric, mullein, nettle, parsley, ginseng, watercress, and dandelion.

 Food Sources:
- Fortified breakfast cereals
- Oysters
- White beans
- Beef liver
- Lentils
- Spinach
- Tofu

Consider cooking with iron pans.

Additional investigations: Complete iron panel (ferritin, hematocrit, hemoglobin, TIBC, % saturation, etc.)

Nutritional support:
- Iron (Ferrous Bisglycinate Chelate)
- Vitamin C
- Copper
- Vitamin A
- Vitamin D3
- Vitamin E
- Vitamin K
- Vitamin B1 (Thiamine)
- Vitamin B2 (Riboflavin)
- Vitamin B3 (Niacin)
- Vitamin B5 (Pantothenic acid)
- Vitamin B6 (Pyridoxine)
- Vitamin B7 (Biotin)
- Vitamin B9 (Folate)
- Vitamin B12 (Cobalamin)
- Magnesium
- Taurine
- L-carnitine
- Coenzyme Q10
- L-glutathione
- L-glutamine
- N-acetyl-L-cysteine (NAC)
- Curcumin
- Zinc
- Selenium

If **HIGH** or > 158 ug/dL:

Clinical Manifestations of Excess or Risk for Toxicity Iron levels are usually evaluated alongside other iron tests or a complete anemia panel. High serum iron levels can result from multiple blood transfusions, excessive iron supplementation or injections, lead poisoning, liver or kidney disease, or genetic conditions like hemochromatosis, where excessive iron accumulation damages organs.

Factors contributing to high iron levels include:
- Multiple blood transfusions.
- Excessive iron supplementation or injections.
- High iron levels from dietary or supplementation are more common in men and postmenopausal women since they don't lose iron through menstruation.
- Lead poisoning.
- Liver or kidney disease.
- Genetic conditions like hemochromatosis, where excessive iron accumulation damages organs.

Considerations for Support:
- Assess if diet or supplements are affecting iron levels and reduce them as needed.
- Discontinue using iron cooking pots.
- If hemochromatosis is a possibility, consider referring the patient to a specialist.

Additional Investigations:
- Perform a comprehensive iron panel (including ferritin, hematocrit, hemoglobin, TIBC, and % saturation) to evaluate iron levels.
- Conduct genetic testing to determine if hemochromatosis is the underlying cause.

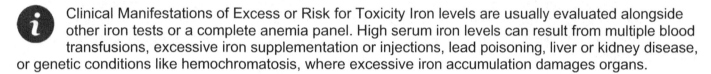

Iron (Cellular)

Iron is essential for producing red blood cells (hematopoiesis) and is a component of hemoglobin, the pigment that gives red blood cells their characteristic red color. Hemoglobin binds to oxygen and facilitates its transport from the lungs to all cells in the body through the arteries. Once oxygen is delivered, the iron (part of hemoglobin) binds to carbon dioxide, which is then transported back to the lungs for exhalation. Iron also plays a role in converting blood sugar into energy. Additionally, the production of enzymes, which are crucial for producing new cells, amino acids, hormones, and neurotransmitters, depends on iron. This aspect becomes particularly important during recovery from illnesses or strenuous exercise. Furthermore, the immune system relies on iron for its efficient functioning. Sufficient iron levels are essential for physical and mental growth, especially during childhood and pregnancy, when the developing fetus solely depends on its mother's iron supply.

Optimal Range	88.9 - 117.0 mg/dL

If **LOW** or < 88.9 mg/dL:

Inadequate iron intake can lead to iron deficiency, which can cause various symptoms. Iron is essential for producing hemoglobin, a protein in red blood cells that carries oxygen throughout the body. When iron stores are low, hemoglobin production slows down, reducing oxygen transport and causing fatigue, dizziness, lowered immunity, and reduced athletic performance.

Since our bodies can't produce iron, it's crucial to consume sufficient amounts through diet. Iron is lost from the body through various processes, including urination, defecation, sweating, and exfoliation of old skin cells. Bleeding further contributes to iron loss, explaining why women have a higher iron demand than men.

To prevent or correct iron deficiency, it's important to eat iron-rich foods and cook in iron skillets. Iron is found in various foods, including heme-iron sources like red meat and poultry, which are easily absorbed, and non-heme sources like lentils, beans, leafy vegetables, pistachios, tofu, fortified bread, and fortified breakfast cereals.

However, iron from different foods is absorbed and processed differently by the body. Heme iron from meat is more easily absorbed than non-heme iron from grains and vegetables. Additionally, heme iron from red meat may increase the risk of colorectal cancer. Minerals and chemicals in one food type can also inhibit the absorption of iron from another food consumed simultaneously. For instance, oxalates and phytic acid form insoluble complexes that bind iron in the gut, preventing its absorption. Iron from plant sources, such as legumes and dark-green leafy vegetables like broccoli, kale, and oriental greens, is less easily absorbed than heme-bound iron from animal sources. Therefore, vegetarians and vegans should consume slightly more iron daily than meat-eaters, fish-eaters, and poultry-eaters. However, spinach and Swiss chard contain oxalates that bind iron, making it almost entirely unavailable for absorption.

To enhance iron absorption from nonheme sources, it's best to consume them with foods containing heme-bound iron or vitamin C. Iron deficiency can manifest even before iron deficiency anemia develops. Iron deficiency symptoms aren't exclusive to anemia; they arise because iron is essential for many enzymes to function normally. Consequently, a wide range of symptoms may eventually emerge, either as secondary effects of anemia or as primary results of iron deficiency.

Common iron deficiency symptoms include fatigue, dizziness, pale skin, hair loss, twitches, irritability, weakness, pica, brittle or grooved nails, and nausea.

Common forms of iron in supplements include ferrous and ferric iron salts, such as ferrous sulfate, ferrous gluconate, ferric citrate, and ferric sulfate. Ferrous iron in dietary supplements is more bioavailable than ferric iron. However, high doses of supplemental iron (45 mg or more daily) may cause gastrointestinal side effects like nausea and constipation.

Other forms of supplemental iron, such as heme iron polypeptides, carbonyl iron, iron amino-acid chelates, and polysaccharide-iron complexes, may have fewer gastrointestinal side effects than ferrous or ferric salts.

Many medicinal herbs can boost iron levels in individuals with iron deficiency. These herbs can be easily assimilated into the bloodstream by making a hot water infusion (tea). Iron-enhancing herbs include yellow dock, red raspberry leaf, gentian, yellow root, turmeric, mullein, nettle, parsley, ginseng, watercress, and dandelion.

Food Sources:
- Fortifiedbreakfast cereals
- Oysters
- White beans
- Beef liver
- Lentils
- Spinach
- Tofu

Consider cooking with iron pans.

Additional investigations: Complete iron panel (ferritin, hematocrit, hemoglobin, TIBC, % saturation, etc.)

Nutritional support:
- Iron (Ferrous Bisglycinate Chelate)
- Vitamin C
- Copper
- Vitamin A
- Vitamin D3
- Vitamin E
- Vitamin K
- Vitamin B1 (Thiamine)
- Vitamin B2 (Riboflavin)
- Vitamin B3 (Niacin)
- Vitamin B5 (Pantothenic acid)
- Vitamin B6 (Pyridoxine)
- Vitamin B7 (Biotin)
- Vitamin B9 (Folate)
- Vitamin B12 (Cobalamin)
- Magnesium
- Taurine
- L-carnitine
- Coenzyme Q10
- L-glutathione
- L-glutamine
- N-acetyl-L-cysteine (NAC)
- Curcumin
- Zinc
- Selenium

If **HIGH** or > 117.0 mg/dL:

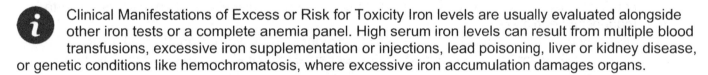

Clinical Manifestations of Excess or Risk for Toxicity Iron levels are usually evaluated alongside other iron tests or a complete anemia panel. High serum iron levels can result from multiple blood transfusions, excessive iron supplementation or injections, lead poisoning, liver or kidney disease, or genetic conditions like hemochromatosis, where excessive iron accumulation damages organs.

Factors contributing to high iron levels include:
- Multiple blood transfusions.
- Excessive iron supplementation or injections.
- High iron levels from dietary or supplementation are more common in men and postmenopausal women since they don't lose iron through menstruation.
- Lead poisoning.
- Liver or kidney disease.
- Genetic conditions like hemochromatosis, where excessive iron accumulation damages organs.

Considerations for Support:
- Assess if diet or supplements are affecting iron levels and reduce them as needed.
- Discontinue using iron cooking pots.
- If hemochromatosis is a possibility, consider referring the patient to a specialist.

Additional Investigations:
- Perform a comprehensive iron panel (including ferritin, hematocrit, hemoglobin, TIBC, and % saturation) to evaluate iron levels.
- Conduct genetic testing to determine if hemochromatosis is the underlying cause.

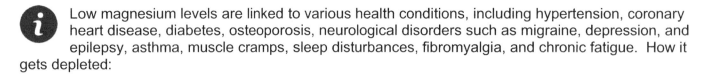

Magnesium (Serum)

Magnesium is essential for over 300 enzymatic reactions and plays a pivotal role in nerve function, muscle contraction, heartbeat regulation, and bone health. Deficiencies can lead to a range of health issues, including muscle weakness, cramps, arrhythmias, and neurological symptoms. The Micronutrient panel by Vibrant America, featuring this test, is particularly valuable for individuals experiencing symptoms of magnesium deficiency or those with conditions like diabetes, heart disease, or gastrointestinal disorders. It's also crucial for athletes and those with high physical demands. By accurately assessing intracellular magnesium levels, healthcare providers can better diagnose and manage conditions related to magnesium imbalance. This test is an indispensable tool in preventive healthcare, aiding in the early detection and treatment of magnesium-related health issues, thereby contributing to overall health and well-being.

| Optimal Range | 1.6 - 2.6 mg/dL |

If **LOW** or < 1.6 mg/dL:

Low magnesium levels are linked to various health conditions, including hypertension, coronary heart disease, diabetes, osteoporosis, neurological disorders such as migraine, depression, and epilepsy, asthma, muscle cramps, sleep disturbances, fibromyalgia, and chronic fatigue. How it gets depleted:

- Alcohol consumption leads to increased excretion in urine.
- Prolonged use of diuretics also results in increased urinary excretion.
- Excessive sweating and prolonged bouts of endurance exercise can contribute to magnesium depletion.
- Certain medical conditions, such as hyperparathyroidism, chronic renal failure, malabsorptive conditions like celiac disease, Crohn's disease, and partial bowel resection, can also lead to magnesium depletion.
- Diabetes (approximately 30% of patients show signs of depletion) is another risk factor.
- Age is a risk factor for magnesium depletion because intestinal absorption of magnesium declines with age.
- High doses of zinc supplements taken in excess can interfere with magnesium absorption.

Hypomagnesemia can be secondary to decreased intake, as seen in the following conditions:
- Starvation
- Alcohol use disorder (with a reported prevalence of 30%)
- Anorexia nervosa
- Terminal cancer
- Critically ill patients receiving total parenteral nutrition

Medications:
- Certain medications, including loop and thiazide diuretics, proton pump inhibitors, aminoglycoside antibiotics, amphotericin B, pentamidine, digitalis, chemotherapeutic drugs like cisplatin, cyclosporine, and antibodies that bind to epidermal growth factor (EGF) receptors (cetuximab, matuzumab, panitumumab), can also contribute to magnesium depletion.

- Laxative abuse can lead to magnesium depletion.

Redistribution from the extracellular to the intracellular compartment:
- Treatment of diabetic ketoacidosis with insulin, refeeding syndrome, correction of metabolic acidosis, acute pancreatitis, and ethanol withdrawal syndrome can also cause magnesium depletion.

Gastrointestinal and renal losses:
- Acute diarrhea and chronic diarrhea (Crohn's disease, ulcerative colitis) can also lead to magnesium depletion.
- Hungry bone syndrome (an increased need for calcium) can also occur. Magnesium uptake by the body to renew bone after parathyroidectomy or thyroidectomy leads to a decrease in serum magnesium levels. Several conditions can cause magnesium deficiency, including acute pancreatitis, gastric bypass surgery, genetic disorders, Gitelman syndrome, Bartter syndrome, familial hypomagnesemia with hypercalciuria and nephrocalcinosis, renal malformations and early-onset diabetes mellitus caused by HNF1-beta mutation, autosomal recessive isolated hypomagnesemia caused by EGF mutation, and autosomal dominant isolated hypomagnesemia caused by Na-K-ATPase gamma subunit, Kv1.1, and cyclin M2 mutations. Intestinal hypomagnesemia with secondary hypocalcemia can also occur.

Acquired tubular dysfunction, such as post-kidney transplant, recovery from acute tubular necrosis, and post-obstructive diuresis, can also lead to magnesium depletion.

The clinical manifestations of magnesium deficiency include weakness, heart irregularities, muscle cramps and twitches, insomnia, mental confusion, fatigue, and irritability. Magnesium deficiency can impair the absorption of Vitamin D and calcium, increasing the risk of bone mineral density disorders. Magnesium depletion is often associated with other disease states, including both type 1 and type 2 diabetes, hypertension, endothelial dysfunction, asthma, and migraine headaches.

Drug interactions with magnesium include:
- Magnesium interferes with the absorption of digoxin (a heart medication), nitrofurantoin (an antibiotic), and other anti-malarial drugs.
- Bisphosphates and magnesium supplements should be taken approximately 2 hours apart to prevent interference with bisphosphate absorption.
- High-dose magnesium supplementation may decrease the effectiveness of some antibiotics and anticoagulant medications.
- High-dose/long-term diuretic use, including furosemide (Lasix) and some thiazide diuretics, can cause magnesium depletion and increase the risk of hypomagnesemia. This is also true for any drug that increases urinary output through the kidneys.
- Long-term (more than 3 months) use of proton pump inhibitors (PPIs) can also cause magnesium depletion.

 Magnesium, a component of chlorophyll, is abundant in leafy greens. Other food sources include pumpkin seeds, chia seeds, almonds, spinach, and cashews.

Supplemental magnesium options are limited to 350 milligrams per day due to the risk of diarrhea. Severe toxicity can lead to confusion, kidney failure, difficulty breathing, and even cardiac arrest. Individuals with kidney disease are particularly vulnerable to magnesium toxicity.

Therapeutic use of supraphysiological magnesium doses is possible. Magnesium supplements are available in various forms, each with unique absorption, bioavailability, and therapeutic value.

- Magnesium oxide and magnesium citrate are commonly recommended for their ability to draw water into the gastrointestinal tract and induce bowel movements. They also alleviate acid reflux.
- Magnesium citrate has higher bioavailability and is generally preferred over magnesium oxide. Citrates have been shown to bind oxalates, making them a suitable choice for individuals following a low oxalate diet.
- Magnesium glycinate is well-absorbed and recommended for increasing magnesium levels without causing gastrointestinal side effects.
- Magnesium malate has been studied for its potential positive effects on depression, chronic fatigue, diabetes, and cardiovascular disease.
- Magnesium threonate has recently gained attention for its ability to cross the blood-brain barrier and enhance memory and brain function. It may also alleviate headaches and migraines.

Numerous studies have demonstrated that supplemental magnesium at doses of approximately 400 milligrams per day can reduce blood pressure in mildly hypertensive patients and pregnant women with preeclampsia.

Nutritional support:
- Magnesium Taurinate
- Magnesium Glycinate
- Magnesium Malate
- Magnesium Citrate
- Multivitamin and Mineral (iron/copper-free)
- Minerals (including calcium, magnesium, zinc, selenium, and others)

If **HIGH** or > 2.6 mg/dL:

Common causes of high magnesium levels (hypermagnesemia) include overuse of medications or supplements containing magnesium, adrenal disorders like Addison's disease, dehydration, hyperparathyroidism, hypothyroidism, kidney failure, and electrolyte imbalances caused by chemotherapy. Elevated magnesium levels can lead to symptoms like nausea, vomiting, lethargy, headaches, flushing, bradycardia, hypotension, and cardiac abnormalities.

Excessive magnesium intake from food is generally safe for healthy individuals as the kidneys efficiently eliminate excess in the urine. However, high doses of magnesium from dietary supplements or medications can cause diarrhea, nausea, and abdominal cramping. Magnesium salts that cause diarrhea include magnesium carbonate, chloride, gluconate, and oxide. The laxative effects of magnesium salts are attributed to the osmotic activity of unabsorbed salts in the intestine and colon, as well as the stimulation of gastric motility.

The Upper Limit (UL) for magnesium only applies to supplemental magnesium. The ULs are as follows: 1-3 years, 65 mg; 4-8 years, 110 mg; 9-18 years, and adults, 350 mg.

Very large doses of magnesium-containing laxatives and antacids (typically providing more than 5,000 mg/day magnesium) have been associated with magnesium toxicity, including fatal hypermagnesemia. Symptoms of magnesium toxicity can include hypotension, nausea, vomiting, facial flushing, urine retention, ileus, depression, and lethargy, progressing to muscle weakness, difficulty breathing, extreme hypotension, irregular heartbeat, and cardiac arrest. The risk of magnesium toxicity increases with impaired renal function or kidney failure, as the ability to remove excess magnesium is compromised.

Considerations for Support:
- Evaluate if dietary changes or supplements are affecting magnesium levels and adjust as required.

- Conduct additional investigations to assess electrolyte levels, thyroid function, parathyroid hormone, kidney function, and adrenal function.

Magnesium (Cellular)

Magnesium is essential for over 300 enzymatic reactions and plays a pivotal role in nerve function, muscle contraction, heartbeat regulation, and bone health. Deficiencies can lead to a range of health issues, including muscle weakness, cramps, arrhythmias, and neurological symptoms. The Micronutrient panel by Vibrant America, featuring this test, is particularly valuable for individuals experiencing symptoms of magnesium deficiency or those with conditions like diabetes, heart disease, or gastrointestinal disorders. It's also crucial for athletes and those with high physical demands. By accurately assessing intracellular magnesium levels, healthcare providers can better diagnose and manage conditions related to magnesium imbalance. This test is an indispensable tool in preventive healthcare, aiding in the early detection and treatment of magnesium-related health issues, thereby contributing to overall health and well-being.

Optimal Range	3.6 - 7.7 mg/dL

If LOW or < 3.6 mg/dL:

Low magnesium levels are linked to various health conditions, including hypertension, coronary heart disease, diabetes, osteoporosis, neurological disorders such as migraine, depression, and epilepsy, asthma, muscle cramps, sleep disturbances, fibromyalgia, and chronic fatigue. How it gets depleted:

- Alcohol consumption leads to increased excretion in urine.
- Prolonged use of diuretics also results in increased urinary excretion.
- Excessive sweating and prolonged bouts of endurance exercise can contribute to magnesium depletion.
- Certain medical conditions, such as hyperparathyroidism, chronic renal failure, malabsorptive conditions like celiac disease, Crohn's disease, and partial bowel resection, can also lead to magnesium depletion.
- Diabetes (approximately 30% of patients show signs of depletion) is another risk factor.
- Age is a risk factor for magnesium depletion because intestinal absorption of magnesium declines with age.
- High doses of zinc supplements taken in excess can interfere with magnesium absorption.

Hypomagnesemia can be secondary to decreased intake, as seen in the following conditions:
- Starvation
- Alcohol use disorder (with a reported prevalence of 30%)
- Anorexia nervosa
- Terminal cancer
- Critically ill patients receiving total parenteral nutrition

Medications:
- Certain medications, including loop and thiazide diuretics, proton pump inhibitors, aminoglycoside antibiotics, amphotericin B, pentamidine, digitalis, chemotherapeutic drugs like cisplatin, cyclosporine, and antibodies that bind to epidermal growth factor (EGF) receptors (cetuximab, matuzumab, panitumumab), can also contribute to magnesium depletion.
- Laxative abuse can lead to magnesium depletion.

Redistribution from the extracellular to the intracellular compartment:

- Treatment of diabetic ketoacidosis with insulin, refeeding syndrome, correction of metabolic acidosis, acute pancreatitis, and ethanol withdrawal syndrome can also cause magnesium depletion.

Gastrointestinal and renal losses:
- Acute diarrhea and chronic diarrhea (Crohn's disease, ulcerative colitis) can also lead to magnesium depletion.
- Hungry bone syndrome (an increased need for calcium) can also occur. Magnesium uptake by the body to renew bone after parathyroidectomy or thyroidectomy leads to a decrease in serum magnesium levels. Several conditions can cause magnesium deficiency, including acute pancreatitis, gastric bypass surgery, genetic disorders, Gitelman syndrome, Bartter syndrome, familial hypomagnesemia with hypercalciuria and nephrocalcinosis, renal malformations and early-onset diabetes mellitus caused by HNF1-beta mutation, autosomal recessive isolated hypomagnesemia caused by EGF mutation, and autosomal dominant isolated hypomagnesemia caused by Na-K-ATPase gamma subunit, Kv1.1, and cyclin M2 mutations. Intestinal hypomagnesemia with secondary hypocalcemia can also occur.

Acquired tubular dysfunction, such as post-kidney transplant, recovery from acute tubular necrosis, and post-obstructive diuresis, can also lead to magnesium depletion.

The clinical manifestations of magnesium deficiency include weakness, heart irregularities, muscle cramps and twitches, insomnia, mental confusion, fatigue, and irritability. Magnesium deficiency can impair the absorption of Vitamin D and calcium, increasing the risk of bone mineral density disorders. Magnesium depletion is often associated with other disease states, including both type 1 and type 2 diabetes, hypertension, endothelial dysfunction, asthma, and migraine headaches.

Drug interactions with magnesium include:
- Magnesium interferes with the absorption of digoxin (a heart medication), nitrofurantoin (an antibiotic), and other anti-malarial drugs.
- Bisphosphates and magnesium supplements should be taken approximately 2 hours apart to prevent interference with bisphosphate absorption.
- High-dose magnesium supplementation may decrease the effectiveness of some antibiotics and anticoagulant medications.
- High-dose/long-term diuretic use, including furosemide (Lasix) and some thiazide diuretics, can cause magnesium depletion and increase the risk of hypomagnesemia. This is also true for any drug that increases urinary output through the kidneys.
- Long-term (more than 3 months) use of proton pump inhibitors (PPIs) can also cause magnesium depletion.

 Magnesium, a component of chlorophyll, is abundant in leafy greens. Other food sources include pumpkin seeds, chia seeds, almonds, spinach, and cashews.

Supplemental magnesium options are limited to 350 milligrams per day due to the risk of diarrhea. Severe toxicity can lead to confusion, kidney failure, difficulty breathing, and even cardiac arrest. Individuals with kidney disease are particularly vulnerable to magnesium toxicity.

Therapeutic use of supraphysiological magnesium doses is possible. Magnesium supplements are available in various forms, each with unique absorption, bioavailability, and therapeutic value.

- Magnesium oxide and magnesium citrate are commonly recommended for their ability to draw water into the gastrointestinal tract and induce bowel movements. They also alleviate acid reflux.
- Magnesium citrate has higher bioavailability and is generally preferred over magnesium oxide. Citrates have been shown to bind oxalates, making them a suitable choice for individuals following a low oxalate diet.

- Magnesium glycinate is well-absorbed and recommended for increasing magnesium levels without causing gastrointestinal side effects.
- Magnesium malate has been studied for its potential positive effects on depression, chronic fatigue, diabetes, and cardiovascular disease.
- Magnesium threonate has recently gained attention for its ability to cross the blood-brain barrier and enhance memory and brain function. It may also alleviate headaches and migraines.

Numerous studies have demonstrated that supplemental magnesium at doses of approximately 400 milligrams per day can reduce blood pressure in mildly hypertensive patients and pregnant women with preeclampsia.

Nutritional support:
- Magnesium Taurinate
- Magnesium Glycinate
- Magnesium Malate
- Magnesium Citrate
- Multivitamin and Mineral (iron/copper-free)
- Minerals (including calcium, magnesium, zinc, selenium, and others)

If **HIGH** or **> 7.7 mg/dL:**

Common causes of high magnesium levels (hypermagnesemia) include overuse of medications or supplements containing magnesium, adrenal disorders like Addison's disease, dehydration, hyperparathyroidism, hypothyroidism, kidney failure, and electrolyte imbalances caused by chemotherapy. Elevated magnesium levels can lead to symptoms like nausea, vomiting, lethargy, headaches, flushing, bradycardia, hypotension, and cardiac abnormalities.

Excessive magnesium intake from food is generally safe for healthy individuals as the kidneys efficiently eliminate excess in the urine. However, high doses of magnesium from dietary supplements or medications can cause diarrhea, nausea, and abdominal cramping. Magnesium salts that cause diarrhea include magnesium carbonate, chloride, gluconate, and oxide. The laxative effects of magnesium salts are attributed to the osmotic activity of unabsorbed salts in the intestine and colon, as well as the stimulation of gastric motility.

The Upper Limit (UL) for magnesium only applies to supplemental magnesium. The ULs are as follows: 1-3 years, 65 mg; 4-8 years, 110 mg; 9-18 years, and adults, 350 mg.

Very large doses of magnesium-containing laxatives and antacids (typically providing more than 5,000 mg/day magnesium) have been associated with magnesium toxicity, including fatal hypermagnesemia. Symptoms of magnesium toxicity can include hypotension, nausea, vomiting, facial flushing, urine retention, ileus, depression, and lethargy, progressing to muscle weakness, difficulty breathing, extreme hypotension, irregular heartbeat, and cardiac arrest. The risk of magnesium toxicity increases with impaired renal function or kidney failure, as the ability to remove excess magnesium is compromised.

Considerations for Support:
- Evaluate if dietary changes or supplements are affecting magnesium levels and adjust as required.
- Conduct additional investigations to assess electrolyte levels, thyroid function, parathyroid hormone, kidney function, and adrenal function.

Manganese (Serum)

Manganese is important in many enzyme-mediated chemical reactions including enzymes involved in antioxidant actions in mitochondria and enzymes involved in the synthesis of cartilage in skin and bone. Manganese also activates enzymes that participate in metabolism of carbohydrates, amino acids, and cholesterol. In addition, enzymes that incorporate manganese convert the neuro-excitatory glutamate to glutamine. The Manganese (Mn) content in the adult human is 11.0 to 23 ng/mL. About 25% is stored in the skeleton. Within each cell, Manganese is concentrated in the mitochondria. Bone, liver, and pancreas tend to have the highest concentrations. Mn is an important part of the anti-oxidant enzyme super oxidase dismutase.

| Optimal Range | 0.3 - 2.0 ng/mL |

If LOW or < 0.3 ng/mL:

Manganese deficiency is quite rare, and there's more concern about toxicity from excessive manganese exposure. Here are some ways manganese can be depleted:
- Iron supplementation may decrease the absorption of dietary manganese.
- Intestinal absorption of manganese is reduced when iron stores (ferritin levels) are higher and tends to be lower in men than women.
- Magnesium supplementation has been shown to decrease manganese levels by reducing intestinal absorption or increasing urinary excretion.

Clinical manifestations of manganese deficiency are rare, but they may include impaired growth, particularly skeletal abnormalities, and possibly glucose tolerance abnormalities. There may also be blood clotting defects, hypocholesterolemia, elevated serum calcium, phosphorus, and alkaline phosphatase, loss of muscle tone, diabetes, and heart disease.

Drug interactions with manganese include:
- Some antacids, laxatives, and tetracycline antibiotics can decrease absorption if taken simultaneously with manganese-containing food or supplements.

Considerations for Support:
- Assess if dietary changes, such as excessive intake of iron or magnesium supplements, are affecting manganese levels. If necessary, reduce these supplements.
- Identify food sources that are rich in manganese. Tea and coffee are significant sources in the American diet. Other sources include nuts, whole grains, legumes, and certain fruits and vegetables, including leafy greens.

Specific food sources include:
- Blue mussels
- Hazelnuts
- Pecans
- Brown rice
- Oysters
- Calms (a type of mushroom)
- Chickpeas
- Spinach
- Pineapple
- Soybean
- Wholewheat bread
- Oatmeal

Nutritional support:
- Manganese Bisglycinate
- Multivitamin (iron and copper-free)
- Magnesium Taurinate
- Magnesium Glycinate
- Magnesium Malate

If HIGH or > 2.0 ng/mL:

Manganese Toxicity: Symptoms of manganese toxicity closely resemble those of Parkinson's disease, leading to permanent neurological damage. It can also trigger hypertension in individuals over 40 and cause significant elevations in manganese levels in patients with hepatitis, cirrhosis, dialysis patients, and those who have experienced heart attacks. Early signs of toxicity include a loss of appetite, impaired memory, and mask-like facial expressions. Excess manganese can also reduce iron absorption.

Clinical Manifestations of Excess or Toxicity:
- Toxicity is relatively uncommon and is most commonly caused by exposure to airborne manganese dust.
- Symptoms of toxicity include a range of neurological problems that are similar to those seen in Parkinson's disease.
- In children, exposure to elevated levels of manganese in drinking water has been linked to an increased risk of attention deficit hyperactivity disorder (ADHD), cognitive decline, and behavioral problems.
- Individuals with liver failure are particularly vulnerable to the neurological symptoms associated with manganese toxicity.

Stop or reduce manganese supplementation or sources. In severe cases, chelation therapy may be considered to remove excess manganese from the body. However, this treatment option is usually reserved for extreme cases and should be administered under the supervision of a qualified healthcare professional.

Manganese (Cellular)

Manganese is important in many enzyme-mediated chemical reactions including enzymes involved in antioxidant actions in mitochondria and enzymes involved in the synthesis of cartilage in skin and bone. Manganese also activates enzymes that participate in metabolism of carbohydrates, amino acids, and cholesterol. In addition, enzymes that incorporate manganese convert the neuro-excitatory glutamate to glutamine. The Manganese (Mn) content in the adult human is 11.0 to 23 ng/mL. About 25% is stored in the skeleton. Within each cell, Manganese is concentrated in the mitochondria. Bone, liver, and pancreas tend to have the highest concentrations. Mn is an important part of the anti-oxidant enzyme super oxidase dismutase.

Optimal Range	2.0 - 75.0 pg/MM WBC

If LOW or < 2.0 pg/MM WBC:

Manganese deficiency is quite rare, and there's more concern about toxicity from excessive manganese exposure. Here are some ways manganese can be depleted:
- Iron supplementation may decrease the absorption of dietary manganese.

- Intestinal absorption of manganese is reduced when iron stores (ferritin levels) are higher and tends to be lower in men than women.
- Magnesium supplementation has been shown to decrease manganese levels by reducing intestinal absorption or increasing urinary excretion.

Clinical manifestations of manganese deficiency are rare, but they may include impaired growth, particularly skeletal abnormalities, and possibly glucose tolerance abnormalities. There may also be blood clotting defects, hypocholesterolemia, elevated serum calcium, phosphorus, and alkaline phosphatase, loss of muscle tone, diabetes, and heart disease.

Drug interactions with manganese include:
- Some antacids, laxatives, and tetracycline antibiotics can decrease absorption if taken simultaneously with manganese-containing food or supplements.

Considerations for Support:
- Assess if dietary changes, such as excessive intake of iron or magnesium supplements, are affecting manganese levels. If necessary, reduce these supplements.
- Identify food sources that are rich in manganese. Tea and coffee are significant sources in the American diet. Other sources include nuts, whole grains, legumes, and certain fruits and vegetables, including leafy greens.

Specific food sources include:
- Blue mussels
- Hazelnuts
- Pecans
- Brown rice
- Oysters
- Calms (a type of mushroom)
- Chickpeas
- Spinach
- Pineapple
- Soybean
- Wholewheat bread
- Oatmeal

Nutritional support:
- Manganese Bisglycinate
- Multivitamin (iron and copper-free)
- Magnesium Taurinate
- Magnesium Glycinate
- Magnesium Malate

If HIGH or > 75.0 pg/MM WBC:

Manganese Toxicity: Symptoms of manganese toxicity closely resemble those of Parkinson's disease, leading to permanent neurological damage. It can also trigger hypertension in individuals over 40 and cause significant elevations in manganese levels in patients with hepatitis, cirrhosis, dialysis patients, and those who have experienced heart attacks. Early signs of toxicity include a loss of appetite, impaired memory, and mask-like facial expressions. Excess manganese can also reduce iron absorption.

Clinical Manifestations of Excess or Toxicity:
- Toxicity is relatively uncommon and is most commonly caused by exposure to airborne manganese dust.

- Symptoms of toxicity include a range of neurological problems that are similar to those seen in Parkinson's disease.
- In children, exposure to elevated levels of manganese in drinking water has been linked to an increased risk of attention deficit hyperactivity disorder (ADHD), cognitive decline, and behavioral problems.
- Individuals with liver failure are particularly vulnerable to the neurological symptoms associated with manganese toxicity.

Stop or reduce manganese supplementation or sources. In severe cases, chelation therapy may be considered to remove excess manganese from the body. However, this treatment option is usually reserved for extreme cases and should be administered under the supervision of a qualified healthcare professional.

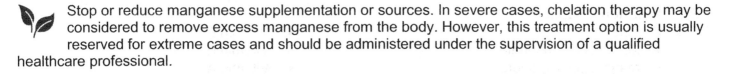

Zinc (Serum)

Zinc is essential for normal growth and sexual maturation. It plays a crucial role in the immune system and is vital for the proper functioning of at least 300 enzymes. Zinc is also involved in the structure of proteins and cell membranes. Additionally, it regulates gene function, influences cell signaling, hormone release, and nerve signaling.

Optimal Range	0.5 - 1.0 mcg/mL

If LOW or < 0.5 mcg/mL:

Inadequate intake of zinc can occur due to several factors. One common reason is insufficient consumption, especially in diets lacking meat intake. Excess phytates, found in legumes, seeds, soy products, and whole grains, and oxalates, present in spinach, okra, nuts, and tea, can also hinder zinc absorption.

Chronic illnesses can also contribute to zinc deficiency. Conditions such as chronic gastrointestinal diseases, diabetes, liver disease, sickle cell disease, kidney disease, excessive alcohol consumption, and HIV infection can all lead to zinc deficiency. Additionally, chronic infections can further impair zinc absorption.

Furthermore, there are specific nutrient interactions that can affect zinc absorption. Supplementation of elemental iron may decrease the absorption of zinc. Therefore, pregnant women and individuals with anemia who supplement iron should consider taking supplemental zinc separately from iron supplementation.

On the other hand, higher doses of supplementary zinc intake can impair the absorption of copper. However, copper intake does not affect zinc absorption unless zinc status is already marginally deficient.

It's important to note that medication interactions with zinc can also occur. Certain antibiotics, such as tetracycline and quinolones, when administered simultaneously with zinc supplements, may decrease the absorption of both zinc and the medication. Therefore, it's advisable to administer these two medications two hours apart.

Therapeutic use of metal-chelating agents, which bind to metals and prevent their absorption, can also lead to severe zinc deficiency. Additionally, anticonvulsant drugs and prolonged use of diuretics can cause zinc deficiency due to increased excretion.

Food Sources
- Oysters
- Beef
- Blue crab
- Fortified breakfast cereal
- Pumpkin seeds

Nutritional support:
- Zinc
- Magnesium Taurinate
- Magnesium Glycinate
- Magnesium Malate
- Calcium
- Potassium
- Magnesium
- Manganese
- Vitamin D
- Vitamin E
- Vitamin A
- Vitamin C
- B-Vitamins
- Copper
- Iron

If **HIGH** or **> 1.0 mcg/mL:**

Contamination: Isolated outbreaks of acute zinc toxicity have occurred due to consuming food or beverages contaminated with zinc released from galvanized containers. Metal fume fever has also been reported after inhaling zinc oxide fumes.

Excess Supplementation: Milder gastrointestinal distress has been reported at doses of 50 to 150 mg/day of supplemental zinc.

Zinc and Copper: The primary consequence of long-term excessive zinc consumption is copper deficiency. For instance, consuming 60 mg/day (50 mg supplemental and 10 mg dietary zinc) for up to 10 weeks has been found to lead to signs of copper deficiency. To prevent copper deficiency, the US Food and Nutrition Board established the tolerable upper intake level (UL) for adults at 40 mg/day, encompassing dietary and supplemental zinc.

Stop or reduce zinc supplementation, and look at your copper levels. If they're low, consider supplementing with copper.

Nutritional support:
- Copper (Glycinate)
- Multi-vitamin/mineral
- Magnesium taurinate
- Magnesium glycinate
- Magnesium malate

Zinc (Cellular)

Zinc is essential for normal growth and sexual maturation. It plays a crucial role in the immune system and is vital for the proper functioning of at least 300 enzymes. Zinc is also involved in the structure of proteins and cell membranes. Additionally, it regulates gene function, influences cell signaling, hormone release, and nerve signaling.

Optimal Range	4.0 - 15.0 ng/MM WBC

If LOW or < 4.0 ng/MM WBC:

 Inadequate intake of zinc can occur due to several factors. One common reason is insufficient consumption, especially in diets lacking meat intake. Excess phytates, found in legumes, seeds, soy products, and whole grains, and oxalates, present in spinach, okra, nuts, and tea, can also hinder zinc absorption.

Chronic illnesses can also contribute to zinc deficiency. Conditions such as chronic gastrointestinal diseases, diabetes, liver disease, sickle cell disease, kidney disease, excessive alcohol consumption, and HIV infection can all lead to zinc deficiency. Additionally, chronic infections can further impair zinc absorption.

Furthermore, there are specific nutrient interactions that can affect zinc absorption. Supplementation of elemental iron may decrease the absorption of zinc. Therefore, pregnant women and individuals with anemia who supplement iron should consider taking supplemental zinc separately from iron supplementation.

On the other hand, higher doses of supplementary zinc intake can impair the absorption of copper. However, copper intake does not affect zinc absorption unless zinc status is already marginally deficient.

It's important to note that medication interactions with zinc can also occur. Certain antibiotics, such as tetracycline and quinolones, when administered simultaneously with zinc supplements, may decrease the absorption of both zinc and the medication. Therefore, it's advisable to administer these two medications two hours apart.

Therapeutic use of metal-chelating agents, which bind to metals and prevent their absorption, can also lead to severe zinc deficiency. Additionally, anticonvulsant drugs and prolonged use of diuretics can cause zinc deficiency due to increased excretion.

Food Sources
- Oysters
- Beef
- Blue crab
- Fortified breakfast cereal
- Pumpkin seeds

Nutritional support:
- Zinc
- Magnesium Taurinate
- Magnesium Glycinate
- Magnesium Malate
- Calcium
- Potassium
- Magnesium
- Manganese
- Vitamin D
- Vitamin E
- Vitamin A
- Vitamin C
- B-Vitamins
- Copper
- Iron

If HIGH or > 15.0 ng/MM WBC:

 Contamination: Isolated outbreaks of acute zinc toxicity have occurred due to consuming food or beverages contaminated with zinc released from galvanized containers. Metal fume fever has also been reported after inhaling zinc oxide fumes.

Excess Supplementation: Milder gastrointestinal distress has been reported at doses of 50 to 150 mg/day of supplemental zinc.

Zinc and Copper: The primary consequence of long-term excessive zinc consumption is copper deficiency. For instance, consuming 60 mg/day (50 mg supplemental and 10 mg dietary zinc) for up to 10 weeks has been found to lead to signs of copper deficiency. To prevent copper deficiency, the US Food and Nutrition Board established the tolerable upper intake level (UL) for adults at 40 mg/day, encompassing dietary and supplemental zinc.

 Stop or reduce zinc supplementation, and look at your copper levels. If they're low, consider supplementing with copper.

 Nutritional support:
- Copper (Glycinate)
- Multi-vitamin/mineral
- Magnesium taurinate
- Magnesium glycinate
- Magnesium malate

Carnitine (Serum)

Carnitine, an essential cofactor in lipid metabolism and cellular energy production, plays a crucial role in neuroprotection. Its antioxidant properties and ability to modulate and promote synaptic neurotransmission contribute to its protective effects. Carnitine acts as a rate-limiting factor in ketone body uptake by brain astrocytes and also helps reduce oxidative stress.

In energy production, carnitine facilitates the transport of long-chain fatty acids into the mitochondria for oxidation and energy release. It is naturally found in animal-based foods and synthesized in the liver, kidneys, and brain from lysine and methionine. Approximately 95% of the body's carnitine is stored in the heart and skeletal muscles.

When dietary fatty acids are metabolized into fuel sources through beta-oxidation, carnitine shuttle transports them across the mitochondrial membrane. However, when beta-oxidation is impaired, fats are metabolized using an alternate pathway called omega-oxidation. This process results in elevated levels of dicarboxylic acids, such as adipic acid and suberic acid.

Impaired beta-oxidation can occur due to carnitine deficiency or enzymatic dysfunction caused by a lack of nutrient cofactors. Vitamin B_2 and magnesium play a vital role in optimizing beta-oxidation.

Optimal Range	11.6 - 43.4 nmol/mL

If LOW or < 11.6 nmol/mL:

 Nutritional carnitine deficiencies have not been observed in healthy individuals without metabolic disorders, implying that most people can synthesize sufficient L-carnitine.

Dietary Intake:
Dietary intake serves as the primary source of carnitine, accounting for nearly three-fourths of the body's total stores. The remaining one-fourth is produced endogenously from lysine and methionine, primarily by the liver and kidneys. Carnitine is primarily obtained from the diet, particularly animal products such as meat, fish, and dairy. A diet lacking these sources can lead to carnitine deficiency, although this is relatively

uncommon. Individuals following strict vegan or vegetarian diets may be at higher risk of carnitine deficiency since plant-based diets typically provide lower amounts of carnitine. Iron and vitamin C are essential for endogenous carnitine synthesis, and severe liver disorders can also impair this process. Additionally, there may be an increased demand for carnitine during ketosis.

Medical Conditions:
Chronic kidney disease and hemodialysis can impair carnitine metabolism or excretion, leading to deficiencies. Malabsorption disorders like celiac disease, Crohn's disease, and other gastrointestinal disorders can also hinder the absorption of nutrients, including carnitine, resulting in deficiencies. Certain medications, such as antibiotics, may interfere with carnitine metabolism or excretion, potentially leading to deficiency. Long-term treatment with pivalic acid antibiotics has been associated with a decrease in serum carnitine concentration.

Genetics:
Primary carnitine deficiency is a genetic disorder of the cellular carnitine transporter system that results in a shortage of carnitine within cells. This disorder is caused by an autosomal-recessive defect in the SLC22A5 gene, which leads to a lack of OCTN2, a high-affinity carnitine-uptake transporter expressed in muscle, kidney, and heart. Secondary carnitine deficiency can arise from various conditions, including chronic renal failure, end-stage renal disease, renal Fanconi syndrome, Lowe syndrome, cystinosis, and valproate therapy. These conditions impair carnitine reuptake from the kidneys. Carnitine-free diets, organic acidurias, and urea-cycle defects can also cause deficiency.

Medications that lower carnitine levels include some anticonvulsant drugs and HIV medications.

Food Sources:
- Beefsteak
- Ground beef
- Milk, whole
- Codfish
- Chicken breast

Support Considerations:
- Increase food sources.
- Consider l-carnitine supplementation.
- Ensure adequate protein intake and digestion.
- Consider supplementing co-factors of beta-oxidation of fatty acids: vitamin B2, B3, B5, magnesium.
- Consider supplementing co-factors of carnitine synthesis: L-lysine, iron, vitamins C, B6.

Additional Investigations:
- OAT (organic acid test) to assess other metabolites around the Krebs cycle and beta-oxidation.
- Stool test to assess gut and digestive health and rule out IBD.
- Celiac testing.

Nutritional support:
- Carnitine
- Riboflavin (Vitamin B2)
- Niacin (Vitamin B3)
- Pantothenic Acid (Vitamin B5)
- Magnesium Citrate
- Magnesium (from tri-mag formula)
- B Vitamins

Carnitine Synthesis Support:

- L-Lysine
- Iron (Ferrous Bisglycinate Chelate)
- Vitamin C
- Vitamin B6 (Pyridoxine)

Digestive Support:
- Digestive enzymes
- Betaine HCl
- Ox Bile
- L-taurine
- Gentian extract
- Dandelion extract
- Fennel
- Amylase
- Protease SP
- Protease
- Diastase
- Lactase
- Glucoamylase
- Alpha-galactosidase
- Beta-glucanase
- Acid protease
- Phytase
- Cellulase
- Hemicellulase
- Invertase
- Lipase
- Bromelain
- Papain
- Pepsin
- Triphala (Emblica officinalis, Terminalia bellirica, Terminalia chebula)
- Magnesium Hydroxide
- Mastic Gum
- DGL (Deglycyrrhizinated Licorice)
- Methylmethionine Sulfonium Chloride (MMSC)
- Zinc L-Carnosine
- Vitamin C
- Berberine
- Ginger
- Bismuth

If **HIGH** or > 43.4 nmol/mL:

Carnitine lacks an established tolerable upper intake level. However, consuming approximately 3 grams of carnitine supplements daily can lead to nausea, vomiting, abdominal cramps, diarrhea, and a distinct fishy body odor. L-carnitine, on the other hand, generally appears well-tolerated, with no reported toxic effects associated with high doses. Nevertheless, L-carnitine supplementation may cause mild gastrointestinal symptoms, including nausea, vomiting, abdominal cramps, and diarrhea. Supplemental doses exceeding 3 grams per day may result in a "fishy" body odor. Elevated levels of total carnitine could indicate several factors:

- Increased Dietary Intake: A diet rich in carnitine-containing foods may temporarily elevate blood levels.
- Supplementation: Carnitine supplements can raise blood levels.
- Liver Dysfunction: Since the liver plays a crucial role in carnitine synthesis and regulation, liver disorders can affect carnitine levels.
- Kidney Dysfunction: Normally, the kidneys regulate carnitine levels by excreting excess carnitine. Impaired kidney function can lead to elevated carnitine levels.
- Metabolic Disorders: Certain metabolic disorders can cause an accumulation of carnitine.
- Increased Muscle Mass or Physical Activity: Since carnitine is involved in energy metabolism, individuals with high muscle mass or those engaged in intense physical activity may have higher levels.
- Medications: Some medications can increase carnitine levels.

Carnitine levels are typically highest during a well-fed state (e.g., not in a state of starvation or catabolism).

Carnitine Palmitoyltransferase 1 (CPT-1) deficiency: Elevated carnitine levels are associated with carnitine palmitoyltransferase 1 (CPT-1) deficiency. CPT-1 is a protein that conjugates carnitine to long-chain fatty acids. Mutations in the CPT1A gene (expressed in liver cells) can lead to encephalopathy, seizures, and hypoketotic hypoglycemia in children younger than 18 months, usually triggered by a minor viral illness or fasting. Blood testing reveals low levels of long-chain acylcarnitines, which are linked to carnitine, and elevated ratios of carnitine: C16+C18. Prevention involves avoiding fasting (with nighttime feedings of cornstarch) and enriching the diet with medium-chain triglycerides, which don't require conjugation to enter the mitochondrial matrix for oxidation. Elevated carnitine levels alone don't diagnose a condition but may prompt further investigation or evaluation by a healthcare provider. If you have concerns about the results, it's advisable to discuss them with a healthcare professional who can offer personalized insights and recommendations.

Stop or reduce carnitine supplementation or sources. Conduct additional investigations, including:
- Organic acid test (OAT) to assess other metabolites in the Krebs cycle and beta-oxidation.
- Evaluate kidney and liver function.
- Consider genetic testing.

Carnitine (Cellular)

Carnitine, an essential cofactor in lipid metabolism and cellular energy production, plays a crucial role in neuroprotection. Its antioxidant properties and ability to modulate and promote synaptic neurotransmission contribute to its protective effects. Carnitine acts as a rate-limiting factor in ketone body uptake by brain astrocytes and also helps reduce oxidative stress.

In energy production, carnitine facilitates the transport of long-chain fatty acids into the mitochondria for oxidation and energy release. It is naturally found in animal-based foods and synthesized in the liver, kidneys, and brain from lysine and methionine. Approximately 95% of the body's carnitine is stored in the heart and skeletal muscles.

When dietary fatty acids are metabolized into fuel sources through beta-oxidation, carnitine shuttle transports them across the mitochondrial membrane. However, when beta-oxidation is impaired, fats are metabolized using an alternate pathway called omega-oxidation. This process results in elevated levels of dicarboxylic acids, such as adipic acid and suberic acid.

Impaired beta-oxidation can occur due to carnitine deficiency or enzymatic dysfunction caused by a lack of nutrient cofactors. Vitamin B_2 and magnesium play a vital role in optimizing beta-oxidation.

Optimal Range	0.3 - 1.5 ng/MM WBC

If LOW or < 0.3 ng/MM WBC:

Nutritional carnitine deficiencies have not been observed in healthy individuals without metabolic disorders, implying that most people can synthesize sufficient L-carnitine.

Dietary Intake:
Dietary intake serves as the primary source of carnitine, accounting for nearly three-fourths of the body's total stores. The remaining one-fourth is produced endogenously from lysine and methionine, primarily by the liver and kidneys. Carnitine is primarily obtained from the diet, particularly animal products such as meat, fish, and dairy. A diet lacking these sources can lead to carnitine deficiency, although this is relatively uncommon. Individuals following strict vegan or vegetarian diets may be at higher risk of carnitine deficiency since plant-based diets typically provide lower amounts of carnitine. Iron and vitamin C are essential for endogenous carnitine synthesis, and severe liver disorders can also impair this process. Additionally, there may be an increased demand for carnitine during ketosis.

Medical Conditions:
Chronic kidney disease and hemodialysis can impair carnitine metabolism or excretion, leading to deficiencies. Malabsorption disorders like celiac disease, Crohn's disease, and other gastrointestinal disorders can also hinder the absorption of nutrients, including carnitine, resulting in deficiencies. Certain medications, such as antibiotics, may interfere with carnitine metabolism or excretion, potentially leading to deficiency. Long-term treatment with pivalic acid antibiotics has been associated with a decrease in serum carnitine concentration.

Genetics:
Primary carnitine deficiency is a genetic disorder of the cellular carnitine transporter system that results in a shortage of carnitine within cells. This disorder is caused by an autosomal-recessive defect in the SLC22A5 gene, which leads to a lack of OCTN2, a high-affinity carnitine-uptake transporter expressed in muscle, kidney, and heart. Secondary carnitine deficiency can arise from various conditions, including chronic renal failure, end-stage renal disease, renal Fanconi syndrome, Lowe syndrome, cystinosis, and valproate therapy. These conditions impair carnitine reuptake from the kidneys. Carnitine-free diets, organic acidurias, and urea-cycle defects can also cause deficiency.

Medications that lower carnitine levels include some anticonvulsant drugs and HIV medications.

Food Sources:
- Beefsteak
- Ground beef
- Milk, whole
- Codfish
- Chicken breast

Support Considerations:
- Increase food sources.
- Consider l-carnitine supplementation.
- Ensure adequate protein intake and digestion.
- Consider supplementing co-factors of beta-oxidation of fatty acids: vitamin B2, B3, B5, magnesium.
- Consider supplementing co-factors of carnitine synthesis: L-lysine, iron, vitamins C, B6.

Additional Investigations:
- OAT (organic acid test) to assess other metabolites around the Krebs cycle and beta-oxidation.
- Stool test to assess gut and digestive health and rule out IBD.
- Celiac testing.

Nutritional support:
- Carnitine
- Riboflavin (Vitamin B2)
- Niacin (Vitamin B3)
- Pantothenic Acid (Vitamin B5)
- Magnesium Citrate
- Magnesium (from tri-mag formula)
- B Vitamins

Carnitine Synthesis Support:
- L-Lysine
- Iron (Ferrous Bisglycinate Chelate)
- Vitamin C
- Vitamin B6 (Pyridoxine)

Digestive Support:
- Digestive enzymes
- Betaine HCl
- Ox Bile
- L-taurine
- Gentian extract
- Dandelion extract
- Fennel
- Amylase
- Protease SP
- Protease
- Diastase
- Lactase
- Glucoamylase
- Alpha-galactosidase
- Beta-glucanase
- Acid protease
- Phytase
- Cellulase
- Hemicellulase
- Invertase
- Lipase
- Bromelain
- Papain
- Pepsin
- Triphala (Emblica officinalis, Terminalia bellirica, Terminalia chebula)
- Magnesium Hydroxide
- Mastic Gum
- DGL (Deglycyrrhizinated Licorice)
- Methylmethionine Sulfonium Chloride (MMSC)
- Zinc L-Carnosine
- Vitamin C
- Berberine
- Ginger
- Bismuth

If **HIGH** or **> 1.5 ng/MM WBC:**

Carnitine lacks an established tolerable upper intake level. However, consuming approximately 3 grams of carnitine supplements daily can lead to nausea, vomiting, abdominal cramps, diarrhea, and a distinct fishy body odor. L-carnitine, on the other hand, generally appears well-tolerated, with no reported toxic effects associated with high doses. Nevertheless, L-carnitine supplementation may cause mild gastrointestinal symptoms, including nausea, vomiting, abdominal cramps, and diarrhea. Supplemental doses exceeding 3 grams per day may result in a "fishy" body odor. Elevated levels of total carnitine could indicate several factors:
- Increased Dietary Intake: A diet rich in carnitine-containing foods may temporarily elevate blood levels.
- Supplementation: Carnitine supplements can raise blood levels.
- Liver Dysfunction: Since the liver plays a crucial role in carnitine synthesis and regulation, liver disorders can affect carnitine levels.
- Kidney Dysfunction: Normally, the kidneys regulate carnitine levels by excreting excess carnitine. Impaired kidney function can lead to elevated carnitine levels.
- Metabolic Disorders: Certain metabolic disorders can cause an accumulation of carnitine.
- Increased Muscle Mass or Physical Activity: Since carnitine is involved in energy metabolism, individuals with high muscle mass or those engaged in intense physical activity may have higher levels.
- Medications: Some medications can increase carnitine levels.

Carnitine levels are typically highest during a well-fed state (e.g., not in a state of starvation or catabolism).

Carnitine Palmitoyltransferase 1 (CPT-1) deficiency: Elevated carnitine levels are associated with carnitine palmitoyltransferase 1 (CPT-1) deficiency. CPT-1 is a protein that conjugates carnitine to long-chain fatty acids. Mutations in the CPT1A gene (expressed in liver cells) can lead to encephalopathy, seizures, and hypoketotic hypoglycemia in children younger than 18 months, usually triggered by a minor viral illness or fasting. Blood testing reveals low levels of long-chain acylcarnitines, which are linked to carnitine, and elevated ratios of carnitine: C16+C18. Prevention involves avoiding fasting (with nighttime feedings of cornstarch) and enriching the diet with medium-chain triglycerides, which don't require conjugation to enter the mitochondrial matrix for oxidation. Elevated carnitine levels alone don't diagnose a condition but may prompt further investigation or evaluation by a healthcare provider. If you have concerns about the results, it's advisable to discuss them with a healthcare professional who can offer personalized insights and recommendations.

 Stop or reduce carnitine supplementation or sources. Conduct additional investigations, including:
- Organic acid test (OAT) to assess other metabolites in the Krebs cycle and beta-oxidation.
- Evaluate kidney and liver function.
- Consider genetic testing.

Choline (Serum)

Choline, an essential nutrient, plays a crucial role in various metabolic functions. It's involved in the synthesis of phosphatidylcholine and sphingomyelin, two vital phospholipids that make up cell membranes. Choline is also essential for the production of acetylcholine, a neurotransmitter that plays a key role in memory, mood, muscle control, and other nervous system functions. Furthermore, choline contributes to modulating gene expression, cell membrane signaling, lipid transport, and metabolism.

Choline is metabolized within cellular mitochondria, resulting in the production of trimethylglycine (TMG). TMG supports methyl donation processes, either directly by methylating homocysteine or indirectly by supporting the production of S-adenosyl methionine (SAMe). Choline is ultimately converted into acetylcholine (ACh).

Food sources rich in choline include meat, poultry, fish, dairy products, eggs, whole grains, and cruciferous vegetables. A deficiency in choline can lead to muscle damage, liver damage, and nonalcoholic fatty liver disease (NAFLD or hepatosteatosis).

Optimal Range	6.8 - 31.0 nmol/mL

If **LOW** or < 6.8 nmol/mL:

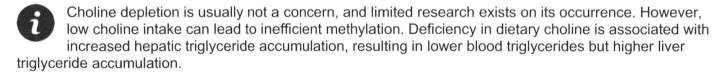 Choline depletion is usually not a concern, and limited research exists on its occurrence. However, low choline intake can lead to inefficient methylation. Deficiency in dietary choline is associated with increased hepatic triglyceride accumulation, resulting in lower blood triglycerides but higher liver triglyceride accumulation.

Individuals following strict vegan or vegetarian diets may be at higher risk of choline deficiency due to the lower choline content in plant-based diets. Excessive alcohol consumption can also interfere with choline metabolism and increase the risk of deficiency.

Several medical conditions can contribute to choline deficiency. Malabsorption disorders, such as celiac disease and Crohn's disease, can affect nutrient absorption and lead to deficiency. Specific medical conditions, growth, pregnancy, and breastfeeding can also increase the body's demand for choline, potentially leading to deficiency if dietary intake doesn't meet these increased requirements.

Genetics can also play a role. A single nucleotide polymorphism (SNP) in the PEMT gene is believed to increase the susceptibility to choline deficiency-induced organ dysfunction, potentially altering the body's choline requirements and increasing the likelihood of developing signs of deficiency when choline intake is inadequate.

Medications, such as anticholinergic drugs, can also interfere with choline utilization or metabolism.

Clinical manifestations of choline depletion include increased hepatic triglyceride accumulation, which leads to lower blood triglycerides but higher liver triglyceride accumulation. Individuals with mutations in the MTHFR enzyme seem to place a greater burden on choline in methylation cycles. Choline depletion can also lead to muscle damage.

Food Sources:
- Beef liver
- Egg
- Soybeans
- Chicken breast
- Codfish
- Potatoes (red)
- Wheat germ
- Beans (kidney)
- Quinoa
- Milk (1% fat)

Correlation between serum and cellular levels:
Serum levels deficient, cellular levels normal: Long-term nutrient status is optimal, but short-term needs improvement.

Possible interventions:
- Increase dietary intake of nutrients
- Increase supplementation dosage
- Medications may have an effect on depletion

Serum levels deficient and cellular levels deficient:
Short-term and long-term status of micronutrients is not optimal, suggesting low dietary intake and both intestinal and cellular malabsorption as possible causes.

Possible interventions:
- Increase dietary intake of nutrients
- Increase supplementation dosage
- Medications may have an effect on depletion
- Consider follow-up testing to identify the source of malabsorption

Additional investigations:
- Stool test to assess gut and digestive health and rule out IBD
- Celiac testing

Nutritional support:
- Phosphatidylcholine
- Multivitamin (iron/copper-free)
- Magnesium Taurinate
- Magnesium Glycinate
- Magnesium Malate

If **HIGH** or > 31.0 nmol/mL:

The recommended daily intake of choline for women is 425 mg, while for men, it's 550 mg. Excessive supplementation, however, should be approached with caution. The tolerable upper intake level (UL) for adults aged 19 and above is set at 3,500 mg daily, based on the amount that can lead to side effects. It's important to note that reaching such high levels is more likely due to excessive intake from supplements rather than a balanced diet. High choline consumption can result in low blood pressure (hypotension) and liver toxicity. Additionally, it may cause the excessive production of TMAO, which is associated with an increased risk of cardiovascular disease. Other potential symptoms include excessive sweating, fishy body odor, or nausea/vomiting.

Stop or reduce choline supplementation or sources. Serum levels are normal or excessive, while cellular levels are deficient. In the short term, micronutrient status is optimal, but cellular absorption may be an issue. Possible interventions include increasing dietary intake of the nutrient, increasing supplementation dosage, considering the status of synergistic nutrients for cellular absorption, assessing levels of oxidative stress on nutrient depletion, and considering follow-up testing to identify the source of malabsorption.

Choline (Cellular)

Choline, an essential nutrient, plays a crucial role in various metabolic functions. It's involved in the synthesis of phosphatidylcholine and sphingomyelin, two vital phospholipids that make up cell membranes. Choline is also essential for the production of acetylcholine, a neurotransmitter that plays a key role in memory, mood, muscle control, and other nervous system functions. Furthermore, choline contributes to modulating gene expression, cell membrane signaling, lipid transport, and metabolism.

Choline is metabolized within cellular mitochondria, resulting in the production of trimethylglycine (TMG). TMG supports methyl donation processes, either directly by methylating homocysteine or indirectly by supporting the production of S-adenosyl methionine (SAMe). Choline is ultimately converted into acetylcholine (ACh).

Food sources rich in choline include meat, poultry, fish, dairy products, eggs, whole grains, and cruciferous vegetables. A deficiency in choline can lead to muscle damage, liver damage, and nonalcoholic fatty liver disease (NAFLD or hepatosteatosis).

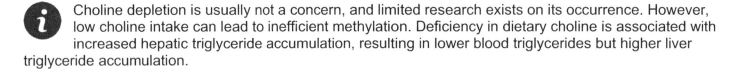

| Optimal Range | 0.2 - 1.5 ng/MM WBC |

If LOW or < 0.2 ng/MM WBC:

Choline depletion is usually not a concern, and limited research exists on its occurrence. However, low choline intake can lead to inefficient methylation. Deficiency in dietary choline is associated with increased hepatic triglyceride accumulation, resulting in lower blood triglycerides but higher liver triglyceride accumulation.

Individuals following strict vegan or vegetarian diets may be at higher risk of choline deficiency due to the lower choline content in plant-based diets. Excessive alcohol consumption can also interfere with choline metabolism and increase the risk of deficiency.

Several medical conditions can contribute to choline deficiency. Malabsorption disorders, such as celiac disease and Crohn's disease, can affect nutrient absorption and lead to deficiency. Specific medical conditions, growth, pregnancy, and breastfeeding can also increase the body's demand for choline, potentially leading to deficiency if dietary intake doesn't meet these increased requirements.

Genetics can also play a role. A single nucleotide polymorphism (SNP) in the PEMT gene is believed to increase the susceptibility to choline deficiency-induced organ dysfunction, potentially altering the body's choline requirements and increasing the likelihood of developing signs of deficiency when choline intake is inadequate.

Medications, such as anticholinergic drugs, can also interfere with choline utilization or metabolism.

Clinical manifestations of choline depletion include increased hepatic triglyceride accumulation, which leads to lower blood triglycerides but higher liver triglyceride accumulation. Individuals with mutations in the MTHFR enzyme seem to place a greater burden on choline in methylation cycles. Choline depletion can also lead to muscle damage.

Food Sources:
- Beef liver
- Egg
- Soybeans
- Chicken breast
- Codfish
- Potatoes (red)
- Wheat germ
- Beans (kidney)
- Quinoa
- Milk (1% fat)

Correlation between serum and cellular levels:
Serum levels deficient, cellular levels normal: Long-term nutrient status is optimal, but short-term needs improvement.

Possible interventions:
- Increase dietary intake of nutrients
- Increase supplementation dosage
- Medications may have an effect on depletion

Serum levels deficient and cellular levels deficient:
Short-term and long-term status of micronutrients is not optimal, suggesting low dietary intake and both intestinal and cellular malabsorption as possible causes.

Possible interventions:
- Increase dietary intake of nutrients
- Increase supplementation dosage
- Medications may have an effect on depletion
- Consider follow-up testing to identify the source of malabsorption

Additional investigations:
- Stool test to assess gut and digestive health and rule out IBD
- Celiac testing

Nutritional support:
- Phosphatidylcholine
- Multivitamin (iron/copper-free)
- Magnesium Taurinate
- Magnesium Glycinate
- Magnesium Malate

If **HIGH** or > 1.5 ng/MM WBC:

The recommended daily intake of choline for women is 425 mg, while for men, it's 550 mg. Excessive supplementation, however, should be approached with caution. The tolerable upper intake level (UL) for adults aged 19 and above is set at 3,500 mg daily, based on the amount that can lead to side effects. It's important to note that reaching such high levels is more likely due to excessive intake from supplements rather than a balanced diet. High choline consumption can result in low blood pressure (hypotension) and liver toxicity. Additionally, it may cause the excessive production of TMAO, which is associated with an increased risk of cardiovascular disease. Other potential symptoms include excessive sweating, fishy body odor, or nausea/vomiting.

Stop or reduce choline supplementation or sources. Serum levels are normal or excessive, while cellular levels are deficient. In the short term, micronutrient status is optimal, but cellular absorption may be an issue. Possible interventions include increasing dietary intake of the nutrient, increasing supplementation dosage, considering the status of synergistic nutrients for cellular absorption, assessing levels of oxidative stress on nutrient depletion, and considering follow-up testing to identify the source of malabsorption.

Inositol (Serum)

Inositol derivatives play a crucial role in cellular signaling after the insulin receptor is activated. They are essential for the development of peripheral nerves, aid in fat removal from the liver, promote lecithin production, and exhibit antiarteriosclerotic and anti-atherogenic properties. Inositol can be released from phytate compounds by intestinal bacteria that produce phytate-degrading enzymes, such as Lactobacillus plantarum, Lactobacillus brevis, Lactobacillus curvatus, L. gasseri B. subtilis, and Saccharomyces cerevisiae. Additionally, inositol is stored in the liver, spinal cord nerves, brain, and cerebral spinal fluid. As an essential nutrient, inositol is found in cell membranes and is necessary for the proper functioning of hormones. Inositol, similar to choline, is a component of phospholipids (phosphatidyl inositols). Phosphatidyl inositols serve as cell membrane components and regulate cell membrane transport by acting as a calcium-mobilizing system, known as the "PI effect." Consequently, inositol status interacts with a diverse range of hormonal and regulatory events within cells. Inositol's lipotropic activity, which involves reducing blood or tissue lipid levels, primarily relies on the role of phosphatidyl inositols in lipoproteins. Since inositol is readily available from dietary sources, as well as endogenous synthesis and gut microbial synthesis, it is not classified as a vitamin. However, it has been considered a component of the B vitamin complex.

Optimal Range	20.5 - 60.7 nmol/mL

If LOW or < 20.5 nmol/mL:

Inositol, a naturally occurring compound, can be depleted through various mechanisms. One such way is through intestinal bacteria breaking down phytate compounds, which are found in plant-based foods. These bacteria produce phytate-degrading enzymes, such as those found in Lactobacillus plantarum, Lactobacillus brevis, Lactobacillus curvatus, L. gasseri B. subtilis, and Saccharomyces cerevisiae. However, prolonged use of antibiotics can lead to a depletion of inositol from the microbiome conversion process.

In addition to its role in the microbiome, inositol is also stored in various tissues, including the liver, spinal cord nerves, and the brain and cerebral spinal fluid. Therefore, an inadequate intake of inositol can lead to various medical conditions. These conditions include metabolic syndrome, type 2 diabetes, polycystic ovary syndrome (PCOS), insulin resistance, and obesity.

It's important to note that while inositol depletion may occur due to antibiotic use, there are currently no known clinical manifestations associated with it. However, inositol deficiency has been linked to certain conditions, such as depression, anxiety, PCOS, diabetes, cardiovascular disease (CVD), and obesity.

Interestingly, urinary levels of inositol derivatives, particularly D-chiro-inositols and myo-inositols, have been identified as biomarkers for insulin resistance. This suggests that inositol may play a crucial role in regulating insulin sensitivity and metabolic processes.

Food sources include meat, fruits, corn, beans, grains, and legumes.

Nutritional support:
- Inositol
- Multivitamin (iron/copper-free)
- Magnesium Taurinate
- Magnesium Glycinate
- Magnesium Malate

If HIGH or > 60.7 nmol/mL:

There is currently no established RDA, AI, or UL for inositol.

Stop or reduce inositol supplementation / sources

Inositol (Cellular)

Inositol derivatives play a crucial role in cellular signaling after the insulin receptor is activated. They are essential for the development of peripheral nerves, aid in fat removal from the liver, promote lecithin production, and exhibit antiarteriosclerotic and anti-atherogenic properties. Inositol can be released from phytate compounds by intestinal bacteria that produce phytate-degrading enzymes, such as Lactobacillus plantarum, Lactobacillus brevis, Lactobacillus curvatus, L. gasseri B. subtilis, and Saccharomyces cerevisiae. Additionally, inositol is stored in the liver, spinal cord nerves, brain, and cerebral spinal fluid. As an essential nutrient, inositol is found in cell membranes and is necessary for the proper functioning of hormones. Inositol, similar to choline, is a component of phospholipids (phosphatidyl inositols). Phosphatidyl inositols serve as cell membrane components and regulate cell membrane transport by acting as a calcium-mobilizing system, known as the "PI effect." Consequently, inositol status interacts with a diverse range of hormonal and regulatory events within cells. Inositol's lipotropic activity, which involves reducing blood or tissue lipid levels, primarily relies on the role of phosphatidyl inositols in lipoproteins. Since inositol is readily available from dietary sources, as well as endogenous synthesis and gut microbial synthesis, it is not classified as a vitamin. However, it has been considered a component of the B vitamin complex.

Optimal Range	0.10 - 2.50 ng/MM WBC

If LOW or < 0.1 ng/MM WBC:

Inositol, a naturally occurring compound, can be depleted through various mechanisms. One such way is through intestinal bacteria breaking down phytate compounds, which are found in plant-based foods. These bacteria produce phytate-degrading enzymes, such as those found in Lactobacillus plantarum, Lactobacillus brevis, Lactobacillus curvatus, L. gasseri B. subtilis, and Saccharomyces cerevisiae. However, prolonged use of antibiotics can lead to a depletion of inositol from the microbiome conversion process.

In addition to its role in the microbiome, inositol is also stored in various tissues, including the liver, spinal cord nerves, and the brain and cerebral spinal fluid. Therefore, an inadequate intake of inositol can lead to various medical conditions. These conditions include metabolic syndrome, type 2 diabetes, polycystic ovary syndrome (PCOS), insulin resistance, and obesity.

It's important to note that while inositol depletion may occur due to antibiotic use, there are currently no known clinical manifestations associated with it. However, inositol deficiency has been linked to certain conditions, such as depression, anxiety, PCOS, diabetes, cardiovascular disease (CVD), and obesity.

Interestingly, urinary levels of inositol derivatives, particularly D-chiro-inositols and myo-inositols, have been identified as biomarkers for insulin resistance. This suggests that inositol may play a crucial role in regulating insulin sensitivity and metabolic processes.

 Food sources include meat, fruits, corn, beans, grains, and legumes.

 Nutritional support:
- Inositol
- Multivitamin (iron/copper-free)
- Magnesium Taurinate
- Magnesium Glycinate
- Magnesium Malate

If **HIGH** or **> 2.5 ng/MM WBC:**

 There is currently no established RDA, AI, or UL for inositol.

 Stop or reduce inositol supplementation / sources

MMA (Methylmalonic Acid) (Serum)

Methylmalonic acid (MMA) is a metabolite associated with vitamin B12 and serves as the most sensitive indicator of vitamin B12 status. MMA is formed when vitamin B12 reacts with methylmalonic acid to produce coenzyme A (CoA), which is crucial for normal cellular function. CoA participates in hundreds of reactions and is essential for metabolizing fatty acids, carbohydrates, amino acids, and ketone bodies. When vitamin B12 deficiencies occur, MMA levels rise. The methylmalonic acid test can help your doctor identify existing vitamin deficiencies, particularly mild or early-stage deficiencies.

Optimal Range	0.10 - 0.50 nmol/mL

If **LOW** or **< 0.1 nmol/mL:**

Lower-than-normal levels of MMA are uncommon and not considered a health issue. MMA, a substance naturally found in the body, is produced during specific metabolic pathways, including the breakdown of certain amino acids and fatty acids. The enzyme methylmalonyl-CoA mutase converts MMA to succinate, requiring vitamin B12 (cobalamin) as a cofactor. Generally, low MMA levels in the blood or urine are considered normal and pose no significant health concerns.

If **HIGH** or **> 0.5 nmol/mL:**

 Vitamin B-12 deficiencies can lead to elevated methylmalonic acid levels. The methylmalonic acid test can help doctors identify existing vitamin deficiencies, especially mild or early-stage B-12 deficiencies.

Several factors can contribute to B-12 depletion. Age is a risk factor due to a natural decline in intrinsic factor. Chronic use of proton pump inhibitors (PPIs) may reduce stomach acid (HCl) levels, potentially leading to sub-clinical deficiencies. Certain genetic single nucleotide polymorphisms (SNPs), such as MTHFR, can affect the absorption of active B12 (methylcobalamin).

Clinical manifestations of B12 depletion include pernicious anemia, often caused by a lack of intrinsic factor. Megoblastic anemia, another form of anemia associated with B12 deficiency, occurs when folate levels are high and insufficient B12 is present, creating a 'folate trap.' Dementia can also be a symptom of B12 deficiency due to the degeneration of myelin.

Methylmalonyl CoA is metabolized to methylmalonic acid (MMA), making MMA the definitive marker for B12 deficiency. Achlorhydria (insufficient stomach acid) can also lead to B12 deficiency because HCl is necessary for releasing B12 from intrinsic factor.

Several medications can reduce the absorption of B12, including:
- Proton pump inhibitors (PPIs) (indirectly by reducing HCl required for Vitamin B12 release from food, but not supplements)
- Metformin (used to treat type 2 diabetes)
- Histamine 2 receptor antagonists
- Bile acid sequestrants (cholestyramine)
- Neomycin

 Food sources include beef liver, clams, nutritional yeast, Atlantic salmon, canned chunk light tuna, ground beef, milk, plain yogurt, and fortified breakfast cereals.

 Nutritional support
- Vitamin B12
- Folate
- B Vitamins (B1, B2, B3, B5, B6, B7, B9, B12)
- Magnesium Taurinate
- Magnesium Glycinate
- Magnesium Malate
- Multivitamin and Mineral (iron/copper-free)
- Magnesium

Coenzyme Q10 (Serum)

CoQ10, a fat-soluble compound, is primarily synthesized by the body and consumed in the diet. It's found in virtually all cell membranes and plays a crucial role in mitochondria, converting carbohydrates and fatty acids into ATP. CoQ10 also supports various cellular functions, including cell signaling, gene expression, cell growth stimulation, apoptosis inhibition, thiol group control, hydrogen peroxide formation, and membrane channel regulation.

While foods are considered poor sources of CoQ10, organ meats from red meat sources are considered better sources. Nuts are considered a moderate source but require extreme consumption to meet daily requirements.

CoQ10 acts as an antioxidant and is essential for basic cell functions, particularly in energy production. Its primary function is to transfer electrons through the electron transport chain in the mitochondrial inner membrane. Electrons are received directly from succinate or indirectly from various substrates like pyruvate, acyl-CoA, and alpha–ketoglutarate in the form of NADH (Nicotinamide adenine dinucleotide). CoQ10 moves from one electron carrier complex to the next, ultimately delivering electrons one at a time. While electrons are delivered one at a time, they leave in pairs to form ATP and H2O.

Optimal Range	0.56 - 2.78 µg/mL

If **LOW** or < 0.56 µg/mL:

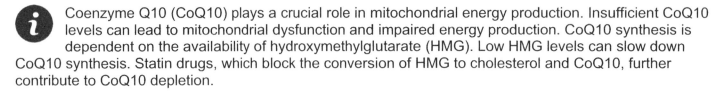

Coenzyme Q10 (CoQ10) plays a crucial role in mitochondrial energy production. Insufficient CoQ10 levels can lead to mitochondrial dysfunction and impaired energy production. CoQ10 synthesis is dependent on the availability of hydroxymethylglutarate (HMG). Low HMG levels can slow down CoQ10 synthesis. Statin drugs, which block the conversion of HMG to cholesterol and CoQ10, further contribute to CoQ10 depletion.

A functional impairment in mitochondrial CoQ10 electron transfer can also lead to elevations of succinate, malate, fumarate, and pyruvate, which are energy pathway intermediates. The direct transfer of electrons from succinate in the electron transport system is slowed when CoQ10's electron shuttle action is inadequate to meet the demands.

Research studies have shown that CoQ10 can inhibit LDL-oxidation and atherosclerosis, with the effect enhanced by co-supplementation of vitamin E. However, inadequate intake of CoQ10 can lead to its depletion.

Endogenous CoQ10 supplies are generated in the liver, but they can also be found in organ meat, soy oil, sardines, and peanuts. Aging naturally leads to a decrease in CoQ10 levels due to decreased synthesis and increased degradation, which cannot be adequately compensated for by diet alone.

Medications, particularly statins, are the most common cause of CoQ10 depletion. Genetics also play a role, with primary deficiency associated with defects in genes directly involved in CoQ10 biosynthesis. CoQ10 and idebenone supplementation are the only treatments for primary deficiency, with early detection leading to better prognosis.

Secondary deficiency can result from mutations in genes not directly involved in CoQ10 biosynthesis (APTX, ETFDH, BRAF, ANO10), impaired CoQ10 synthesis, insufficient dietary intake, or excessive cellular usage of CoQ10.

Medication interactions with CoQ10 include:
- Statins, which are HMG-CoA reductase inhibitors, work on the same pathway as CoQ10, leading to simultaneous depletion of the body's CoQ10 production.
- Simultaneous administration of warfarin (Coumadin) and CoQ10 supplements has been reported to decrease the anticoagulant effect of warfarin.

 Supplement with CoQ10

 Nutritional support:
- Coenzyme Q10 (Ubiquinol)

Lipid Support (high):
- Red Yeast Rice (Monascus purpureus)
- Coenzyme Q10
- Sweet Orange (Citrus sinensis)
- Quercetin
- Gotu Kola (Centella asiatica)
- Horse Chestnut (Aesculus hippocastanum)
- Grape Seed Extract (Vitis vinifera)
- Vitamin C
- Plant Sterols/Stanols (Beta-Sitosterol, Campesterol, Campestanol, Sitostanol)
- Monostroma nitidum (seaweed) extract

Mitochondrial Support:
- L-Carnitine
- D-Ribose
- Malic Acid
- Succinic Acid
- Coenzyme Q10 (Ubiquinol)
- R-Lipoic Acid
- Trans Resveratrol
- Curcumin
- Manganese
- Pantothenic Acid (Vitamin B5)
- Vitamins B1, B2, B4, B6, B12
- Nicotinamide Riboside Chloride
- Trans-Geranylgeraniol
- Rhodiola Rosea
- Pyrroloquinoline Quinone (PQQ)
- MVM (Multi-vitamin/mineral)
- Magnesium Taurinate
- Magnesium Glycinate
- Magnesium Malate

If **HIGH** or **> 2.78 µg/mL:**

Coenzyme Q10 (CoQ10) is a fat-soluble vitamin that plays a crucial role in energy production. While it's possible to obtain high levels of CoQ10 through supplements, it's important to note that abnormally high levels are only practically achievable through supplementation.

The safety of CoQ10 supplementation varies depending on the dose and duration of use. While there have been no reports of significant adverse side effects at doses as high as 3,000 mg/day for up to eight months, 1,200 mg/day for up to 16 months, and 600 mg/day for up to 30 months, it's essential to consider the lack of established Recommended Dietary Allowances (RDAs), Acceptable Daily Intakes (ADIs), or Upper Limits (ULs) for CoQ10.

Furthermore, there are no reliable data on the safety of CoQ10 supplementation during lactation, as it's not well-studied in this population. Therefore, it's recommended to avoid CoQ10 supplementation during breastfeeding.

 Stop or reduce Coenzyme Q10 supplementation

Coenzyme Q10 (Cellular)

CoQ10, a fat-soluble compound, is primarily synthesized by the body and consumed in the diet. It's found in virtually all cell membranes and plays a crucial role in mitochondria, converting carbohydrates and fatty acids into ATP. CoQ10 also supports various cellular functions, including cell signaling, gene expression, cell growth stimulation, apoptosis inhibition, thiol group control, hydrogen peroxide formation, and membrane channel regulation.

While foods are considered poor sources of CoQ10, organ meats from red meat sources are considered better sources. Nuts are considered a moderate source but require extreme consumption to meet daily requirements.

CoQ10 acts as an antioxidant and is essential for basic cell functions, particularly in energy production. Its primary function is to transfer electrons through the electron transport chain in the mitochondrial inner membrane. Electrons are received directly from succinate or indirectly from various substrates like pyruvate, acyl-CoA, and alpha–ketoglutarate in the form of NADH (Nicotinamide adenine dinucleotide). CoQ10 moves from one electron carrier complex to the next, ultimately delivering electrons one at a time. While electrons are delivered one at a time, they leave in pairs to form ATP and H2O.

Optimal Range	39.6 - 225.3 pg/MM WBC

If LOW or < 39.6 pg/MM WBC:

Coenzyme Q10 (CoQ10) plays a crucial role in mitochondrial energy production. Insufficient CoQ10 levels can lead to mitochondrial dysfunction and impaired energy production. CoQ10 synthesis is dependent on the availability of hydroxymethylglutarate (HMG). Low HMG levels can slow down CoQ10 synthesis. Statin drugs, which block the conversion of HMG to cholesterol and CoQ10, further contribute to CoQ10 depletion.

A functional impairment in mitochondrial CoQ10 electron transfer can also lead to elevations of succinate, malate, fumarate, and pyruvate, which are energy pathway intermediates. The direct transfer of electrons from succinate in the electron transport system is slowed when CoQ10's electron shuttle action is inadequate to meet the demands.

Research studies have shown that CoQ10 can inhibit LDL-oxidation and atherosclerosis, with the effect enhanced by co-supplementation of vitamin E. However, inadequate intake of CoQ10 can lead to its depletion.

Endogenous CoQ10 supplies are generated in the liver, but they can also be found in organ meat, soy oil, sardines, and peanuts. Aging naturally leads to a decrease in CoQ10 levels due to decreased synthesis and increased degradation, which cannot be adequately compensated for by diet alone.

Medications, particularly statins, are the most common cause of CoQ10 depletion. Genetics also play a role, with primary deficiency associated with defects in genes directly involved in CoQ10 biosynthesis. CoQ10 and idebenone supplementation are the only treatments for primary deficiency, with early detection leading to better prognosis.

Secondary deficiency can result from mutations in genes not directly involved in CoQ10 biosynthesis (APTX, ETFDH, BRAF, ANO10), impaired CoQ10 synthesis, insufficient dietary intake, or excessive cellular usage of CoQ10.

Medication interactions with CoQ10 include:
- Statins, which are HMG-CoA reductase inhibitors, work on the same pathway as CoQ10, leading to simultaneous depletion of the body's CoQ10 production.
- Simultaneous administration of warfarin (Coumadin) and CoQ10 supplements has been reported to decrease the anticoagulant effect of warfarin.

Supplement with CoQ10

Nutritional support:
- Coenzyme Q10 (Ubiquinol)

Lipid Support (high):
- Red Yeast Rice (Monascus purpureus)
- Coenzyme Q10
- Sweet Orange (Citrus sinensis)
- Quercetin
- Gotu Kola (Centella asiatica)
- Horse Chestnut (Aesculus hippocastanum)
- Grape Seed Extract (Vitis vinifera)
- Vitamin C
- Plant Sterols/Stanols (Beta-Sitosterol, Campesterol, Campestanol, Sitostanol)
- Monostroma nitidum (seaweed) extract

Mitochondrial Support:
- L-Carnitine
- D-Ribose
- Malic Acid
- Succinic Acid
- Coenzyme Q10 (Ubiquinol)
- R-Lipoic Acid
- Trans Resveratrol
- Curcumin
- Manganese
- Pantothenic Acid (Vitamin B5)
- Vitamins B1, B2, B4, B6, B12
- Nicotinamide Riboside Chloride (NIAGEN™)
- Trans-Geranylgeraniol (GG-Gold™)
- Rhodiola Rosea
- Pyrroloquinoline Quinone (PQQ)
- MVM (Multi-vitamin/mineral)
- Magnesium Taurinate
- Magnesium Glycinate
- Magnesium Malate

If HIGH or > 225.3 pg/MM WBC:

Coenzyme Q10 (CoQ10) is a fat-soluble vitamin that plays a crucial role in energy production. While it's possible to obtain high levels of CoQ10 through supplements, it's important to note that abnormally high levels are only practically achievable through supplementation.

The safety of CoQ10 supplementation varies depending on the dose and duration of use. While there have been no reports of significant adverse side effects at doses as high as 3,000 mg/day for up to eight months, 1,200 mg/day for up to 16 months, and 600 mg/day for up to 30 months, it's essential to consider the lack of established Recommended Dietary Allowances (RDAs), Acceptable Daily Intakes (ADIs), or Upper Limits (ULs) for CoQ10.

Furthermore, there are no reliable data on the safety of CoQ10 supplementation during lactation, as it's not well-studied in this population. Therefore, it's recommended to avoid CoQ10 supplementation during breastfeeding.

Stop or reduce Coenzyme Q10 supplementation

Cysteine (Serum)

Cysteine, an essential amino acid, possesses antioxidant properties and serves as a precursor molecule for glutathione production, the primary antioxidant in the body. Additionally, it plays a crucial role in iron-sulfide metabolism as an essential source of sulfide. Cysteine's ability to readily bind to metals like iron, nickel, copper, zinc, and heavy metals like mercury and lead through its thiol group may provide some chelation benefits. Furthermore, cysteine effectively neutralizes the harmful effects of acetaldehyde, a byproduct of alcohol consumption, potentially reducing the severity of hangovers.

| Optimal Range | 3.4 - 37.0 nmol/mL |

If LOW or < 3.4 nmol/mL:

Cysteine can be synthesized endogenously if sufficient methionine is available in the diet. However, depletion is extremely rare.

Individuals following strict vegan or vegetarian diets may have a higher risk of cysteine deficiency since plant-based diets typically provide lower amounts of cysteine.

Gastrointestinal conditions like celiac disease or Crohn's disease can impair the absorption of nutrients, including cysteine, leading to deficiencies.

Children and adolescents, especially during rapid growth and development periods, may require increased cysteine to support tissue development.

Certain medical conditions can also increase cysteine requirements. Cystinuria, a genetic disorder affecting the transport of cystine, a form of cysteine, in the kidneys, leads to increased cysteine loss in the urine and lower body levels. Chronic inflammatory diseases and chronic kidney disease, which involve oxidative stress, may also increase the body's demand for cysteine. Severe burn injuries can further increase cysteine requirements to support wound healing and tissue repair.

Food Sources:
- Meat
- Poultry
- Eggs
- Dairy
- Red peppers
- Onions
- Broccoli
- Brussels sprouts
- Oats
- Granola
- Wheat germ
- Lentils

Repletion Information:
- Cysteine is found in all proteins. However, some cysteine is oxidized to cystine and other compounds during cooking and storage, reducing its availability to the body. Regardless of dietary protein intake, cysteine supplementation with N-Acetyl-L-Cysteine (NAC) has been found to be safe at doses up to 2000 mg daily.
- Supplementation with cysteine is not recommended due to its poor tolerance by many patients. Additionally, it may be rapidly oxidized to cystine, which is less available for utilization.

Support Considerations:
- Increase food sources of cysteine, such as red peppers, onions, broccoli, Brussels sprouts, oats, granola, wheat germ, and lentils.
- Consider NAC supplementation.
- Ensure adequate protein intake and digestion.

Additional Investigations:
- Perform a stool test to assess gut and digestive health and rule out inflammatory bowel disease (IBD).

Nutritional support
- N-Acetyl-Cysteine (NAC)
- MVM (Multi-vitamin/mineral)
- Magnesium Taurinate
- Magnesium Glycinate
- Magnesium Malate

If **HIGH** or > 37.0 nmol/mL:

There is currently no established Recommended Dietary Allowance (RDA), Adequate Intake (AI), or Upper Limit (UL) for cysteine.

Excess supplementation:
- Cysteine is usually purchased in supplement form as N-acetyl cysteine (NAC).
- For general antioxidant support, doses typically start at 500 mg per day and can be increased based on the medical provider's recommendations.
- However, it's important to avoid D-cysteine or D-cystine, which are toxic.
- A diet rich in cysteine-rich proteins can elevate cysteine levels.

As with all sulfur-containing amino acids, the enzyme sulfite oxidase catabolizes cysteine into sulfite for excretion.

An important cofactor for this enzyme is molybdenum. Insufficient molybdenum can contribute to elevated cysteine levels.

Homocysteine is converted into cysteine through the enzyme cystathionine-beta-synthase (CBS) via the transsulfuration pathway. Cystathionine formation is an intermediate step in this process.

Cysteine levels may be elevated due to a CBS Single Nucleotide Polymorphism (SNP) that results in an upregulation of the enzyme, leading to increased cystathionine and cysteine production.

Zinc is another crucial cofactor downstream from cysteine in the transsulfuration pathway. Consequently, cysteine elevations can also occur in cases of zinc insufficiency.

Vitamin B12 may also play a role in the peripheral utilization of cysteine. Therefore, functional deficiencies of vitamin B12 can contribute to higher cysteine levels.

Stop or reduce cysteine / NAC supplementation
Consider co-factors for trans-sulfuration: molybdenum, zinc, B12

Nutritional support:
- Molybdenum

- Zinc
- Magnesium
- Vitamin B12
- Folate
- B Vitamins (B1, B2, B3, B5, B6, B7, B9)
- Vitamin B complex

Cysteine (Cellular)

Cysteine, an essential amino acid, possesses antioxidant properties and serves as a precursor molecule for glutathione production, the primary antioxidant in the body. Additionally, it plays a crucial role in iron-sulfide metabolism as an essential source of sulfide. Cysteine's ability to readily bind to metals like iron, nickel, copper, zinc, and heavy metals like mercury and lead through its thiol group may provide some chelation benefits. Furthermore, cysteine effectively neutralizes the harmful effects of acetaldehyde, a byproduct of alcohol consumption, potentially reducing the severity of hangovers.

| Optimal Range | 60.0 - 565.0 pg/MM WBC |

If LOW or < 60.0 pg/MM WBC:

 Cysteine can be synthesized endogenously if sufficient methionine is available in the diet. However, depletion is extremely rare.

Individuals following strict vegan or vegetarian diets may have a higher risk of cysteine deficiency since plant-based diets typically provide lower amounts of cysteine.

Gastrointestinal conditions like celiac disease or Crohn's disease can impair the absorption of nutrients, including cysteine, leading to deficiencies.

Children and adolescents, especially during rapid growth and development periods, may require increased cysteine to support tissue development.

Certain medical conditions can also increase cysteine requirements. Cystinuria, a genetic disorder affecting the transport of cystine, a form of cysteine, in the kidneys, leads to increased cysteine loss in the urine and lower body levels. Chronic inflammatory diseases and chronic kidney disease, which involve oxidative stress, may also increase the body's demand for cysteine. Severe burn injuries can further increase cysteine requirements to support wound healing and tissue repair.

 Food Sources:
- Meat
- Poultry
- Eggs
- Dairy
- Red peppers
- Onions
- Broccoli
- Brussels sprouts
- Oats
- Granola
- Wheat germ
- Lentils

Repletion Information:
- Cysteine is found in all proteins. However, some cysteine is oxidized to cystine and other compounds during cooking and storage, reducing its availability to the body. Regardless of dietary protein intake, cysteine supplementation with N-Acetyl-L-Cysteine (NAC) has been found to be safe at doses up to 2000 mg daily.
- Supplementation with cysteine is not recommended due to its poor tolerance by many patients. Additionally, it may be rapidly oxidized to cystine, which is less available for utilization.

Support Considerations:
- Increase food sources of cysteine, such as red peppers, onions, broccoli, Brussels sprouts, oats, granola, wheat germ, and lentils.
- Consider NAC supplementation.
- Ensure adequate protein intake and digestion.

Additional Investigations:
- Perform a stool test to assess gut and digestive health and rule out inflammatory bowel disease (IBD).

Nutritional support
- N-Acetyl-Cysteine (NAC)
- MVM (Multi-vitamin/mineral)
- Magnesium Taurinate
- Magnesium Glycinate
- Magnesium Malate

If HIGH or > 565.0 pg/MM WBC:

There is currently no established Recommended Dietary Allowance (RDA), Adequate Intake (AI), or Upper Limit (UL) for cysteine.

Excess supplementation:
- Cysteine is usually purchased in supplement form as N-acetyl cysteine (NAC).
- For general antioxidant support, doses typically start at 500 mg per day and can be increased based on the medical provider's recommendations.
- However, it's important to avoid D-cysteine or D-cystine, which are toxic.
- A diet rich in cysteine-rich proteins can elevate cysteine levels.

As with all sulfur-containing amino acids, the enzyme sulfite oxidase catabolizes cysteine into sulfite for excretion.

An important cofactor for this enzyme is molybdenum. Insufficient molybdenum can contribute to elevated cysteine levels.

Homocysteine is converted into cysteine through the enzyme cystathionine-beta-synthase (CBS) via the transsulfuration pathway. Cystathionine formation is an intermediate step in this process.

Cysteine levels may be elevated due to a CBS Single Nucleotide Polymorphism (SNP) that results in an upregulation of the enzyme, leading to increased cystathionine and cysteine production.

Zinc is another crucial cofactor downstream from cysteine in the transsulfuration pathway. Consequently, cysteine elevations can also occur in cases of zinc insufficiency.

Vitamin B12 may also play a role in the peripheral utilization of cysteine. Therefore, functional deficiencies of vitamin B12 can contribute to higher cysteine levels.

Stop or reduce cysteine / NAC supplementation
Consider co-factors for trans-sulfuration: molybdenum, zinc, B12

Nutritional support:
- Molybdenum
- Zinc
- Magnesium
- Vitamin B12
- Folate
- B Vitamins (B1, B2, B3, B5, B6, B7, B9)
- Vitamin B complex

Glutathione (Cellular)

Glutathione (GSH) is the master intracellular antioxidant. The only cells in the body that have been found to absorb intact GSH are hepatocytes, intestinal mucosal cells, and retinal cells.

| Optimal Range | 98.7 - 1163.0 pg/MM WBC |

If LOW or < 98.7 pg/MM WBC:

Glutathione levels naturally decline with age. However, this could be linked to reduced protein consumption in older individuals. Pro-inflammatory states and elevated oxidative stress deplete GSH stores, necessitating a conditionally higher intake of high cysteine foods or NAC as a supplement to boost endogenous GSH production. Depleted glutathione is converted back to its active form through an NADPH-dependent enzyme. Therefore, it's plausible that low NAD (or niacin, nicotinic acid) levels could further hinder this conversion back to the active GSH form.

Genetics:
- Glutathione synthetase deficiency.
- To assess if deficiency or depletion is genetically influenced, consider mutations in the GSHPx gene.

Dietary glutathione doesn't necessarily reflect systemic levels of glutathione. However, fruits and vegetables like asparagus, avocado, spinach, broccoli, cantaloupe, tomato, carrot, grapefruit, orange, zucchini, strawberry, watermelon, papaya, red bell peppers, peaches, lemons, mangoes, cauliflower, and cabbage are good sources of glutathione. Consider increasing your intake of cysteine and glutathione, and you may also want to take NAC and vitamin B3 (NAD) supplements. Genetic tests for GSH SNPs can also provide further insights.

Nutritional support
- N-Acetyl-Cysteine (NAC)
- Riboflavin (Vitamin B2)
- B Vitamins

If HIGH or > 1163.0 pg/MM WBC:

There's currently no Recommended Daily Allowance (RDA), Acceptable Daily Intake (ADI), or Upper Limit (UL) established for glutathione intake.

Excess supplementation:
- High-dose supplementation is sometimes used for skin lightening and antioxidant support.
- Glutathione can't enter cells intact; it must be synthesized inside the cell to be effective. Therefore, supplementation usually has minimal benefit.
- Supplementing the building blocks like NAC, glutamic acid, and glycine may increase cellular glutathione production; however, NAC may be most impactful since cysteine, an amino acid, is known to be rate-limiting for glutathione synthesis.
- Direct glutathione supplementation has only been shown to benefit slowing the breakdown of nitric oxide in the bloodstream.

 Stop or reduce glutathione supplementation
Consider support cellular production of glutathione with precursors and co-factors if appropriate (i.e. supplementary glutathione is high but you suspect antioxidant status overall is still poor)

 Nutritional support:
- N-Acetyl-Cysteine (NAC)
- Riboflavin (Vitamin B2)
- B Vitamins

Selenium (Serum)

Selenium, an essential trace element, plays a crucial role in immune function and thyroid hormone synthesis. It works through selenoproteins like iodothyronine deiodinase and directly converts thyroxine (T4) to triiodothyronine (T3). Moreover, selenium aids enzymes in protecting cell membranes from damage and is a vital component of antioxidant reactions. It supports the production of selenoproteins, particularly glutathione peroxidase, which helps regenerate vitamins C and E from their oxidized forms, enhancing their antioxidant activity. Protein-rich food sources are believed to be the most effective in increasing circulating levels of glutathione peroxidase.

Optimal Range	109.8 - 218.4 ng/mL

If LOW or < 109.8 ng/mL:

 Inadequate selenium intake occurs when there's insufficient selenium in the diet, usually due to limited selenium sources in a region. Notably, many selenium deficiency diseases are associated with concurrent vitamin E deficiency. Individuals at risk for low selenium levels or depletion include those who've had bariatric surgery, celiac patients, and Crohn's disease patients. The interaction of selenium with other medications is poorly understood. Only a few interactions have been reported.

 Food Sources:
- Brazil nuts
- Yellowfin tuna
- Halibut
- Sardines
- Ham
- Shrimp
- Beef
- Turkey

- Chicken

Support Considerations:
- Increase food sources of selenium (as little as 2-3 Brazil nuts per day may be beneficial for maintenance).
- Consider selenium and vitamin E supplementation.

Additional Investigations:
- Stool test to assess gut and digestive health and rule out IBD.
- Celiac testing.

Nutritional support
- Selenium
- Vitamin E tocotrienols

If HIGH or > 218.4 ng/mL:

The tolerable upper intake level (UL) for selenium in adults, set at 400 micrograms per day (mcg/day), is based on preventing hair and nail brittleness and loss, as well as the early signs of chronic selenium toxicity. This UL encompasses both selenium obtained from food and supplements. While selenium is essential for health, consuming excessive amounts can lead to toxicity. Acute and even fatal toxicities have been reported in cases of accidental or suicidal ingestion of large quantities of selenium. Chronic selenium toxicity, known as selenosis, can develop with smaller doses over extended periods. The most commonly reported symptoms of selenosis include hair and nail brittleness and loss. Other symptoms may include gastrointestinal disturbances, skin rashes, a garlic breath odor, fatigue, irritability, and neurological disorders.

Stop or reduce selenium supplementation / sources

Selenium (Cellular)

Selenium, an essential trace element, plays a crucial role in immune function and thyroid hormone synthesis. It works through selenoproteins like iodothyronine deiodinase and directly converts thyroxine (T4) to triiodothyronine (T3). Moreover, selenium aids enzymes in protecting cell membranes from damage and is a vital component of antioxidant reactions. It supports the production of selenoproteins, particularly glutathione peroxidase, which helps regenerate vitamins C and E from their oxidized forms, enhancing their antioxidant activity. Protein-rich food sources are believed to be the most effective in increasing circulating levels of glutathione peroxidase.

| Optimal Range | 234.0 - 1050.0 pg/MM WBC |

If LOW or < 234.0 pg/MM WBC:

Inadequate selenium intake occurs when there's insufficient selenium in the diet, usually due to limited selenium sources in a region. Notably, many selenium deficiency diseases are associated with concurrent vitamin E deficiency. Individuals at risk for low selenium levels or depletion include those who've had bariatric surgery, celiac patients, and Crohn's disease patients. The interaction of selenium with other medications is poorly understood. Only a few interactions have been reported.

Food Sources:
- Brazil nuts
- Yellowfin tuna
- Halibut
- Sardines
- Ham
- Shrimp
- Beef
- Turkey
- Chicken

Support Considerations:
- Increase food sources of selenium (as little as 2-3 Brazil nuts per day may be beneficial for maintenance).
- Consider selenium and vitamin E supplementation.

Additional Investigations:
- Stool test to assess gut and digestive health and rule out IBD.
- Celiac testing.

Nutritional support
- Selenium
- Vitamin E tocotrienols

If HIGH or > 1050.0 pg/MM WBC:

The tolerable upper intake level (UL) for selenium in adults, set at 400 micrograms per day (mcg/day), is based on preventing hair and nail brittleness and loss, as well as the early signs of chronic selenium toxicity. This UL encompasses both selenium obtained from food and supplements. While selenium is essential for health, consuming excessive amounts can lead to toxicity. Acute and even fatal toxicities have been reported in cases of accidental or suicidal ingestion of large quantities of selenium. Chronic selenium toxicity, known as selenosis, can develop with smaller doses over extended periods. The most commonly reported symptoms of selenosis include hair and nail brittleness and loss. Other symptoms may include gastrointestinal disturbances, skin rashes, a garlic breath odor, fatigue, irritability, and neurological disorders.

Stop or reduce selenium supplementation / sources

Folate (Serum)

Vitamin B9, also known as folate, is naturally found in foods. Folic acid, a synthetic form of folate, is often used as a supplement. Folate is more bioavailable than folic acid. Once in circulation, folate undergoes methylation, converting to methyl-tetrahydrofolate (5-MTHF), which is the most abundant form in the body. 5-MTHF plays a crucial role in methylation reactions, reducing homocysteine levels and supporting DNA synthesis and red blood cell production. Additionally, it helps mask B12 deficiency and reduces metabolic defects caused by the MTHFR single nucleotide polymorphism (SNP).

| Optimal Range | ≥4.6 ng/mL |

If **LOW** or **< 4.6 ng/mL**:

Folate depletion can occur due to various factors. Inadequate intake is a common cause, as is digestive disorders such as celiac disease, Crohn's disease, and certain gastrointestinal surgeries, which can impair folate absorption. Alcoholism, pregnancy and breastfeeding, growth phases, medications, medical treatments, anemia, hemolytic anemias, excessive stress or infection, and genetic factors like MTHFR gene mutations can also contribute to folate deficiency. Aging: Older adults may be at higher risk of folate deficiency due to reduced dietary intake, reduced absorption, and increased medication use.

Clinical Manifestations of Depletion:
- Folate deficiency can manifest as anemia, particularly megoblastic anemia, which also involves vitamin B12.
- Often, folate deficiency is secondary to vitamin B12 deficiency because the conversion to 5-methyl folate is B12-dependent.
- Symptoms of B12 deficiency can include elevated homocysteine (hyperhomocysteinemia), neural tube defects if the mother is deficient during pregnancy, mood disorders such as anxiety and depression, especially in the elderly, and fatigue, impaired immune function, and cardiovascular disease.

Medications that deplete folate include:
- Methotrexate
- Anticonvulsants
- Antacids
- Oral contraceptives
- Long-term, high doses of NSAIDs

Food Sources:
- Beef liver
- Green leafy vegetables (especially spinach and mustard greens)
- Black-eyed peas
- Fortified breakfast cereals
- White rice
- Asparagus
- Brussels sprouts

Support Considerations:
- Increase food sources
- Reduce alcohol consumption
- Consider supplementation

Correlation between Serum and Cellular Levels:
- Cellular levels are low, and serum levels are normal or excessive.
- In the short term, the status of micro-nutrients is optimal, but cellular absorption may be a problem.
- Recommendations:
- Increase dietary intake of nutrients
- Increase supplementation dosage
- Consider the status of synergistic nutrients for cellular absorption
- Consider levels of oxidative stress on nutrient depletion
- Consider follow-up testing to identify the source of malabsorption.

Cellular levels are low, and serum levels are low as well.

In the short term and long term, the status of micro-nutrients is not optimal, suggesting low dietary intake and possible causes including intestinal and cellular absorption.

Recommendations:
- Increase dietary intake of nutrients
- Increase supplementation dosage
- Medications may have an effect on depletion
- Consider follow-up testing to identify the source of malabsorption.

Additional Investigations:
- Genetic testing
- Impairments in methylation, transsulfuration, and biopterin (neurotransmitter) pathways may impact the need for B6.

Nutritional support
- Folate
- Vitamin B12

Folate (Cellular)

Vitamin B9, also known as folate, is naturally found in foods. Folic acid, a synthetic form of folate, is often used as a supplement. Folate is more bioavailable than folic acid. Once in circulation, folate undergoes methylation, converting to methyl-tetrahydrofolate (5-MTHF), which is the most abundant form in the body. 5-MTHF plays a crucial role in methylation reactions, reducing homocysteine levels and supporting DNA synthesis and red blood cell production. Additionally, it helps mask B12 deficiency and reduces metabolic defects caused by the MTHFR single nucleotide polymorphism (SNP).

Optimal Range	≥95.5 ng/mL

If LOW or < 95.5 ng/mL:

Folate depletion can occur due to various factors. Inadequate intake is a common cause, as is digestive disorders such as celiac disease, Crohn's disease, and certain gastrointestinal surgeries, which can impair folate absorption. Alcoholism, pregnancy and breastfeeding, growth phases, medications, medical treatments, anemia, hemolytic anemias, excessive stress or infection, and genetic factors like MTHFR gene mutations can also contribute to folate deficiency. Aging: Older adults may be at higher risk of folate deficiency due to reduced dietary intake, reduced absorption, and increased medication use.

Clinical Manifestations of Depletion:
- Folate deficiency can manifest as anemia, particularly megoblastic anemia, which also involves vitamin B12.
- Often, folate deficiency is secondary to vitamin B12 deficiency because the conversion to 5-methyl folate is B12-dependent.
- Symptoms of B12 deficiency can include elevated homocysteine (hyperhomocysteinemia), neural tube defects if the mother is deficient during pregnancy, mood disorders such as anxiety and depression, especially in the elderly, and fatigue, impaired immune function, and cardiovascular disease.

Medications that deplete folate include:
- Methotrexate

- Anticonvulsants
- Antacids
- Oral contraceptives
- Long-term, high doses of NSAIDs

Food Sources:
- Beef liver
- Green leafy vegetables (especially spinach and mustard greens)
- Black-eyed peas
- Fortified breakfast cereals
- White rice
- Asparagus
- Brussels sprouts

Support Considerations:
- Increase food sources
- Reduce alcohol consumption
- Consider supplementation

Correlation between Serum and Cellular Levels:
- Cellular levels are low, and serum levels are normal or excessive.
- In the short term, the status of micro-nutrients is optimal, but cellular absorption may be a problem.
- Recommendations:
- Increase dietary intake of nutrients
- Increase supplementation dosage
- Consider the status of synergistic nutrients for cellular absorption
- Consider levels of oxidative stress on nutrient depletion
- Consider follow-up testing to identify the source of malabsorption.

Cellular levels are low, and serum levels are low as well.
In the short term and long term, the status of micro-nutrients is not optimal, suggesting low dietary intake and possible causes including intestinal and cellular absorption.

Recommendations:
- Increase dietary intake of nutrients
- Increase supplementation dosage
- Medications may have an effect on depletion
- Consider follow-up testing to identify the source of malabsorption.

Additional Investigations:
- Genetic testing
- Impairments in methylation, transsulfuration, and biopterin (neurotransmitter) pathways may impact the need for B6.

Nutritional support
- Folate
- Vitamin B12

Vitamin A (Serum)

Vitamin A, a fat-soluble vitamin, plays a crucial role in various bodily functions, including vision, immune function, and cell differentiation. Serum vitamin A levels are measured to assess an individual's nutritional status, typically expressed in micrograms per deciliter (mcg/dL) or international units per deciliter (IU/dL).

Vitamin A is a group of fat-soluble vitamins, including retinol, retinal, retinoic acid, and several provitamin A carotenoids, with beta-carotene being the most significant. It has multiple functions, such as supporting infant, child, and adolescent growth and development, maintaining the immune system, and promoting healthy vision. Vitamin A is essential for both low-light and color vision in the retina of the eye. Additionally, it functions as retinoic acid, a hormone-like growth factor for epithelial and other cells.

Furthermore, vitamin A contributes to gene transcription, hematopoiesis, and antioxidant activity within the body. The upper intake level (UL) for adult vitamin A is set at 3,000 micrograms retinol activity equivalents (mcg RAE) per day.

Optimal Range	43.1 - 107.0 mcg/dL

If **LOW** or < 43.1 mcg/dL:

How Vitamin A Depletion Occurs

Inadequate Intake: Consuming insufficient amounts of vitamin A through diet is a primary cause of depletion.

Malabsorption Disorders: Certain conditions that affect the digestive tract can hinder vitamin A absorption. These include:
- Celiac disease
- Inflammatory bowel disease (IBD)
- Pancreatic insufficiency
- Liver disorders such as cirrhosis and non-alcoholic fatty liver disease (NAFLD)
- Gallbladder disorders, including holecystitis and gallstones
- Short bowel syndrome
- Giardiasis

Alcoholism: Excessive alcohol consumption can interfere with vitamin A utilization.

Zinc Deficiency: Zinc plays a crucial role in converting inactive vitamin A (retinol) into its active form (retinoic acid) within the retina. Adequate zinc is essential for synthesizing retinol binding protein (RAP), which transports vitamin A. Consequently, a zinc deficiency limits the body's ability to mobilize vitamin A stores from the liver.

Hypothyroidism: Retinoids appear to be involved in the development and maturation of thyroid cell phenotypes. Clinical manifestations of vitamin A depletion due to hypothyroidism include:
- Vision loss or night blindness
- Dry, scaly, or itchy skin
- Infertility
- Delayed growth in children
- Respiratory tract infections

Diet/Medication Interactions: Certain medications and dietary factors can interact with vitamin A absorption. These include:

- Oral contraceptives
- Cholesterol-lowering medications
- Agents that cause fat malabsorption, such as orlistat, mineral oil, and the fat substitute olestra, can affect the absorption of all fat-soluble vitamins.

Food sources: Beef liver, sweet potato, spinach, pumpkin, carrots, and herring. Considerations: Increase food sources, reduce alcohol consumption, consider supplementation, and assess zinc status.

Nutritional support
- Vitamin A (Retinol)
- Vitamin D3
- Vitamin K2

If **HIGH** or > 107.0 mcg/dL:

Excessive vitamin A levels, medically referred to as hypervitaminosis A, can develop when the body accumulates 10,000 IU or more of vitamin A daily over an extended period. As a fat-soluble vitamin, the body stores excessive amounts rather than excreting them. Several factors can contribute to the development of hypervitaminosis A:
- High Dietary Intake: Consuming large quantities of vitamin A-rich foods, such as fish liver, eggs, and dairy products, can lead to excessive vitamin A accumulation.
- Chronic Overconsumption of Fortified Foods: Regularly consuming highly fortified foods, particularly certain breakfast cereals, can contribute to elevated vitamin A levels.
- Consumption of Animal Liver: Eating large amounts of animal liver, which is rich in vitamin A, can result in elevated vitamin A levels.
- High-Dose Supplements: Consuming vitamin A supplements at doses significantly higher than the recommended daily allowance (RDA) over an extended period can lead to excessive vitamin A levels.
- Consumption of High-Dose Vitamin A Medications: Certain prescription medications, such as isotretinoin (used to treat severe acne), contain high doses of vitamin A and can lead to elevated levels when used improperly.
- Liver Dysfunction: Liver disorders, including hepatitis or cirrhosis, can impair the liver's ability to metabolize and store vitamin A effectively, resulting in elevated levels.

Excessive vitamin A intake is toxic and must be avoided, especially during pregnancy. Hypervitaminosis A can lead to liver abnormalities, reduced bone density (osteoporosis), and central nervous system disorders. Early signs of toxicity include peeling or itching skin, brittle nails, yellowish skin, hair loss (alopecia), and bone or joint pain. Provitamin A (beta carotene and mixed carotenoids, found in orange and yellow vegetables) is much less toxic and not associated with the commonly observed side effects of excessive vitamin A intake. Therefore, it is advisable to stop or reduce vitamin A supplementation or sources.

Vitamin A (Cellular)

Vitamin A, a fat-soluble vitamin, plays a crucial role in various bodily functions, including vision, immune function, and cell differentiation. Serum vitamin A levels are measured to assess an individual's nutritional status, typically expressed in micrograms per deciliter (mcg/dL) or international units per deciliter (IU/dL).

Vitamin A is a group of fat-soluble vitamins, including retinol, retinal, retinoic acid, and several provitamin A carotenoids, with beta-carotene being the most significant. It has multiple functions, such as supporting infant, child, and adolescent growth and development, maintaining the immune system, and promoting healthy vision. Vitamin A is essential for both low-light and color vision in the retina of the eye. Additionally, it functions as retinoic acid, a hormone-like growth factor for epithelial and other cells.

Furthermore, vitamin A contributes to gene transcription, hematopoiesis, and antioxidant activity within the body. The upper intake level (UL) for adult vitamin A is set at 3,000 micrograms retinol activity equivalents (mcg RAE) per day.

| Optimal Range | 0.9 - 17.3 pg/MM WBC |

If **LOW** or < 0.9 pg/MM WBC:

How Vitamin A Depletion Occurs

Inadequate Intake: Consuming insufficient amounts of vitamin A through diet is a primary cause of depletion.

Malabsorption Disorders: Certain conditions that affect the digestive tract can hinder vitamin A absorption. These include:
- Celiac disease
- Inflammatory bowel disease (IBD)
- Pancreatic insufficiency
- Liver disorders such as cirrhosis and non-alcoholic fatty liver disease (NAFLD)
- Gallbladder disorders, including holecystitis and gallstones
- Short bowel syndrome
- Giardiasis

Alcoholism: Excessive alcohol consumption can interfere with vitamin A utilization.

Zinc Deficiency: Zinc plays a crucial role in converting inactive vitamin A (retinol) into its active form (retinoic acid) within the retina. Adequate zinc is essential for synthesizing retinol binding protein (RAP), which transports vitamin A. Consequently, a zinc deficiency limits the body's ability to mobilize vitamin A stores from the liver.

Hypothyroidism: Retinoids appear to be involved in the development and maturation of thyroid cell phenotypes. Clinical manifestations of vitamin A depletion due to hypothyroidism include:
- Vision loss or night blindness
- Dry, scaly, or itchy skin
- Infertility
- Delayed growth in children
- Respiratory tract infections

Diet/Medication Interactions: Certain medications and dietary factors can interact with vitamin A absorption. These include:
- Oral contraceptives
- Cholesterol-lowering medications
- Agents that cause fat malabsorption, such as orlistat, mineral oil, and the fat substitute olestra, can affect the absorption of all fat-soluble vitamins.

Food sources: Beef liver, sweet potato, spinach, pumpkin, carrots, and herring. Considerations: Increase food sources, reduce alcohol consumption, consider supplementation, and assess zinc status.

Nutritional support
- Vitamin A (Retinol)
- Vitamin D3
- Vitamin K2

If **HIGH** or **> 17.3 pg/MM WBC:**

Excessive vitamin A levels, medically referred to as hypervitaminosis A, can develop when the body accumulates 10,000 IU or more of vitamin A daily over an extended period. As a fat-soluble vitamin, the body stores excessive amounts rather than excreting them. Several factors can contribute to the development of hypervitaminosis A:

- High Dietary Intake: Consuming large quantities of vitamin A-rich foods, such as fish liver, eggs, and dairy products, can lead to excessive vitamin A accumulation.
- Chronic Overconsumption of Fortified Foods: Regularly consuming highly fortified foods, particularly certain breakfast cereals, can contribute to elevated vitamin A levels.
- Consumption of Animal Liver: Eating large amounts of animal liver, which is rich in vitamin A, can result in elevated vitamin A levels.
- High-Dose Supplements: Consuming vitamin A supplements at doses significantly higher than the recommended daily allowance (RDA) over an extended period can lead to excessive vitamin A levels.
- Consumption of High-Dose Vitamin A Medications: Certain prescription medications, such as isotretinoin (used to treat severe acne), contain high doses of vitamin A and can lead to elevated levels when used improperly.
- Liver Dysfunction: Liver disorders, including hepatitis or cirrhosis, can impair the liver's ability to metabolize and store vitamin A effectively, resulting in elevated levels.

Excessive vitamin A intake is toxic and must be avoided, especially during pregnancy. Hypervitaminosis A can lead to liver abnormalities, reduced bone density (osteoporosis), and central nervous system disorders. Early signs of toxicity include peeling or itching skin, brittle nails, yellowish skin, hair loss (alopecia), and bone or joint pain. Provitamin A (beta carotene and mixed carotenoids, found in orange and yellow vegetables) is much less toxic and not associated with the commonly observed side effects of excessive vitamin A intake. Therefore, it is advisable to stop or reduce vitamin A supplementation or sources.

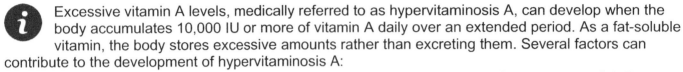

Vitamin B1 (Serum)

Vitamin B1 (Thiamine) is a water-soluble vitamin essential for energy metabolism, nerve function, and maintaining proper heart and muscle function. It acts as a coenzyme in the breakdown and transformation of carbohydrates, fats, and proteins to produce energy in the form of ATP.

| Optimal Range | 188.4 - 428.9 nmol/L |

If **LOW** or **< 188.4 nmol/L:**

How thiamine gets depleted:
- Inadequate intake: Thiamine deficiency can occur due to insufficient consumption of the nutrient.
- Alcohol abuse: Alcohol interferes with thiamine absorption and utilization.
- Malabsorption: Conditions affecting the digestive system, such as gastric bypass surgery, can hinder thiamine absorption.

- Frequent consumption of thiaminases, which are present in higher amounts in raw fish, can lead to thiamine depletion.
- Thiamine can also be lost during cooking.

Clinical manifestations of depletion:
- Thiamine deficiency can cause nervous system and cardiac abnormalities.
- The most severe form of thiamine deficiency is called beriberi, which commonly results in weakness, fatigue, confusion, irritability, weight loss, muscle wasting, and peripheral neuropathy.

There are three classical syndromes of frank thiamin deficiency:
- Beriberi
- Wernicke's Encephalopathy
- Korsakoff's Psychosis

Medications that reduce thiamine levels include:
- Tricyclic antidepressants
- Oral contraceptives
- Diuretics such as furosemide
- Anti-convulsant medications such as phenytoin
- Some cancer medications

Food sources include fortified breakfast cereals, enriched food products, pork, trout, black beans, and mussels. Considerations include increasing food sources, reducing alcohol consumption, considering supplementation, and looking at cooking methods. High, prolonged heat and boiling can deplete B vitamins, so avoid frying. Instead, think "low and slow" for cooking. There is no Upper Limit (UL) for thiamin.

Nutritional support includes:
- Thiamine (Vitamin B1)
- B Vitamins

If HIGH or > 428.9 nmol/L:

Excessive Supplementation The human body excretes excess thiamin in the urine. There is a lack of evidence of toxicity from high thiamin intake from food or supplements.
https://www.ncbi.nlm.nih.gov/books/NBK482360/

Stop or reduce B1 supplementation / sources

Vitamin B1 (Cellular)

Vitamin B1 (Thiamine) is a water-soluble vitamin essential for energy metabolism, nerve function, and maintaining proper heart and muscle function. It acts as a coenzyme in the breakdown and transformation of carbohydrates, fats, and proteins to produce energy in the form of ATP.

Optimal Range	0.10 - 7.00 pg/MM WBC

If LOW or < 0.10 pg/MM WBC:

How thiamine gets depleted:
- Inadequate intake: Thiamine deficiency can occur due to insufficient consumption of the nutrient.
- Alcohol abuse: Alcohol interferes with thiamine absorption and utilization.
- Malabsorption: Conditions affecting the digestive system, such as gastric bypass surgery, can hinder thiamine absorption.
- Frequent consumption of thiaminases, which are present in higher amounts in raw fish, can lead to thiamine depletion.
- Thiamine can also be lost during cooking.

Clinical manifestations of depletion:
- Thiamine deficiency can cause nervous system and cardiac abnormalities.
- The most severe form of thiamine deficiency is called beriberi, which commonly results in weakness, fatigue, confusion, irritability, weight loss, muscle wasting, and peripheral neuropathy.

There are three classical syndromes of frank thiamin deficiency:
- Beriberi
- Wernicke's Encephalopathy
- Korsakoff's Psychosis

Medications that reduce thiamine levels include:
- Tricyclic antidepressants
- Oral contraceptives
- Diuretics such as furosemide
- Anti-convulsant medications such as phenytoin
- Some cancer medications

Food sources include fortified breakfast cereals, enriched food products, pork, trout, black beans, and mussels. Considerations include increasing food sources, reducing alcohol consumption, considering supplementation, and looking at cooking methods. High, prolonged heat and boiling can deplete B vitamins, so avoid frying. Instead, think "low and slow" for cooking. There is no Upper Limit (UL) for thiamin.

Nutritional support includes:
- Thiamine (Vitamin B1)
- B Vitamins

If **HIGH** or **> 7.00 pg/MM WBC**:

Excessive Supplementation The human body excretes excess thiamin in the urine. There is a lack of evidence of toxicity from high thiamin intake from food or supplements.
https://www.ncbi.nlm.nih.gov/books/NBK482360/

Stop or reduce B1 supplementation / sources

Vitamin B12 (Serum)

Vitamin B12, or cobalamin, plays a crucial role as an active coenzyme in its methylcobalamin and adenosyl cobalamin forms. Primarily, it aids in the metabolism of folic acid by acting as a methyl donor. However, its absorption is dependent on intrinsic factor, which is calcium-dependent. Additionally, there's evidence suggesting that vitamin B12 may contribute to the production of certain neurotransmitters, potentially leading to mood imbalances in susceptible individuals.

| Optimal Range | 232 - 1245 pg/mL |

If LOW or < 232 pg/mL:

How does vitamin B12 get depleted?
Age is a risk factor for vitamin B12 deficiency because of a natural decline in intrinsic factor. Chronic use of proton pump inhibitors (PPIs) may reduce stomach acid levels and lead to sub-clinical deficiencies. Certain genetic single nucleotide polymorphisms (SNPs), such as MTHFR, can also cause deficiencies in active vitamin B12 (methylcobalamin).

Other factors that can contribute to vitamin B12 deficiency include:
- Pernicious anemia: An autoimmune condition where the body's immune system attacks cells in the stomach that produce a protein needed for vitamin B12 absorption.
- Celiac disease: A condition that damages the intestines and hinders the absorption of vitamin B12 and other nutrients.
- Atrophic gastritis: Chronic inflammation and thinning of the stomach lining can impair vitamin B12 absorption.
- Hypochlorhydria: Low stomach acid production can also affect vitamin B12 absorption.
- Oral contraceptive pills: Long-term use of these medications can reduce stomach acid levels and hinder vitamin B12 absorption.
- Chronic alcohol dependence: Excessive alcohol consumption can interfere with vitamin B12 absorption.
- Obesity, pregnancy, preeclampsia, and eclampsia: These conditions can also increase the risk of vitamin B12 deficiency.
- Bariatric surgery: Certain weight loss surgeries, such as gastric bypass, can lead to reduced vitamin B12 absorption due to alterations in the digestive tract.
- Medication: Proton pump inhibitors (PPIs) and H2 blockers can also reduce stomach acid levels and hinder vitamin B12 absorption. Metformin, a medication used to manage diabetes, may reduce B12 levels in some individuals. Clinical manifestations of B12 depletion include pernicious anemia, usually due to a lack of intrinsic factor. Megoblastic anemia, another form of anemia associated with B12 deficiency, occurs when folate is in excess and insufficient B12 is present, creating a 'folate trap.' Dementia due to degeneration of myelin is another symptom of B12 deficiency. Methylmalonyl CoA is metabolized to methylmalonic acid (MMA) in B12 deficiency, making MMA the definitive marker for B12 deficiency. Achlorhydria (insufficient stomach acid) can lead to B12 deficiency because hydrochloric acid (HCl) is required to cleave B12 from intrinsic factor.

Many medications reduce the absorption of B12, including:
- Proton pump inhibitors (PPIs) (indirectly by reducing HCl required for Vitamin B12 release from food, but not supplements)
- Metformin (type 2 diabetes medication)
- Histamine 2 receptor antagonists
- Bile acid sequestrants (cholestyramine)
- Neomysin

Food Sources:
- Beef liver
- Clams
- Nutritional yeast
- Atlantic salmon

- Canned chunk light tuna
- Ground beef
- Milk
- Plain yogurt
- Fortified breakfast cereals

It's important to note that the B12 synthesized by gut bacteria may not be a significant source for humans since it's not absorbed in the colon.

Support considerations:
- Look to diet and lifestyle reasons for insufficiency, such as veganism, gastric bypass, celiac disease, medications, poor diet, etc.
- Increase food sources and supplement if appropriate. Preferred versions of B12 are methylcobalamin and adenosylcobalamin, which are metabolically active forms. Hydroxocobalamin may be better tolerated for sensitive clients. Cyanocobalamin is a synthetic form of Vitamin B12 that the body converts into Adenosylcobalamin and Methylcobalamin before it can be used.

Supplement Options:
- The RDA for B12 is 6 mcg/day.
- Consider the upper limit of folate supplementation as a factor for B12 supplementation, as it may lead to folate trap.
- Vitamin B12 is extremely safe. No toxicity from high doses of vitamin B12 has ever been reported.
- Intramuscular injections are often used, particularly in the elderly, to bypass intrinsic factor.
- Humans store large amounts of B12 in the liver, so larger doses can be given at 6-month intervals.
- Supplementation is highly encouraged on a vegan diet. Due to the liver's high storage capacity for B12, it may take years for the body to completely deplete its stores after adopting a vegan diet.

To address this, consider the following:

- Genetic factors: MTHFR genetic mutations and hyperhomocysteinemia may require methyl cobalamin supplementation.
- Methylcobalamin: It's the recommended form of supplementation, but it may be poorly absorbed by individuals taking antacids or those with poor absorption (e.g., celiac disease, intestinal permeability).
- Cyanocobalamin: It's not recommended for patients with MTHFR mutations.
- Hydroxocobalamin: It's recommended for patients with autoimmune diseases and elevated nitric oxide levels.
- Glutathione: It's essential for methylcobalamin to be adequately bound for transport.

Vitamin B12 supplementation may help manage various conditions, including anemia, asthma, fatigue, hepatitis, dementia, epilepsy, depression, psychosis, irritability, ataxia, numbness, tingling, neuropathy, AIDS, multiple sclerosis, tinnitus, and infertility.

Supplemental B12 is typically given in doses of 1000 to 5000 mcg.

Additionally, consider the following tests:
- Stool test to assess gut and digestive health and rule out inflammatory bowel disease (IBD).
- Celiac testing.
- Pernicious anemia testing.
- Genetic testing for MTHFR, MTR, MTRR, and other SNPs involved in methylation.

Nutritional support
- Vitamin B12
- Folate
- B Vitamins (B1, B2, B3, B5, B6, B7, B9)
- Vitamin B complex

If **HIGH** or **> 1245 pg/mL:**

Vitamin B12, when consumed in large quantities from food or supplements, has not been linked to any toxic or adverse effects in healthy individuals. However, when high doses are administered orally, only a small percentage can be absorbed, which may explain the relatively low toxicity associated with vitamin B12. Consequently, the US Food and Nutrition Board has not established a tolerable upper intake level (UL) for vitamin B12 due to its low toxicity.

While cobalamin toxicity can be unexpected and unusual, it's important to remember that the administration of any drug carries inherent risks. A case report serves as a reminder that even seemingly safe practices can have unforeseen consequences.

Excessive vitamin B12 levels are more commonly associated with high-dose supplementation or intravenous injections. A study published in the Journal of the American Medical Association (https://doi.org/10.1093/qjmed/hcz164) found that high or supraphysiological serum B12 levels without supplementation have been linked to various pathological conditions, including renal failure, hematological disorders, cancer, and hepatic or autoimmune diseases. These conditions often exhibit elevated concentrations of B12 transport proteins. Additionally, there may be an increased release of B12 in liver disease due to hepatic cytolysis and/or reduced B12 clearance. Consequently, a high or supraphysiological serum B12 concentration without supplementation could serve as a diagnostic marker for severe underlying disease. Furthermore, very high serum B12 levels have been frequently reported in critically ill patients.

Polycythemia Vera, a rare blood cancer that causes the bone marrow to produce an excessive number of red blood cells, can also lead to elevated B12 levels. Elevated serum B12 levels may also be associated with a functional deficiency of the vitamin due to a failure of cellular uptake, intracellular processing, trafficking, or utilization.

Vitamin B12 (Cellular)

Vitamin B12, or cobalamin, plays a crucial role as an active coenzyme in its methylcobalamin and adenosyl cobalamin forms. Primarily, it aids in the metabolism of folic acid by acting as a methyl donor. However, its absorption is dependent on intrinsic factor, which is calcium-dependent. Additionally, there's evidence suggesting that vitamin B12 may contribute to the production of certain neurotransmitters, potentially leading to mood imbalances in susceptible individuals.

Optimal Range	2.00 - 11.99 pg/MM WBC

If **LOW** or **< 2.00 pg/MM WBC:**

 How does vitamin B12 get depleted?
Age is a risk factor for vitamin B12 deficiency because of a natural decline in intrinsic factor. Chronic use of proton pump inhibitors (PPIs) may reduce stomach acid levels and lead to sub-

clinical deficiencies. Certain genetic single nucleotide polymorphisms (SNPs), such as MTHFR, can also cause deficiencies in active vitamin B12 (methylcobalamin).

Other factors that can contribute to vitamin B12 deficiency include:
- Pernicious anemia: An autoimmune condition where the body's immune system attacks cells in the stomach that produce a protein needed for vitamin B12 absorption.
- Celiac disease: A condition that damages the intestines and hinders the absorption of vitamin B12 and other nutrients.
- Atrophic gastritis: Chronic inflammation and thinning of the stomach lining can impair vitamin B12 absorption.
- Hypochlorhydria: Low stomach acid production can also affect vitamin B12 absorption.
- Oral contraceptive pills: Long-term use of these medications can reduce stomach acid levels and hinder vitamin B12 absorption.
- Chronic alcohol dependence: Excessive alcohol consumption can interfere with vitamin B12 absorption.
- Obesity, pregnancy, preeclampsia, and eclampsia: These conditions can also increase the risk of vitamin B12 deficiency.
- Bariatric surgery: Certain weight loss surgeries, such as gastric bypass, can lead to reduced vitamin B12 absorption due to alterations in the digestive tract.
- Medication: Proton pump inhibitors (PPIs) and H2 blockers can also reduce stomach acid levels and hinder vitamin B12 absorption. Metformin, a medication used to manage diabetes, may reduce B12 levels in some individuals. Clinical manifestations of B12 depletion include pernicious anemia, usually due to a lack of intrinsic factor. Megoblastic anemia, another form of anemia associated with B12 deficiency, occurs when folate is in excess and insufficient B12 is present, creating a 'folate trap.' Dementia due to degeneration of myelin is another symptom of B12 deficiency. Methylmalonyl CoA is metabolized to methylmalonic acid (MMA) in B12 deficiency, making MMA the definitive marker for B12 deficiency. Achlorhydria (insufficient stomach acid) can lead to B12 deficiency because hydrochloric acid (HCl) is required to cleave B12 from intrinsic factor.

Many medications reduce the absorption of B12, including:
- Proton pump inhibitors (PPIs) (indirectly by reducing HCl required for Vitamin B12 release from food, but not supplements)
- Metformin (type 2 diabetes medication)
- Histamine 2 receptor antagonists
- Bile acid sequestrants (cholestyramine)
- Neomysin

Food Sources:
- Beef liver
- Clams
- Nutritional yeast
- Atlantic salmon
- Canned chunk light tuna
- Ground beef
- Milk
- Plain yogurt
- Fortified breakfast cereals

It's important to note that the B12 synthesized by gut bacteria may not be a significant source for humans since it's not absorbed in the colon.

Support considerations:
- Look to diet and lifestyle reasons for insufficiency, such as veganism, gastric bypass, celiac disease, medications, poor diet, etc.
- Increase food sources and supplement if appropriate. Preferred versions of B12 are methylcobalamin and adenosylcobalamin, which are metabolically active forms. Hydroxocobalamin may be better tolerated for sensitive clients. Cyanocobalamin is a synthetic form of Vitamin B12 that the body converts into Adenosylcobalamin and Methylcobalamin before it can be used.

Supplement Options:
- The RDA for B12 is 6 mcg/day.
- Consider the upper limit of folate supplementation as a factor for B12 supplementation, as it may lead to folate trap.
- Vitamin B12 is extremely safe. No toxicity from high doses of vitamin B12 has ever been reported.
- Intramuscular injections are often used, particularly in the elderly, to bypass intrinsic factor.
- Humans store large amounts of B12 in the liver, so larger doses can be given at 6-month intervals.
- Supplementation is highly encouraged on a vegan diet. Due to the liver's high storage capacity for B12, it may take years for the body to completely deplete its stores after adopting a vegan diet.

To address this, consider the following:

- Genetic factors: MTHFR genetic mutations and hyperhomocysteinemia may require methyl cobalamin supplementation.
- Methylcobalamin: It's the recommended form of supplementation, but it may be poorly absorbed by individuals taking antacids or those with poor absorption (e.g., celiac disease, intestinal permeability).
- Cyanocobalamin: It's not recommended for patients with MTHFR mutations.
- Hydroxocobalamin: It's recommended for patients with autoimmune diseases and elevated nitric oxide levels.
- Glutathione: It's essential for methylcobalamin to be adequately bound for transport.

Vitamin B12 supplementation may help manage various conditions, including anemia, asthma, fatigue, hepatitis, dementia, epilepsy, depression, psychosis, irritability, ataxia, numbness, tingling, neuropathy, AIDS, multiple sclerosis, tinnitus, and infertility.

Supplemental B12 is typically given in doses of 1000 to 5000 mcg.

Additionally, consider the following tests:
- Stool test to assess gut and digestive health and rule out inflammatory bowel disease (IBD).
- Celiac testing.
- Pernicious anemia testing.
- Genetic testing for MTHFR, MTR, MTRR, and other SNPs involved in methylation.

Nutritional support
- Vitamin B12
- Folate
- B Vitamins (B1, B2, B3, B5, B6, B7, B9)
- Vitamin B complex

If **HIGH** or **> 11.99 pg/MM WBC:**

Vitamin B12, when consumed in large quantities from food or supplements, has not been linked to any toxic or adverse effects in healthy individuals. However, when high doses are administered orally, only a small percentage can be absorbed, which may explain the relatively low toxicity associated with vitamin B12. Consequently, the US Food and Nutrition Board has not established a tolerable upper intake level (UL) for vitamin B12 due to its low toxicity.

While cobalamin toxicity can be unexpected and unusual, it's important to remember that the administration of any drug carries inherent risks. A case report serves as a reminder that even seemingly safe practices can have unforeseen consequences.

Excessive vitamin B12 levels are more commonly associated with high-dose supplementation or intravenous injections. A study published in the Journal of the American Medical Association (https://doi.org/10.1093/qjmed/hcz164) found that high or supraphysiological serum B12 levels without supplementation have been linked to various pathological conditions, including renal failure, hematological disorders, cancer, and hepatic or autoimmune diseases. These conditions often exhibit elevated concentrations of B12 transport proteins. Additionally, there may be an increased release of B12 in liver disease due to hepatic cytolysis and/or reduced B12 clearance. Consequently, a high or supraphysiological serum B12 concentration without supplementation could serve as a diagnostic marker for severe underlying disease. Furthermore, very high serum B12 levels have been frequently reported in critically ill patients.

Polycythemia Vera, a rare blood cancer that causes the bone marrow to produce an excessive number of red blood cells, can also lead to elevated B12 levels. Elevated serum B12 levels may also be associated with a functional deficiency of the vitamin due to a failure of cellular uptake, intracellular processing, trafficking, or utilization.

Vitamin B2 (Serum)

Two critical coenzymes involved in energy metabolism are derived from riboflavin to participate in oxidation/reduction reactions. Riboflavin is also essential for the enzymes nitric oxide synthase (NOS) and glutathione reductase, the latter of which regenerates glutathione and is crucial for antioxidation/detoxification.

Optimal Range	82.6 - 126.1 mcg/L

If **LOW** or **< 82.6 mcg/L:**

Inadequate intake is the primary cause of riboflavin depletion. Malabsorption disorders, such as celiac disease and Crohn's disease, can hinder absorption due to intestinal inflammation and damage. Alcoholism and certain medications, including antidepressants and antipsychotics, can also interfere with riboflavin absorption and utilization.

While riboflavin deficiency is rare in developed countries, marginal deficiency is common. Deficiency is associated with fatigue and weakness. Dietary deficiency can lead to lesions on the lips and the angles of the mouth, fissured and magenta-colored tongue, corneal vascularization, and normocytic, normochromic anemia. Skin lesions may include red, scaly, greasy patches on the nose, eyelids, scrotum, and labia, as well as seborrheic dermatitis.

Serum levels deficient and cellular normal indicate that long-term nutrient status is optimal, but short-term needs improvement. Conversely, serum levels deficient and cellular deficient suggest that both short-term and long-term micronutrient status is not optimal, implying low dietary intake and either intestinal or cellular malabsorption as possible causes.

To address riboflavin deficiency, interventions can include increasing dietary intake of the nutrient, increasing supplementation dosage, and considering the potential impact of medications on depletion. If serum levels are deficient and cellular deficient, follow-up testing may be necessary to identify the source of malabsorption.

Medications that reduce riboflavin levels include oral contraceptives, tricyclic antidepressants, anti-psychotic medications such as chlorpromazine, anti-malarial medications like quinacrine, and chemotherapy agents like adriamycin.

Food Sources:
- Beef liver
- Fortified breakfast cereals, oats
- Yogurt
- Milk
- Clams
- Almonds
- Swiss cheese

Support Considerations:
- Increase food sources
- Reduce alcohol consumption
- Consider supplementation

Supplement Options:
- The RDA for riboflavin is 1.7 mg/day.
- Common therapeutic levels of riboflavin are 25-50 mg/day.
- There is no UL for riboflavin.

Additional Investigations:
- Stool test to assess gut and digestive health and rule out IBD
- Celiac testing

Nutritional support includes:
- Riboflavin (Vitamin B2)
- B Vitamins
- Vitamin B complex
- Iron
- Copper
- Magnesium

If HIGH or > 126.1 mcg/L:

Most riboflavin is immediately used by the body and not stored, so any excess is excreted in urine. High riboflavin intakes from foods or supplements up to 400 mg daily for at least three months are generally safe and do not cause adverse effects. No cases of riboflavin toxicity in humans have been reported.

However, consuming large quantities of foods fortified with riboflavin, such as breakfast cereals, or taking high doses of riboflavin supplements above the recommended levels can lead to elevated riboflavin levels in the body. Excess dietary riboflavin, usually from supplements, can cause urine to become bright yellow.

For more information, refer to the following reference: https://www.ncbi.nlm.nih.gov/books/NBK525977/

 Stop or reduce B2 supplementation / sources

Vitamin B2 (Cellular)

Two critical coenzymes involved in energy metabolism are derived from riboflavin to participate in oxidation/reduction reactions. Riboflavin is also essential for the enzymes nitric oxide synthase (NOS) and glutathione reductase, the latter of which regenerates glutathione and is crucial for antioxidation/detoxification.

Optimal Range	0.2 - 3.6 pg/MM WBC

If LOW or < 0.2 pg/MM WBC:

Inadequate intake is the primary cause of riboflavin depletion. Malabsorption disorders, such as celiac disease and Crohn's disease, can hinder absorption due to intestinal inflammation and damage. Alcoholism and certain medications, including antidepressants and antipsychotics, can also interfere with riboflavin absorption and utilization.

While riboflavin deficiency is rare in developed countries, marginal deficiency is common. Deficiency is associated with fatigue and weakness. Dietary deficiency can lead to lesions on the lips and the angles of the mouth, fissured and magenta-colored tongue, corneal vascularization, and normocytic, normochromic anemia. Skin lesions may include red, scaly, greasy patches on the nose, eyelids, scrotum, and labia, as well as seborrheic dermatitis.

Serum levels deficient and cellular normal indicate that long-term nutrient status is optimal, but short-term needs improvement. Conversely, serum levels deficient and cellular deficient suggest that both short-term and long-term micronutrient status is not optimal, implying low dietary intake and either intestinal or cellular malabsorption as possible causes.

To address riboflavin deficiency, interventions can include increasing dietary intake of the nutrient, increasing supplementation dosage, and considering the potential impact of medications on depletion. If serum levels are deficient and cellular deficient, follow-up testing may be necessary to identify the source of malabsorption.

Medications that reduce riboflavin levels include oral contraceptives, tricyclic antidepressants, anti-psychotic medications such as chlorpromazine, anti-malarial medications like quinacrine, and chemotherapy agents like adriamycin.

 Food Sources:
- Beef liver
- Fortified breakfast cereals, oats
- Yogurt
- Milk
- Clams
- Almonds
- Swiss cheese

Support Considerations:
- Increase food sources
- Reduce alcohol consumption
- Consider supplementation

Supplement Options:
- The RDA for riboflavin is 1.7 mg/day.
- Common therapeutic levels of riboflavin are 25-50 mg/day.
- There is no UL for riboflavin.

Additional Investigations:
- Stool test to assess gut and digestive health and rule out IBD
- Celiac testing

Nutritional support includes:
- Riboflavin (Vitamin B2)
- B Vitamins
- Vitamin B complex
- Iron
- Copper
- Magnesium

If **HIGH** or **> 3.6 pg/MM WBC:**

Most riboflavin is immediately used by the body and not stored, so any excess is excreted in urine. High riboflavin intakes from foods or supplements up to 400 mg daily for at least three months are generally safe and do not cause adverse effects. No cases of riboflavin toxicity in humans have been reported.

However, consuming large quantities of foods fortified with riboflavin, such as breakfast cereals, or taking high doses of riboflavin supplements above the recommended levels can lead to elevated riboflavin levels in the body. Excess dietary riboflavin, usually from supplements, can cause urine to become bright yellow.

For more information, refer to the following reference: https://www.ncbi.nlm.nih.gov/books/NBK525977/

Stop or reduce B2 supplementation / sources

Vitamin B3 (Serum)

Vitamin B3 (Niacin) plays a crucial role in metabolic reduction reactions through NAD-NADPH pathways. Over 200 enzymes in the human body require niacin for various functions. It is involved in fatty acid synthesis, ATP synthesis, DNA repair, cholesterol/LDL reduction, and circulation enhancement. Niacin is frequently prescribed therapeutically for lipid management. Numerous studies have demonstrated that niacin can lower LDL cholesterol, lipoprotein(a), triglyceride, and fibrinogen levels while simultaneously increasing HDL levels. However, high doses of niacin may cause flushing. Aspirin has been shown to help reduce flushing symptoms. Time-release niacin or no-flush niacin are not recommended for therapeutic treatment due to the risk of flushing. Individuals taking high doses of niacin should closely monitor their liver function.

Optimal Range	2.6 - 36.1 ng/mL

If LOW or < 2.6 ng/mL:

 Niacin, a B vitamin, can be synthesized from tryptophan through the kynurenine pathway. It requires iron, B6, and riboflavin as cofactors. Deficiencies in these nutrients may be underlying causes of niacin depletion. Additionally, inflammation in the kynurenine pathway, driven by high quinolinic acid levels, can decrease NAD synthesis.

Inadequate niacin intake can lead to malabsorption disorders, such as celiac disease and Crohn's disease. Intestinal inflammation and damage can hinder absorption. Medications like isoniazid, used for tuberculosis treatment, can inhibit the conversion of tryptophan to niacin, potentially leading to lower niacin levels. Alcoholism can result in poor dietary intake and impaired niacin absorption, contributing to a deficiency.

Long-term inadequate niacin intake can lead to pellagra, a condition characterized by niacin deficiency. It often occurs in regions with limited dietary diversity and reliance on corn-based diets.

Clinical manifestations of niacin depletion include vomiting, constipation, red tongue, headache, fatigue, and depression. Severe niacin deficiency is called pellagra. Pellagra is commonly accompanied by the four Ds: dermatitis, diarrhea, dementia, and death.

If both cellular and serum levels of niacin are low, it suggests a low dietary intake and possible causes include intestinal and cellular absorption issues.

Recommended interventions include increasing dietary intake of niacin and supplementation dosage. Medications may also have an effect on depletion. Consider follow-up testing to identify the source of malabsorption.

Medications interactions related to niacin include:
- Niacin may reduce the effectiveness of sulfinpyrazone (a medication for gout).
- Oral contraceptives may decrease dietary requirements.
- Long-term chemotherapy use may cause niacin depletion.

 Food Sources:
- Beef liver
- Chicken breast
- Marinara
- Turkey breast
- Salmon
- Tuna
- Pork
- Brown rice
- Peanuts
- Fortified breakfast cereal

Support Considerations:
- Increase food sources
- Reduce alcohol consumption
- Consider supplementation

If serum and cellular levels are low, it suggests low dietary intake and possible causes include intestinal and cellular absorption issues.

Recommended Interventions:
- Increase dietary intake of nutrients
- Increase supplementation dosage
- Reduce alcohol consumption
- Assess iron, B6, and riboflavin (B2) status
- Medications may contribute to depletion
- Consider follow-up testing to identify the source of malabsorption.

Supplement Options:
- The RDA for niacin is 20 mg/day.
- The UL for niacin is 35 mg/day, but oral administration of up to 6g per day has been used without side effects.
- Niacin is often recommended therapeutically for lipid management. It has been shown to lower LDL cholesterol, lipoprotein(a), triglyceride, and fibrinogen levels while raising HDL levels. However, flushing can occur at high doses. Aspirin may help reduce flushing. Time-release niacin or no-flush niacin is not recommended for therapeutic treatment. Monitor liver function carefully with high-dose niacin supplementation.

Additional Investigations:
- Stool test to assess gut and digestive health and rule out IBD
- Celiac testing

Nutritional support
- Niacin (as Nicotinic Acid)
- B Vitamins
- Vitamin B complex

If **HIGH** or > 36.1 ng/mL:

The tolerable upper intake level (UL) for niacin in adults is 35 mg per day, based on flushing as the primary adverse effect. Excessive niacin intake, often exceeding the recommended levels, can lead to elevated niacin levels in the body.

Niacin therapy, where high doses are prescribed for specific medical conditions like high cholesterol, can also result in elevated niacin levels. Additionally, energy drinks often contain significant amounts of vitamins, including niacin.

While the amount of niacin found in food is generally safe and does not cause side effects, taking high doses of niacin as a supplement can lead to adverse effects. These include:
- Flushed or itchy skin
- Nausea
- Vomiting
- Constipation
- Headache
- Rash
- Dizziness

Excess vitamin B-3 can also have the following effects:
- Reduced glucose tolerance and insulin resistance
- Triggered gout attacks in individuals with the condition
- Eye problems
- Gastrointestinal issues
- Increased risk of liver damage

- Lower blood pressure, which can lead to a loss of balance and an increased risk of falls

Flushing can occur at high doses. Aspirin may help reduce flushing. Time-release niacin or no-flush niacin is not recommended for therapeutic treatment.

It's important to monitor liver function carefully when supplementing with high doses of niacin.

Additionally, there's a correlation between serum and cellular levels of niacin. If the cellular level is low while the serum level is normal or excessive, it may indicate an optimal status of micro-nutrients in the short term, but cellular absorption may be a problem.

In such cases, interventions may include:
- Increasing dietary intake of nutrients
- Increasing supplementation dosage
- Considering the status of synergistic nutrients for cellular absorption
- Assessing levels of oxidative stress related to nutrient depletion
- Conducting follow-up testing to identify the source of nutrient absorption issues.

Stop or reduce vitamin B3 supplementation / sources
Monitor liver function carefully with high dose Niacin supplementation

Vitamin B3 (Cellular)

Vitamin B3 (Niacin) plays a crucial role in metabolic reduction reactions through NAD-NADPH pathways. Over 200 enzymes in the human body require niacin for various functions. It is involved in fatty acid synthesis, ATP synthesis, DNA repair, cholesterol/LDL reduction, and circulation enhancement. Niacin is frequently prescribed therapeutically for lipid management. Numerous studies have demonstrated that niacin can lower LDL cholesterol, lipoprotein(a), triglyceride, and fibrinogen levels while simultaneously increasing HDL levels. However, high doses of niacin may cause flushing. Aspirin has been shown to help reduce flushing symptoms. Time-release niacin or no-flush niacin are not recommended for therapeutic treatment due to the risk of flushing. Individuals taking high doses of niacin should closely monitor their liver function.

| Optimal Range | 39.6 - 303.5 pg/MM WBC |

If LOW or < 39.6 pg/MM WBC:

Niacin, a B vitamin, can be synthesized from tryptophan through the kynurenine pathway. It requires iron, B6, and riboflavin as cofactors. Deficiencies in these nutrients may be underlying causes of niacin depletion. Additionally, inflammation in the kynurenine pathway, driven by high quinolinic acid levels, can decrease NAD synthesis.

Inadequate niacin intake can lead to malabsorption disorders, such as celiac disease and Crohn's disease. Intestinal inflammation and damage can hinder absorption. Medications like isoniazid, used for tuberculosis treatment, can inhibit the conversion of tryptophan to niacin, potentially leading to lower niacin levels. Alcoholism can result in poor dietary intake and impaired niacin absorption, contributing to a deficiency.

Long-term inadequate niacin intake can lead to pellagra, a condition characterized by niacin deficiency. It often occurs in regions with limited dietary diversity and reliance on corn-based diets.

Clinical manifestations of niacin depletion include vomiting, constipation, red tongue, headache, fatigue, and depression. Severe niacin deficiency is called pellagra. Pellagra is commonly accompanied by the four Ds: dermatitis, diarrhea, dementia, and death.

If both cellular and serum levels of niacin are low, it suggests a low dietary intake and possible causes include intestinal and cellular absorption issues.

Recommended interventions include increasing dietary intake of niacin and supplementation dosage. Medications may also have an effect on depletion. Consider follow-up testing to identify the source of malabsorption.

Medications interactions related to niacin include:
- Niacin may reduce the effectiveness of sulfinpyrazone (a medication for gout).
- Oral contraceptives may decrease dietary requirements.
- Long-term chemotherapy use may cause niacin depletion.

Food Sources:
- Beef liver
- Chicken breast
- Marinara
- Turkey breast
- Salmon
- Tuna
- Pork
- Brown rice
- Peanuts
- Fortified breakfast cereal

Support Considerations:
- Increase food sources
- Reduce alcohol consumption
- Consider supplementation

If serum and cellular levels are low, it suggests low dietary intake and possible causes include intestinal and cellular absorption issues.

Recommended Interventions:
- Increase dietary intake of nutrients
- Increase supplementation dosage
- Reduce alcohol consumption
- Assess iron, B6, and riboflavin (B2) status
- Medications may contribute to depletion
- Consider follow-up testing to identify the source of malabsorption.

Supplement Options:
- The RDA for niacin is 20 mg/day.
- The UL for niacin is 35 mg/day, but oral administration of up to 6g per day has been used without side effects.
- Niacin is often recommended therapeutically for lipid management. It has been shown to lower LDL cholesterol, lipoprotein(a), triglyceride, and fibrinogen levels while raising HDL levels. However, flushing can occur at high doses. Aspirin may help reduce flushing. Time-release niacin or no-flush niacin is not recommended for therapeutic treatment. Monitor liver function carefully with high-dose niacin supplementation.

Additional Investigations:
- Stool test to assess gut and digestive health and rule out IBD
- Celiac testing

Nutritional support
- Niacin (as Nicotinic Acid)
- B Vitamins
- Vitamin B complex

If **HIGH** or **> 303.5 pg/MM WBC:**

The tolerable upper intake level (UL) for niacin in adults is 35 mg per day, based on flushing as the primary adverse effect. Excessive niacin intake, often exceeding the recommended levels, can lead to elevated niacin levels in the body.

Niacin therapy, where high doses are prescribed for specific medical conditions like high cholesterol, can also result in elevated niacin levels. Additionally, energy drinks often contain significant amounts of vitamins, including niacin.

While the amount of niacin found in food is generally safe and does not cause side effects, taking high doses of niacin as a supplement can lead to adverse effects. These include:
- Flushed or itchy skin
- Nausea
- Vomiting
- Constipation
- Headache
- Rash
- Dizziness

Excess vitamin B-3 can also have the following effects:
- Reduced glucose tolerance and insulin resistance
- Triggered gout attacks in individuals with the condition
- Eye problems
- Gastrointestinal issues
- Increased risk of liver damage
- Lower blood pressure, which can lead to a loss of balance and an increased risk of falls

Flushing can occur at high doses. Aspirin may help reduce flushing. Time-release niacin or no-flush niacin is not recommended for therapeutic treatment.

It's important to monitor liver function carefully when supplementing with high doses of niacin.

Additionally, there's a correlation between serum and cellular levels of niacin. If the cellular level is low while the serum level is normal or excessive, it may indicate an optimal status of micro-nutrients in the short term, but cellular absorption may be a problem.

In such cases, interventions may include:
- Increasing dietary intake of nutrients
- Increasing supplementation dosage
- Considering the status of synergistic nutrients for cellular absorption
- Assessing levels of oxidative stress related to nutrient depletion
- Conducting follow-up testing to identify the source of nutrient absorption issues.

Stop or reduce vitamin B3 supplementation / sources
Monitor liver function carefully with high dose Niacin supplementation

Vitamin B5 (Serum)

Vitamin B5 (Pantothenic Acid) plays a crucial role in the structural composition of coenzyme A. It is also essential for the synthesis of red blood cells, sex hormones, adrenal hormones, and vitamin D. Notably, B5 significantly contributes to the collaboration of carnitine and CoQ10 in fatty acid oxidation and metabolism.

| Optimal Range | 22.7 - 429.2 mcg/L |

If **LOW** or **< 22.7 mcg/L:**

How Vitamin B5 Depletion Occurs:
- Inadequate intake: Deficiency of B5 is very rare, however, in a diet that is high in biotin, or if high dose biotin supplementation occurs, B5 may become conditionally deficient due to competition for the same uptake receptor in the intestine.
- Malabsorption Disorders (e.g., celiac disease, Crohn's): intestinal inflammation and damage can hinder absorption.
- Alcoholism can lead to poor dietary intake and impaired B5 absorption, contributing to a deficiency.
- Clinical Manifestations of Depletion: Rare but may include fatigue, insomnia, depression, irritability, vomiting, stomach pains, burning feet, and upper respiratory infections.
- Diet/Medication Interactions: Medications that reduce pantothenic acid include oral contraceptives

Food Sources:
- Beef liver
- Fortified breakfast cereal
- Shiitake mushrooms
- Sunflower seeds
- Chicken breast
- Tuna
- Avocado

Support Considerations:
- Increase food sources
- Reduce alcohol consumption
- Consider supplementation

There is currently no Recommended Dietary Allowance (RDA) established for B5. The Adequate Intake (AI) for B5 is 5 mg/day in adults, 6 mg/day during pregnancy, and 7 mg/day during lactation. Since the breakdown of B5 is slow, and deficiency is rare, supplementation is rarely necessary.

Serum levels deficient and cellular levels are normal: Long-term nutrient status is optimal, but short-term needs improvement.

Serum levels deficient and cellular levels are deficient: Short-term and long-term status of micronutrients is not optimal, suggesting low dietary intake and both intestinal and cellular malabsorption as possible causes.

Possible interventions:
- Increase dietary intake of the nutrient
- Increase supplementation dosage
- Medications may have an effect on depletion
- Consider follow-up testing to identify the source of malabsorption

Additional Investigations:
- Stool test to assess gut and digestive health and rule out Inflammatory Bowel Disease (IBD)
- Celiac testing

Nutritional support:
- Pantothenic Acid (Vitamin B5)
- Vitamin B Complex
- Magnesium Taurinate
- Magnesium Glycinate
- Magnesium Malate

If **HIGH** or > 429.2 mcg/L:

There are currently no upper limits established for vitamin B5 intake since there have been no reports of toxicity in humans with high consumption. However, some individuals taking large doses of pantothenic acid supplements (e.g., 10 to 20 g/day) may experience mild diarrhea and gastrointestinal distress. The mechanism behind this effect is still unknown.

Additionally, excessive consumption of fortified foods or pantothenic acid-containing supplements can lead to elevated pantothenic acid levels in the body. Similarly, taking high doses of pantothenic acid supplements, often exceeding the recommended levels, can also result in elevated levels.

In medical settings, high doses of pantothenic acid may be used for specific conditions, which can also lead to elevated levels. Furthermore, certain rare genetic conditions (e.g., Pantothenate Kinase-Associated Neurodegeneration) can disrupt pantothenic acid metabolism, potentially causing elevated levels.

Stop or reduce vitamin B5 supplementation or sources. With very large daily doses of 10 grams, stomach upset or mild diarrhea has been reported. However, this is rare, and a Tolerable Upper Intake Level for pantothenic acid has not been established.

Correlation between serum and WBC ("Cellular") levels: Serum levels are normal or excess, while WBC levels are deficient. In the short term, micronutrient status is optimal, but cellular absorption may be a problem.

Possible interventions:
- Increase dietary intake of the nutrient
- Increase supplementation dosage
- Consider the status of synergistic nutrients for cellular absorption
- Consider levels of oxidative stress on nutrient depletion
- Consider follow-up testing to identify the source of malabsorption

Vitamin B5 (Cellular)

Vitamin B5 (Pantothenic Acid) plays a crucial role in the structural composition of coenzyme A. It is also essential for the synthesis of red blood cells, sex hormones, adrenal hormones, and vitamin D. Notably, B5 significantly contributes to the collaboration of carnitine and CoQ10 in fatty acid oxidation and metabolism.

Optimal Range	2.5 - 32.8 pg/MM WBC

If LOW or < 2.5 pg/MM WBC:

How Vitamin B5 Depletion Occurs:
- Inadequate intake: Deficiency of B5 is very rare, however, in a diet that is high in biotin, or if high dose biotin supplementation occurs, B5 may become conditionally deficient due to competition for the same uptake receptor in the intestine.
- Malabsorption Disorders (e.g., celiac disease, Crohn's): intestinal inflammation and damage can hinder absorption.
- Alcoholism can lead to poor dietary intake and impaired B5 absorption, contributing to a deficiency.
- Clinical Manifestations of Depletion: Rare but may include fatigue, insomnia, depression, irritability, vomiting, stomach pains, burning feet, and upper respiratory infections.
- Diet/Medication Interactions: Medications that reduce pantothenic acid include oral contraceptives

Food Sources:
- Beef liver
- Fortified breakfast cereal
- Shiitake mushrooms
- Sunflower seeds
- Chicken breast
- Tuna
- Avocado

Support Considerations:
- Increase food sources
- Reduce alcohol consumption
- Consider supplementation

There is currently no Recommended Dietary Allowance (RDA) established for B5. The Adequate Intake (AI) for B5 is 5 mg/day in adults, 6 mg/day during pregnancy, and 7 mg/day during lactation. Since the breakdown of B5 is slow, and deficiency is rare, supplementation is rarely necessary.

Serum levels deficient and cellular levels are normal: Long-term nutrient status is optimal, but short-term needs improvement.

Serum levels deficient and cellular levels are deficient: Short-term and long-term status of micronutrients is not optimal, suggesting low dietary intake and both intestinal and cellular malabsorption as possible causes.

Possible interventions:
- Increase dietary intake of the nutrient
- Increase supplementation dosage
- Medications may have an effect on depletion

- Consider follow-up testing to identify the source of malabsorption

Additional Investigations:
- Stool test to assess gut and digestive health and rule out Inflammatory Bowel Disease (IBD)
- Celiac testing

Nutritional support:
- Pantothenic Acid (Vitamin B5)
- Vitamin B Complex
- Magnesium Taurinate
- Magnesium Glycinate
- Magnesium Malate

If HIGH or > 32.8 pg/MM WBC:

There are currently no upper limits established for vitamin B5 intake since there have been no reports of toxicity in humans with high consumption. However, some individuals taking large doses of pantothenic acid supplements (e.g., 10 to 20 g/day) may experience mild diarrhea and gastrointestinal distress. The mechanism behind this effect is still unknown.

Additionally, excessive consumption of fortified foods or pantothenic acid-containing supplements can lead to elevated pantothenic acid levels in the body. Similarly, taking high doses of pantothenic acid supplements, often exceeding the recommended levels, can also result in elevated levels.

In medical settings, high doses of pantothenic acid may be used for specific conditions, which can also lead to elevated levels. Furthermore, certain rare genetic conditions (e.g., Pantothenate Kinase-Associated Neurodegeneration) can disrupt pantothenic acid metabolism, potentially causing elevated levels.

Stop or reduce vitamin B5 supplementation or sources. With very large daily doses of 10 grams, stomach upset or mild diarrhea has been reported. However, this is rare, and a Tolerable Upper Intake Level for pantothenic acid has not been established.

Correlation between serum and WBC ("Cellular") levels: Serum levels are normal or excess, while WBC levels are deficient. In the short term, micronutrient status is optimal, but cellular absorption may be a problem.

Possible interventions:
- Increase dietary intake of the nutrient
- Increase supplementation dosage
- Consider the status of synergistic nutrients for cellular absorption
- Consider levels of oxidative stress on nutrient depletion
- Consider follow-up testing to identify the source of malabsorption

Vitamin B6 (Serum)

Vitamin B6, also known as Pyrodoxine, is a water-soluble vitamin that plays a crucial role in various metabolic functions. It is involved in the production of 117 known vitamin B6-dependent enzymes, most of which are aminotransferase reactions essential for protein metabolism. Additionally, Vitamin B6 aids in the absorption of Vitamin B12 and converts tryptophan into serotonin, which can regulate steroid hormone activity. Furthermore, Vitamin B6 participates in the methylation cycle and helps clear homocysteine, along with folate and B12.

| Optimal Range | 2.8 - 76.2 ng/mL |

If LOW or < 2.8 ng/mL:

 Inadequate intake is the most common cause of vitamin B6 depletion. Malabsorption disorders, such as celiac disease and Crohn's disease, can also contribute to low levels due to intestinal inflammation and damage that hinders absorption. Certain medications, including isoniazid used for tuberculosis treatment and penicillamine used for Wilson's disease, can interfere with vitamin B6 metabolism and lead to low levels. Renal impairment, particularly in chronic renal failure patients on hemodialysis or peritoneal dialysis, can also cause low serum pyridoxal-5'-phosphate (PLP) concentrations and symptoms of vitamin B6 deficiency. Autoimmune disorders, such as rheumatoid arthritis, increase the body's need for vitamin B6 due to increased catabolism.

Other factors that can contribute to vitamin B6 depletion include malabsorption in the gastrointestinal tract due to gastrointestinal diseases, diabetes, chronic alcoholism, sickle cell disease, kidney stones containing oxalates, kidney dialysis, rheumatoid arthritis, and liver cancer.

Clinical manifestations of vitamin B6 depletion include irritability, depression, confusion, an inflamed tongue, skin disorders, mouth sores, sores at the corners of the mouth, morning sickness in pregnant mothers, and premenstrual syndrome (PMS). Chronic inflammation, which can occur when vitamin B6 levels are low, may be associated with various conditions, including cancer, heart disease, PMS, carpal tunnel syndrome, and dementia. When there is a vitamin B6 deficiency, homocysteine levels rise, increasing the risk of heart disease.

Diet and medication interactions can also affect vitamin B6 levels. Oral contraceptives may interfere with vitamin B6 metabolism, while anti-tuberculosis medications (isoniazid and cycloserine) and metal chelators and anti-Parkinson's drugs (L-Dopa) can form complexes with B6 and reduce its bioavailability. Long-term use of nonsteroidal anti-inflammatory drugs (NSAIDs) may also deplete vitamin B6 levels. High doses of vitamin B6 supplementation can decrease the effectiveness of certain medications, such as phenobarbital, phenytoin, and L-Dopa anticonvulsant therapy.

Food Sources:
- Chickpeas
- Beef liver
- Yellowfin tuna
- Sockeye salmon
- Chicken breast
- Fortified breakfast cereal
- Potatoes
- Turkey
- Banana

Support Considerations:
- Increase food sources.
- Consider supplementation.

Supplement Options:
- The recommended daily intake of vitamin B6 for adults is 1.4 mg for women and 1.6 mg for men.
- Daily vitamin B6 intake should not exceed 25 mg. An intake of 50 mg/day is associated with neurological side effects.

Additional Investigations:
- Stool test to assess gut and digestive health and rule out IBD.
- Celiac testing.
- Genetic testing.
- Impairments in methylation, transsulfuration, and biopterin (neurotransmitter) pathways may impact the need for B6.

Nutritional support
- Vitamin B6
- B Vitamins
- Magnesium

If HIGH or > 76.2 ng/mL:

A major metabolite of vitamin B6. High pyridoxic acid indicates high recent intake of vitamin B6. Because some individuals may require very high doses of vitamin B6, high values do not necessarily indicate the need to reduce vitamin B6 intake.

Stop or reduce vitamin B6 supplementation / sources
Daily vitamin B6 intake should not exceed 25 mg as an intake of 50 mg/day is associated with neurological side effects. Elevated plasma vitamin B6 levels are associated with sensory and peripheral neuropathy, leading to progressive sensory ataxia, unstable gait, numbness of the hands and absent tendon reflexes.

Vitamin B6 (Cellular)

Vitamin B6, also known as Pyrodoxine, is a water-soluble vitamin that plays a crucial role in various metabolic functions. It is involved in the production of 117 known vitamin B6-dependent enzymes, most of which are aminotransferase reactions essential for protein metabolism. Additionally, Vitamin B6 aids in the absorption of Vitamin B12 and converts tryptophan into serotonin, which can regulate steroid hormone activity. Furthermore, Vitamin B6 participates in the methylation cycle and helps clear homocysteine, along with folate and B12.

Optimal Range	0.5 - 9.7 pg/MM WBC

If LOW or < 0.5 pg/MM WBC:

Inadequate intake is the most common cause of vitamin B6 depletion. Malabsorption disorders, such as celiac disease and Crohn's disease, can also contribute to low levels due to intestinal inflammation and damage that hinders absorption. Certain medications, including isoniazid used for tuberculosis treatment and penicillamine used for Wilson's disease, can interfere with vitamin B6 metabolism and lead to low levels. Renal impairment, particularly in chronic renal failure patients on hemodialysis or peritoneal dialysis, can also cause low serum pyridoxal-5'-phosphate (PLP) concentrations and symptoms of vitamin B6 deficiency. Autoimmune disorders, such as rheumatoid arthritis, increase the body's need for vitamin B6 due to increased catabolism.

Other factors that can contribute to vitamin B6 depletion include malabsorption in the gastrointestinal tract due to gastrointestinal diseases, diabetes, chronic alcoholism, sickle cell disease, kidney stones containing oxalates, kidney dialysis, rheumatoid arthritis, and liver cancer.

Clinical manifestations of vitamin B6 depletion include irritability, depression, confusion, an inflamed tongue, skin disorders, mouth sores, sores at the corners of the mouth, morning sickness in pregnant mothers, and premenstrual syndrome (PMS). Chronic inflammation, which can occur when vitamin B6 levels are low, may be associated with various conditions, including cancer, heart disease, PMS, carpal tunnel syndrome, and dementia. When there is a vitamin B6 deficiency, homocysteine levels rise, increasing the risk of heart disease.

Diet and medication interactions can also affect vitamin B6 levels. Oral contraceptives may interfere with vitamin B6 metabolism, while anti-tuberculosis medications (isoniazid and cycloserine) and metal chelators and anti-Parkinson's drugs (L-Dopa) can form complexes with B6 and reduce its bioavailability. Long-term use of nonsteroidal anti-inflammatory drugs (NSAIDs) may also deplete vitamin B6 levels. High doses of vitamin B6 supplementation can decrease the effectiveness of certain medications, such as phenobarbital, phenytoin, and L-Dopa anticonvulsant therapy.

Food Sources:
- Chickpeas
- Beef liver
- Yellowfin tuna
- Sockeye salmon
- Chicken breast
- Fortified breakfast cereal
- Potatoes
- Turkey
- Banana

Support Considerations:
- Increase food sources.
- Consider supplementation.

Supplement Options:
- The recommended daily intake of vitamin B6 for adults is 1.4 mg for women and 1.6 mg for men.
- Daily vitamin B6 intake should not exceed 25 mg. An intake of 50 mg/day is associated with neurological side effects.

Additional Investigations:
- Stool test to assess gut and digestive health and rule out IBD.
- Celiac testing.
- Genetic testing.
- Impairments in methylation, transsulfuration, and biopterin (neurotransmitter) pathways may impact the need for B6.

Nutritional support
- Vitamin B6
- B Vitamins
- Magnesium

If HIGH or > 9.7 pg/MM WBC:

A major metabolite of vitamin B6. High pyridoxic acid indicates high recent intake of vitamin B6. Because some individuals may require very high doses of vitamin B6, high values do not necessarily indicate the need to reduce vitamin B6 intake.

Stop or reduce vitamin B6 supplementation / sources
Daily vitamin B6 intake should not exceed 25 mg as an intake of 50 mg/day is associated with neurological side effects. Elevated plasma vitamin B6 levels are associated with sensory and peripheral neuropathy, leading to progressive sensory ataxia, unstable gait, numbness of the hands and absent tendon reflexes.

Vitamin C (Serum)

Vitamin C, or Ascorbic Acid, plays a crucial role as an antioxidant. It enhances immunity by increasing the production of white blood cells and supports the regeneration of vitamin E. Additionally, Vitamin C helps reduce the risk of atherosclerosis, stroke, high blood pressure, and inflammation. Furthermore, it is essential for optimal collagen production, as it contributes to the generation of connective tissue. Vitamin C is also an integral component of L-carnitine, which is crucial for metabolizing fats into energy.

| Optimal Range | 0.8 - 1.7 mg/dL |

If LOW or < 0.8 mg/dL:

Vitamin C is most commonly depleted due to inadequate dietary intake. The body's vitamin C pool typically depletes within 4 to 12 days. Ascorbic acid is affected by various factors that can impair its absorption and functions. Regular consumption of fruits and vegetables is the most effective way to prevent vitamin C deficiency. Vitamin C levels can also be depleted during severe oxidative stress, as it is a cofactor required for both catecholamine biosynthesis and adrenal steroidogenesis.

Clinical manifestations of vitamin C depletion include reduced bone density, bleeding gums, easy bruising, anemia, fatigue, weakness, and joint pain. These symptoms result from weakened or deficient connective tissues throughout the body. Severe cases of vitamin C deficiency are known as scurvy.

Medications that can lower vitamin C levels include oral contraceptives and aspirin, especially when used frequently.

Food Sources:
- Red and green sweet peppers
- Oranges
- Grapefruit
- Kiwifruit
- Broccoli
- Strawberries
- Brussels sprouts
- Tomatoes
- Cantaloupe
- Cabbage
- Cauliflower

Support Considerations:
- Increase food sources.
- Consider supplementation.

Supplement Options:
- The recommended daily intake of vitamin C is 75 mg for women and 90 mg for men. During pregnancy and lactation, the intake should be 120 mg/day.

- Vitamin C has a half-life of about 30 minutes in circulation after supplementation, so large, single doses may not be as effective as smaller, more frequent doses.
- In addition to taking supplemental vitamin C, α-Lipoic acid can help restore vitamin C levels when depleted.

Correlation between Serum and Cellular Levels:
- Serum levels are deficient, but cellular levels are normal.
- Long-term nutrient status is optimal, but short-term needs improvement.
- Possible interventions include increasing dietary intake of nutrients, increasing supplementation dosage, and considering medications that may have an effect on depletion.

Serum levels are deficient and cellular levels are deficient:
- Short-term and long-term status of micronutrients is not optimal, suggesting low dietary intake and both intestinal and cellular malabsorption as possible causes.
- Possible interventions include increasing dietary intake of nutrients, increasing supplementation dosage, considering medications that may have an effect on depletion, and considering follow-up testing to identify the source of malabsorption.

Nutritional support:
- Vitamin C
- Magnesium taurinate
- Magnesium glycinate
- Magnesium malate

If **HIGH** or **> 1.7 mg/dL:**

Vitamin C, a water-soluble vitamin, is not considered toxic and lacks a known toxic level. It is commonly administered intravenously to treat various conditions without causing any adverse effects. To ensure the safety of generally healthy adults, a tolerable upper intake level (UL) of 2 grams (2,000 milligrams) per day has been established. This level is set to prevent diarrhea and gastrointestinal disturbances, which are usually not severe and resolve with temporary discontinuation of vitamin C supplementation.

While several potential adverse health effects of extremely high vitamin C doses have been suggested, primarily based on in vitro experiments or isolated case reports, none have been conclusively proven. These effects include genetic mutations, congenital disabilities, cancer, atherosclerosis, kidney stones (and possibly increased oxalates), "rebound scurvy," increased oxidative stress, excess iron absorption, vitamin B12 deficiency, and dental enamel erosion.

However, it's important to note that none of these alleged adverse effects have been consistently replicated in subsequent studies. Therefore, there is no reliable scientific evidence to support the claim that doses of vitamin C up to 10 grams per day in adults are toxic or detrimental to health.

Vitamin C supplementation or sources should be stopped or reduced. Intake of more than 1-2 grams of vitamin C can cause loose stools in some individuals. In those with a glucose-6-phosphatase deficiency, high vitamin C levels can lead to blood cell fragility, causing bruising or hemorrhaging. The correlation between serum and cellular levels is significant. When serum levels are normal or excessive, cellular levels may be deficient. In such cases, the short-term status of micronutrients is optimal, but cellular absorption may be a problem. Possible interventions include increasing dietary intake of the nutrient, increasing supplementation dosage, considering the status of synergistic nutrients for cellular absorption, assessing levels of oxidative stress on nutrient depletion, and considering follow-up testing to identify the source of malabsorption.

Vitamin C (Cellular)

Vitamin C, or Ascorbic Acid, plays a crucial role as an antioxidant. It enhances immunity by increasing the production of white blood cells and supports the regeneration of vitamin E. Additionally, Vitamin C helps reduce the risk of atherosclerosis, stroke, high blood pressure, and inflammation. Furthermore, it is essential for optimal collagen production, as it contributes to the generation of connective tissue. Vitamin C is also an integral component of L-carnitine, which is crucial for metabolizing fats into energy.

Optimal Range	0.5 - 9.7 ng/MM WBC

If LOW or < 0.5 ng/MM WBC:

Vitamin C is most commonly depleted due to inadequate dietary intake. The body's vitamin C pool typically depletes within 4 to 12 days. Ascorbic acid is affected by various factors that can impair its absorption and functions. Regular consumption of fruits and vegetables is the most effective way to prevent vitamin C deficiency. Vitamin C levels can also be depleted during severe oxidative stress, as it is a cofactor required for both catecholamine biosynthesis and adrenal steroidogenesis.

Clinical manifestations of vitamin C depletion include reduced bone density, bleeding gums, easy bruising, anemia, fatigue, weakness, and joint pain. These symptoms result from weakened or deficient connective tissues throughout the body. Severe cases of vitamin C deficiency are known as scurvy.

Medications that can lower vitamin C levels include oral contraceptives and aspirin, especially when used frequently.

Food Sources:
- Red and green sweet peppers
- Oranges
- Grapefruit
- Kiwifruit
- Broccoli
- Strawberries
- Brussels sprouts
- Tomatoes
- Cantaloupe
- Cabbage
- Cauliflower

Support Considerations:
- Increase food sources.
- Consider supplementation.

Supplement Options:
- The recommended daily intake of vitamin C is 75 mg for women and 90 mg for men. During pregnancy and lactation, the intake should be 120 mg/day.
- Vitamin C has a half-life of about 30 minutes in circulation after supplementation, so large, single doses may not be as effective as smaller, more frequent doses.
- In addition to taking supplemental vitamin C, α-Lipoic acid can help restore vitamin C levels when depleted.

Correlation between Serum and Cellular Levels:
- Serum levels are deficient, but cellular levels are normal.
- Long-term nutrient status is optimal, but short-term needs improvement.
- Possible interventions include increasing dietary intake of nutrients, increasing supplementation dosage, and considering medications that may have an effect on depletion.

Serum levels are deficient and cellular levels are deficient:
- Short-term and long-term status of micronutrients is not optimal, suggesting low dietary intake and both intestinal and cellular malabsorption as possible causes.
- Possible interventions include increasing dietary intake of nutrients, increasing supplementation dosage, considering medications that may have an effect on depletion, and considering follow-up testing to identify the source of malabsorption.

Nutritional support:
- Vitamin C
- Magnesium taurinate
- Magnesium glycinate
- Magnesium malate

If **HIGH** or > 9.7 ng/MM WBC:

Vitamin C, a water-soluble vitamin, is not considered toxic and lacks a known toxic level. It is commonly administered intravenously to treat various conditions without causing any adverse effects. To ensure the safety of generally healthy adults, a tolerable upper intake level (UL) of 2 grams (2,000 milligrams) per day has been established. This level is set to prevent diarrhea and gastrointestinal disturbances, which are usually not severe and resolve with temporary discontinuation of vitamin C supplementation.

While several potential adverse health effects of extremely high vitamin C doses have been suggested, primarily based on in vitro experiments or isolated case reports, none have been conclusively proven. These effects include genetic mutations, congenital disabilities, cancer, atherosclerosis, kidney stones (and possibly increased oxalates), "rebound scurvy," increased oxidative stress, excess iron absorption, vitamin B12 deficiency, and dental enamel erosion.

However, it's important to note that none of these alleged adverse effects have been consistently replicated in subsequent studies. Therefore, there is no reliable scientific evidence to support the claim that doses of vitamin C up to 10 grams per day in adults are toxic or detrimental to health.

Vitamin C supplementation or sources should be stopped or reduced. Intake of more than 1-2 grams of vitamin C can cause loose stools in some individuals. In those with a glucose-6-phosphatase deficiency, high vitamin C levels can lead to blood cell fragility, causing bruising or hemorrhaging. The correlation between serum and cellular levels is significant. When serum levels are normal or excessive, cellular levels may be deficient. In such cases, the short-term status of micronutrients is optimal, but cellular absorption may be a problem. Possible interventions include increasing dietary intake of the nutrient, increasing supplementation dosage, considering the status of synergistic nutrients for cellular absorption, assessing levels of oxidative stress on nutrient depletion, and considering follow-up testing to identify the source of malabsorption.

Vitamin D, 25-OH (Serum)

25-OH-D3, a standard laboratory test, measures the inactive precursor to 1,25-OH-D3, a combination of two forms of vitamin D in the body: vitamin D2 and D3. Unlike 1,25-OH-D3, 25-OH-D3 has a longer half-life in the blood, which can lead to differences in levels between the two forms. Since 25-OH-D3 is a precursor to active forms of vitamin D (calcitriol), it's crucial to understand that it doesn't directly reflect overall active D3 levels but rather the amount available for conversion if cofactors are sufficient. The conversion of 25-OHD to 1,25-OHD occurs in the kidneys and is regulated by parathyroid hormone (PTH). When blood calcium levels drop, PTH signals the kidneys to convert more 25-OHD to 1,25-OHD, which enhances intestinal calcium absorption and reduces bone demineralization. Upon conversion to 1,25-OHD, it also regulates the function of hundreds of genes, supports the immune system, aids in the production and function of endocrine hormones, is essential for normal bone and tooth growth and development, tightly regulates the absorption and release of calcium and phosphorus from the intestines and bones, regulates cell differentiation and growth, and may play a role in regulating mood. Patients with hypercalcemia, hyperphosphatemia, and low PTH may experience unregulated conversion of 25-OH-VitD to 1,25-OHD.

| Optimal Range | 30.0 - 108.0 ng/mL |

If LOW or < 30.0 ng/mL:

Vitamin D deficiency is quite common in the United States. Several factors contribute to this deficiency.
- Inadequate intake: The elderly population tends to have lower oral intake of vitamin D.
- Malabsorption disorders: Certain malabsorption syndromes, such as celiac disease, short bowel syndrome, gastric bypass, inflammatory bowel disease, chronic pancreatic insufficiency, and cystic fibrosis, can lead to vitamin D deficiency.
- Decreased sun exposure: About 50% to 90% of vitamin D is produced in the skin from sunlight. Twenty minutes of sun exposure daily with over 40% of the skin exposed is sufficient to prevent deficiency. However, this can be reduced in individuals who use sunscreen consistently, institutionalized individuals, or those with prolonged hospitalizations.
- Decreased endogenous synthesis: Chronic liver disease, such as cirrhosis, can lead to defective 25-hydroxylation, resulting in a deficiency of active vitamin D. Defects in 1-alpha 25-hydroxylation can also occur in hyperparathyroidism, renal failure, and 1-alpha hydroxylase deficiency.
- Increased hepatic catabolism: Certain medications, such as phenobarbital, carbamazepine, dexamethasone, nifedipine, spironolactone, clotrimazole, and rifampin, induce hepatic cytochrome P450 enzymes that activate the degradation of vitamin D.
- End-organ resistance to vitamin D: Hereditary vitamin D-resistant rickets is an example of end-organ resistance to vitamin D. Clinical manifestations of depletion conditions associated with low vitamin D status include Alzheimer's disease, asthma, autism, cancer, cavities, colds and flus, cystic fibrosis, dementia, depression, diabetes 1 and 2, eczema and psoriasis, hearing loss, heart disease, hypertension, infertility, inflammatory bowel disease, insomnia, macular degeneration, migraines, multiple sclerosis, Crohn's disease, muscle pain, obesity, osteomalacia, osteoporosis, periodontal disease, preeclampsia, rheumatoid arthritis, schizophrenia, seizures, septicemia, and tuberculosis.

Specifically, reasons for suboptimal 25-OHD levels include lack of sun exposure (especially in northern latitudes and during the winter season), malabsorption due to Celiac disease or other inflammatory digestive disorders, inadequate hepatic vitamin D 25-hydroxylase enzyme activity, and certain prescription medications such as antiepileptic drugs, including phenytoin, phenobarbital, and carbamazepine, which increase 25-OHD metabolism.

PTH levels may be high-normal or elevated in sub-clinical and frank vitamin D deficiency.

Medications that can lower Vitamin D levels include epileptic/anticonvulsant medications, medications that decrease intestinal absorption of Vitamin D, including bile acid sequestrants (cholestyramine), and some laxatives, agents that cause fat malabsorption, such as orlistat, mineral oil, and the fat substitute olestra, which can affect the absorption of all fat-soluble vitamins.

Food Sources:
- Cod liver oil
- Rainbow trout
- Sockeye salmon
- White mushrooms
- Fortified milk

Naturally occurring sources of vitamin D3, such as cod liver oil and rainbow trout, contain the active form of vitamin D. Fortified sources, like baker's yeast, typically contain vitamin D2.

Support Considerations:
- Increase food sources of vitamin D.
- Consider supplementation, especially if you're not getting enough vitamin D from your diet or sun exposure.
- Supplement with vitamin K2 alongside vitamin D to maintain healthy blood calcium levels and prevent excessive bone demineralization caused by high vitamin D intake.
- Increase safe sun exposure.

Supplement Options:
- The recommended daily intake of vitamin D (RDA) of 400 IU/day is insufficient for therapeutic needs. Common doses range from 1000 to 10,000 IU/day.
- Vitamin D comes in two forms: D2 (ergocalciferol) and D3 (cholecalciferol). Both forms can be converted to the active form of vitamin D in the body (25-hydroxyvitamin D).
- Vitamin D is produced when the skin is exposed to ultraviolet light from the sun.
- Supplementation with vitamin D is almost always necessary because it's challenging to meet needs through diet and sun exposure alone. Consult your practitioner for supplement recommendations and target serum levels.
- Obese individuals and pregnant women have higher vitamin D requirements due to the body's ability to store or trap vitamin D in adipose tissue (fat cells).
- Obtaining too much vitamin D from sun exposure is not possible, but it's possible to get too much from supplementation.
- Taking too much vitamin D in supplement form can lead to an increase in blood calcium levels (hypercalcemia) due to increased intestinal absorption of calcium when serum vitamin D levels are high.
- Vitamin D toxicity has been observed in individuals taking more than 50,000 IU/day, but intake levels less than 10,000 IU/day are unlikely to cause toxicity.

Additional Investigations:
- Stool test to assess gut and digestive health and rule out inflammatory bowel disease (IBD).
- Celiac testing
- Liver function tests
- Parathyroid function tests
- Levels of parathyroid hormone (PTH) may be high-normal or elevated in individuals with subclinical or frank vitamin D deficiency.

Nutritional support
- Vitamin D3
- Vitamin K2
- Vitamin A
- Magnesium taurinate
- Magnesium glycinate
- Magnesium malate

If **HIGH** or **> 108.0 ng/mL:**

Stop or reduce vitamin D3 supplementation / sources

Excessive vitamin D intake, often resulting from misuse of over-the-counter supplements or erroneous prescriptions, can lead to hypervitaminosis D. Intake levels below 10,000 IU/day are unlikely to cause toxicity. However, individuals taking over 50,000 IU/day for a few months have been observed to develop vitamin D toxicity. This condition causes abnormally high serum calcium concentration (hypercalcemia), which can lead to bone loss, kidney stones, and calcification of organs like the heart and kidneys if left untreated for an extended period. To prevent excess bone demineralization, it is recommended to supplement vitamin K2 alongside vitamin D. Less commonly, poisoning from exposure to rodenticides containing cholecalciferol can also cause vitamin D toxicity. Notably, vitamin D toxicity (hypervitaminosis D) has not been associated with sun exposure.

Vitamin D3 (Serum)

Vitamin D3 is also referred to as 1,25-hydroxyvitamin D3 (1,25-OHD3). 1,25-OHD3 has a shorter half-life in the blood than 25-OHD (what most standard labs run, and what is most commonly used to assess total vitamin D status), and, therefore, levels may differ from what is measured as 25-OHD. The conversion of 25-OHD to 1,25-OHD is performed in D the kidneys and regulated by parathyroid hormone (PTH). When blood calcium levels fall, PTH signals the kidneys to convert more 25-OHD to 1,25-OHD, which increases intestinal absorption of calcium, and reduces bone demineralization of calcium. Vitamin D3 also regulates the function of hundreds of genes, supports the immune system, supports production and function of endocrine hormones, is important for normal growth and development of bones and teeth, tightly regulates the levels of calcium and phosphorus being absorbed intestinally as well as released from bone, regulates cell differentiation and growth, and may play an important role in regulating mood.

Optimal Range	0.4 - 1.8 ng/mL

If **LOW** or **< 0.4 ng/mL:**

Vitamin D deficiency is quite common in the United States. Several factors contribute to this deficiency.

- Inadequate intake: The elderly population tends to have lower oral intake of vitamin D.
- Malabsorption disorders: Certain malabsorption syndromes, such as celiac disease, short bowel syndrome, gastric bypass, inflammatory bowel disease, chronic pancreatic insufficiency, and cystic fibrosis, can lead to vitamin D deficiency.
- Decreased sun exposure: About 50% to 90% of vitamin D is produced in the skin from sunlight. Twenty minutes of sun exposure daily with over 40% of the skin exposed is sufficient to prevent deficiency. However, this can be reduced in individuals who use sunscreen consistently, institutionalized individuals, or those with prolonged hospitalizations.

- Decreased endogenous synthesis: Chronic liver disease, such as cirrhosis, can lead to defective 25-hydroxylation, resulting in a deficiency of active vitamin D. Defects in 1-alpha 25-hydroxylation can also occur in hyperparathyroidism, renal failure, and 1-alpha hydroxylase deficiency.
- Increased hepatic catabolism: Certain medications, such as phenobarbital, carbamazepine, dexamethasone, nifedipine, spironolactone, clotrimazole, and rifampin, induce hepatic cytochrome P450 enzymes that activate the degradation of vitamin D.
- End-organ resistance to vitamin D: Hereditary vitamin D-resistant rickets is an example of end-organ resistance to vitamin D. Clinical Manifestations of Vitamin D Deficiency: Conditions associated with low vitamin D levels include Alzheimer's disease, asthma, autism, cancer, cavities, colds and flus, cystic fibrosis, dementia, depression, diabetes 1 and 2, eczema and psoriasis, hearing loss, heart disease, hypertension, infertility, inflammatory bowel disease, insomnia, macular degeneration, migraines, multiple sclerosis, Crohn's disease, muscle pain, obesity, osteomalacia, osteoporosis, periodontal disease, preeclampsia, rheumatoid arthritis, schizophrenia, seizures, septicemia, and tuberculosis.

Medications that can lower vitamin D levels include epileptic/anticonvulsant medications, medications that can decrease intestinal absorption of vitamin D, such as bile acid sequestrants (cholestyramine) and some laxatives, and agents that cause fat malabsorption, such as orlistat, mineral oil, and the fat substitute olestra, which can affect the absorption of all fat-soluble vitamins.

Food Sources:
- Cod liver oil
- Rainbow trout
- Sockeye salmon
- White mushrooms
- Fortified milk

Naturally occurring sources of vitamin D3 include cod liver oil, rainbow trout, sockeye salmon, and white mushrooms. Fortified milk, on the other hand, typically contains vitamin D2.

Support Considerations:
- Increase food sources of vitamin D.
- Consider supplementation, including K2. Supplementing vitamin K2 alongside vitamin D is recommended to maintain blood calcium levels in homeostasis and prevent excessive bone demineralization of calcium with higher vitamin D intake.
- Increase safe sun exposure.

Supplement Options:
- The previously established RDA of 400IU/day has been found to be insufficient for therapeutic needs. Common doses range from 1000 to 10,000 IU/day.
- Vitamin D exists in two forms: D2 (ergocalciferol) and D3 (cholecalciferol). Both forms can be used as active vitamin D3 in the body. D2 can be converted to D3 when needed, but this is a tightly controlled metabolic process to prevent excessive D2 to D3 conversion.
- Vitamin D is produced endogenously when the skin is exposed to ultraviolet light from the sun.
- Supplementation with vitamin D is almost always necessary because it is challenging to meet needs through diet and sun exposure alone. Consult your practitioner for supplement recommendations and target serum levels.
- Obese individuals and pregnant women have higher vitamin D requirements due to the storage or trapping of vitamin D in adipose tissue (fat cells).
- Obtaining too much vitamin D from sun exposure is not possible, but it is possible to obtain too much from supplementation.
- Taking too much vitamin D in supplement form can lead to hypercalcemia (high blood calcium levels) due to increased intestinal absorption of calcium when serum vitamin D levels are high.

- Supplementing vitamin K2 alongside vitamin D is recommended to maintain blood calcium levels in homeostasis and prevent excessive bone demineralization of calcium with higher vitamin D intake. Additional investigations include a stool test to evaluate gut and digestive health and rule out inflammatory bowel disease (IBD), celiac testing, liver function tests, and parathyroid function tests. Levels of parathyroid hormone (PTH) may be high-normal or elevated in individuals with sub-clinical or frank vitamin D deficiency.

Nutritional support
- Vitamin D3
- Vitamin K2
- Vitamin A
- Magnesium taurinate
- Magnesium glycinate
- Magnesium malate

If **HIGH** or **> 1.8 ng/mL:**

Excessive vitamin D intake, often resulting from misuse of over-the-counter supplements or erroneous prescriptions, can lead to hypervitaminosis D. Intake levels below 10,000 IU/day are unlikely to cause toxicity. However, individuals taking over 50,000 IU/day for a few months have been observed to develop vitamin D toxicity. This condition causes abnormally high serum calcium concentration (hypercalcemia), which can lead to bone loss, kidney stones, and calcification of organs like the heart and kidneys if left untreated for an extended period. To prevent excess bone demineralization, it is recommended to supplement vitamin K2 alongside vitamin D. Less commonly, poisoning from exposure to rodenticides containing cholecalciferol can also cause vitamin D toxicity. Notably, vitamin D toxicity (hypervitaminosis D) has not been associated with sun exposure.

Stop or reduce vitamin D3 supplementation / sources

Vitamin D3 (Cellular)

Vitamin D3 is also referred to as 1,25-hydroxyvitamin D3 (1,25-OHD3). 1,25-OHD3 has a shorter half-life in the blood than 25-OHD (what most standard labs run, and what is most commonly used to assess total vitamin D status), and, therefore, levels may differ from what is measured as 25-OHD. The conversion of 25-OHD to 1,25-OHD is performed in D the kidneys and regulated by parathyroid hormone (PTH). When blood calcium levels fall, PTH signals the kidneys to convert more 25-OHD to 1,25-OHD, which increases intestinal absorption of calcium, and reduces bone demineralization of calcium. Vitamin D3 also regulates the function of hundreds of genes, supports the immune system, supports production and function of endocrine hormones, is important for normal growth and development of bones and teeth, tightly regulates the levels of calcium and phosphorus being absorbed intestinally as well as released from bone, regulates cell differentiation and growth, and may play an important role in regulating mood.

Optimal Range	25.9 - 246.6 pg/MM WBC

If **LOW** or **< 25.9 pg/MM WBC:**

Vitamin D deficiency is quite common in the United States. Several factors contribute to this deficiency.

- Inadequate intake: The elderly population tends to have lower oral intake of vitamin D.

- Malabsorption disorders: Certain malabsorption syndromes, such as celiac disease, short bowel syndrome, gastric bypass, inflammatory bowel disease, chronic pancreatic insufficiency, and cystic fibrosis, can lead to vitamin D deficiency.
- Decreased sun exposure: About 50% to 90% of vitamin D is produced in the skin from sunlight. Twenty minutes of sun exposure daily with over 40% of the skin exposed is sufficient to prevent deficiency. However, this can be reduced in individuals who use sunscreen consistently, institutionalized individuals, or those with prolonged hospitalizations.
- Decreased endogenous synthesis: Chronic liver disease, such as cirrhosis, can lead to defective 25-hydroxylation, resulting in a deficiency of active vitamin D. Defects in 1-alpha 25-hydroxylation can also occur in hyperparathyroidism, renal failure, and 1-alpha hydroxylase deficiency.
- Increased hepatic catabolism: Certain medications, such as phenobarbital, carbamazepine, dexamethasone, nifedipine, spironolactone, clotrimazole, and rifampin, induce hepatic cytochrome P450 enzymes that activate the degradation of vitamin D.
- End-organ resistance to vitamin D: Hereditary vitamin D-resistant rickets is an example of end-organ resistance to vitamin D. Clinical Manifestations of Vitamin D Deficiency: Conditions associated with low vitamin D levels include Alzheimer's disease, asthma, autism, cancer, cavities, colds and flus, cystic fibrosis, dementia, depression, diabetes 1 and 2, eczema and psoriasis, hearing loss, heart disease, hypertension, infertility, inflammatory bowel disease, insomnia, macular degeneration, migraines, multiple sclerosis, Crohn's disease, muscle pain, obesity, osteomalacia, osteoporosis, periodontal disease, preeclampsia, rheumatoid arthritis, schizophrenia, seizures, septicemia, and tuberculosis.

Medications that can lower vitamin D levels include epileptic/anticonvulsant medications, medications that can decrease intestinal absorption of vitamin D, such as bile acid sequestrants (cholestyramine) and some laxatives, and agents that cause fat malabsorption, such as orlistat, mineral oil, and the fat substitute olestra, which can affect the absorption of all fat-soluble vitamins.

Food Sources:
- Cod liver oil
- Rainbow trout
- Sockeye salmon
- White mushrooms
- Fortified milk

Naturally occurring sources of vitamin D3 include cod liver oil, rainbow trout, sockeye salmon, and white mushrooms. Fortified milk, on the other hand, typically contains vitamin D2.

Support Considerations:
- Increase food sources of vitamin D.
- Consider supplementation, including K2. Supplementing vitamin K2 alongside vitamin D is recommended to maintain blood calcium levels in homeostasis and prevent excessive bone demineralization of calcium with higher vitamin D intake.
- Increase safe sun exposure.

Supplement Options:
- The previously established RDA of 400IU/day has been found to be insufficient for therapeutic needs. Common doses range from 1000 to 10,000 IU/day.
- Vitamin D exists in two forms: D2 (ergocalciferol) and D3 (cholecalciferol). Both forms can be used as active vitamin D3 in the body. D2 can be converted to D3 when needed, but this is a tightly controlled metabolic process to prevent excessive D2 to D3 conversion.
- Vitamin D is produced endogenously when the skin is exposed to ultraviolet light from the sun.

- Supplementation with vitamin D is almost always necessary because it is challenging to meet needs through diet and sun exposure alone. Consult your practitioner for supplement recommendations and target serum levels.
- Obese individuals and pregnant women have higher vitamin D requirements due to the storage or trapping of vitamin D in adipose tissue (fat cells).
- Obtaining too much vitamin D from sun exposure is not possible, but it is possible to obtain too much from supplementation.
- Taking too much vitamin D in supplement form can lead to hypercalcemia (high blood calcium levels) due to increased intestinal absorption of calcium when serum vitamin D levels are high.
- Supplementing vitamin K2 alongside vitamin D is recommended to maintain blood calcium levels in homeostasis and prevent excessive bone demineralization of calcium with higher vitamin D intake. Additional investigations include a stool test to evaluate gut and digestive health and rule out inflammatory bowel disease (IBD), celiac testing, liver function tests, and parathyroid function tests. Levels of parathyroid hormone (PTH) may be high-normal or elevated in individuals with sub-clinical or frank vitamin D deficiency.

Nutritional support
- Vitamin D3
- Vitamin K2
- Vitamin A
- Magnesium taurinate
- Magnesium glycinate
- Magnesium malate

If **HIGH** or **> 246.6 pg/MM WBC:**

Excessive vitamin D intake, often resulting from misuse of over-the-counter supplements or erroneous prescriptions, can lead to hypervitaminosis D. Intake levels below 10,000 IU/day are unlikely to cause toxicity. However, individuals taking over 50,000 IU/day for a few months have been observed to develop vitamin D toxicity. This condition causes abnormally high serum calcium concentration (hypercalcemia), which can lead to bone loss, kidney stones, and calcification of organs like the heart and kidneys if left untreated for an extended period. To prevent excess bone demineralization, it is recommended to supplement vitamin K2 alongside vitamin D. Less commonly, poisoning from exposure to rodenticides containing cholecalciferol can also cause vitamin D toxicity. Notably, vitamin D toxicity (hypervitaminosis D) has not been associated with sun exposure.

Stop or reduce vitamin D3 supplementation / sources

Vitamin E (Serum)

Vitamin E (Tocopherol or alpha-tocopherol) is a fat-soluble vitamin and is an important antioxidant that reduces the formation of reactive oxygen species (ROS) that result from fat oxidation. Vitamin E also regulates cell signaling, influences immune function, and inhibits coagulation, which can playa role in reducing atherosclerosis and lowering rates of ischemic heart disease.

| Optimal Range | 7.4 - 30.6 mg/L |

If **LOW** or **< 7.4 mg/L:**

 Vitamin E depletion, though rare in developed countries due to adequate diet intake, can occur through various factors. In infants, premature low birth weight (less than 1500 grams or 3.3 pounds) and malabsorption disorders are common causes. Malabsorption occurs when the small intestine, which requires fat for vitamin E absorption, is disrupted. Conditions like cystic fibrosis, short-bowel syndrome, surgical resection, mesenteric vascular thrombosis, and pseudo-obstruction can lead to this issue. Chronic cholestatic hepatobiliary disease, Crohn's disease, exocrine pancreatic insufficiency, and liver disease can also impair fat absorption. Genetic mutations in the tocopherol transfer protein and autosomal-recessive diseases like abetalipoproteinemia and isolated vitamin E deficiency syndrome can cause impaired fat metabolism.

In developing countries, inadequate vitamin E intake is the primary cause of depletion. Smoking also contributes to vitamin E depletion.

Vitamin E deficiency can manifest in peripheral neuropathy, ataxia, muscle weakness, skeletal myopathy, retinopathy, and an increased risk of cardiovascular disease, red blood cell destruction, prostate cancer, and cataracts.

Medications can interact with vitamin E, affecting its absorption. Epileptic and anticonvulsant drugs, cholesterol-lowering medications, and agents that cause fat malabsorption, such as orlistat, mineral oil, and olestra, can interfere with vitamin E absorption, impacting the absorption of all fat-soluble vitamins.

Food Sources:
- Wheatgerm oil
- Sunflower seeds
- Almonds
- Sunflower oil
- Safflower oil
- Hazelnuts

Support Considerations:
- Increase food sources
- Reduce or cease smoking
- Consider supplementation

Supplement Options:
- The RDA for vitamin E is 15 mg/day.
- The UL for vitamin E is set at 1000 mg/day to prevent interference in vitamin K clotting pathways.
- The only supplementary form of vitamin E that reverses deficiency symptoms is α-tocopherol.
- In addition, α-Lipoic acid is an important cofactor that can aid in restoring vitamin E levels when depleted.

Correlation between Serum and Cellular Levels:
- Cellular levels are low, and serum levels are normal or excessive.
- In the short term, the status of micro-nutrients is optimal, but cellular absorption may be a problem.

Recommendations:
- Increase dietary intake of nutrients
- Increase supplementation dosage
- Consider the status of synergistic nutrients for cellular absorption
- Consider levels of oxidative stress on nutrient depletion

- Consider follow-up testing to identify the source of malabsorption.

Cellular levels are low, and serum levels are low as well.
In the short term and long term, the status of micro-nutrients is not optimal, suggesting low dietary intake and both intestinal and cellular absorption as possible causes.

Recommended interventions:
- Increase dietary intake of nutrients
- Increase supplementation dosage
- Medications may have an effect on depletion
- Consider follow-up testing to identify the source of malabsorption.

Additional Investigations:
- Stool test to assess gut and digestive health and rule out IBD
- Celiac testing

Nutritional support
- Vitamin E tocotrienols
- Magnesium taurinate
- Magnesium glycinate
- Magnesium malate

If HIGH or > 30.6 mg/L:

Vitamin E, a fat-soluble nutrient, plays a vital role in maintaining the immune system and acting as an antioxidant, protecting cells from free radical damage. While few side effects have been observed in adults taking supplements of less than 2,000 mg of a-tocopherol daily (natural or synthetic), the most concerning possibility is impaired blood clotting, which may increase the risk of hemorrhage in some individuals.

The Upper Limit (UL) of 1,000 mg/day of atocopherol in any supplemental form (equivalent to 1,500 IU/day of RRR-atocopherol or 1,100 IU/day of all-rac-atocopherol) represents the highest dose unlikely to cause hemorrhage in almost all adults. Elevated Vitamin E levels are uncommon and often result from excessive intake of supplements rather than dietary sources. The body efficiently regulates Vitamin E obtained from food, but high doses from supplements can lead to accumulation in the body.

Potential implications of high serum Vitamin E levels include:
- Increased Risk of Bleeding: Vitamin E has anticoagulant properties, which can thin the blood. High levels may elevate the risk of bleeding, especially when combined with blood-thinning medications.
- Vitamin E Toxicity: Although rare, extremely high doses of Vitamin E can lead to toxicity, manifesting in symptoms such as nausea, diarrhea, stomach cramps, fatigue, weakness, headache, blurred vision, rash, and bruising.
- Interference with Other Nutrients: High levels of Vitamin E may interfere with the absorption or metabolism of other fat-soluble vitamins (A, D, and K).

It is crucial to interpret high serum Vitamin E levels in the context of clinical symptoms, dietary intake, and supplement usage.

 Vitamin E supplementation may be causing low WBC levels despite normal serum levels. Increase dietary intake, supplementation dosage, and consider cellular absorption factors.

Vitamin E (Cellular)

Vitamin E (Tocopherol or alpha-tocopherol) is a fat-soluble vitamin and is an important antioxidant that reduces the formation of reactive oxygen species (ROS) that result from fat oxidation. Vitamin E also regulates cell signaling, influences immune function, and inhibits coagulation, which can playa role in reducing atherosclerosis and lowering rates of ischemic heart disease.

| Optimal Range | 18.4 - 1031.1 pg/MM WBC |

If LOW or < 18.4 pg/MM WBC:

 Vitamin E depletion, though rare in developed countries due to adequate diet intake, can occur through various factors. In infants, premature low birth weight (less than 1500 grams or 3.3 pounds) and malabsorption disorders are common causes. Malabsorption occurs when the small intestine, which requires fat for vitamin E absorption, is disrupted. Conditions like cystic fibrosis, short-bowel syndrome, surgical resection, mesenteric vascular thrombosis, and pseudo-obstruction can lead to this issue. Chronic cholestatic hepatobiliary disease, Crohn's disease, exocrine pancreatic insufficiency, and liver disease can also impair fat absorption. Genetic mutations in the tocopherol transfer protein and autosomal-recessive diseases like abetalipoproteinemia and isolated vitamin E deficiency syndrome can cause impaired fat metabolism.

In developing countries, inadequate vitamin E intake is the primary cause of depletion. Smoking also contributes to vitamin E depletion.

Vitamin E deficiency can manifest in peripheral neuropathy, ataxia, muscle weakness, skeletal myopathy, retinopathy, and an increased risk of cardiovascular disease, red blood cell destruction, prostate cancer, and cataracts.

Medications can interact with vitamin E, affecting its absorption. Epileptic and anticonvulsant drugs, cholesterol-lowering medications, and agents that cause fat malabsorption, such as orlistat, mineral oil, and olestra, can interfere with vitamin E absorption, impacting the absorption of all fat-soluble vitamins.

Food Sources:
- Wheatgerm oil
- Sunflower seeds
- Almonds
- Sunflower oil
- Safflower oil
- Hazelnuts

Support Considerations:
- Increase food sources
- Reduce or cease smoking
- Consider supplementation

Supplement Options:
- The RDA for vitamin E is 15 mg/day.
- The UL for vitamin E is set at 1000 mg/day to prevent interference in vitamin K clotting pathways.
- The only supplementary form of vitamin E that reverses deficiency symptoms is α-tocopherol.

- In addition, α-Lipoic acid is an important cofactor that can aid in restoring vitamin E levels when depleted.

Correlation between Serum and Cellular Levels:
- Cellular levels are low, and serum levels are normal or excessive.
- In the short term, the status of micro-nutrients is optimal, but cellular absorption may be a problem.

Recommendations:
- Increase dietary intake of nutrients
- Increase supplementation dosage
- Consider the status of synergistic nutrients for cellular absorption
- Consider levels of oxidative stress on nutrient depletion
- Consider follow-up testing to identify the source of malabsorption.

Cellular levels are low, and serum levels are low as well.
In the short term and long term, the status of micro-nutrients is not optimal, suggesting low dietary intake and both intestinal and cellular absorption as possible causes.

Recommended interventions:
- Increase dietary intake of nutrients
- Increase supplementation dosage
- Medications may have an effect on depletion
- Consider follow-up testing to identify the source of malabsorption.

Additional Investigations:
- Stool test to assess gut and digestive health and rule out IBD
- Celiac testing

Nutritional support
- Vitamin E tocotrienols
- Magnesium taurinate
- Magnesium glycinate
- Magnesium malate

If HIGH or > 1031.1 pg/MM WBC:

Vitamin E, a fat-soluble nutrient, plays a vital role in maintaining the immune system and acting as an antioxidant, protecting cells from free radical damage. While few side effects have been observed in adults taking supplements of less than 2,000 mg of a-tocopherol daily (natural or synthetic), the most concerning possibility is impaired blood clotting, which may increase the risk of hemorrhage in some individuals.

The Upper Limit (UL) of 1,000 mg/day of atocopherol in any supplemental form (equivalent to 1,500 IU/day of RRR-atocopherol or 1,100 IU/day of all-rac-atocopherol) represents the highest dose unlikely to cause hemorrhage in almost all adults. Elevated Vitamin E levels are uncommon and often result from excessive intake of supplements rather than dietary sources. The body efficiently regulates Vitamin E obtained from food, but high doses from supplements can lead to accumulation in the body.

Potential implications of high serum Vitamin E levels include:
- Increased Risk of Bleeding: Vitamin E has anticoagulant properties, which can thin the blood. High levels may elevate the risk of bleeding, especially when combined with blood-thinning medications.

- Vitamin E Toxicity: Although rare, extremely high doses of Vitamin E can lead to toxicity, manifesting in symptoms such as nausea, diarrhea, stomach cramps, fatigue, weakness, headache, blurred vision, rash, and bruising.
- Interference with Other Nutrients: High levels of Vitamin E may interfere with the absorption or metabolism of other fat-soluble vitamins (A, D, and K).

It is crucial to interpret high serum Vitamin E levels in the context of clinical symptoms, dietary intake, and supplement usage.

 Vitamin E supplementation may be causing low WBC levels despite normal serum levels. Increase dietary intake, supplementation dosage, and consider cellular absorption factors.

Vitamin K1 (Serum)

Vitamin K1 (phylloquinone) is a fat-soluble vitamin and is present primarily in green leafy vegetables and is the main dietary form of vitamin K1. Vitamin K assists with blood clotting, supports the K1 formation of bone and bone matrix, and aids in glucose to glycogen conversion for storage in the liver.

Optimal Range	0.10 - 8.10 ng/mL

If LOW or < 0.10 ng/mL:

Vitamin K1 deficiency is extremely rare unless there's significant damage to the intestinal lining, such as in inflammatory bowel disorders like Crohn's and ulcerative colitis, liver disease, cystic fibrosis, and fat malabsorption disorders. Taking broad-spectrum antibiotics can also reduce vitamin K1 production in the gut. Individuals with chronic kidney disease and those with the ApoE4 genotype may be at higher risk for vitamin K1 deficiency. Since vitamin K1 is a fat-soluble vitamin, a chronically low-fat diet can inhibit its absorption.

Symptoms of vitamin K depletion or deficiency include excessive bleeding, menorrhagia, bruises that form easily, or the appearance of ruptured capillaries.

Medications that can interfere with vitamin K include:
- Broad-spectrum antibiotics
- Amiodarone used for cardiac arrhythmias, which can enhance the anticoagulant effect of warfarin
- Cholesterol-lowering medications
- Agents that cause fat malabsorption, such as orlistat, mineral oil, and the fat substitute olestra, which can affect the absorption of all fat-soluble vitamins.

 Food sources include natto, collards, turnip greens, spinach, kale, broccoli, soybeans, and carrot juice.

The best sources of Vitamin K1 are plant foods, especially dark green leafy vegetables.

Note: the absorption of vitamin K1 from food is extremely low. Only 10 percent of the vitamin K, which is found in green leafy vegetables, is absorbed in your body. There's no variable or modification of the consumption that will significantly increase the absorption

 Nutritional support:
- Vitamin K1

- Vitamin K2
- Vitamin D3
- Vitamin A
- Magnesium taurinate
- Magnesium glycinate
- Magnesium malate

If **HIGH** or **> 8.10 ng/mL:**

 Currently, there is no evidence of toxicity associated with high doses of vitamin K1 or vitamin K2. Consequently, there is no established upper intake level (UL) for these vitamins. While allergic reactions are possible, there is no known toxicity associated with high doses (dietary or supplemental) of the phylloquinone (vitamin K1) or menaquinone (vitamin K2) forms of vitamin K. No tolerable upper intake level (UL) has been determined for vitamin K1.

Stop or reduce vitamin K supplementation / sources

Vitamin K1 (Cellular)

Vitamin K1 (phylloquinone) is a fat-soluble vitamin and is present primarily in green leafy vegetables and is the main dietary form of vitamin K1. Vitamin K assists with blood clotting, supports the K1 formation of bone and bone matrix, and aids in glucose to glycogen conversion for storage in the liver.

| Optimal Range | 0.10 - 0.71 pg/MM WBC |

If **LOW** or **< 0.10 pg/MM WBC:**

Vitamin K1 deficiency is extremely rare unless there's significant damage to the intestinal lining, such as in inflammatory bowel disorders like Crohn's and ulcerative colitis, liver disease, cystic fibrosis, and fat malabsorption disorders. Taking broad-spectrum antibiotics can also reduce vitamin K1 production in the gut. Individuals with chronic kidney disease and those with the ApoE4 genotype may be at higher risk for vitamin K1 deficiency. Since vitamin K1 is a fat-soluble vitamin, a chronically low-fat diet can inhibit its absorption.

Symptoms of vitamin K depletion or deficiency include excessive bleeding, menorrhagia, bruises that form easily, or the appearance of ruptured capillaries.

Medications that can interfere with vitamin K include:
- Broad-spectrum antibiotics
- Amiodarone used for cardiac arrhythmias, which can enhance the anticoagulant effect of warfarin
- Cholesterol-lowering medications
- Agents that cause fat malabsorption, such as orlistat, mineral oil, and the fat substitute olestra, which can affect the absorption of all fat-soluble vitamins.

 Food sources include natto, collards, turnip greens, spinach, kale, broccoli, soybeans, and carrot juice.

The best sources of Vitamin K1 are plant foods, especially dark green leafy vegetables.

Note: the absorption of vitamin K1 from food is extremely low. Only 10 percent of the vitamin K, which is found in green leafy vegetables, is absorbed in your body. There's no variable or modification of the consumption that will significantly increase the absorption

Nutritional support:
- Vitamin K1
- Vitamin K2
- Vitamin D3
- Vitamin A
- Magnesium taurinate
- Magnesium glycinate
- Magnesium malate

If HIGH or > 0.71 pg/MM WBC:

Currently, there is no evidence of toxicity associated with high doses of vitamin K1 or vitamin K2. Consequently, there is no established upper intake level (UL) for these vitamins. While allergic reactions are possible, there is no known toxicity associated with high doses (dietary or supplemental) of the phylloquinone (vitamin K1) or menaquinone (vitamin K2) forms of vitamin K. No tolerable upper intake level (UL) has been determined for vitamin K1.

Stop or reduce vitamin K supplementation / sources

Vitamin K2 (Serum)

Vitamin K2 (a series of menaquinones) are predominantly of bacterial origin and are present in modest amounts in various animal-based and fermented foods. Vitamin K2 is the primary storage form of vitamin K in animals. Bacteria, e.g., Bacillus subtilis, in the colon, can convert K1 (from K plant-based foods) into vitamin K2. Vitamin K2 is necessary to prevent arterial calcification, which is done by activating matrix GLA protein (MGP). MGP in blood vessels inhibits soft tissue calcification. MGP needs to be carboxylated to work properly, and vitamin K2-MK7 plays a significant role in this carboxylation.

Optimal Range	0.10 - 5.19 ng/mL

If LOW or < 0.10 ng/mL:

Vitamin K1 deficiency is extremely rare unless there's significant damage to the intestinal lining, such as in inflammatory bowel disorders like Crohn's and ulcerative colitis, liver disease, cystic fibrosis, or fat malabsorption disorders. Oral blood-thinning medications and some antibiotics can also interfere with vitamin K absorption. Individuals with chronic kidney disease and those with the ApoE4 genotype may be at higher risk for vitamin K deficiency. Since Vitamin K is a fat-soluble vitamin, a chronically low-fat diet can hinder its absorption.

Inadequate levels of both Vitamin K1 and K2 significantly increase the risk of heart disease and stroke. Chronically low vitamin K levels can lead to uncontrolled bleeding, while marginally low levels are associated with osteoporosis in some studies. Vitamin K2 also helps regulate calcium homeostasis, so low or deficient levels can cause unregulated calcium release from bone tissue sources when vitamin D3 is supplemented. However, Vitamin D2 supplementation doesn't typically lead to this issue. It's recommended to supplement Vitamin K2 when Vitamin D3 is also taken. Levels of K2 are inversely related to cardiovascular disease and coronary calcification.

Medications that can interfere with Vitamin K include broad-spectrum antibiotics, amiodarone used for cardiac arrhythmias, cholesterol-lowering medications, agents that cause fat malabsorption like orlistat, mineral oil, and the fat substitute olestra, which can affect the absorption of all fat-soluble vitamins.

Food Sources:
- Natto
- Collards
- Turnip greens
- Spinach
- Kale
- Broccoli
- Soybeans
- Carrot juice

The best sources of vitamin K2 include fermented foods, such as natto and some rare fermented cheeses, and liver. Minor amounts are also found in egg yolks and butter.

Support Considerations:
- Increase food sources of vitamin K2, including fermented foods and liver.
- Consider vitamin K2 supplementation.

Supplement Options:
- Studies suggest daily therapeutic doses of about 360-500 micrograms (mcg) of vitamin K2.
- Fermented foods contain a variety of bacteria, and only certain ones, such as Bacillus subtilis, produce vitamin K2. Regular consumption of fermented foods can enhance dietary vitamin K2 intake.
- You can make fermented foods yourself by using a starter culture specifically designed to optimize vitamin K2 production.
- Vitamin K2 supplements come in 'MK' varieties, and MK-4 is the form that all forms of vitamin K2 are converted into in the body. If you take an MK-7 variety, your body will convert it to MK-4. However, MK-4 supplements are available commercially to bypass activation after absorption.

Additional Investigations:
- Stool test to assess gut and digestive health and rule out inflammatory bowel disease (IBD) and fat malabsorption.
- Celiac testing
- Liver function tests
- Kidney function tests
- Genetic testing for ApoE4

Nutritional support:
- Vitamin K1
- Vitamin K2
- Vitamin D3
- Vitamin A
- Magnesium taurinate
- Magnesium glycinate
- Magnesium malate

If **HIGH** or **> 5.19 ng/mL:**

Currently, there is no known toxicity is associated with high doses of vitamin K1 or vitamin K2. Therefore, there is no designated upper intake level (UL). Although allergic reactions are possible, there is no known toxicity associated with high doses (dietary or supplemental) of the phylloquinone (vitamin K1) or menaquinone (vitamin K2) forms of vitamin K). No tolerable upper intake level (UL) has been established for vitamin K

 Stop or reduce vitamin K supplementation / sources

Vitamin K2 (Cellular)

Vitamin K2 (a series of menaquinones) are predominantly of bacterial origin and are present in modest amounts in various animal-based and fermented foods. Vitamin K2 is the primary storage form of vitamin K in animals. Bacteria, e.g., Bacillus subtilis, in the colon, can convert K1 (from K plant-based foods) into vitamin K2. Vitamin K2 is necessary to prevent arterial calcification, which is done by activating matrix GLA protein (MGP). MGP in blood vessels inhibits soft tissue calcification. MGP needs to be carboxylated to work properly, and vitamin K2-MK7 plays a significant role in this carboxylation.

Optimal Range	0.10 - 0.89 pg/MM WBC

If LOW or < 0.10 pg/MM WBC:

Vitamin K1 deficiency is extremely rare unless there's significant damage to the intestinal lining, such as in inflammatory bowel disorders like Crohn's and ulcerative colitis, liver disease, cystic fibrosis, or fat malabsorption disorders. Oral blood-thinning medications and some antibiotics can also interfere with vitamin K absorption. Individuals with chronic kidney disease and those with the ApoE4 genotype may be at higher risk for vitamin K deficiency. Since Vitamin K is a fat-soluble vitamin, a chronically low-fat diet can hinder its absorption.

Inadequate levels of both Vitamin K1 and K2 significantly increase the risk of heart disease and stroke. Chronically low vitamin K levels can lead to uncontrolled bleeding, while marginally low levels are associated with osteoporosis in some studies. Vitamin K2 also helps regulate calcium homeostasis, so low or deficient levels can cause unregulated calcium release from bone tissue sources when vitamin D3 is supplemented. However, Vitamin D2 supplementation doesn't typically lead to this issue. It's recommended to supplement Vitamin K2 when Vitamin D3 is also taken. Levels of K2 are inversely related to cardiovascular disease and coronary calcification.

Medications that can interfere with Vitamin K include broad-spectrum antibiotics, amiodarone used for cardiac arrhythmias, cholesterol-lowering medications, agents that cause fat malabsorption like orlistat, mineral oil, and the fat substitute olestra, which can affect the absorption of all fat-soluble vitamins.

 Food Sources:
- Natto
- Collards
- Turnip greens
- Spinach
- Kale
- Broccoli
- Soybeans
- Carrot juice

The best sources of vitamin K2 include fermented foods, such as natto and some rare fermented cheeses, and liver. Minor amounts are also found in egg yolks and butter.

Support Considerations:

- Increase food sources of vitamin K2, including fermented foods and liver.
- Consider vitamin K2 supplementation.

Supplement Options:
- Studies suggest daily therapeutic doses of about 360-500 micrograms (mcg) of vitamin K2.
- Fermented foods contain a variety of bacteria, and only certain ones, such as Bacillus subtilis, produce vitamin K2. Regular consumption of fermented foods can enhance dietary vitamin K2 intake.
- You can make fermented foods yourself by using a starter culture specifically designed to optimize vitamin K2 production.
- Vitamin K2 supplements come in 'MK' varieties, and MK-4 is the form that all forms of vitamin K2 are converted into in the body. If you take an MK-7 variety, your body will convert it to MK-4. However, MK-4 supplements are available commercially to bypass activation after absorption.

Additional Investigations:
- Stool test to assess gut and digestive health and rule out inflammatory bowel disease (IBD) and fat malabsorption.
- Celiac testing
- Liver function tests
- Kidney function tests
- Genetic testing for ApoE4

Nutritional support:
- Vitamin K1
- Vitamin K2
- Vitamin D3
- Vitamin A
- Magnesium taurinate
- Magnesium glycinate
- Magnesium malate

If **HIGH** or **> 0.89 pg/MM WBC:**

Currently, there is no known toxicity is associated with high doses of vitamin K1 or vitamin K2. Therefore, there is no designated upper intake level (UL). Although allergic reactions are possible, there is no known toxicity associated with high doses (dietary or supplemental) of the phylloquinone (vitamin K1) or menaquinone (vitamin K2) forms of vitamin K). No tolerable upper intake level (UL) has been established for vitamin K

Stop or reduce vitamin K supplementation / sources

Potassium (Serum)

Potassium is one of the main bodily electrolytes (a substance that carries an electrical charge). Potassium helps regulate blood pressure and heart contractions and is needed for muscle contractions. It also helps control intracellular and extracellular fluid balance in an appropriate ratio with sodium.

| Optimal Range | 3.5 - 5.1 mmol/L |

VIBRANT MICRONUTRIENT

If **LOW** or < 3.5 mmol/L:

 Blood electrolyte levels are not usually considered indicators of nutritional status. Deviations from the normal range are usually not caused by dietary factors. In isolation, decreased potassium intake rarely leads to hypokalemia because the kidneys can effectively minimize potassium excretion. However, reduced intake can contribute to hypokalemia when combined with other causes, such as malnutrition or diuretic therapy.

Increased potassium loss (skin, gastrointestinal, and renal losses): When potassium levels are low, it's important to consider body fluid losses first because most cases of hypokalemia result from gastrointestinal (GI) or renal losses.

Magnesium deficiency can contribute to potassium loss, and potassium repletion is more difficult when magnesium levels are inadequate.

Diabetes can cause excessive potassium loss through urine.

Excessive alcohol use, excessive laxative use, excessive sweating, diabetic ketoacidosis, folic acid deficiency, and certain antibiotic use can also cause potassium deficiency.

Potassium-wasting diuretics are a class of drugs known to cause potassium depletion.

Transcellular shifts (increased intracellular uptake): Cellular uptake of potassium is promoted by alkalemia, insulin, beta-adrenergic stimulation, aldosterone, and xanthines, such as caffeine.

 Apricots, lentils, squash, prunes, raisins, potato, kidney beans, and orange juice are food sources.

 Nutritional support
- Multi-mineral
- Potassium
- Sodium
- Chloride
- Magnesium
- Vitamin C
- Zinc

If **HIGH** or > 5.1 mmol/L:

 Currently, there is no known toxicity is associated with high doses of vitamin K1 or vitamin K2. Therefore, there is no designated upper intake level (UL). Although allergic reactions are possible, there is no known toxicity associated with high doses (dietary or supplemental) of the phylloquinone (vitamin K1) or menaquinone (vitamin K2) forms of vitamin K). No tolerable upper intake level (UL) has been established for vitamin K

 Stop or reduce potassium supplementation. Consider other causes of hyperkalemia besides diet and supplements. Also, test electrolytes and kidney function.

Sodium (Serum)

Sodium is one of the main bodily electrolytes (a substance that carries an electrical charge). Sodium helps maintain extracellular and intracellular fluid balance, is needed for muscle contractions, and helps with nerve signaling.

Optimal Range	136.0 - 145.0 mmol/L

If LOW or < 136.0 mmol/L:

Inadequate intake of sodium can occur due to dietary changes that eliminate or reduce processed foods. This can lead to a significant reduction in sodium intake and, in some cases, acute depletion of sodium levels and loss of stored water from liver and muscle glycogen stores.

Several medical conditions can also contribute to sodium depletion. For instance, diarrhea, vomiting, and excessive sweating can cause significant fluid loss, leading to sodium depletion. Additionally, Addison's disease, a condition characterized by the lack of production of mineralocorticoids from the adrenal glands, can result in excessive electrolyte loss, including sodium.

Furthermore, certain medications can increase the risk of hyponatremia. These include diuretics, non-steroidal anti-inflammatory drugs (NSAIDs), opiate derivatives, phenothiazines, serotonin-reuptake inhibitors (SSRIs), and tricyclic antidepressants.

Reduce sodium sources: deli meat sandwiches, pizza, burritos, tacos, soups, savory snacks, poultry, pasta dishes, burgers.

Additional investigations: electrolytes.

Nutritional support
- Potassium
- Sodium
- Chloride
- Magnesium
- Vitamin C
- Zinc

If HIGH or > 145.0 mmol/L:

Hypernatremia generally develops from excess water loss (e.g., burns, respiratory infections, renal loss, osmotic diarrhea, hypothalamic disorders) or reduced water intake, frequently accompanied by an impaired thirst mechanism.

Stop or reduce sodium supplementation from food sources like deli meat sandwiches, pizza, burritos, tacos, soups, savory snacks, poultry, pasta dishes, burgers, and more.

Bibliography

Research Articles

Lab companies

Books

Trainings/teachers/seminars

Other digital source material

Drug-Nutrient Interactions and Depletions resources

Unit Conversion Links

Get LabDx Online Here:

Research Articles

Abdelwahab, M. G., et al. (2012). The ketogenic diet is an effective adjuvant to radiation therapy for the treatment of malignant glioma. PloS One, 7(5), e36197. https://doi.org/10.1371/journal.pone.0036197

Ackermans, L., et al. (1991). Anti-IgG antibodies in rheumatic diseases cross-react with Streptococcus mutans SR antigen. Clinical and Experimental Immunology, 85, 265–269.

Adal, K. A., et al. (1994). Cat scratch disease, bacillary angiomatosis, and other infections due to Rochalimaea. The New England Journal of Medicine, 330, 1509–1515.

Ahmadi, S., Mirzaei, K., Hossein-Nezhad, A., & Shariati, G. (2012). Vitamin D receptor FokI genotype may modify the susceptibility to schizophrenia and bipolar mood disorder by regulation of dopamine D1 receptor gene expression. Minerva Medica, 103(5), 383–391. [PMID: 23042374].

Al Shamsi, B., et al. (2022). Hypoketotic hypoglycemia without neuromuscular complications in patients with SLC25A32 deficiency. European Journal of Human Genetics, 30(8), 976–979. https://doi.org/10.1038/s41431-021-00995-7

Alesci, S., De Martino, M. U., & Kino, T. (2004). L-carnitine is a modulator of the glucocorticoid receptor alpha. Annals of the New York Academy of Sciences, 1024, 147–152. https://doi.org/10.1196/annals.1321.012

Alesci, S., De Martino, M. U., Mirani, M., Benvenga, S., Trimarchi, F., Kino, T., & Chrousos, G. P. (2003). L-carnitine: A nutritional modulator of glucocorticoid receptor functions. FASEB Journal, 17(11), 1553–1555. https://doi.org/10.1096/fj.02-1024fje

Allen, R. H., Stabler, S. P., & Lindenbaum, J. (1993). Serum betaine, N,N-dimethylglycine, and N-methylglycine levels in patients with cobalamin and folate deficiency and related inborn errors of metabolism. Metabolism, 42(11), 1448–1460.

Allos, B. M. (2001). Campylobacter jejuni infections: Update on emerging issues and trends. Clinical Infectious Diseases, 32, 1201–1206.

Amar, S., et al. (2009). Is Porphyromonas gingivalis cell invasion required for atherogenesis? Pharmacotherapeutic implications. Journal of Immunology, 182, 1584–1592.

Amelio, I., Cutruzzolà, F., Antonov, A., Agostini, M., & Melino, G. (2014). Serine and glycine metabolism in cancer. Trends in Biochemical Sciences, 39(4), 191–198.

Anderson, C. A., et al. (2009). Investigation of Crohn's disease risk loci in ulcerative colitis further defines their molecular relationship. Gastroenterology, 136(2), 523–529.e3. https://doi.org/10.1053/j.gastro.2008.10.032

Ang, C. W., et al. (2004). The Guillain-Barré syndrome: A true case of molecular mimicry. Trends in Immunology, 25(2), 61–66.

Anstee, Q. M., & Day, C. P. (2012). S-adenosylmethionine (SAMe) therapy in liver disease: A review of current evidence and clinical utility. Journal of Hepatology, 57(5), 1097-109. https://doi.org/10.1016/j.jhep.2012.04.041

Aras, O., Hanson, N. Q., Yang, F., & Tsai, M. Y. (2000). Influence of 699C-->T and 1080C-->T polymorphisms of the cystathionine beta-synthase gene on plasma homocysteine levels. Clinical Genetics, 58(6), 455–459. https://doi.org/10.1034/j.1399-0004.2000.580605.x

Arici, M., & Özhan, G. (2017). CYP2C9, CYP2C19, and CYP2D6 gene profiles and gene susceptibility to drug response and toxicity in the Turkish population. Saudi Pharmaceutical Journal, 25(3), 376–380. https://doi.org/10.1016/j.jsps.2016.09.003

Arnold, R., & Richter, W. (2001). Is obsessive–compulsive disorder an autoimmune disease? Canadian Medical Association Journal, 165(10), 1353–1358.

Ashton, K. A., et al. (2009). Polymorphisms in TP53 and MDM2 combined are associated with high grade endometrial cancer. Gynecologic Oncology, 113(1), 109–114. https://doi.org/10.1016/j.ygyno.2008.12.036

RESEARCH ARTICLES

Avila, M. A., Corrales, F. J., Ruiz, F., Sánchez-Góngora, E., Mingorance, J., Carretero, M. V., & Mato, I. M. (1998). Specific interaction of methionine adenosyltransferase with free radicals. *Biofactors, 8*(1-2), 27–32. https://doi.org/10.1002/biof.5520080106

Ayala, C., García, R., Cruz, E., Prieto, K., & Bermúdez, M. (2010). Niveles de homocisteína y polimorfismos de los genes de la MTHFR y la CBS en pacientes colombianos con trombosis venosa superficial y profunda [Homocysteine levels and polymorphisms of MTHFR and CBS genes in Colombian patients with superficial and deep venous thrombosis]. *Biomedica, 30*(2), 259–267. [PMID: 20890573].

Babic, M., Krmpotic, A., & Jonjic, S. (2011). All is fair in virus-host interactions: NK cells and cytomegalovirus. *Trends in Molecular Medicine, 17*(11), 677–685. https://doi.org/10.1016/j.molmed.2011.07.003

Baker, S. E. (2006). Aspergillus niger genomics: Past, present and into the future. *Medical Mycology, 44*(Suppl 1), S17–S21. https://doi.org/10.1080/13693780600921037

Ball, J. K., Tarr, A. W., & McKeating, J. A. (2014). The past, present, and future of neutralizing antibodies for hepatitis C virus. *Antiviral Research, 105*, 100–111. https://doi.org/10.1016/j.antiviral.2014.02.013

Barnes, C., Buckley, S., Pacheco, F., & Portnoy, J. (2002). IgE-reactive proteins from *Stachybotrys chartarum*. *Annals of Allergy, Asthma & Immunology, 89*(1), 29–33. https://doi.org/10.1016/S1081-1206(10)61907-4

Bartlett, J. G. (2006). Narrative review: The new epidemic of *Clostridium difficile*-associated enteric disease. *Annals of Internal Medicine, 145*(10), 758-764. https://doi.org/10.7326/0003-4819-145-10-200611210-00008

Bartlett, J. G., Chang, T. W., Gurwith, M., Gorbach, S. L., & Onderdonk, A. B. (1978). Antibiotic-associated pseudomembranous colitis due to toxin-producing clostridia. *New England Journal of Medicine, 298*(10), 531-534. https://doi.org/10.1056/NEJM197803092981003

Baseman, J. B., & Tully, J. G. (1997). Mycoplasmas: Sophisticated, reemerging, and burdened by their notoriety. *Emerging Infectious Diseases, 3*(1), 21-32. https://doi.org/10.3201/eid0301.970103

Bashir, M. E., Ismail, E. A., & Ahmed, S. H. (2014). Serological versus antigen detection methods for *Giardia duodenalis* diagnosis. *Journal of the Egyptian Society of Parasitology, 44*(3), 709-718.

Bason, C., Corrocher, R., Lunardi, C., Puccetti, P., Olivieri, O., Girelli, D., Navone, R., Beri, R., Millo, E., Margonato, A., Martinelli, N., & Puccetti, A. (2003). Interaction of antibodies against cytomegalovirus with heat-shock protein 60 in pathogenesis of atherosclerosis. *The Lancet, 362*(9400), 1971-1977. https://doi.org/10.1016/S0140-6736(03)15016-7

Beagle, B., Yang, T. L., Hung, J., Cogger, E. A., Moriarty, D. J., & Jacobsen, D. W. (2000). Biochemistry and metabolism. In *Homocysteine and vascular disease* (pp. 15-39). Springer.

Beagle, B., Yang, T. L., Hung, J., Cogger, E. A., Moriarty, D. J., & Caudill, M. A. (2005). The glycine N-methyltransferase (GNMT) 1289 C->T variant influences plasma total homocysteine concentrations in young women after restricting folate intake. *The Journal of Nutrition, 135*(12), 2780-2785. https://doi.org/10.1093/jn/135.12.2780

Beaver, K. M., Barnes, J. C., & Boutwell, B. B. (2014). The 2-repeat allele of the MAOA gene confers an increased risk for shooting and stabbing behaviors. *Psychiatric Quarterly, 85*(3), 257-265. https://doi.org/10.1007/s11126-013-9287-x

Behera, J., Bala, J., Nuru, M., Tyagi, S. C., & Tyagi, N. (2017). Homocysteine as a pathological biomarker for bone disease. *Journal of Cellular Physiology, 232*(10), 2704-2709. https://doi.org/10.1002/jcp.25693

Benvenga, S., Guarneri, F., Vaccaro, M., Santarpia, L., & Trimarchi, F. (2004). Homologies between proteins of *Borrelia burgdorferi* and thyroid autoantigens. *Thyroid, 14*(11), 964-966. https://doi.org/10.1089/thy.2004.14.964

Bergner-Rabinowitz, S., Ofek, I., & Fleiderman, S. (1973). Evaluation of streptozyme and antistreptolysin O tests in streptococcal pyodermal nephritis. *Applied Microbiology, 26*(1), 56-58.

Berigan, T. R. (2002). A case report of a manic episode triggered by S-Adenosylmethionine (SAMe). *Primary Care Companion to the Journal of Clinical Psychiatry, 4*(4), 159.

Bermejo, J. L., Garcia-Ahonen, O., & Harth, V. (2009). Representation of genetic association via attributable familial relative risks in order to identify polymorphisms functionally relevant to rheumatoid arthritis. *BMC Proceedings, 3*(Suppl 7), S10. https://doi.org/10.1186/1753-6561-3-S7-S10

RESEARCH ARTICLES

Bertolo, R. F., & McBreairty, L. E. (2013). The nutritional burden of methylation reactions. *Current Opinion in Clinical Nutrition and Metabolic Care, 16*(1), 102-108. https://doi.org/10.1097/MCO.0b013e32835ad2ee

Bertram, L., McQueen, M. B., Mullin, K., Blacker, D., & Tanzi, R. E. (2007). Systematic meta-analyses of Alzheimer disease genetic association studies: The AlzGene database. *Nature Genetics, 39*(1), 17-23. https://doi.org/10.1038/ng1934

Beumer, W., van Exel, E., Gussekloo, J., Ligthart, G. J., & Westendorp, R. G. (2010). Detection of *Mycobacterium avium* subsp. *paratuberculosis* in drinking water and biofilms by quantitative PCR. *Applied and Environmental Microbiology, 76*(21), 7367-7370. https://doi.org/10.1128/AEM.00906-10

Biberfeld, G. (1971). Antibodies to brain and other tissues in cases of *Mycoplasma pneumoniae* infection. *Clinical and Experimental Immunology, 8*(2), 319-333.

Binkley, P. F., Cooke, G. E., Lesinski, A., Taylor, M., Chen, M., Laskowski, B., Waldman, W. J., Ariza, M. E., Williams, M. V., Knight, D. A., & Glaser, R. (2013). Evidence for the role of Epstein-Barr virus infections in the pathogenesis of acute coronary events. *PLoS ONE, 8*(1), e54008. https://doi.org/10.1371/journal.pone.0054008

Blair, C., Sulik, M., Willoughby, M., Mills-Koonce, R., Petrill, S., Bartlett, C., Greenberg, M., & Family Life Project Investigators. (2015). Catechol-O-methyltransferase Val158met polymorphism interacts with early experience to predict executive functions in early childhood. *Developmental Psychobiology, 57*(7), 833-841. https://doi.org/10.1002/dev.21332

Blaser, M. J. (2006). Who are we? Indigenous microbes and the ecology of human diseases. *EMBO Reports, 7*(10), 956-960. https://doi.org/10.1038/sj.embor.7400812

Blom, H. J., & Smulders, Y. (2011). Overview of homocysteine and folate metabolism. With special references to cardiovascular disease and neural tube defects. *Journal of Inherited Metabolic Disease, 34*(1), 75-81. https://doi.org/10.1007/s10545-010-9177-4

Bogdanos, D. P., Choudhuri, K., & Vergani, D. (2000). Virus/self double reactivity characterises the humoral immune response in autoimmune hepatitis-2. *Journal of Hepatology, 32*(Suppl 2), 45.

Borges, M., Barreira-Silva, P., Flórido, M., Jordan, M. B., Correia-Neves, M., & Appelberg, R. (2012). Molecular and cellular mechanisms of *Mycobacterium avium*-induced thymic atrophy. *The Journal of Immunology, 189*(7), 3600-3608. https://doi.org/10.4049/jimmunol.1201525

Bottiglieri, T. (2002). S-Adenosyl-L-methionine (SAMe): From the bench to the bedside—molecular basis of a pleiotrophic molecule. *The American Journal of Clinical Nutrition, 76*(5), 1151S-1157S. https://doi.org/10.1093/ajcn/76.5.1151S

Bottone, E. J. (1997). *Yersinia enterocolitica*: The charisma continues. *Clinical Microbiology Reviews, 10*(2), 257-276. https://doi.org/10.1128/CMR.10.2.257

Bouzid, M., Hunter, P. R., Chalmers, R. M., & Tyler, K. M. (2013). Cryptosporidium pathogenicity and virulence. *Clinical Microbiology Reviews, 26*(1), 115-134. https://doi.org/10.1128/CMR.00076-12

Braiteh, F., & Golden, M. P. (2007). Cryptogenic invasive *Klebsiella pneumoniae* liver abscess syndrome. *International Journal of Infectious Diseases, 11*(1), 16-22. https://doi.org/10.1016/j.ijid.2005.10.006

Brasel, T. L., Martin, J. M., Carriker, C. G., Wilson, S. C., & Straus, D. C. (2005). Detection of airborne *Stachybotrys chartarum* macrocyclic trichothecene mycotoxins on particulates smaller than conidia. *Applied and Environmental Microbiology, 71*(1), 114-122. https://doi.org/10.1128/AEM.71.1.114-122.2005

Bronze, M. S., & Dale, J. B. (1993). Epitopes of streptococcal M proteins that evoke antibodies that cross-react with human brain. *The Journal of Immunology, 151*(5), 2820-2828.

Brosnan, J. T., Jacobs, R. L., Stead, L. M., & Brosnan, M. E. (2004). Methylation demand: A key determinant of homocysteine metabolism. *Acta Biochimica Polonica, 51*(2), 405-414. https://doi.org/10.18388/abp.2004_3516

Bruckbauer, H. R., Preac-Mursic, V., Fuchs, R., & Wilske, B. (1992). Crossreactive proteins of *Borrelia burgdorferi*. *European Journal of Clinical Microbiology & Infectious Diseases, 11*(3), 224-232. https://doi.org/10.1007/BF02098084

Brunham, R. C. (1985). *Chlamydia trachomatis*: Its role in tubal infertility. *The Journal of Infectious Diseases, 152*(6), 1275-1282. https://doi.org/10.1093/infdis/152.6.1275

Burazor, I., Vojdani, A., & Burazor, M. (2006). *Porhyromonas gingivalis* and acute myocardial infarction. *Acta Facultatis Medicae Naissensis, 23*(2), 69-74.

Byard, R. W., Jimenez, C. L., Carpenter, B. F., & Hsu, E. (1987). Aspergillus-related aortic thrombosis. *Canadian Medical Association Journal, 136*(2), 155-156.

Caesar, R., Tremaroli, V., Kovatcheva-Datchary, P., Cani, P. D., & Bäckhed, F. (2015). Crosstalk between gut microbiota and dietary lipids aggravates WAT inflammation through TLR signaling. *Cell Metabolism, 22*, 658–668. https://doi.org/10.1016/j.cmet.2015.07.026

Campbell, L. A., Kuo, C. C., Grayston, J. T., & Daling, J. R. (1998). *Chlamydia pneumoniae* and cardiovascular disease. *Emerging Infectious Diseases, 4*(4), 571-579.

Campos-Rodríguez, R., & Jarillo-Luna, A. (2005). The pathogenicity of *Entamoeba histolytica* is related to the capacity of evading innate immunity. *Parasite Immunology, 17*, 1-8.

Cannon, J., et al. (2010). Review of cytomegalovirus seroprevalence and demographic characteristics associated with infection. *Review of Medical Virology, 20*(4), 202-213.

Capdevila, A., Burk, R. F., Freedman, J., Frantzen, F., Alfheim, I., & Wagner, C. (2007). A simple rapid immunoassay for S-adenosylhomocysteine in plasma. *Journal of Nutritional Biochemistry, 18*(12), 827-831.

Casas, J. P., Bautista, L. E., Humphries, S. E., & Hingorani, A. D. (2004). Endothelial nitric oxide synthase genotype and ischemic heart disease: Meta-analysis of 26 studies involving 23,028 subjects. *Circulation, 109*(11), 1359-1365. https://doi.org/10.1161/01.CIR.0000121357.76910.A3

Cassinadane, A. V., & Ramasamy, R. (n.d.). Association of BHMT (RS 3733890) gene polymorphism with biochemical markers of B12 deficiency in T2DM patients on metformin therapy. *International Research Journal on Advanced Science Hub*. Retrieved from https://rspsciencehub.com/index.php/journal/article/view/413

Castro, R., Rivera, I., Blom, H. J., Jakobs, C., & Tavares de Almeida, I. (2006). Homocysteine metabolism, hyperhomocysteinaemia and vascular disease: An overview. *Journal of Inherited Metabolic Disease, 29*(1), 3-20.

Catry, E., Bindels, L. B., Tailleux, A., Lestavel, S., Neyrinck, A. M., Goossens, J. F., Lobysheva, I., Plovier, H., Essaghir, A., Demoulin, J. B., Bouzin, C., Pachikian, B. D., Cani, P. D., Staels, B., Dessy, C., & Delzenne, N. M. (2018). Targeting the gut microbiota with inulin-type fructans: Preclinical demonstration of a novel approach in the management of endothelial dysfunction. *Gut, 67*(2), 271-283. https://doi.org/10.1136/gutjnl-2016-313316

Cavalieri, E. L., Stack, D. E., Devanesan, P. D., Todorovic, R., Dwivedy, I., Higginbotham, S., Johansson, S. L., Patil, K. D., Gross, M. L., Gooden, J. K., Ramanathan, R., Cerny, R. L., & Rogan, E. G. (1997). Molecular origin of cancer: Catechol estrogen-3,4-quinones as endogenous tumor initiators. *Proceedings of the National Academy of Sciences of the United States of America, 94*(20), 10937-10942.

Centers for Disease Control and Prevention. (2012). Cryptosporidiosis surveillance—United States, 2009–2010 and giardiasis surveillance—United States, 2009–2010. *MMWR, 61*(5), 1-28.

Chang, P. Y., Lu, S. C., & Chen, C. H. (2010). S-adenosylhomocysteine: A better marker of the development of Alzheimer's disease than homocysteine? *Journal of Alzheimer's Disease: JAD, 21*(1), 65–66. https://doi.org/10.3233/JAD-2010-100144

Chattopadhyay, M. K., Chen, W., & Tabor, H. (2013). Escherichia coli glutathionylspermidine synthetase/amidase: Phylogeny and effect on regulation of gene expression. *FEMS Microbiology Letters, 338*(2), 132–140. https://doi.org/10.1111/1574-6968.12035

Chen, C. H., Ferreira, J. C., Gross, E. R., & Mochly-Rosen, D. (2014). Targeting aldehyde dehydrogenase 2: New therapeutic opportunities. *Physiological Reviews, 94*(1), 1-34. https://doi.org/10.1152/physrev.00017.2013

Chen, M., Huang, Y. L., Huang, Y. C., Shui, I. M., Giovannucci, E., Chen, Y. C., & Chen, Y. M. (2014, May 6). Genetic polymorphisms of the glycine N-methyltransferase and prostate cancer risk in the health professionals follow-up study. *PLOS ONE, 9*(5), e94683. https://doi.org/10.1371/journal.pone.0094683

Chen, S. L., & Morgan, T. R. (2006). The natural history of hepatitis C virus (HCV) infection. *International Journal of Medical Sciences, 3*(2), 47–52. https://doi.org/10.7150/ijms.3.47

Cheng, M., & Kang, N. (2019, February). Stereotypes about Enterotype: The Old and New Ideas. *Genomics, Proteomics & Bioinformatics, 17*(1), 4–12. https://doi.org/10.1016/j.gpb.2018.02.004

Chien, Y. H., Abdenur, J. E., Baronio, F., Bannick, A. A., Corrales, F., Couce, M., Donner, M. G., Ficicioglu, C., Freehauf, C., Frithiof, D., Gotway, G., Hirabayashi, K., Hofstede, F., Hoganson, G., Hwu, W. L., James, P., Kim, S., Korman, S. H., Lachmann, R., Levy, H., Lindner, M., Lykopoulou, L., Mayatepek, E., Muntau, A., Okano, Y., Raymond, K., Rubio-Gozalbo, E., Scholl-Bürgi, S., Schulze, A., Singh, R., Stabler, S., Stuy, M., Thomas, J., Wagner, C., Wilson, W. G., Wortmann, S., Yamamoto, S., Pao, M., & Blom, H. J. (2015). Mudd's disease (MAT I/III deficiency): A survey of data for MAT1A homozygotes and compound heterozygotes. *Orphanet Journal of Rare Diseases, 10*, 99. https://doi.org/10.1186/s13023-015-0321-y

Chomel, B., et al. (2009). Ecological fitness and strategies of adaptation of *Bartonella* species to their hosts and vectors. *Veterinary Research, 40*, 29.

Christakos, S., Dhawan, P., Liu, Y., Peng, X., & Porta, A. (2003). New insights into the mechanisms of vitamin D action. *Journal of Cellular Biochemistry, 88*(4), 695-705.

Chung, K. H., Lee, S. H., Park, J. Y., Kim, S. H., & Kim, S. K. (2005). Dose-dependent allergic responses to an extract of *Penicillium chrysogenum* in BALB/c mice. *Toxicology, 209*(1), 77-89.

Chung, M. R., Kim, H. B., Kim, S. H., Kim, S. J., Kim, Y. H., Lee, K. H., & Kim, C. U. (2007). Emerging invasive liver abscess caused by K1 serotype *Klebsiella pneumoniae* in Korea. *Journal of Infection, 54*, 578–583.

Cimolai, N., Kenny, G. E., & Krause, D. C. (1987). Immunological cross-reactivity of a *Mycoplasma pneumoniae* membrane-associated protein antigen with *Mycoplasma genitalium* and *Acholeplasma laidlawii*. *Journal of Clinical Microbiology, 25*(11), 2136–2139.

Cishek, M. B., Yost, B., & Schaefer, S. (1996). Cardiac aspergillosis presenting as myocardial infarction. *Clinical Cardiology, 19*(10), 824–827. https://doi.org/10.1002/clc.4960191012

Claeys, G., et al. (1998). The gastric H+,K+-ATPase is a major autoantigen in chronic *Helicobacter pylori* gastritis with body mucosa atrophy. *Gastroenterology, 115*, 340–347.

Claussnitzer, M., Dankel, S. N., Kim, K. H., Quon, G., Meuleman, W., Haugen, C., Glunk, V., Sousa, I. S., Beaudry, J. L., Puviindran, V., Abdennur, N. A., Liu, J., Svensson, P. A., Hsu, Y. H., Drucker, D. J., Mellgren, G., Hui, C. C., Hauner, H., & Kellis, M. (2015). FTO obesity variant circuitry and adipocyte browning in humans. *The New England Journal of Medicine, 373*(10), 895–907. https://doi.org/10.1056/NEJMoa1502214

Cohen, A., et al. (1947). The treatment of acute gold and arsenic poisoning; Use of BAL (2,3-Dimercaptopropanol, British Anti-Lewisite). *Journal of the American Medical Association, 133*(11), 749–752. https://doi.org/10.1001/jama.1947.02880110015004

Coker, R. J., et al. (2001). *Helicobacter pylori* seropositivity in children with diabetes mellitus type 1. *Journal of Tropical Pediatrics, 47*, 123–124.

Cole, B. C., Aho, K., & Ward, J. R. (1976). Arthritis of mice induced by *Mycoplasma arthritidis*. *Annals of the Rheumatic Diseases, 35*, 14–22.

Cole, D. C., Talley, N. J., Creedon, P. H., Aziz, Q., & Stanghellini, V. (2006). Migraine, fibromyalgia, and depression among people with IBS: A prevalence study. *BMC Gastroenterology, 6*, 26.

Collin, S. M., Metcalfe, C., Refsum, H., Lewis, S. J., Zuccolo, L., Smith, G. D., Chen, L., Harris, R., Davis, M., Marsden, G., Johnston, C., Lane, J. A., Ebbing, M., Bønaa, K. H., Nygård, O., Ueland, P. M., Grau, M. V., Baron, J. A., Donovan, J. L., Neal, D. E., Hamdy, F. C., Smith, A. D., & Martin, R. M. (2010). Circulating folate, vitamin B12, homocysteine, vitamin B12 transport proteins, and risk of prostate cancer: A case-control study, systematic review, and meta-analysis. *Cancer Epidemiology, Biomarkers & Prevention, 19*(6), 1632–1642. https://doi.org/10.1158/1055-9965.EPI-10-0180

Corouge, A., et al. (2015). Humoral immunity links *Candida albicans* infection and celiac disease. *PLOS ONE, 10*(3), e0121776.

Cossu, M., et al. (2013). Association of *Mycobacterium avium* subsp. *paratuberculosis* and SLC11A1 polymorphisms in Sardinian multiple sclerosis patients. *Journal of Infection in Developing Countries, 7*(3), 203–207.

Costa, L. G., Cole, T. B., Vitalone, A., & Furlong, C. E. (2005). Measurement of paraoxonase (PON1) status as a potential biomarker of susceptibility to organophosphate toxicity. *Clinica Chimica Acta; International Journal of Clinical Chemistry, 352*(1-2), 37–47. https://doi.org/10.1016/j.cccn.2004.09.019

Costa, L. G., Giordano, G., & Furlong, C. E. (2011). Pharmacological and dietary modulators of paraoxonase 1 (PON1) activity and expression: The hunt goes on. *Biochemical Pharmacology, 81*(3), 337–344. https://doi.org/10.1016/j.bcp.2010.11.008

Costa, L. G., Vitalone, A., Cole, T. B., & Furlong, C. E. (2005). Modulation of paraoxonase (PON1) activity. *Biochemical Pharmacology, 69*(4), 541–550. https://doi.org/10.1016/j.bcp.2004.08.027

Costenbader, K. H., & Karlson, E. W. (2006). Epstein–Barr virus and rheumatoid arthritis: Is there a link? *Arthritis Research & Therapy, 8*, 204.

Cryz, S. J., Jr., Robbins, J. B., Schneerson, R., Shiloach, J., & Vann, W. F. (1990). Immunological cross-reactivity between *Enterobacter aerogenes* and *Klebsiella* capsular polysaccharides. *Microbial Pathogenesis, 9*(2), 127–130.

Cullen, C. E., Carter, G. T., Weiss, M. D., Grant, P. A., & Saperstein, D. S. (2012). Hypohomocysteinemia: A potentially treatable cause of peripheral neuropathology? *Physical Medicine and Rehabilitation Clinics of North America, 23*(1), 59–65. https://doi.org/10.1016/j.pmr.2011.11.001

Cunningham, M. W. (2000). Pathogenesis of group A streptococcal infections. *Clinical Microbiology Reviews, 13*(5), 470–511.

Cunningham, M. W., Turner, W. E., & Musser, J. M. (1997). Molecular analysis of human cardiac myosin-cross-reactive B- and T-cell epitopes of the group A streptococcal M5 protein. *Infection and Immunity, 65*(9), 3913–3923.

Current, W. L., & Reese, C. S. (1986). A comparison of endogenous development of three isolates of *Cryptosporidium* in suckling mice. *The Journal of Protozoology, 33*, 98–108.

da Costa, K. A., Corbin, K. D., Niculescu, M. D., Galanko, J. A., & Zeisel, S. H. (2014). Identification of new genetic polymorphisms that alter the dietary requirement for choline and vary in their distribution across ethnic and racial groups. *FASEB Journal, 28*(7), 2970–2978. https://doi.org/10.1096/fj.14-255000

Dagenais, T. R., & Keller, N. P. (2009). Pathogenesis of *Aspergillus fumigatus* in invasive aspergillosis. *Clinical Microbiology Reviews, 22*(3), 447–465. https://doi.org/10.1128/CMR.00055-08

Dammacco, F., Sansonno, D., Piccoli, C., Racanelli, V., D'Amore, F. P., & Lauletta, G. (2000). The lymphoid system in hepatitis C virus infection: Autoimmunity, mixed cryoglobulinemia, and overt B-cell malignancy. *Seminars in Liver Disease, 20*(2), 143–157.

Danesh, J., Collins, R., & Peto, R. (1997). Chronic infections and coronary heart disease: Is there a link? *The Lancet, 350*(9075), 430–436.

Danesh, J., Youngman, L., Clark, S., Parish, S., Peto, R., & Collins, R. (1999). Helicobacter pylori infection and early onset myocardial infarction: Case-control and sibling pairs study. *BMJ, 319*(7210), 1157–1162. https://doi.org/10.1136/bmj.319.7210.1157

Darby, C., Chakraborti, A., Polotsky, V. Y., Kosek, M. N., Cheng, L., Montague, M. G., Fitzpatrick, S. K., Blanchard, T. G., & Nataro, J. P. (2014). Cytotoxic and pathogenic properties of *Klebsiella oxytoca* isolated from laboratory animals. *PLOS ONE, 9*(7), e100542. https://doi.org/10.1371/journal.pone.0100542

De Bolle, L., Naesens, L., & De Clercq, E. (2005). Update on human herpesvirus 6 biology, clinical features, and therapy. *Clinical Microbiology Reviews, 18*(1), 217–245. https://doi.org/10.1128/CMR.18.1.217-245.2005

de Luis, D. A., Aller, R., Izaola, O., Primo, D., Urdiales, S., & Romero, E. (2015). Effects of a high-protein/low-carbohydrate diet versus a standard hypocaloric diet on weight and cardiovascular risk factors: Role of a genetic variation in the rs9939609 FTO gene variant. *Journal of Nutrigenetics and Nutrigenomics, 8*(3), 128–136. https://doi.org/10.1159/000441142

De Stefano, V., Dekou, V., Nicaud, V., Chasse, J. F., London, J., Stansbie, D., Humphries, S. E., & Gudnason, V. (1998). Linkage disequilibrium at the cystathionine beta synthase (CBS) locus and the association between genetic variation at the CBS locus and plasma levels of homocysteine. *Annals of Human Genetics, 62*(6), 481–490. https://doi.org/10.1046/j.1469-1809.1998.6260481.x

Denning, D. W. (1998). Invasive aspergillosis. *Clinical Infectious Diseases, 26*(4), 781–803. https://doi.org/10.1086/513943

Di Luca, D., Zorzenon, M., Mirandola, P., Colle, R., Botta, G. A., & Cassai, E. (1995). Human herpesvirus 6 and human herpesvirus 7 in chronic fatigue syndrome. *Journal of Clinical Microbiology, 33*(6), 1660–1661.

RESEARCH ARTICLES

Di Prisco, M. C., Hagel, I., Lynch, N. R., Jiménez, J. C., Rojas, R., Gil, M., & Mata, E. (1993). Possible relationship between allergic disease and infection by *Giardia lamblia*. *Annals of Allergy, 70*(3), 210–213.

di Somma, C., Fiore, R., Dolei, A., Cipriani, P., Rossi, P., & Pini, C. (2003). Cross-reactivity between the major *Parietaria* allergen and rotavirus VP4 protein. *Allergy, 58*(6), 503–510. https://doi.org/10.1034/j.1398-9995.2003.00162.x

Dileepan, T., Smith, E. D., Knowland, D., Hsu, M., Platt, M., Bittner-Eddy, P., Cohen, B., Southern, P., Latimer, E., Harley, E., Agalliu, D., & Cleary, P. P. (2016). Group A Streptococcus intranasal infection promotes CNS infiltration by streptococcal-specific Th17 cells. *Journal of Clinical Investigation, 126*(1), 303–317. https://doi.org/10.1172/JCI80792

Dinleyici, E. C., Eren, M., Dogan, N., Reyhanioglu, S., Yargic, Z. A., & Vandenplas, Y. (2011). Clinical efficacy of *Saccharomyces boulardii* or metronidazole in symptomatic children with *Blastocystis hominis* infection. *Parasitology Research, 108*(3), 541–545. https://doi.org/10.1007/s00436-010-2095-4

Diuk-Wasser, M. A., Hoen, A. G., Cislo, P., Brinkerhoff, R., Hamer, S. A., Rowland, M., Cortinas, R., Vourc'h, G., Melton, F., Hickling, G. J., Tsao, J. I., Bunikis, J., Barbour, A. G., Kitron, U., Piesman, J., & Fish, D. (2012). Human risk of infection with *Borrelia burgdorferi*, the Lyme disease agent, in eastern United States. *The American Journal of Tropical Medicine and Hygiene, 86*(2), 320–327. https://doi.org/10.4269/ajtmh.2012.11-0395

Dix, B. A., & Lambooy, J. P. (1981). Brain monoamine oxidase and replacement of its coenzyme flavin in rats. *Journal of Nutrition, 111*(8), 1397–1402. https://doi.org/10.1093/jn/111.8.1397

Dolcino, M., Zanoni, G., Bason, C., Tinazzi, E., Boccola, E., Valletta, E., Contreas, G., Lunardi, C., & Puccetti, A. (2013). A subset of anti-rotavirus antibodies directed against the viral protein VP7 predicts the onset of celiac disease and induces typical features of the disease in the intestinal epithelial cell line T84. *Immunologic Research, 56*(2–3), 465–476. https://doi.org/10.1007/s12026-013-8420-0

Donofry, S. D., Roecklein, K. A., Wildes, J. E., Miller, M. A., Flory, J. D., & Manuck, S. B. (2014). COMT met allele differentially predicts risk versus severity of aberrant eating in a large community sample. *Psychiatry Research, 220*(1–2), 513–518. https://doi.org/10.1016/j.psychres.2014.08.037

Doolin, M. T., Barbaux, S., McDonnell, M., Hoess, K., Whitehead, A. S., & Mitchell, L. E. (2002). Maternal genetic effects, exerted by genes involved in homocysteine remethylation, influence the risk of spina bifida. *American Journal of Human Genetics, 71*(5), 1222–1226. https://doi.org/10.1086/344209

Drancourt, M., Brouqui, P., & Raoult, D. (1997). *Afipia clevelandensis* antibodies and cross-reactivity with *Brucella* spp. and *Yersinia enterocolitica* O:9. *Clinical and Diagnostic Laboratory Immunology, 4*(6), 748–752.

Dunn, B. E., Cohen, H., & Blaser, M. J. (1997). Helicobacter pylori. *Clinical Microbiology Reviews, 10*(4), 720–741. https://doi.org/10.1128/CMR.10.4.720

Ebringer, A., Brezinschek, R. P., & Ebringer, R. L. (1978). Sequential studies in ankylosing spondylitis. Association of *Klebsiella pneumoniae* with active disease. *Annals of the Rheumatic Diseases, 37*(2), 146–151.

Ebringer, A., Brezinschek, R. P., & Ebringer, R. L. (2012). The role of *Acinetobacter* in the pathogenesis of multiple sclerosis examined by using Popper sequences. *Medical Hypotheses, 78*, 763–769.

Edman, U., Akiyoshi, D. E., McLaughlin, J., & Gillin, F. D. (1987). Genomic and cDNA actin sequences from a virulent strain of *Entamoeba histolytica*. *Proceedings of the National Academy of Sciences of the United States of America, 84*(9), 3024–3028.

El Wakil, S. S. (2007). Evaluation of the in vitro effect of *Nigella sativa* aqueous extract on *Blastocystis hominis* isolates. *Journal of the Egyptian Society of Parasitology, 37*(3), 801–813. https://doi.org/10.1016/j.jpes.2007.03.002

Elshorbagy, A. K., Jernerén, F., Samocha-Bonet, D., Refsum, H., & Heilbronn, L. K. (2016). Serum S-adenosylmethionine, but not methionine, increases in response to overfeeding in humans. *Nutrition & Diabetes, 6*(1), e192. https://doi.org/10.1038/nutd.2015.44

Elshorbagy, A. K., Nijpels, G., Valdivia-Garcia, M., Stehouwer, C. D., Ocke, M., Refsum, H., & Dekker, J. M. (2013). S-adenosylmethionine is associated with fat mass and truncal adiposity in older adults. *The Journal of Nutrition, 143*(12), 1982–1988. https://doi.org/10.3945/jn.113.179192

Emin Erdal, M., Herken, H., Yilmaz, M., & Bayazit, Y. A. (2001). Significance of the catechol-O-methyltransferase gene polymorphism in migraine. *Brain Research. Molecular Brain Research, 94*(1–2), 193–196.

Eschete, B., Foos, R. Y., & Robinson, N. M. (1981). *Penicillium chrysogenum* endophthalmitis. *Mycopathologia, 74*(2), 125–127.

Esposito, S., Putignani, L., Sette, C., Sette, G., & Trojano, M. (1999). Human transaldolase and cross-reactive viral epitopes identified by autoantibodies of multiple sclerosis patients. *The Journal of Immunology, 163*, 4027–4032.

Everard, A., Belzer, C., Geurts, L., Ouwerkerk, J. P., Druart, C., Bindels, L. B., Guiot, Y., Derrien, M., Muccioli, G. G., Delzenne, N. M., de Vos, W. M., & Cani, P. D. (2013). Cross-talk between *Akkermansia muciniphila* and intestinal epithelium controls diet-induced obesity. *Proceedings of the National Academy of Sciences, 110*(22), 9066–9071. https://doi.org/10.1073/pnas.1219451110

Ewen, S. W., & Pusztai, A. (1999). Effect of diets containing genetically modified potatoes expressing *Galanthus nivalis* lectin on rat small intestine. *The Lancet, 354*(9187), 1353–1354. https://doi.org/10.1016/S0140-6736(99)00246-0

Fahey, L. M., et al. (2018). Food allergen triggers are increased in children with the TSLP risk allele and eosinophilic esophagitis. *Clinical and Translational Gastroenterology, 9*(3), 139. https://doi.org/10.1038/s41424-018-0003-x

Falgier, B., et al. (2011). *Candida* species differ in their interactions with immature human gastrointestinal epithelial cells. *Pediatric Research, 69*(5 Pt 1), 384–389.

Feng, J., Leone, J., Schweig, S., & Zhang, Y. (2020). Evaluation of natural and botanical medicines for activity against growing and non-growing forms of *B. burgdorferi*. *Frontiers in Medicine (Lausanne), 7*, 6. https://doi.org/10.3389/fmed.2020.00006

Fernando, M. M., Stevens, C. R., Sabeti, P. C., Walsh, E. C., McWhinnie, A. J., Shah, A., Green, T., Rioux, J. D., & Vyse, T. J. (2007). Identification of two independent risk factors for lupus within the MHC in United Kingdom families. *PLoS Genetics, 3*(11), e192. https://doi.org/10.1371/journal.pgen.0030192

Ferretti, J. J., et al. (1980). Cross-reactivity of *Streptococcus mutans* antigens and human heart tissue. *Infection and Immunity, 30*(1), 69–73.

Finkelstein, J. D. (2000). Pathways and regulation of homocysteine metabolism in mammals. *Seminars in Thrombosis and Hemostasis, 26*(3), 219–225.

Ford, P. J., et al. (2005). Cross-reactivity of GroEL antibodies with human heat shock protein 60 and quantification of pathogens in atherosclerosis. *Oral Microbiology and Immunology, 20*, 296–302.

Fournier, P. E., & Richet, H. (2006). The epidemiology and control of *Acinetobacter baumannii* in health care facilities. *Clinical Infectious Diseases, 42*, 692–699.

Francis, M. B., et al. (2013). Bile acid recognition by the *Clostridium difficile* germinant receptor, CspC, is important for establishing infection. *PLoS Pathogens, 9*, e1003356.

Frulloni, L., et al. (2009). Identification of a novel antibody associated with autoimmune pancreatitis. *The New England Journal of Medicine, 361*(22), 2135–2142.

Fujiya, M., et al. (2010). Fulminant type 1 diabetes mellitus associated with a reactivation of Epstein–Barr virus that developed in the course of chemotherapy for multiple myeloma. *Journal of Diabetes Investigation, 1*(6), 286–289.

Gammazza, A. M., et al. (2014). Elevated blood Hsp60, its structural similarities and cross-reactivity with thyroid molecules, and its presence on the plasma membrane of oncocytes point to the chaperonin as an immunopathogenic factor in Hashimoto's thyroiditis. *Cell Stress and Chaperones, 19*(3), 343–353.

Garcia, L. S., Arrowood, M., Kokoskin, E., Paltridge, G. P., Pillai, D. R., Procop, G. W., Ryan, N., Shimizu, R. Y., & Visvesvara, G. (2017). Practical guidance for clinical microbiology laboratories: Laboratory diagnosis of parasites from the gastrointestinal tract. *Clinical Microbiology Reviews, 31*(1), e00025-17. https://doi.org/10.1128/CMR.00025-17

Gariballa, S. (2011). Testing homocysteine-induced neurotransmitter deficiency and depression of mood hypothesis in clinical practice. *Age and Ageing, 40*(6), 702–705.

Garibotto, G., Valli, A., Anderstam, B., et al. (2009). The kidney is the major site of S-adenosylhomocysteine disposal in humans. *Kidney International, 76*(3), 293–296.

Gateva, V., et al. (2009). A large-scale replication study identifies TNIP1, PRDM1, JAZF1, UHRF1BP1, and IL10 as risk loci for systemic lupus erythematosus. *Nature Genetics, 41*(11), 1228–1233. https://doi.org/10.1038/ng.468

Gaughan, D. J., Kluijtmans, L. A., Barbaux, S., McMaster, D., Young, I. S., Yarnell, J. W., Evans, A., & Whitehead, A. S. (2001). The methionine synthase reductase (MTRR) A66G polymorphism is a novel genetic determinant of plasma homocysteine concentrations. *Atherosclerosis, 157*(2), 451–456. https://doi.org/10.1016/S0021-9150(00)00739-5

Gaulton, K. J., et al. (2008). Comprehensive association study of type 2 diabetes and related quantitative traits with 222 candidate genes. *Diabetes, 57*(11), 3136–3144. https://doi.org/10.2337/db07-1731

Gautam, Y., et al. (2020). Comprehensive functional annotation of susceptibility variants associated with asthma. *Human Genetics, 139*(8), 1037–1053. https://doi.org/10.1007/s00439-020-02151-5

Gavino, A. C., Chung, J. S., Sato, K., Ariizumi, K., & Cruz, P. D., Jr. (2005). Identification and expression profiling of a human C-type lectin, structurally homologous to mouse dectin-2. *Experimental Dermatology, 14*(4), 281–288.

Ghose, C. (2013). *Clostridium difficile* infection in the twenty-first century. *Emerging Microbes & Infections, 2*(9), e62. https://doi.org/10.1038/emi.2013.62

Girschick, H. J., et al. (2009). Treatment of Lyme borreliosis. *Arthritis Research & Therapy, 11*, 258. https://doi.org/10.1186/ar2853

Goldstein, I. J., & Poretz, R. D. (2012). Isolation, physicochemical characterization, and carbohydrate-binding specificity of lectins. In I. E. Liener, N. Sharon, & I. J. Goldstein (Eds.), *The Lectins: Properties, Functions, and Applications in Biology and Medicine* (pp. 33–247). Elsevier.

Goodman, A. D., et al. (2003). Human herpesvirus 6 genome and antigen in acute multiple sclerosis lesions. *Journal of Infectious Diseases, 187*, 1365–1376.

Goodman, J. E., Lavigne, J. A., Wu, K., et al. (2001). COMT genotype, micronutrients in the folate metabolic pathway, and breast cancer risk. *Carcinogenesis, 22*(10), 1661–1665.

Gran, J. T., et al. (1983). HLA DR antigens and gold toxicity. *Annals of the Rheumatic Diseases, 42*(1), 63–66. https://doi.org/10.1136/ard.42.1.63

Green, T. J., Skeaff, C. M., McMahon, J. A., et al. (2010). Homocysteine-lowering vitamins do not lower plasma S-adenosylhomocysteine in older people with elevated homocysteine concentrations. *British Journal of Nutrition, 103*(11), 1629–1634.

Greenfield, J. (2021). *Don't fall into the methyl trap!* Retrieved from http://datapunk.net/opus23blog/2016/02/20/dont-fall-into-the-methyl-trap/

Gross, A. J., et al. (2005). EBV and systemic lupus erythematosus: A new perspective. *Journal of Immunology, 174*, 6599–6607.

Gu, H. F., & Zhang, X. (2017). Zinc deficiency and epigenetics. In V. Preedy & V. Patel (Eds.), *Handbook of famine, starvation, and nutrient deprivation*. Springer, Cham. https://doi.org/10.1007/978-3-319-40007-5_80-1

Guarneri, F., Guarneri, B., Borgia, F., & Guarneri, C. (2011). Potential role of molecular mimicry between human U1-70 kDa and fungal proteins in the development of T-cell mediated anti-U1-70 kDa autoimmunity. *Immunopharmacology and Immunotoxicology, 33*(4), 620–625. https://doi.org/10.3109/08923973.2011.553722

Guerra-Shinohara, E. M., Morita, O. E., Pagliusi, R. A., Blaia-d'Avila, V. L., Allen, R. H., & Stabler, S. P. (2007). Elevated serum S-adenosylhomocysteine in cobalamin-deficient megaloblastic anemia. *Metabolism, 56*(3), 339–347.

Gugnani, H. C. (2003). Ecology and taxonomy of pathogenic aspergilli. *Frontiers in Bioscience, 8*, s346–s357. https://doi.org/10.2741/1002

Guimarães, S., & Sogayar, M. I. L. (2002). Detection of anti-*Giardia lamblia* serum antibody among children of day care centers. *Revista de Saúde Pública, 36*(1), 63–68.

Guo, Q. N., Wang, H. D., Tie, L. Z., Li, T., Xiao, H., Long, J. G., & Liao, S. X. (2017). Parental genetic variants, MTHFR 677C>T and MTRR 66A>G, associated differently with fetal congenital heart defect. *BioMed Research International, 2017*, 3043476. https://doi.org/10.1155/2017/3043476

Gursoy, S., Erdal, E., Herken, H., Madenci, E., Alasehirli, B., & Erdal, N. (2003). Significance of catechol-O-methyltransferase gene polymorphism in fibromyalgia syndrome. *Rheumatology International, 23*(3), 104–107.

Haas, H., Falcone, F. H., Schramm, G., Haisch, K., Gibbs, B. F., Klaucke, J., Pöppelmann, M., Becker, W. M., Gabius, H. J., & Schlaak, M. (1999). Dietary lectins can induce in vitro release of IL-4 and IL-13 from human basophils. *European Journal of Immunology, 29*(3), 918–927. https://doi.org/10.1002/(SICI)1521-4141(199903)29:03<918::AID-IMMU918>3.0.CO;2-T

Haerian, M. S., Haerian, B. S., Molanaei, S., Kosari, F., Sabeti, S., Bidari-Zerehpoosh, F., & Abdolali, E. (2017). MTRR rs1801394 and its interaction with MTHFR rs1801133 in colorectal cancer: A case-control study and meta-analysis. *Pharmacogenomics, 18*(11), 1075–1084. https://doi.org/10.2217/pgs-2017-0030

Hagen, T. M., Wierzbicka, G. T., Sillau, A., Bowman, B. B., & Jones, D. P. (1990). Bioavailability of dietary glutathione: Effect on plasma concentration. *American Journal of Physiology - Gastrointestinal and Liver Physiology, 259*(4), G524–G529.

Hahn, Y. W., Kim, J. H., Bae, Y. S., Kim, Y. O., & Hwang, Y. J. (2000). Cytokine induction by *Streptococcus mutans* and pulpal pathogenesis. *Infection and Immunity, 68*(12), 6785–6789.

Hajishengallis, G. (2015). Periodontitis: From microbial immune subversion to systemic inflammation. *Nature Reviews Immunology, 15*, 30–44.

Hall, K. T., Nelson, C. P., Davis, R. B., et al. (2014). Polymorphisms in catechol-O-methyltransferase modify treatment effects of aspirin on risk of cardiovascular disease. *Arteriosclerosis, Thrombosis, and Vascular Biology, 34*(9), 2160–2167. https://doi.org/10.1161/ATVBAHA.114.303845

Han, Y., Wang, Q., Song, P., Zhu, Y., & Zou, M. H. (2010). Redox regulation of the AMP-activated protein kinase. *PLOS ONE, 5*(11), e15420. https://doi.org/10.1371/journal.pone.0015420

Hao, X., Huang, Y., Qiu, M., Yin, C., Ren, H., Gan, H., Li, H., Zhou, Y., Xia, J., Li, W., Guo, L., & Angres, I. A. (2016). Immunoassay of S-adenosylmethionine and S-adenosylhomocysteine: The methylation index as a biomarker for disease and health status. *BMC Research Notes, 9*(1), 498. https://doi.org/10.1186/s13104-016-2296-8

Haque, R., Huston, C. D., Hughes, M., Houpt, E., & Petri, C. A. (2002). Innate and acquired resistance to amebiasis in Bangladeshi children. *The Journal of Infectious Diseases, 186*(4), 547–552.

Harel, M., Aharoni, A., Gaidukov, L., Brumshtein, B., Khersonsky, O., Meged, R., Dvir, H., Ravelli, R. B., McCarthy, A., Toker, L., Silman, I., Sussman, J. L., & Tawfik, D. S. (2004). Structure and evolution of the serum paraoxonase family of detoxifying and anti-atherosclerotic enzymes. *Nature Structural & Molecular Biology, 11*(5), 412–419. https://doi.org/10.1038/nsmb767

Hashimoto, K. (2006). Glycine transporter inhibitors as therapeutic agents for schizophrenia. *Recent Patents on CNS Drug Discovery, 1*(1), 43–53.

Hassan, F. M., Khattab, A. A., Abo El Fotoh, W. M. M., & Zidan, R. S. (2017). A66G and C524T polymorphisms of methionine synthase reductase gene are linked to the development of acyanotic congenital heart diseases in Egyptian children. *Gene, 629*, 59–63. https://doi.org/10.1016/j.gene.2017.07.081

Hassoun, B. S., Lindeque, P., & Bjorkhem, L. (1995). Selenium detoxification by methylation. *Research Communications in Molecular Pathology and Pharmacology, 90*(1), 133–142. Retrieved from https://www.ncbi.nlm.nih.gov/pubmed/8581338

Hayes, K. C. (1985). Taurine requirement in primates. *Nutrition Reviews, 43*(3), 65–70.

Hedayati, M. T., Pasqualotto, A. C., Warn, P. A., Bowyer, P., & Denning, D. W. (2007). *Aspergillus flavus*: Human pathogen, allergen and mycotoxin producer. *Microbiology* (Reading, England), 153(Pt 6), 1677–1692. https://doi.org/10.1099/mic.0.2007/007641-0

Hei, G., Pang, L., Chen, X., et al. (2014). [Association of serum folic acid and homocysteine levels and 5, 10-methylenetetrahydrofolate reductase gene polymorphism with schizophrenia]. *Zhonghua yi xue za zhi, 94*(37), 2897–2901.

Hendrix, P., Foreman, P. M., Harrigan, M. R., Fisher, W. S., Vyas, N. A., Lipsky, R. H., Lin, M., Walters, B. C., Tubbs, R. S., Shoja, M. M., Pittet, J. F., Mathru, M., & Griessenauer, C. J. (2018). Association of cystathionine beta-synthase polymorphisms and aneurysmal subarachnoid hemorrhage. *Journal of Neurosurgery, 128*(6), 1771–1777. https://doi.org/10.3171/2017.2.JNS162933

Hermon-Taylor, A., Buller, N., Vaughan, J., & Sanderson, J. D. (2000). Causation of Crohn's disease by *Mycobacterium avium* subspecies *paratuberculosis*. *Canadian Journal of Gastroenterology, 14*(6), 521–539.

RESEARCH ARTICLES

Hershey, G. K., Friedrich, M. F., Esswein, L. A., Thomas, M. L., & Chatila, T. A. (1997). The association of atopy with a gain-of-function mutation in the alpha subunit of the interleukin-4 receptor. *The New England Journal of Medicine, 337*(24), 1720–1725. https://doi.org/10.1056/NEJM199712113372403

Heuser, R., & Bacher, P. (1993). Candida albicans and migraine headaches: A possible link. *Journal of Advancement in Medicine, 5*(3), 177–187.

Heyma, P., Wiersinga, W. M., Roos, A., & Habib, F. A. (1986). Thyrotrophin (TSH) binding sites on *Yersinia enterocolitica* recognized by immunoglobulins from humans with Graves' disease. *Clinical and Experimental Immunology, 64*, 249–254.

Hiborn, C., et al. (2006). Persistence of nontuberculous mycobacteria in a drinking water system after addition of filtration treatment. *Applied and Environmental Microbiology, 72*(9), 5864–5869.

Hiemstra, H., et al. (2001). Cytomegalovirus in autoimmunity: T cell crossreactivity to viral antigen and autoantigen glutamic acid decarboxylase. *Proceedings of the National Academy of Sciences of the United States of America, 98*(7), 3988–3991.

Hirata, H., Hinoda, Y., Okayama, N., et al. (2008). COMT polymorphisms affecting protein expression are risk factors for endometrial cancer. *Molecular Carcinogenesis, 47*(10), 768–774. https://doi.org/10.1002/mc.20432

Ho, V., Massey, T. E., & King, W. D. (2013). Effects of methionine synthase and methylenetetrahydrofolate reductase gene polymorphisms on markers of one-carbon metabolism. *Genes and Nutrition, 8*(6), 571–580. https://doi.org/10.1007/s12263-013-0358-2

Hobgood, D. K. (2011). Personality traits of aggression-submissiveness and perfectionism associate with ABO blood groups through catecholamine activities. *Medical Hypotheses, 77*(2), 294–300. https://doi.org/10.1016/j.mehy.2011.04.039

Hoffmann, J. A., et al. (1999). Phylogenetic perspectives in innate immunity. *Science, 284*(5418), 1313–1318.

Högenauer, C., et al. (2006). *Klebsiella oxytoca* as a causative organism of antibiotic-associated hemorrhagic colitis. *New England Journal of Medicine, 355*(23), 2418–2426.

Hom, G., et al. (2008). Association of systemic lupus erythematosus with C8orf13-BLK and ITGAM-ITGAX. *New England Journal of Medicine, 358*(9), 900–909. https://doi.org/10.1056/NEJMoa0707865

Homer, M. J., et al. (2000). Babesiosis. *Clinical Microbiology Reviews, 13*(3), 451–469.

Honeyman, M. C., et al. (2010). Evidence for molecular mimicry between human T cell epitopes in rotavirus and pancreatic islet autoantigens. *Journal of Immunology, 184*(4), 2204–2210.

Hosseini, M. (2013). Role of polymorphism of methyltetrahydrofolate-homocysteine methyltransferase (MTR) A2756G and breast cancer risk. *Polish Journal of Pathology, 64*(3), 191–195. https://doi.org/10.5114/pjp.2013.38138

Howard, A., et al. (2012). *Acinetobacter baumannii*: An emerging opportunistic pathogen. *Virulence, 3*(3), 243–250.

Hu, K., et al. (2005). Immunoglobulin mimicry by Hepatitis C virus envelope protein E2. *Virology, 332*(2), 538–549.

Huang, C. S., Chern, H. D., Chang, K. J., Cheng, C. W., Hsu, S. M., & Shen, C. Y. (1999). Breast cancer risk associated with genotype polymorphism of the estrogen-metabolizing genes CYP17, CYP1A1, and COMT: A multigenic study on cancer susceptibility. *Cancer Research, 59*(19), 4870–4875.

Huang, T., Tucker, K., Lee, Y., et al. (2012). MAT1A variants modulate the effect of dietary fatty acids on plasma homocysteine concentrations. *Nutrition, Metabolism and Cardiovascular Diseases, 22*(4), 362–368.

Hughes, L. E., et al. (2003). Cross-reactivity between related sequences found in *Acinetobacter spp.*, *Pseudomonas aeruginosa*, myelin basic protein, and myelin oligodendrocyte glycoprotein in multiple sclerosis. *Journal of Neuroimmunology, 144*(1–2), 105–115.

Huizinga, R., et al. (2013). Sialylation of *Campylobacter jejuni* endotoxin promotes dendritic cell-mediated B cell responses through CD14-dependent production of IFN-β and TNF-α. *Journal of Immunology, 191*(11), 5636–5645.

Hukin, J., et al. (1998). Case-control study of primary human herpesvirus 6 infection in children with febrile seizures. *Pediatrics, 101*(2), e5.

Humphreys, B. D., Forman, J. P., Zandi-Nejad, K., Bazari, H., Seifter, J., & Magee, C. C. (2005). Acetaminophen-induced anion gap metabolic acidosis and 5-oxoprolinuria (pyroglutamic aciduria) acquired in hospital. *American Journal of Kidney Diseases, 46*(1), 143–146. https://doi.org/10.1053/j.ajkd.2005.04.010

Hunter, P. R., & Nichols, G. (2002). Epidemiology and clinical features of *Cryptosporidium* infection in immunocompromised patients. *Clinical Microbiology Reviews, 15*(1), 145–154.

Hussain, R., et al. (1997). Significantly increased IgG2 subclass antibody levels to *Blastocystis hominis* in patients with irritable bowel syndrome. *American Journal of Tropical Medicine and Hygiene, 56*(3), 301–306.

Inoue-Choi, M., Nelson, H. H., Robien, K., Arning, E., Bottiglieri, T., Koh, W. P., & Yuan, J. M. (2012). One-carbon metabolism nutrient status and plasma S-adenosylmethionine concentrations in middle-aged and older Chinese in Singapore. *International Journal of Molecular Epidemiology and Genetics, 3*(2), 160–173. Epub 2012 May 15. PMID: 22724053; PMCID: PMC3376917.

Jamerson, B. D., Payne, M. E., Garrett, M. E., Ashley-Koch, A. E., Speer, M. C., & Steffens, D. C. (2013). Folate metabolism genes, dietary folate, and response to antidepressant medications in late-life depression. *International Journal of Geriatric Psychiatry, 28*(9), 925–932. https://doi.org/10.1002/gps.3899

James, S. J., Melnyk, S., Pogribna, M., Pogribny, I. P., & Caudill, M. A. (2002). Elevation in S-adenosylhomocysteine and DNA hypomethylation: Potential epigenetic mechanism for homocysteine-related pathology. *The Journal of Nutrition, 132*(8), 2361S–2366S.

Janeff, A., et al. (1971). A screening test for streptococcal exoenzymes. *Laboratory Medicine, 2*, 38–40.

Janegova, A., et al. (2015). The role of Epstein-Barr virus infection in the development of autoimmune thyroid diseases. *Endokrynologia Polska, 66*(2), 132–136.

Jankovic, J. (2008). Parkinson's disease: Clinical features and diagnosis. *Journal of Neurology, Neurosurgery & Psychiatry, 79*(4), 368–376.

Jentzmik, F., Stephan, C., Miller, K., et al. (2010). Sarcosine in urine after digital rectal examination fails as a marker in prostate cancer detection and identification of aggressive tumours. *European Urology, 58*(1), 12–18.

Jiang, R., et al. (2009). Genome-wide association study of rheumatoid arthritis by a score test based on wavelet transformation. *BMC Proceedings, 3*(Suppl 7), S8. https://doi.org/10.1186/1753-6561-3-s7-s8

Jin, J., Liu, L., Gao, Q., Chan, R. C., Li, H., Chen, Y., Wang, Y., & Qian, Q. (2016). The divergent impact of COMT Val158Met on executive function in children with and without attention-deficit/hyperactivity disorder. *Genes, Brain and Behavior, 15*(2), 271–279. https://doi.org/10.1111/gbb.12270

Johnson, N., Fletcher, O., Palles, C., Rudd, M., Webb, E., Sellick, G., dos Santos Silva, I., McCormack, V., Gibson, L., Fraser, A., Leonard, A., Gilham, C., Tavtigian, S. V., Ashworth, A., Houlston, R., & Peto, J. (2007). Counting potentially functional variants in BRCA1, BRCA2, and ATM predicts breast cancer susceptibility. *Human Molecular Genetics, 16*(9), 1051–1057. https://doi.org/10.1093/hmg/ddm050

Jones, D. P., Coates, R. J., Flagg, E. W., et al. (1992). Glutathione in foods listed in the National Cancer Institute's health habits and history food frequency questionnaire. *Journal of Nutrition Research, 12*(1), 23–27.

Kagnoff, M. F., et al. (1984). Possible role for a human adenovirus in the pathogenesis of celiac disease. *Journal of Experimental Medicine, 160*, 1544–1557.

Kalhan, S. C., & Hanson, R. W. (2012). Resurgence of serine: An often neglected but indispensable amino acid. *Journal of Biological Chemistry, 287*(24), 19786–19791.

Kanome, T., Watanabe, T., Nishio, K., Takahashi, K., Hongo, S., & Miyazaki, A. (2008). Angiotensin II upregulates acyl-CoA:cholesterol acyltransferase-1 via the angiotensin II type 1 receptor in human monocyte-macrophages. *Hypertension Research, 31*(9), 1801–1810.

Karra, E., O'Daly, O. G., Choudhury, A. I., Yousseif, A., Millership, S., Neary, M. T., Scott, W. R., Chandarana, K., Manning, S., Hess, M. E., Iwakura, H., Akamizu, T., Millet, Q., Gelegen, C., Drew, M. E., Rahman, S., Emmanuel, J. J., Williams, S. C., Rüther, U. U., Brüning, J. C., Withers, D. J., Zelaya, F. O., & Batterham, R. L. (2013). A link between FTO, ghrelin, and impaired brain food-cue responsivity. *Journal of Clinical Investigation, 123*(8), 3539–3551. https://doi.org/10.1172/JCI44403

Kashyap, B., & Sarkar, M. (2010). Mycoplasma pneumonia: Clinical features and management. *Lung India, 27*(2), 75–85.

Kawakami, Y., Ohuchi, S., Morita, T., & Sugiyama, K. (2009). Hypohomocysteinemic effect of cysteine is associated with increased plasma cysteine concentration in rats fed diets low in protein and methionine levels. *Journal of Nutritional Science and Vitaminology (Tokyo), 55*(1), 66–74. https://doi.org/10.3177/jnsv.55.66

Kemp, J. A., & McKernan, R. M. (2002). NMDA receptor pathways as drug targets. *Nature Neuroscience, 5*(11), 1039–1042.

Kendall, R. V., & Lawson, J. W. (2000). Recent findings on N, N-dimethylglycine (DMG): A nutrient for the new millennium. *Townsend Letter for Doctors and Patients, 2000*, 75–85.

Kenneson, A., & Cannon, M. J. (2007). Review and meta-analysis of the epidemiology of congenital cytomegalovirus (CMV) infection. *Reviews in Medical Virology, 17*(4), 253–276.

Kerins, D. M., Koury, M. J., Capdevila, A., Rana, S., & Wagner, C. (2001). Plasma S-adenosylhomocysteine is a more sensitive indicator of cardiovascular disease than plasma homocysteine. *American Journal of Clinical Nutrition, 74*(6), 723–729.

Kerkar, N., et al. (2003). Cytochrome P4502D6(193-212): A new immunodominant epitope and target of virus/self cross-reactivity in liver kidney microsomal autoantibody type 1-positive liver disease. *Journal of Immunology, 170*(3), 1481–1489.

Kevere, L., Purvina, S., Bauze, D., et al. (2012). Elevated serum levels of homocysteine as an early prognostic factor of psychiatric disorders in children and adolescents. *Schizophrenia Research and Treatment, 2012*, Article 373261. https://doi.org/10.1155/2012/373261

Khanna, S., & Pardi, D. S. (2010). The growing incidence and severity of *Clostridium difficile* infection in inpatient and outpatient settings. *Expert Review of Gastroenterology & Hepatology, 4*(4), 409–416.

Khersonsky, O., & Tawfik, D. S. (2005). Structure-reactivity studies of serum paraoxonase PON1 suggest that its native activity is lactonase. *Biochemistry, 44*(16), 6371–6382. https://doi.org/10.1021/bi047440d

Kirchhoff, C., et al. (1989). Pathogenetic mechanisms in the *Mycoplasma arthritidis* polyarthritis of rats. *Rheumatology International, 9*(3–5), 193–196.

Klein, K., Winter, S., Turpeinen, M., Schwab, M., & Zanger, U. M. (2010). Pathway-targeted pharmacogenomics of CYP1A2 in human liver. *Frontiers in Pharmacology, 1*, Article 129. https://doi.org/10.3389/fphar.2010.00129

Klerk, M., Lievers, K. J., Kluijtmans, L. A., Blom, H. J., den Heijer, M., Schouten, E. G., Kok, F. J., & Verhoef, P. (2003). The 2756A>G variant in the gene encoding methionine synthase: Its relation with plasma homocysteine levels and risk of coronary heart disease in a Dutch case-control study. *Thrombosis Research, 110*(2–3), 87–91. https://doi.org/10.1016/s0049-3848(03)00341-4

Klotz, S. A., et al. (2011). Cat-scratch disease. *American Family Physician, 83*(2), 152–155.

Ko, S., et al. (1997). Monoclonal antibodies against *Helicobacter pylori* cross-react with human tissue. *Helicobacter, 2*(4), 210–215.

Koch, S., et al. (2006). Human cytomegalovirus infection and T cell immunosenescence: A mini review. *Mechanisms of Ageing and Development, 127*(6), 538–543.

Koh, W. J., & Kwon, O. J. (2005). *Mycobacterium avium* complex lung disease and panhypopituitarism. *Mayo Clinic Proceedings, 80*(7), 960–962.

Krause, P. J., et al. (2003). Increasing health burden of human babesiosis in endemic sites. *American Journal of Tropical Medicine and Hygiene, 68*(4), 431–436.

Kruger, W. D., Evans, A. A., Wang, L., Malinow, M. R., Duell, P. B., Anderson, P. H., Block, P. C., Hess, D. L., Graf, E. E., & Upson, B. (2000). Polymorphisms in the CBS gene associated with decreased risk of coronary artery disease and increased responsiveness to total homocysteine lowering by folic acid. *Molecular Genetics and Metabolism, 70*(1), 53–60. https://doi.org/10.1006/mgme.2000.2993

Kumamoto, C. A. (2011). Inflammation and gastrointestinal *Candida* colonization. *Current Opinion in Microbiology, 14*(4), 386–391.

Kuo, C. C., et al. (1995). *Chlamydia pneumoniae* (TWAR). *Clinical Microbiology Reviews, 8*(4), 451–461. https://doi.org/10.1128/CMR.8.4.451

Kusters, J. G., et al. (2006). Pathogenesis of *Helicobacter pylori* infection. *Clinical Microbiology Reviews, 19*(3), 449–490.

Lachman, H. M., Papolos, D. F., Saito, T., Yu, Y. M., Szumlanski, C. L., & Weinshilboum, R. M. (1996). Human catechol-O-methyltransferase pharmacogenetics: Description of a functional polymorphism and its potential application to neuropsychiatric disorders. *Pharmacogenetics, 6*(3), 243–250.

Lai, C. Q., Parnell, L. D., Troen, A. M., et al. (2010). MAT1A variants are associated with hypertension, stroke, and markers of DNA damage and are modulated by plasma vitamin B-6 and folate. *American Journal of Clinical Nutrition, 91*(5), 1377–1386.

Lansdown, A. B. G. (2018). GOLD: Human exposure and update on toxic risks. *Critical Reviews in Toxicology, 48*(7), 596–614. https://doi.org/10.1080/10408444.2018.1513991

LaPenta, F. A., et al. (1994). Group A streptococci efficiently invade human respiratory epithelial cells. *Proceedings of the National Academy of Sciences USA, 91*, 12115–12119.

Larizza, D., et al. (2006). Helicobacter pylori infection and autoimmune thyroid disease in young patients: The disadvantage of carrying the human leukocyte antigen-DRB1*0301 allele. *The Journal of Clinical Endocrinology and Metabolism, 91*(1), 176–179.

Larone, D. H. (1995). Thermally monomorphic molds. In *Medically Important Fungi: A Guide to Identification* (3rd ed., pp. 103–206). ASM Press.

Larsen, F. O., Clementsen, P., Hansen, M., Maltbaek, N., Gravesen, S., Skov, P. S., & Norn, S. (1996). The indoor microfungus *Trichoderma viride* potentiates histamine release from human bronchoalveolar cells. *APMIS, 104*(9), 673–679. https://doi.org/10.1111/j.1600-0463.1996.tb00342.x

Larsson, S. C., Hakansson, N., & Wolk, A. (2015). Dietary cysteine and other amino acids and stroke incidence in women. *Stroke, 46*(4), 922–926.

LaRue, R. S., et al. (2007). Chlamydial Hsp60-2 is iron responsive in *Chlamydia trachomatis* serovar E-infected human endometrial epithelial cells in vitro. *Infection and Immunity, 75*(5), 2374–2380. https://doi.org/10.1128/IAI.01476-06

LaVerda, D., et al. (1999). Chlamydial heat shock proteins and disease pathology: New paradigms for old problems? *Infectious Diseases in Obstetrics and Gynecology, 7*, 64–71.

Lavigne, J. A., Helzlsouer, K. J., Huang, H. Y., et al. (1997). An association between the allele coding for a low activity variant of catechol-O-methyltransferase and the risk for breast cancer. *Cancer Research, 57*(24), 5493–5497.

Lavoie-Charland, E., et al. (2016). Asthma susceptibility variants are more strongly associated with clinically similar subgroups. *The Journal of Asthma: Official Journal of the Association for the Care of Asthma, 53*(9), 907–913. https://doi.org/10.3109/02770903.2016.1165699

Lawson, S. K., et al. (1992). Mouse cytomegalovirus infection induces antibodies which cross-react with virus and cardiac myosin: A model for the study of molecular mimicry in the pathogenesis of viral myocarditis. *Immunology, 75*, 513–519.

Lederman, R. J., & Crum, S. M. (2005). Pyogenic liver abscess with a focus on *Klebsiella pneumoniae* as a primary pathogen: An emerging disease with unique clinical characteristics. *American Journal of Gastroenterology, 100*, 322–331. https://doi.org/10.1111/j.1572-0241.2005.41709.x

Lee, M. Y., Lin, Y. R., Tu, Y. S., Tseng, Y. J., Chan, M. H., & Chen, H. H. (2017). Effects of sarcosine and N, N-dimethylglycine on NMDA receptor-mediated excitatory field potentials. *Journal of Biomedical Science, 24*(1), 18. https://doi.org/10.1186/s12929-017-0334-0

Lehtonen, J. M., et al. (1984). Amount and avidity of salivary and serum antibodies against *Streptococcus mutans* in two groups of human subjects with different dental caries susceptibility. *Infection and Immunity, 43*(1), 308–313.

Lejeune, M., et al. (2009). Recent discoveries in the pathogenesis and immune response toward *Entamoeba histolytica*. *Future Microbiology, 4*(1), 105–118. https://doi.org/10.2217/fmb.09.102

Lepczyńska, M., Białkowska, J., Dzika, E., Piskorz-Ogórek, K., & Korycińska, J. (2017). Blastocystis: How do specific diets and human gut microbiota affect its development and pathogenicity? *European Journal of Clinical Microbiology and Infectious Diseases, 36*(6), 1123–1132. https://doi.org/10.1007/s10096-017-2932-9

RESEARCH ARTICLES

Lepidi, H., et al. (2000). Comparative pathology and immunohistology associated with clinical illness after *Ehrlichia phagocytophila*-group infections. *American Journal of Tropical Medicine and Hygiene, 62*(1), 29–37. https://doi.org/10.4269/ajtmh.2000.62.29

Lever, M., & Slow, S. (2010). The clinical significance of betaine, an osmolyte with a key role in methyl group metabolism. *Clinical Biochemistry, 43*(9), 732–744. https://doi.org/10.1016/j.clinbiochem.2010.03.009

Li, Q., Lan, Q., Zhang, Y., Bassig, B. A., Holford, T. R., Leaderer, B., Boyle, P., Zhu, Y., Qin, Q., Chanock, S., Rothman, N., & Zheng, T. (2013). Role of one-carbon metabolizing pathway genes and gene-nutrient interaction in the risk of non-Hodgkin lymphoma. *Cancer Causes & Control, 24*(10), 1875–1884. https://doi.org/10.1007/s10552-013-0264-3

Li, Y., Guo, B., Zhang, L., Han, J., Wu, B., & Xiong, H. (2008). Association between C-589T polymorphisms of interleukin-4 gene promoter and asthma: A meta-analysis. *Respiratory Medicine, 102*(7), 984–992. https://doi.org/10.1016/j.rmed.2008.02.008

Lin, C.-L., et al. (2014). Disease caused by rotavirus infection. *The Open Virology Journal, 8*, 14–19. https://doi.org/10.2174/1874357901408010014

Lindholt, J. S., et al. (2004). Serum antibodies against *Chlamydia pneumoniae* outer membrane protein cross-react with the heavy chain of immunoglobulin in the wall of abdominal aortic aneurysms. *Circulation, 109*, 2097–2102. https://doi.org/10.1161/01.CIR.0000123739.41777.8F

Liu, X.-Y., et al. (2013). The effect of apigenin on pharmacokinetics of imatinib and its metabolite N-desmethyl imatinib in rats. *BioMed Research International, 2013*, 789184. https://doi.org/10.1155/2013/789184

Liu, Y., et al. (2008). A genome-wide association study of psoriasis and psoriatic arthritis identifies new disease loci. *PLoS Genetics, 4*(3), e1000041. https://doi.org/10.1371/journal.pgen.1000041

Locasale, J. W. (2013). Serine, glycine, and one-carbon units: Cancer metabolism in full circle. *Nature Reviews Cancer, 13*(8), 572–583. https://doi.org/10.1038/nrc3557

Lu, S. C. (2013). Glutathione synthesis. *Biochimica et Biophysica Acta, 1830*(5), 3143–3153. https://doi.org/10.1016/j.bbagen.2012.09.008

Lucarelli, G., Fanelli, M., Larocca, A. M. V., et al. (2012). Serum sarcosine increases the accuracy of prostate cancer detection in patients with total serum PSA less than 4.0 ng/ml. *Prostate, 72*(15), 1611–1621. https://doi.org/10.1002/pros.22546

Luka, Z., Mudd, S. H., & Wagner, C. (2009). Glycine N-methyltransferase and regulation of S-adenosylmethionine levels. *Journal of Biological Chemistry, 284*(15), 9492–9499. https://doi.org/10.1074/jbc.R109.019273

Lunardi, C., et al. (2006). Antibodies against human cytomegalovirus in the pathogenesis of systemic sclerosis: A gene array approach. *PLoS Medicine, 3*(1), e2. https://doi.org/10.1371/journal.pmed.0030002

Lundberg, M., et al. (2008). Antibodies to citrullinated α-enolase peptide 1 are specific bacterial enolase. *Arthritis & Rheumatism, 58*(10), 3009–3019. https://doi.org/10.1002/art.23728

Lünemann, J. D., et al. (2010). Dysregulated Epstein-Barr virus infection in patients with CIDP. *Journal of Neuroimmunology, 218*, 107–111. https://doi.org/10.1016/j.jneuroim.2010.08.001

Lynch, B. (2017). SHEICON 2017 Conference Proceedings and Pathway Planner v5. Seattle.

Lyons, J., Rauh-Pfeiffer, A., Yu, Y., et al. (2000). Blood glutathione synthesis rates in healthy adults receiving a sulfur amino acid-free diet. *Proceedings of the National Academy of Sciences, 97*(10), 5071–5076. https://doi.org/10.1073/pnas.97.10.5071

Lyratzopoulos, G., et al. (2002). Invasive infection due to *Penicillium* species other than *P. marneffei*. *Journal of Infection, 45*, 184–207. https://doi.org/10.1053/jinf.2002.1061

Mackness, B., Durrington, P. N., & Mackness, M. I. (1998). Human serum paraoxonase. *General Pharmacology, 31*(3), 329–336. https://doi.org/10.1016/s0306-3623(98)00028-7

Maclean, K. N., Greiner, L. S., Evans, J. R., et al. (2012). Cystathionine protects against endoplasmic reticulum stress-induced lipid accumulation, tissue injury, and apoptotic cell death. *Journal of Biological Chemistry, 287*(38), 31994–32005. https://doi.org/10.1074/jbc.M112.394719

RESEARCH ARTICLES

Madsen, L., et al. (1986). Species-specific monoclonal antibody to a 43,000-molecular weight membrane protein of *Mycoplasma pneumoniae*. *Journal of Clinical Microbiology, 24*, 680–683. https://doi.org/10.1128/JCM.24.4.680-683.1986

Magnarelli, L. A., et al. (1987). Cross-reactivity in serological tests for Lyme disease and other spirochetal infections. *Journal of Infectious Diseases, 156*(1), 183–188. https://doi.org/10.1093/infdis/156.1.183

Mahmood, N., Cheishvili, D., Arakelian, A., Tanvir, I., Khan, H. A., Pépin, A. S., Szyf, M., & Rabbani, S. A. (2017). Methyl donor S-adenosylmethionine (SAM) supplementation attenuates breast cancer growth, invasion, and metastasis in vivo; therapeutic and chemopreventive applications. *Oncotarget, 9*(4), 5169–5183. https://doi.org/10.18632/oncotarget.23704

Makishima, M., Lu, T. T., Xie, W., Whitfield, G. K., Domoto, H., Evans, R. M., Haussler, M. R., & Mangelsdorf, D. J. (2002). Vitamin D receptor as an intestinal bile acid sensor. *Science, 296*(5571), 1313–1316. https://doi.org/10.1126/science.1070174

Malik, R., Rannikmae, K., Traylor, M., et al. (2018). Genome-wide meta-analysis identifies 3 novel loci associated with stroke. *Annals of Neurology, 84*(6), 934–939. https://doi.org/10.1002/ana.25369

Malovini, A., Illario, M., Iaccarino, G., Villa, F., Ferrario, A., Roncarati, R., et al. (2011). Association study on long-living individuals from Southern Italy identifies rs10491334 in the CAMKIV gene that regulates survival proteins. *Rejuvenation Research, 14*(3), 283–291. https://doi.org/10.1089/rej.2010.1114

Mameli, G., et al. (2014). Epstein-Barr virus and Mycobacterium avium subsp. paratuberculosis peptides are cross recognized by anti-myelin basic protein antibodies in multiple sclerosis patients. *Journal of Neuroimmunology, 270*(1-2), 51-55.

Mandelli, L., & Serretti, A. (2013). Gene-environment interaction studies in depression and suicidal behavior: An update. *Neuroscience & Biobehavioral Reviews, 37*(10 Pt 1), 2375–2397. https://doi.org/10.1016/j.neubiorev.2013.07.011

Mangin, M., Sinha, R., & Fincher, K. (2014). Inflammation and vitamin D: The infection connection. *Inflammation Research, 63*(10), 803–819. https://doi.org/10.1007/s00011-014-0755-z

Mann, A., et al. (2012). The neuroprotective enzyme CYP2D6 increases in the brain with age and is lower in Parkinson's disease patients. *Neurobiology of Aging, 33*(9), 2160–2171. https://doi.org/10.1016/j.neurobiolaging.2011.08.014

Mannisto, P. T., & Kaakkola, S. (1999). Catechol-O-methyltransferase (COMT): Biochemistry, molecular biology, pharmacology, and clinical efficacy of the new selective COMT inhibitors. *Pharmacological Reviews, 51*(4), 593-628.

Manns, M., & Obermayer-Straub, P. (1997). Cytochromes P450 and uridine triphosphate-glucuronosyltransferases: Model autoantigens to study drug-induced, virus-induced, and autoimmune liver disease. *Hepatology, 26*(4), 1054-1066.

Manoli, I., De Martino, U. M., Kino, T., & Alesci, S. (2004). Modulatory effects of L-carnitine on glucocorticoid receptor activity. *Annals of the New York Academy of Sciences, 1033*, 147-157. https://doi.org/10.1196/annals.1320.014

Mansoory, D., Roozbahany, N. A., Mazinany, H., & Samimagam, A. (2003). Chronic Fusarium infection in an adult patient with undiagnosed chronic granulomatous disease. *Clinical Infectious Diseases, 37*(7), e107–e108. https://doi.org/10.1086/377608

Manthey, K., et al. (1997). Cryptosporidiosis and inflammatory bowel disease: Experience from the Milwaukee outbreak. *Digestive Diseases and Sciences, 42*(8), 1580–1586.

Maric, M., et al. (2004). Human herpesvirus-6-associated acute lymphadenitis in immunocompetent adults. *Modern Pathology, 17*, 1427–1433.

Marr, K. A., Patterson, T., & Denning, D. (2002). Aspergillosis: Pathogenesis, clinical manifestations, and therapy. *Infectious Disease Clinics of North America, 16*(4), 875–894, vi. https://doi.org/10.1016/s0891-5520(02)00035-1

Masala, G., et al. (2011). Antibodies recognizing *Mycobacterium avium* paratuberculosis epitopes cross-react with the beta-cell antigen ZnT8 in Sardinian type 1 diabetic patients. *PLoS ONE, 6*(10), e26931. https://doi.org/10.1371/journal.pone.0026931

Massei, F., et al. (2003). High prevalence of antibodies to *Bartonella henselae* among Italian children without evidence of cat scratch disease. *Clinical Infectious Diseases, 38*, 145–148.

Mato, J. M., Martínez-Chantar, M. L., & Lu, S. C. (2013). S-adenosylmethionine metabolism and liver disease. *Annals of Hepatology, 12*(2), 183–189. PMID: 23396728; PMCID: PMC4027041

Mayer, F. L., et al. (2013). *Candida albicans* pathogenicity mechanisms. *Virulence, 4*(2), 119–128.

McCarty, M. F., O'Keefe, J. H., & DiNicolantonio, J. J. (2018). Dietary glycine is rate-limiting for glutathione synthesis and may have broad potential for health protection. *Ochsner Journal, 18*(1), 81–87. PMID: 29559876; PMCID: PMC5855430

McCormack, M., et al. (2011). HLA-A*3101 and carbamazepine-induced hypersensitivity reactions in Europeans. *The New England Journal of Medicine, 364*(12), 1134–1143. https://doi.org/10.1056/NEJMoa1013297

McDonald, D., et al. (2018). American Gut: An open platform for citizen science microbiome research. *mSystems, 3*(3), e00031–18. https://doi.org/10.1128/mSystems.00031-18

McKinnon, E., Morahan, G., Nolan, D., James, I., & Diabetes Genetics Consortium. (2009). Association of MHC SNP genotype with susceptibility to type 1 diabetes: A modified survival approach. *Diabetes, Obesity and Metabolism, 11*(Suppl 1), 92–100. https://doi.org/10.1111/j.1463-1326.2008.01009.x

Michalek, J. E., et al. (2017). Genetic predisposition to advanced biological ageing increases risk for childhood-onset recurrent major depressive disorder in a large UK sample. *Journal of Affective Disorders, 213*, 207–213. https://doi.org/10.1016/j.jad.2017.01.017

Mikuls, T. R., et al. (2012). *Porphyromonas gingivalis* and disease-related autoantibodies in individuals at increased risk of rheumatoid arthritis. *Arthritis & Rheumatism, 64*(11), 3522–3530.

Miller, J. D., et al. (2003). Stachybotrys chartarum: Cause of human disease or media darling? *Medical Mycology, 41*, 271–291.

Miné, M., & da Rosa, P. A. (2008). Frequency of *Blastocystis hominis* and other intestinal parasites in stool samples examined at the Parasitology Laboratory of the School of Pharmaceutical Sciences at the São Paulo State University, Araraquara. *Revista da Sociedade Brasileira de Medicina Tropical, 41*(6), 565–569.

Mischoulon, D., & Fava, M. (2002). Role of S-adenosyl-L-methionine in the treatment of depression: A review of the evidence. *American Journal of Clinical Nutrition, 76*(5), 1158S–1161S. https://doi.org/10.1093/ajcn/76/5.1158S

Mishori, R., et al. (2012). Chlamydia trachomatis infections: Screening, diagnosis, and management. *American Family Physician, 86*(12), 1127–1132.

Mohapatra, S., Singh, D. P., Alcid, D., & Pitchumoni, C. S. (2018). Beyond O&P Times Three. *American Journal of Gastroenterology, 113*(6), 805–818. https://doi.org/10.1038/s41395-018-0083-y

Moonah, S., et al. (2013). Host immune response to intestinal amebiasis. *PLoS Pathogens, 9*, e100349. https://doi.org/10.1371/journal.ppat.100349

Mortimer, L., et al. (2015). The NLRP3 inflammasome is a pathogen sensor for invasive *Entamoeba histolytica* via activation of α5β1 integrin at the macrophage-amebae intercellular junction. *PLoS Pathogens, 11*, e1004887. https://doi.org/10.1371/journal.ppat.1004887

Moye, Z. D., et al. (2014). Fueling the caries process: Carbohydrate metabolism and gene regulation by *Streptococcus mutans*. *Journal of Oral Microbiology, 6*, 24878. https://doi.org/10.3402/jom.v6.24878

Mudd, S. H. (2011). Hypermethioninemias of genetic and non-genetic origin: A review. *American Journal of Medical Genetics Part C: Seminars in Medical Genetics, 157C*(1), 3–32. https://doi.org/10.1002/ajmg.c.30293

Mudd, S. H., & Levy, H. L. (1995). Plasma homocyst(e)ine or homocysteine? *The New England Journal of Medicine, 333*(5), 325. https://doi.org/10.1056/NEJM199508033330520

Müller, N., et al. (2001). Increased titers of antibodies against streptococcal M12 and M19 proteins in patients with Tourette's syndrome. *Psychiatry Research, 101*(2), 187–193. https://doi.org/10.1016/S0165-1781(01)00346-5

Musa, L. M., et al. (2010). *Clostridium difficile* infection and liver disease. *Journal of Gastrointestinal and Liver Diseases, 19*(3), 303–310.

Nagel, R. E., et al. (2015). *Blastocystis* specific serum immunoglobulin in patients with irritable bowel syndrome (IBS) versus healthy controls. *Parasites & Vectors, 8*, 453. https://doi.org/10.1186/s13071-015-1000-0

Nair, R., & Maseeh, A. (2012). Vitamin D: The 'sunshine' vitamin. *Journal of Pharmacology and Pharmacotherapeutics, 3*(2), 118–126. https://doi.org/10.4103/0976-500X.95506

Nakajima, M., et al. (2010). New sequence variants in HLA Class II/III region associated with susceptibility to knee osteoarthritis identified by genome-wide association study. *PLoS ONE, 5*(3), e9723. https://doi.org/10.1371/journal.pone.0009723

Nakanishi, K., & Shima, Y. (2010). Capture of type 1 diabetes-susceptible HLA DR-DQ haplotypes in Japanese subjects using a tag single nucleotide polymorphism. *Diabetes Care, 33*(1), 162–164. https://doi.org/10.2337/dc09-1210

Nakano, T., et al. (2011). Sudden death from systemic rotavirus infection and detection of nonstructural rotavirus proteins. *Journal of Clinical Microbiology, 49*(12), 4382–4385. https://doi.org/10.1128/JCM.05482-11

Nermes, E., et al. (1995). Nitro-cellulose-RAST analysis of allergenic cross-reactivity of *Candida albicans* and *Saccharomyces cerevisiae* mannans. *International Archives of Allergy and Immunology, 106*(1), 118-123.

Newman, A. B., et al. (2010). A meta-analysis of four genome-wide association studies of survival to age 90 years or older: The Cohorts for Heart and Aging Research in Genomic Epidemiology Consortium. *The Journals of Gerontology: Series A, Biological Sciences and Medical Sciences, 65*(5), 478–487. https://doi.org/10.1093/gerona/glq028

Niedoszytko, M., Chełmińska, M., Jassem, E., & Czestochowska, E. (2007). Association between sensitization to *Aureobasidium pullulans* (Pullularia sp) and severity of asthma. *Annals of Allergy, Asthma & Immunology, 98*(2), 153-156. https://doi.org/10.1016/S1081-1206(10)60688-6

Nielen, M. M., et al. (2004). Specific autoantibodies precede the symptoms of rheumatoid arthritis: A study of serial measurements in blood donors. *Arthritis & Rheumatism, 50*(2), 380-386.

Nieuwenhuizen, N., et al. (2003). Is *Candida albicans* a trigger in the onset of coeliac disease? *Lancet, 361*(9372), 2152–2154.

Nijhout, H. F., Reed, M. C., Budu, P., & Ulrich, C. M. (2004). A mathematical model of the folate cycle: New insights into folate homeostasis. *The Journal of Biological Chemistry, 279*(53), 55008-55016. https://doi.org/10.1074/jbc.M406394200

Nishiuchi, Y., et al. (2007). The recovery of *Mycobacterium avium*-intracellulare complex (MAC) from the residential bathrooms of patients with pulmonary MAC. *Clinical Infectious Diseases, 45*(3), 347-351. https://doi.org/10.1086/519986

Nociti, F., et al. (2010). Epstein-Barr virus antibodies in serum and cerebrospinal fluid from multiple sclerosis, chronic inflammatory demyelinating polyradiculoneuropathy, and amyotrophic lateral sclerosis. *Journal of Neuroimmunology, 225*(1-2), 149-152. https://doi.org/10.1016/j.jneuroim.2010.06.016

O'Callaghan, P., European Cg, Meleady, R., et al. (2002). Smoking and plasma homocysteine. *European Heart Journal, 23*(20), 1580-1586.

Obeid, R. (2013). The metabolic burden of methyl donor deficiency with focus on the betaine homocysteine methyltransferase pathway. *Nutrients, 5*(9), 3481-3495. https://doi.org/10.3390/nu5093481

Obeid, R., Schadt, A., Dillmann, U., Kostopoulos, P., Fassbender, K., & Herrmann, W. (2009). Methylation status and neurodegenerative markers in Parkinson disease. *Clinical Chemistry, 55*(10), 1852-1860. https://doi.org/10.1373/clinchem.2009.129447

O'Hara, A. & Lin, R. (2006). Accumulation of tropomyosin isoform 5 at the infection sites of host cells during *Cryptosporidium* invasion. *Parasitology Research, 99*(1), 45-54. https://doi.org/10.1007/s00436-006-0146-4

Ohlsson, C., et al. (2011). Genetic determinants of serum testosterone concentrations in men. *PLoS Genetics, 7*(10), e1002313. https://doi.org/10.1371/journal.pgen.1002313

Ohuchi, S., Matsumoto, Y., Morita, T., & Sugiyama, K. (2008). High-casein diet suppresses guanidinoacetic acid-induced hyperhomocysteinemia and potentiates the hypohomocysteinemic effect of serine in rats. *Bioscience, Biotechnology, and Biochemistry, 72*(12), 3258-3264. https://doi.org/10.1271/bbb.80543

Olteanu, H., Munson, T., & Banerjee, R. (2002). Differences in the efficiency of reductive activation of methionine synthase and exogenous electron acceptors between the common polymorphic variants of human methionine synthase reductase. *Biochemistry, 41*(45), 13378-13385. https://doi.org/10.1021/bi020536s

Onuma, E. K., Amenta, P. S., Ramaswamy, K., Lin, J. J., & Das, K. M. (2000). Autoimmunity in ulcerative colitis (UC): A predominant colonic mucosal B cell response against human tropomyosin isoform 5. *Clinical and Experimental Immunology, 121*(3), 466-471. https://doi.org/10.1046/j.1365-2249.2000.01330.x

Ordi-Ros, J., et al. (2000). Anticardiolipin antibodies in patients with chronic hepatitis C virus infection: Characterization in relation to antiphospholipid syndrome. *Clinical and Diagnostic Laboratory Immunology, 7*(2), 241-244.

Osada Oka, M., Kita, H., Yagi, S., Sato, T., Izumi, Y., & Iwao, H. (2012). Angiotensin AT1 receptor blockers suppress oxidized low-density lipoprotein derived formation of foam cells. *European Journal of Pharmacology, 679*(1-3), 9-15. https://doi.org/10.1016/j.ejphar.2012.04.001

Ozanne, S. E., & Lefebvre, P. (1991). Specificity of the microimmunofluorescence assay for the serodiagnosis of Chlamydia pneumoniae infections. *Canadian Journal of Microbiology, 38*(11), 1185-1189. https://doi.org/10.1139/m91-173

Paffen, E., Medina, P., de Visser, M. C., van Wijngaarden, A., Zorio, E., Estellés, A., Rosendaal, F. R., España, F., Bertina, R. M., & Doggen, C. J. (2008). The -589C>T polymorphism in the interleukin-4 gene (IL-4) is associated with a reduced risk of myocardial infarction in young individuals. *Journal of Thrombosis and Haemostasis, 6*(10), 1633-1638. https://doi.org/10.1111/j.1538-7836.2008.03096.x

Påhlman, L., et al. (2006). Streptococcal M protein: A multipotent and powerful inducer of inflammation. *Journal of Immunology, 177*(2), 1221-1228.Pak, et al. Association of cytomegalovirus infection with autoimmune type 1 diabetes. Lancet, 1988; 2(8601):1-4.

Panza, F., et al. (2014). Immunoglobulin G subclass profile of anticitrullinated peptide antibodies specific for Epstein-Barr virus-derived and histone-derived citrullinated peptides. *Journal of Rheumatology, 41*, 407-408.

Papakostas, G. I., Cassiello, C. F., & Iovieno, N. (2012). Folates and S-adenosylmethionine for major depressive disorder. *Canadian Journal of Psychiatry, 57*(7), 406-413. https://doi.org/10.1177/070674371205700703

Papaleo, F., Crawley, J. N., Song, J., Lipska, B. K., Pickel, J., Weinberger, D. R., & Chen, J. (2008). Genetic dissection of the role of catechol-O-methyltransferase in cognition and stress reactivity in mice. *Journal of Neuroscience, 28*(35), 8709-8723. https://doi.org/10.1523/JNEUROSCI.2077-08.2008

Papolos, D. F., Veit, S., Faedda, G. L., Saito, T., & Lachman, H. M. (1998). Ultra-ultra rapid cycling bipolar disorder is associated with the low activity catecholamine-O-methyltransferase allele. *Molecular Psychiatry, 3*(4), 346-349.

Pardini, B., Kumar, R., Naccarati, A., Prasad, R. B., Forsti, A., Polakova, V., Vodickova, L., Novotny, J., Hemminki, K., & Vodicka, P. (2011). MTHFR and MTRR genotype and haplotype analysis and colorectal cancer susceptibility in a case-control study from the Czech Republic. *Mutation Research, 721*(1), 74-80. https://doi.org/10.1016/j.mrgentox.2010.12.008

Pathak, S., Hatam, L. J., Bonagura, V., & Vambutas, A. (2013). Innate immune recognition of molds and homology to the inner ear protein, cochlin, in patients with autoimmune inner ear disease. *Journal of Clinical Immunology, 33*(7), 1204-1215. https://doi.org/10.1007/s10875-013-9926-x

Patil, A. A., et al. (2013). Possible significance of anti-heat shock protein (HSP-65) antibodies in autoimmune myasthenia gravis. *Journal of Neuroimmunology, 257*(1-2), 107-109.

Peattie, R. A., et al. (1989). Ultrastructural localization of giardins to the edges of disk microribbons of *Giardia lamblia* and the nucleotide and deduced protein sequence of alpha giardin. *Journal of Cell Biology, 109*(5), 2323-2335.

Peeling, R. W., et al. (1998). Antibody response to the 60-kDa chlamydial heat-shock protein is associated with scarring trachoma. *Journal of Infectious Diseases, 177*, 256-259.

Peñas-Lledó, E. M., & Llerena, A. (2014). CYP2D6 variation, behaviour and psychopathology: Implications for pharmacogenomics-guided clinical trials. *British Journal of Clinical Pharmacology, 77*(4), 673-683. https://doi.org/10.1111/bcp.12227

Persat, F., et al. (2017). Aspergillus antibody detection: Diagnostic strategy and technical considerations from the Société Française de Mycologie Médicale (French Society for Medical Mycology) expert committee. *Medical Mycology, 55*(3), 302-307. https://doi.org/10.1093/mmy/myw078

Petri, W. A., Jr., & Singh, U. (1999). Diagnosis and management of amebiasis. *Clinical Infectious Diseases, 29*(5), 1117-1125. https://doi.org/10.1086/313493

Petrovec, M., et al. (1997). Human disease in Europe caused by a granulocytic Ehrlichia species. *Journal of Clinical Microbiology, 35*(6), 1556-1559. https://doi.org/10.1128/jcm.35.6.1556-1559.1997

Pierce, E. S. (2010). Ulcerative colitis and Crohn's disease: Is *Mycobacterium avium* subspecies paratuberculosis the common villain? *Gut Pathogens, 2*(1), 21. https://doi.org/10.1186/1757-4749-2-21

Pietroiusti, A., et al. (2002). Cytotoxin-associated gene-A–positive *Helicobacter pylori* strains are associated with atherosclerotic stroke. *Circulation, 106*(5), 580-584. https://doi.org/10.1161/01.cir.0000023894.10871.2f

Piolot, A., et al. (2003). Effect of fish oil on LDL oxidation and plasma homocysteine concentrations in health. *The Journal of Laboratory and Clinical Medicine, 141*(1), 41-49. https://doi.org/10.1067/mlc.2003.3

Pogribna, M., Melnyk, S., Pogribny, I., Chango, A., Yi, P., & James, S. J. (2001). Homocysteine metabolism in children with Down syndrome: In vitro modulation. *American Journal of Human Genetics, 69*(1), 88-95. PMID: 11391481

Pohjalainen, T., et al. (1998). The A1 allele of the human D2 dopamine receptor gene predicts low D2 receptor availability in healthy volunteers. *Molecular Psychiatry, 3*(3), 256-260. https://doi.org/10.1038/sj.mp.4000350

Poirier, L. A., Brown, A. T., Fink, L. M., et al. (2001). Blood S-adenosylmethionine concentrations and lymphocyte methylenetetrahydrofolate reductase activity in diabetes mellitus and diabetic nephropathy. *Metabolism, 50*(9), 1014-1018.

Polymeros, D., et al. (2006). Does cross-reactivity between *Mycobacterium avium* paratuberculosis and human intestinal antigens characterize Crohn's disease? *Gastroenterology, 131*, 85-96.

Pool, L. D., et al. (2006). Epstein-Barr virus and molecular mimicry in systemic lupus erythematosus. *Autoimmunity, 39*(1), 63-70.

Popp, J., Lewczuk, P., Linnebank, M., Cvetanovska, G., Smulders, Y., & Kölsch, H. (2009). Homocysteine metabolism and cerebrospinal fluid markers for Alzheimer's disease. *Journal of Alzheimer's Disease, 18*.

Powers, H. J., et al. (2011). Correcting a marginal riboflavin deficiency improves hematologic status in young women in the United Kingdom (RIBOFEM). *The American Journal of Clinical Nutrition, 93*(6), 1274–1284. https://doi.org/10.3945/ajcn.110.008409

Pratesi, F., et al. (2006). Deiminated Epstein-Barr virus nuclear antigen 1 is a target of anti–citrullinated protein antibodies in rheumatoid arthritis. *Arthritis & Rheumatism, 54*(3), 733-741.

Prohászka, Z., et al. (n.d.). Antibodies against human heat-shock protein (Hsp) 60 and mycobacterial Hsp65 differ in their antigen specificity and complement-activating ability.

Pusztai, A. (1992). *Plant lectins (Chemistry and pharmacology of natural products)*. Cambridge University Press. https://doi.org/10.1017/CBO9780511895371

Qin, X., Peng, Q., Qin, A., et al. (2012). Association of COMT Val158Met polymorphism and breast cancer risk: An updated meta-analysis. *Diagnostic Pathology, 7*, 136. https://doi.org/10.1186/1746-1596-7-136

Quinn, J., et al. (1998). Immunological relationship between the class I epitope of streptococcal M protein and myosin. *Infection and Immunity, 66*(9), 4418-4424.

Rafatian, N., Milne, R. W., Leenen, F. H., & Whitman, S. C. (2013). Role of renin-angiotensin system in activation of macrophages by modified lipoproteins. *American Journal of Physiology-Heart and Circulatory Physiology, 305*(9), H1309–H1320.

Rajagopalan, K. V. (1988). Molybdenum: An essential trace element in human nutrition. *Annual Review of Nutrition, 8*, 401–427.

Ramasamy, A., et al. (2011). A genome-wide meta-analysis of genetic variants associated with allergic rhinitis and grass sensitization and their interaction with birth order. *The Journal of Allergy and Clinical Immunology, 128*(5), 996–1005. https://doi.org/10.1016/j.jaci.2011.08.030

Ramesh, G., et al. (2013). The Lyme disease spirochete *Borrelia burgdorferi* induces inflammation and apoptosis in cells from dorsal root ganglia. *Journal of Neuroinflammation, 10*, 88.

Ramos, P. S., et al. (2013). Variable association of reactive intermediate genes with systemic lupus erythematosus in populations with different African ancestry. *The Journal of Rheumatology, 40*(6), 842–849. https://doi.org/10.3899/jrheum.120989

Rand, T. G., et al. (2005). Inflammatory and cytotoxic responses in mouse lungs exposed to purified toxins from building-isolated *Penicillium brevicompactum* Dierckx and *P. chrysogenum* Thom. *Toxicological Sciences, 87*(1), 213-222.

Rani, M., et al. (2010). *Mycobacterium avium* subsp. *paratuberculosis* as a trigger of type-1 diabetes: Destination Sardinia, or beyond? *Gut Pathogens, 2*, 1. https://doi.org/10.1186/1757-4749-2-1

Rawlins, M., et al. (2005). Evaluation of a Western blot method for the detection of *Yersinia* antibodies: Evidence of serological cross-reactivity between *Yersinia* outer membrane proteins and *Borrelia burgdorferi*. *Clinical and Diagnostic Laboratory Immunology, 12*(11), 1269-1274.

Reid, J. D., & Chiodini, R. J. (1993). Serologic reactivity against *Mycobacterium paratuberculosis* antigens in patients with sarcoidosis. *Sarcoidosis, 10*(1), 32-35.

Retnoningrum, D. S., & Cleary, P. P. (1994). M12 protein from *Streptococcus pyogenes* is a receptor for immunoglobulin G3 and human albumin. *Infection and Immunity, 62*(6), 2387–2394.

Reynolds, K. K., et al. (2016). Clinical utility and economic impact of CYP2D6 genotyping. *Clinics in Laboratory Medicine, 36*(3), 525–542. https://doi.org/10.1016/j.cll.2016.05.008

Riario Sforza, G. G., & Marinou, A. (2017). Hypersensitivity pneumonitis: A complex lung disease. *Clinical and Molecular Allergy, 15*, 6. https://doi.org/10.1186/s12948-017-0062-7

Richie, J. P., Jr., Nichenametla, S., Neidig, W., et al. (2015). Randomized controlled trial of oral glutathione supplementation on body stores of glutathione. *European Journal of Nutrition, 54*(2), 251-263.

Rider, L. G., et al. (1997). Human cytomegalovirus infection and systemic lupus erythematosus. *Clinical and Experimental Rheumatology, 15*(4), 405-409.

Ridlon, J. M., & Bajaj, J. S. (2015). The human gut sterolbiome: Bile acid-microbiome endocrine aspects and therapeutics. *Acta Pharmaceutica Sinica B, 5*(2), 99-105. https://doi.org/10.1016/j.apsb.2015.01.006

Ripps, H., & Shen, W. (2012). Taurine: A "very essential" amino acid. *Molecular Vision, 18*, 2673.

Rodriguez, Y., et al. (2012). *Porphyromonas gingivalis* strain-specific interactions with human coronary artery endothelial cells: A comparative study. *PLoS ONE, 7*(12), e52606. https://doi.org/10.1271/journal.pone.0052606

Ropper, A. H. (1988). *Campylobacter* diarrhea and Guillain-Barré syndrome. *Archives of Neurology, 45*(6), 655-656.

Roush, J. F., et al. (2019). Experiential avoidance, cognitive fusion, and suicide ideation among psychiatric inpatients: The role of thwarted interpersonal needs. *Psychotherapy Research, 29*(4), 514–523. https://doi.org/10.1080/10503307.2017.1395923

Routsias, J. G., et al. (2011). Autopathogenic correlation of periodontitis and rheumatoid arthritis. *Rheumatology, 50*, 1189-1193.

Rudolph, M. J., Johnson, J. L., Rajagopalan, K. V., et al. (2003). The 1.2 Å structure of the human sulfite oxidase cytochrome b5 domain. *Acta Crystallographica Section D: Structural Biology, 59*, 1183–1191. https://doi.org/10.1107/S0907444903009934

Ruebush, T. K., et al. (1977). Human babesiosis on Nantucket Island: Clinical features. *Annals of Internal Medicine, 86*, 6–9.

Ruhnke, M. (2002). Skin and mucous membrane infections. In R. A. Calderone (Ed.), *Candida and Candidiasis* (pp. 307–325). ASM Press.

Rujescu, D., Giegling, I., Gietl, A., Hartmann, A. M., & Moller, H. J. (2003). A functional single nucleotide polymorphism (V158M) in the COMT gene is associated with aggressive personality traits. *Biological Psychiatry, 54*(1), 34–39.

Rupnik, M., et al. (2009). *Clostridium difficile* infection: New developments in epidemiology and pathogenesis. *Nature Reviews Microbiology, 7*, 526–536.

Sabina, M., et al. (2001). *Yersinia enterocolitica*: Mode of transmission, molecular insights of virulence, and pathogenesis of infection. *Journal of Pathogens, 2001*, Article ID 429069.

Sabine, K., Liebers, V., Maryska, S., Meurer, U., Litzenberger, C., Merget, R., & Raulf, M. (2022). What should be tested in patients with suspected mold exposure? Usefulness of serological markers for the diagnosis. *Allergologie Select, 6*, 118–132. https://doi.org/10.5414/ALX02298E

Sal, E., Stemler, J., Salmanton-García, J., Falces-Romero, I., Kredics, L., Meyer, E., Würstl, B., Lass-Flörl, C., Racil, Z., Klimko, N., Cesaro, S., Kindo, A. J., Wisplinghoff, H., Koehler, P., Cornely, O. A., & Seidel, D. (2022). Invasive *Trichoderma* spp. infections: Clinical presentation and outcome of cases from the literature and the FungiScope® registry. *Journal of Antimicrobial Chemotherapy, 77*(10), 2850–2858. https://doi.org/10.1093/jac/dkac235

Salardi, S., et al. (1999). Helicobacter pylori and type 1 diabetes mellitus in children. *Journal of Pediatric Gastroenterology and Nutrition, 28*, 307–309.

Samocha-Bonet, D., Justo, D., Rogowski, O., Saar, N., Abu-Abeid, S., Shenkerman, G., Shapira, I., Berliner, S., & Tomer, A. (2008). Platelet counts and platelet activation markers in obese subjects. *Mediators of Inflammation, 2008*, Article ID 834153. https://doi.org/10.1155/2008/834153

Sanders, L. M., & Zeisel, S. H. (2007). Choline: Dietary requirements and role in brain development. *Nutrition Today, 42*(4), 181–186. https://doi.org/10.1097/01.NT.0000286155.55343.fa

Santos, S. R., & Rivera, W. L. (2009). Kinetic analysis of antibody responses to *Blastocystis hominis* in sera and intestinal secretions of orally infected mice. *Parasitology Research, 105*(5), 1303–1310.

Santulli, G., Cipolletta, E., Sorriento, D., Del Giudice, C., Anastasio, A., Monaco, S., Maione, A. S., Condorelli, G., Puca, A., Trimarco, B., Illario, M., & Iaccarino, G. (2012). CaMK4 gene deletion induces hypertension. *Journal of the American Heart Association, 1*(4), e001081. https://doi.org/10.1161/JAHA.112.001081

Sarubin, N., et al. (2017). The sex-dependent role of the glucocorticoid receptor in depression: Variations in the NR3C1 gene are associated with major depressive disorder in women but not in men. *European Archives of Psychiatry and Clinical Neuroscience, 267*(2), 123–133. https://doi.org/10.1007/s00406-016-0722-5

Savioli, L., et al. (2006). Giardia and Cryptosporidium join the 'neglected diseases initiative'. *Trends in Parasitology, 22*, 203–208.

Schaffer, S. W., Jong, C. J., Ito, T., & Azuma, J. (2014). Effect of taurine on ischemia–reperfusion injury. *Amino Acids, 46*(1), 21–30.

Schalinske, K. L., & Smazal, A. L. (2012). Homocysteine imbalance: A pathological metabolic marker. *Advances in Nutrition, 3*(6), 755–762.

Schmidt, J. A., Rinaldi, S., Scalbert, A., Ferrari, P., Achaintre, D., Gunter, M. J., Appleby, P. N., Key, T. J., & Travis, R. C. (2016). Plasma concentrations and intakes of amino acids in male meat-eaters, fish-eaters, vegetarians, and vegans: A cross-sectional analysis in the EPIC-Oxford cohort. *European Journal of Clinical Nutrition, 70*(3), 306–312. https://doi.org/10.1038/ejcn.2015.144

Schønheyder, H., Andersen, I., & Andersen, P. (1983). Serum antibodies to *Aspergillus fumigatus* in patients with rheumatic diseases. *Sabouraudia, 21*(2), 149–157. https://doi.org/10.1080/00362178385380241

Schwab, C., et al. (2004). Allergic inflammation induced by a *Penicillium chrysogenum* conidia-associated allergen extract in a murine model. *Allergy, 59*, 758–765.

Scriver, C. R., Beaudet, A. L., Sly, W. S., et al. (2000). *Metabolic and molecular bases of inherited disease* (4-volume set). McGraw-Hill Professional Publishing.

Selden, R., et al. (1971). Nosocomial *Klebsiella* infections: Intestinal colonization as a reservoir. *Annals of Internal Medicine, 74*, 657–664.

Shakir, R. M., et al. (2012). Determination of serum antibodies to *Clostridium difficile* toxin B in patients with inflammatory bowel disease. *Gastroenterology & Hepatology, 8*(5), 313–317.

Shaw, G. M., Lu, W., Zhu, H., et al. (2009). 118 SNPs of folate-related genes and risks of spina bifida and conotruncal heart defects. *BMC Medical Genetics, 10*, 49. https://doi.org/10.1186/1471-2350-10-49

Shea, T. B., & Chan, A. (2008). S-adenosyl methionine: A natural therapeutic agent effective against multiple hallmarks and risk factors associated with Alzheimer's disease. *Journal of Alzheimer's Disease, 13*(1), 67–70. https://doi.org/10.3233/JAD-2008-13107

Shen, J., Tong, X., Sud, N., Khound, R., Song, Y., Maldonado-Gomez, M. X., Walter, J., & Su, Q. (2016). Low-density lipoprotein receptor signaling mediates the triglyceride-lowering action of *Akkermansia muciniphila* in genetic-induced hyperlipidemia. *Arteriosclerosis, Thrombosis, and Vascular Biology, 36*(7), 1448–1456. https://doi.org/10.1161/ATVBAHA.116.307597

Shumay, E., Logan, J., Volkow, N. D., & Fowler, J. S. (2012). Evidence that the methylation state of the monoamine oxidase A (MAOA) gene predicts brain activity of MAO A enzyme in healthy men. *Epigenetics, 7*(10), 1151–1160. https://doi.org/10.4161/epi.21976

Silverberg, M. S., et al. (2009). Ulcerative colitis-risk loci on chromosomes 1p36 and 12q15 found by genome-wide association study. *Nature Genetics, 41*(2), 216–220. https://doi.org/10.1038/ng.275

Simmons, R. B., Price, D. L., Noble, J. A., Crow, S. A., & Ahearn, D. G. (1997). Fungal colonization of air filters from hospitals. *American Industrial Hygiene Association Journal, 58*(12), 900–904. https://doi.org/10.1080/15428119791012252

Simon-Nobbe, B., Denk, U., Pöll, V., Rid, R., & Breitenbach, M. (2008). The spectrum of fungal allergy. *International Archives of Allergy and Immunology, 145*(1), 58–86. https://doi.org/10.1159/000107578

Sinha, R., Sinha, I., Calcagnotto, A., et al. (2018). Oral supplementation with liposomal glutathione elevates body stores of glutathione and markers of immune function. *European Journal of Clinical Nutrition, 72*(1), 105–111. https://doi.org/10.1038/ejcn.2017.165

Siński, E., & Behnke, J. M. (2004). Apicomplexan parasites: Environmental contamination and transmission. *Polish Journal of Microbiology, 53*, 67–73.

Skwor, T., et al. (2010). Characterization of humoral immune responses to chlamydial HSP60, CPAF, and CT795 in inflammatory and severe trachoma. *Investigative Ophthalmology & Visual Science, 51*, 5128–5136. https://doi.org/10.1167/iovs.09-4936

Smith, S. B., Reenilä, I., Männistö, P. T., Slade, G. D., Maixner, W., Diatchenko, L., & Nackley, A. G. (2014). Epistasis between polymorphisms in COMT, ESR1, and GCH1 influences COMT enzyme activity and pain. *Pain, 155*(11), 2390–2399. https://doi.org/10.1016/j.pain.2014.09.009

Smulders, Y. M., Smith, D. E., Kok, R. M., Teerlink, T., Swinkels, D. W., Stehouwer, C. D., & Jakobs, C. (2006). Cellular folate vitamer distribution during and after correction of vitamin B12 deficiency: A case for the methylfolate trap. *British Journal of Haematology, 132*(5), 623–629.

Sokol, C. L., Chu, N. Q., Yu, S., Nish, S., Laufer, T., & Medzhitov, R. (2009). Basophils function as antigen-presenting cells for an allergen-induced T helper type 2 response. *Nature Immunology, 10*(7), 713–720. https://doi.org/10.1038/ni.1738

Song, C. S., Echchgadda, I., Seo, Y. K., Oh, T., Kim, S., Kim, S. A., Cho, S., Shi, L., & Chatterjee, B. (2006). An essential role of the CAAT/enhancer binding protein-alpha in the vitamin D-induced expression of the human steroid/bile acid sulfotransferase (SULT2A1). *Molecular Endocrinology, 20*(4), 795–808. https://doi.org/10.1210/me.2005-0346

Sorenson, W. G., & Lewis, D. M. (1996). Organic dust toxic syndrome. In D. Howard & J. D. Miller (Eds.), *The Mycota* (Vol. VII, pp. 159–172). Springer-Verlag.

Sreekumar, A., Poisson, L. M., Rajendiran, T. M., et al. (2009). Metabolomic profiles delineate potential role for sarcosine in prostate cancer progression. *Nature, 457*(7231), 910. https://doi.org/10.1038/nature07762

Stabler, S. P., Allen, R. H., Dolce, E. T., & Johnson, M. A. (2006). Elevated serum S-adenosylhomocysteine in cobalamin-deficient elderly and response to treatment. *American Journal of Clinical Nutrition, 84*(6), 1422–1429.

Stabler, S. P., Lindenbaum, J., Savage, D. G., & Allen, R. H. (1993). Elevation of serum cystathionine levels in patients with cobalamin and folate deficiency. *Blood, 81*(12), 3404–3413.

Steele, C., et al. (1969). Mycoplasma pneumoniae as a determinant of the Guillain-Barré syndrome. *The Lancet, 2*(7614), 710.

Steere, A. C. (1989). Lyme disease. *The New England Journal of Medicine, 321*(9), 586–596. https://doi.org/10.1056/NEJM198908313210906

Stenzel, D. J., & Boreham, P. F. (1996). *Blastocystis hominis* revisited. *Clinical Microbiology Reviews, 9*(4), 563–584.

Stevenson, J., et al. (2010). The role of histamine degradation gene polymorphisms in moderating the effects of food additives on children's ADHD symptoms. *The American Journal of Psychiatry, 167*(9), 1108–1115. https://doi.org/10.1176/appi.ajp.2010.09101529

Stipanuk, M. H., & Ueki, I. (2011). Dealing with methionine/homocysteine sulfur: Cysteine metabolism to taurine and inorganic sulfur. *Journal of Inherited Metabolic Disease, 34*(1), 17–32. https://doi.org/10.1007/s10545-009-9006-6

Stipanuk, M. H., Coloso, R. M., Garcia, R. A. G., & Banks, M. F. (1992). Cysteine concentration regulates cysteine metabolism to glutathione, sulfate, and taurine in rat hepatocytes. *Journal of Nutrition, 122*(3), 420–427. https://doi.org/10.1093/jn/122.3.420

Strzelecki, D., Podgorski, M., Kaluzynska, O., et al. (2015). Supplementation of antipsychotic treatment with the amino acid sarcosine influences proton magnetic resonance spectroscopy parameters in left frontal white matter in patients with schizophrenia. *Nutrients, 7*(10), 8767–8782. https://doi.org/10.3390/nu7105439

Sun, S., Lui, Q., Han, L., et al. (2018). Identification and characterization of *Fusarium proliferatum*, a new species of fungi that cause fungal keratitis. *Scientific Reports, 8*, 4859. https://doi.org/10.1038/s41598-018-23255-z

Symes, A. L., Missala, K., & Sourkes, T. L. (1971). Iron- and riboflavin-dependent metabolism of a monoamine in the rat in vivo. *Science, 174*(4005), 153–155. https://doi.org/10.1126/science.174.4005.153

Talley, N. J., Holtmann, G., Walker, M. M., Burns, G., Potter, M., Shah, A., Jones, M., Koloski, N. A., & Keely, S. (2019). Circulating anti-cytolethal distending toxin B and anti-vinculin antibodies as biomarkers in community and healthcare populations with functional dyspepsia and irritable bowel syndrome. *Clinical and Translational Gastroenterology, 10*(7), e00064. https://doi.org/10.14309/ctg.0000000000000064

Tatchou-Nyamsi-König, J. A., et al. (2009). Survival of *Mycobacterium avium* attached to polyethylene terephthalate (PET) water bottles. *Journal of Applied Microbiology, 106*(3), 825–832. https://doi.org/10.1111/j.1365-2672.2008.04046.x

Tavares, P., et al. (2005). Roles of cell adhesion and cytoskeleton activity in *Entamoeba histolytica* pathogenesis: A delicate balance. *Infection and Immunity, 73*(3), 1771–1778. https://doi.org/10.1128/IAI.73.3.1771-1778.2005

Tchidjou, H., et al. (2015). Celiac disease in an adoptive child with recurrent *Giardia* infection. *International Journal of Health Sciences (Qassim), 9*(2), 193–197.

Tejada-Simon, M. V., et al. (2003). Cross-reactivity with myelin basic protein and human herpesvirus-6 in multiple sclerosis. *Annals of Neurology, 53*, 189–197. https://doi.org/10.1002/ana.10431

Thöny, B., & Blau, N. (2006). Mutations in the BH4-metabolizing genes GTP cyclohydrolase I, 6-pyruvoyl-tetrahydropterin synthase, sepiapterin reductase, carbinolamine-4a-dehydratase, and dihydropteridine reductase. *Human Mutation, 27*(9), 870–878. https://doi.org/10.1002/humu.20355

Tiihonen, K., Ouwehand, A. C., & Rautonen, N. (2010). Effect of overweight on gastrointestinal microbiology and immunology: Correlation with blood biomarkers. *British Journal of Nutrition, 103*(7), 1070–1078. https://doi.org/10.1017/S0007114509992750

Tisman, G., & Garcia, A. (2011). Control of prostate cancer associated with withdrawal of a supplement containing folic acid, L-methyltetrahydrofolate, and vitamin B12: A case report. *Journal of Medical Case Reports, 5*, 413. https://doi.org/10.1186/1752-1947-5-413

Tleyjeh, I. M., et al. (2012). Association between proton pump inhibitor therapy and *Clostridium difficile* infection: A contemporary systematic review and meta-analysis. *PLoS ONE, 7*(e50836). https://doi.org/10.1371/journal.pone.0050836

Tomer, Y., & Davies, T. F. (1993). Infection, thyroid disease, and autoimmunity. *Endocrine Reviews, 14*, 107–120. https://doi.org/10.1210/edrv-14-1-107

Townsend, D. M., Tew, K. D., & Tapiero, H. (2003). The importance of glutathione in human disease. *Biomedicine & Pharmacotherapy, 57*(3-4), 145–155. https://doi.org/10.1016/S0753-3322(03)00043-X

Tupchong, L., et al. (1999). Beaver fever—a rare cause of reactive arthritis. *Journal of Rheumatology, 26*, 2701–2702.

Turner, M. A., Yang, X., Yin, D., Kuczera, K., Borchardt, R. T., & Howell, P. L. (2000). Structure and function of S-adenosylhomocysteine hydrolase. *Cell Biochemistry and Biophysics, 33*(2), 101–125. https://doi.org/10.1385/CBB:33:2:101

Ueland, P. M. (2011). Choline and betaine in health and disease. *Journal of Inherited Metabolic Disease, 34*(1), 3–15. https://doi.org/10.1007/s10545-010-9088-4

Ushida, Y., & Talalay, P. (2013). Sulforaphane accelerates acetaldehyde metabolism by inducing aldehyde dehydrogenases: Relevance to ethanol intolerance. *Alcohol, 48*(5), 526–534. https://doi.org/10.1093/alcalc/agt063

Valdimarsson, H., et al. (1995). Psoriasis: A T-cell-mediated autoimmune disease induced by streptococcal superantigens. *Immunology Today, 16*(3), 145–149. https://doi.org/10.1016/0167-5699(95)80145-0

van der Gaag, M. S., Ubbink, J. B., Sillanaukee, P., Nikkari, S., & Hendriks, H. F. (2000). Effect of consumption of red wine, spirits, and beer on serum homocysteine. *The Lancet, 355*(9214), 1522. https://doi.org/10.1016/S0140-6736(00)02131-1

Van Dongen, A. M. (Ed.). (2009). *Biology of the NMDA receptor.* CRC Press/Taylor & Francis. https://doi.org/10.1201/9781420044157

van Driel, L. M., Eijkemans, M. J., de Jonge, R., de Vries, J. H., van Meurs, J. B., Steegers, E. A., & Steegers-Theunissen, R. P. (2009). Body mass index is an important determinant of methylation biomarkers in women of reproductive ages. *Journal of Nutrition, 139*(12), 2315–2321. https://doi.org/10.3945/jn.109.109710

van Goozen, S. H., Langley, K., Northover, C., Hubble, K., Rubia, K., Schepman, K., O'Donovan, M. C., & Thapar, A. (2016). Identifying mechanisms that underlie links between COMT genotype and aggression in male adolescents with ADHD. *Journal of Child Psychology and Psychiatry, 57*(4), 472–480. https://doi.org/10.1111/jcpp.12464

Van Heel, D. A., et al. (2007). A genome-wide association study for celiac disease identifies risk variants in the region harboring IL2 and IL21. *Nature Genetics, 39*(7), 827–829. https://doi.org/10.1038/ng2058

Van Meurs, J. B. J., et al. (2008). Large-scale analysis of association between LRP5 and LRP6 variants and osteoporosis. *JAMA, 299*(11), 1277–1290. https://doi.org/10.1001/jama.299.11.1277

Van Sechel, A. C., et al. (1999). EBV-induced expression and HLA-DR-restricted presentation by human B cells of alpha B-crystallin, a candidate autoantigen in multiple sclerosis. *Journal of Immunology, 162*(1), 129–135.

Vanitha, M., Baskaran, K., Periyasamy, K., et al. (2015). A review on the biomedical importance of taurine. *International Journal of Pharmacy Research and Health Sciences, 3*(3), 680–686.

Vatrella, A., Fabozzi, I., Calabrese, C., Maselli, R., & Pelaia, G. (2014). Dupilumab: A novel treatment for asthma. *Journal of Asthma and Allergy, 7*, 123–130. https://doi.org/10.2147/JAA.S52387

Veatch, O. J., Pendergast, J. S., Allen, M. J., Leu, R. M., Johnson, C. H., Elsea, S. H., & Malow, B. A. (2015). Genetic variation in melatonin pathway enzymes in children with autism spectrum disorder and comorbid sleep onset delay. *Journal of Autism and Developmental Disorders, 45*(1), 100–110.

Vidrascu, E. M., et al. (2019). Effects of early- and mid-life stress on DNA methylation of genes associated with subclinical cardiovascular disease and cognitive impairment: A systematic review. *BMC Medical Genetics, 20*(1), 39. https://doi.org/10.1186/s12881-019-0764-4

Vojdani, A. (2004). Cross-reactivity of Aspergillus, Penicillium, and Stachybotrys antigens using affinity-purified antibodies and immunoassay. *Archives of Environmental Health, 59*(5), 256–265. https://doi.org/10.3200/AEOH.59.5.256-265

Vojdani, A. (2014). A potential link between environmental triggers and autoimmunity. *Autoimmune Diseases, 2014*, 437231. https://doi.org/10.1155/2014/437231

Vojdani, A. (2015). Reaction of monoclonal and polyclonal antibodies made against infectious agents with various food antigens. *Journal of Clinical & Cellular Immunology, 6*(5). https://doi.org/10.4172/2155-9899.1000359

Vojdani, A. (2017, October 16). OCD: Non-autoimmune versus autoimmune (PANDAS) versions. *ACN Latitudes.* https://latitudes.org/ocd-non-autoimmune-versus-autoimmune-pandas-versions/

Vojdani, A., et al. (1996). Immunological cross-reactivity between Candida albicans and human tissue. *Journal of Clinical & Laboratory Immunology, 48*(1), 1–15.

Vojdani, A., et al. (2002). Antibodies to neuron-specific antigens in children with autism: Possible cross-reaction with encephalitogenic proteins from milk, *Chlamydia pneumoniae,* and *Streptococcus* group A. *Journal of Neuroimmunology, 129*(1–2), 168–177. https://doi.org/10.1016/s0165-5728(02)00180-7

Vojdani, A., et al. (2009). Novel diagnosis of Lyme disease: Potential for CAM intervention. *Evidence-Based Complementary and Alternative Medicine, 6*(3), 283–295. https://doi.org/10.1093/ecam/nem138

Vollbracht, C., McGregor, G. P., & Kraft, K. (2020). Supraphysiological vitamin B12 serum concentrations without supplementation: The pitfalls of interpretation. *QJM: An International Journal of Medicine, 113*(9), 619–620. https://doi.org/10.1093/qjmed/hcz164

Wageningen University and Research Centre. (2013, May 15). Intestinal bacterium Akkermansia curbs obesity. *ScienceDaily.*

Wagner, C., & Koury, M. J. (2007). S-Adenosylhomocysteine—a better indicator of vascular disease than homocysteine? *American Journal of Clinical Nutrition, 86*(6), 1581–1585.

Waites, K. B., & Talkington, D. F. (2004). Mycoplasma pneumoniae and its role as a human pathogen. *Clinical Microbiology Reviews, 17*(4), 697–728.

Wald, D. S., Bishop, L., Wald, N. J., et al. (2001). Randomized trial of folic acid supplementation and serum homocysteine levels. *Archives of Internal Medicine, 161*(5), 695–700.

Walker, B. C., & Mittal, S. (2020). Antitumor activity of curcumin in glioblastoma. *International Journal of Molecular Sciences, 21*(24), 9435. https://doi.org/10.3390/ijms21249435

Wang, W., Jiao, X. H., Wang, X. P., Sun, X. Y., & Dong, C. (2016). MTR, MTRR, and MTHFR gene polymorphisms and susceptibility to nonsyndromic cleft lip with or without cleft palate. *Genetic Testing and Molecular Biomarkers, 20*(6), 297–303. https://doi.org/10.1089/gtmb.2015.0186

Wang, W., Wu, Z., Dai, Z., Yang, Y., Wang, J., & Wu, G. (2013). Glycine metabolism in animals and humans: Implications for nutrition and health. *Amino Acids, 45*(3), 463–477.

Wang, Y., et al. (2013). Meta-analysis on the association between the TF gene Rs1049296 and AD. *The Canadian Journal of Neurological Sciences, 40*(5), 691–697. https://doi.org/10.1017/s0317167100014931

Wardle, J., Carnell, S., Haworth, C. M., Farooqi, I. S., O'Rahilly, S., & Plomin, R. (2008). Obesity-associated genetic variation in FTO is associated with diminished satiety. *Journal of Clinical Endocrinology & Metabolism, 93*(9), 3640–3643. https://doi.org/10.1210/jc.2008-0472

Wedemeyer, H., et al. (2001). Cross-reactivity between Hepatitis C virus and influenza A virus determinant-specific cytotoxic T cells. *Journal of Virology, 75*(23), 11392–11400.

Weidinger, S., et al. (2008). Genome-wide scan on total serum IgE levels identifies FCER1A as a novel susceptibility locus. *PLoS Genetics, 4*(8), e1000166. https://doi.org/10.1371/journal.pgen.1000166

Wensaas, K. A., et al. (2010). Post-infectious gastrointestinal symptoms after acute giardiasis: A 1-year follow-up in general practice. *Family Practice, 27*(3), 255–259.

Wensaas, K. A., et al. (2012). Irritable bowel syndrome and chronic fatigue 3 years after acute giardiasis: A historic cohort study. *Gut, 61*(2), 214–219.

Wenzel, B. E., et al. (1988). Antibodies to plasmid-encoded proteins of enteropathogenic Yersinia in patients with autoimmune thyroid disease. *The Lancet, 1*(8575–6), 56.

Whitney, C., et al. (1992). Serum immunoglobulin G antibody to *Porphyromonas gingivalis* in rapidly progressive periodontitis: Titer, avidity, and subclass distribution. *Infection and Immunity, 60*(6), 2194–2200.

Widerström, M., et al. (2014). Large outbreak of *Cryptosporidium hominis* infection transmitted through the public water supply, Sweden. *Emerging Infectious Diseases, 20*(4). https://doi.org/10.3201/eid2004.121415

Wildner, G., & Diedrichs-Möhring, M. (2003). Autoimmune uveitis induced by molecular mimicry of peptides from rotavirus, bovine casein, and retinal S-antigen. *European Journal of Immunology, 33*(10), 2577–2587.

Wilking, H., et al. (2015). Antibodies against *Borrelia burgdorferi* sensu lato among adults, Germany, 2008–2011. *Emerging Infectious Diseases, 21*(1), 107–110.

Williams, A. L., Girard, C., Jui, D., Sabina, A., & Katz, D. L. (2005). S-adenosylmethionine (SAMe) as treatment for depression: A systematic review. *Clinical and Investigative Medicine, 28*(3), 132–139.

Williams, K. T., & Schalinske, K. L. (2007). New insights into the regulation of methyl group and homocysteine metabolism. *Journal of Nutrition, 137*(2), 311–314.

Wilson, A. S., Power, B. E., & Molloy, P. L. (2007). DNA hypomethylation and human diseases. *Biochimica et Biophysica Acta (BBA) - Reviews on Cancer, 1775*(1), 138–162.

Wink, D. A., & Schmitz, J. A. (1980). Cytomegalovirus myocarditis. *American Heart Journal, 100*, 667.

RESEARCH ARTICLES

Wojcik, O. P., Koenig, K. L., Zeleniuch-Jacquotte, A., Costa, M., & Chen, Y. (2010). The potential protective effects of taurine on coronary heart disease. *Atherosclerosis, 208*(1), 19–25. https://doi.org/10.1016/j.atherosclerosis.2009.10.035

Wojdani, A., et al. (1986). Measurements of humoral and cellular immunity for the diagnosis of candidiasis. *Clinical Ecology, 3*(4), 201–207.

Woo, J. M., Yoon, K. S., & Yu, B. H. (2002). Catechol O-methyltransferase genetic polymorphism in panic disorder. *American Journal of Psychiatry, 159*(10), 1785–1787.

Woods, J. S., et al. (2014). Genetic polymorphisms of catechol-O-methyltransferase modify the neurobehavioral effects of mercury in children. *Journal of Toxicology and Environmental Health, Part A, 77*(6), 293–312. https://doi.org/10.1080/15287394.2014.867210

Worda, C., Sator, M. O., Schneeberger, C., Jantschev, T., Ferlitsch, K., & Huber, J. C. (2003). Influence of the catechol-O-methyltransferase (COMT) codon 158 polymorphism on estrogen levels in women. *Human Reproduction, 18*(2), 262–266.

Wouters, M. M., et al. (2014). Genetic variants in CDC42 and NXPH1 as susceptibility factors for constipation and diarrhea predominant irritable bowel syndrome. *Gut, 63*(7), 1103–1111. https://doi.org/10.1136/gutjnl-2013-304570

Wu, D. F., Yin, R. X., Cao, X. L., & Chen, W. X. (2014). Association between single nucleotide polymorphism rs1044925 and the risk of coronary artery disease and ischemic stroke. *International Journal of Molecular Sciences, 15*(3), 3546–3559.

Wu, G., Fang, Y.-Z., Yang, S., Lupton, J. R., & Turner, N. D. (2004). Glutathione metabolism and its implications for health. *The Journal of Nutrition, 134*(3), 489–492.

Wu, X., Zou, T., Cao, N., Ni, J., Xu, W., Zhou, T., & Wang, X. (2014). Plasma homocysteine levels and genetic polymorphisms in folate metabolism are associated with breast cancer risk in Chinese women. *Heredity Cancer Clinical Practice, 12*(1), 2. https://doi.org/10.1186/1897-4287-12-2

Wu, X.-Y., & Lu, L. (2012). Vitamin B6 deficiency, genome instability and cancer. *Asian Pacific Journal of Cancer Prevention, 13*(11), 5333–5338.

Wucherpfennig, K. W., & Strominger, J. L. (1995). Molecular mimicry in T cell-mediated autoimmunity: Viral peptides activate human T cell clones specific for myelin basic protein. *Cell, 80*(5), 695–705.

Wyatt, L. S., et al. (1991). Human herpesvirus 7: Antigenic properties and prevalence in children and adults. *Journal of Virology, 65*, 6260–6265.

Xiang, L., Wu, H., Pan, A., Patel, B., Xiang, G., Qi, L., Kaplan, R. C., Hu, F., Wylie-Rosett, J., & Qi, Q. (2016). FTO genotype and weight loss in diet and lifestyle interventions: A systematic review and meta-analysis. *American Journal of Clinical Nutrition, 103*(4), 1162–1170. https://doi.org/10.3945/ajcn.115.123448

Xiao, Y., Su, X., Huang, W., Zhang, J., Peng, C., Huang, H., Wu, X., Huang, H., Xia, M., & Ling, W. (2015). Role of S-adenosylhomocysteine in cardiovascular disease and its potential epigenetic mechanism. *International Journal of Biochemistry and Cell Biology, 67*, 158–166. https://doi.org/10.1016/j.biocel.2015.06.015

Xiao, Y., Zhang, Y., Wang, M., et al. (2013). Plasma S-adenosylhomocysteine is associated with the risk of cardiovascular events in patients undergoing coronary angiography: A cohort study. *American Journal of Clinical Nutrition, 98*(5), 1162–1169.

Xiong, D. H., Shen, H., Zhao, L. J., Xiao, P., Yang, T. L., Guo, Y., Wang, W., Guo, Y. F., Liu, Y. J., Recker, R. R., & Deng, H. W. (2006). Robust and comprehensive analysis of 20 osteoporosis candidate genes by very high-density single-nucleotide polymorphism screen among 405 white nuclear families identified significant association and gene-gene interaction. *Journal of Bone and Mineral Research, 21*(11), 1678–1695. https://doi.org/10.1359/jbmr.060808

Xu, Q., et al. (1993). Association of serum antibodies to heat-shock protein 65 with carotid atherosclerosis. *Lancet, 341*(8840), 255–259. https://doi.org/10.1016/0140-6736(93)92613-x

Yakoob, J., et al. (2004). Irritable bowel syndrome: In search of an etiology: Role of *Blastocystis hominis*. *American Journal of Tropical Medicine and Hygiene, 70*(4), 383–385.

Yi, P., Melnyk, S., Pogribna, M., Pogribny, I. P., Hine, R. J., & James, S. J. (2000). Increase in plasma homocysteine associated with parallel increases in plasma S-adenosylhomocysteine and lymphocyte DNA hypomethylation. *Journal of Biological Chemistry, 275*(38), 29318–29323.

Yokota, T., et al. (2000). Autoantibodies against chaperonin CCT in human sera with rheumatic autoimmune diseases: Comparison with antibodies against other Hsp60 family proteins. *Cell Stress and Chaperones, 5*(4), 337–346.

Yoshikawa, T., et al. (2001). Comparison of specific serological assays for diagnosing human herpesvirus 6 infection after liver transplantation. *Clinical and Diagnostic Laboratory Immunology, 8*(1), 170–173.

Yu, R. K., et al. (2006). Ganglioside molecular mimicry and its pathological roles in Guillain-Barré syndrome and related diseases. *Infection and Immunity, 74*(12), 6517–6527. https://doi.org/10.1128/IAI.00967-06

Yuki, N., & Koga, M. (2006). Bacterial infections in Guillain–Barré and Fisher syndromes. *Current Opinion in Neurology, 19*, 451–457.

Yuki, N., et al. (1993). A bacterium lipopolysaccharide that elicits Guillain-Barré syndrome has a GM1 ganglioside–like structure. *Journal of Experimental Medicine, 178*, 1771–1775.

Zain, M. E. (2011). Impact of mycotoxins on humans and animals. *Journal of the Saudi Chemical Society, 15*, 129–144. https://doi.org/10.1016/j.jscs.2010.06.006

Zbinden, R., et al. (1998). IgM to *Bartonella henselae* in cat scratch disease during acute Epstein-Barr virus infection. *Medical Microbiology and Immunology, 186*, 167–170.

Zhang, J., Chen, Y., Zhang, K., Yang, H., Sun, Y., Fang, Y., Shen, Y., & Xu, Q. (2010). A cis-phase interaction study of genetic variants within the MAOA gene in major depressive disorder. *Biological Psychiatry, 68*(9), 795–800. https://doi.org/10.1016/j.biopsych.2010.06.004

Zhang, X. J., et al. (2009). Psoriasis genome-wide association study identifies susceptibility variants within LCE gene cluster at 1q21. *Nature Genetics, 41*(2), 205–210. https://doi.org/10.1038/ng.310

Zheng, Y., & Zhang, M. (2014). Cross-reactivity between human cytomegalovirus peptide 981–1003 and myelin oligodendroglia glycoprotein peptide 35–55 in experimental autoimmune encephalomyelitis in Lewis rats. *Biochemical and Biophysical Research Communications, 443*(3), 1118–1123.

Zheng, Y., et al. (2015). Dietary fat modifies the effects of FTO genotype on changes in insulin sensitivity. *The Journal of Nutrition, 145*(5), 977–982. https://doi.org/10.3945/jn.115.210005

Zhernakova, A., Alizadeh, B. Z., Bevova, M., van Leeuwen, M. A., Coenen, M. J., Franke, B., Franke, L., Posthumus, M. D., van Heel, D. A., van der Steege, G., Radstake, T. R., Barrera, P., Roep, B. O., Koeleman, B. P., & Wijmenga, C. (2007). Novel association in chromosome 4q27 region with rheumatoid arthritis and confirmation of type 1 diabetes point to a general risk locus for autoimmune diseases. *American Journal of Human Genetics, 81*(6), 1284–1288. https://doi.org/10.1086/522037

Zhou, S. F., Wang, B., Yang, L. P., & Liu, J. P. (2010). Structure, function, regulation and polymorphism and the clinical significance of human cytochrome P450 1A2. *Drug Metabolism Reviews, 42*(2), 268–354. https://doi.org/10.3109/03602530903286476

Zhu, H., et al. (2001). Antibodies to human heat-shock protein 60 are associated with the presence and severity of coronary artery disease. *Circulation, 103*, 1071–1075.

Zollner-Schwetz, I., et al. (2008). Role of *Klebsiella oxytoca* in antibiotic-associated diarrhea. *Clinical Infectious Diseases, 47*, e74–e78.

Zunszain, P. A., Anacker, C., Cattaneo, A., Carvalho, L. A., & Pariante, C. M. (2011). Glucocorticoids, cytokines and brain abnormalities in depression. *Progress in Neuropsychopharmacology & Biological Psychiatry, 35*(3), 722–729. https://doi.org/10.1016/j.pnpbp.2010.04.011

Lab Companies

- 3x4 Genetics
- Alletess Medical Labs
- Analytical Research Labs
- BiomeFx™
- BioReference Health ®
- Boston Heart Diagnostics ®
- Cyrex ® Labs
- Designs For Health ® (DFH Spotlight testing)
- Diagnostic Solutions Laboratory
- Doctor's Data
- Gemelli Biotech
- Genova Diagnostics
- Immunosciences Lab
- Invivo ® Healthcare
- LabCorp
- Life Extension ® (GX Sciences)
- Lifecode Gx ®
- Mosaic™ Diagnostics (formerly Great Plains Labs)
- MTHFR Genetics UK & Europe
- myDNAHealth
- Nordic ® Labs
- Nutrigenomix ®
- Optimal DX
- Precision Analytical (DUTCH test) ®
- Precision Point Diagnostics
- Pure Encapsulations ®
- Quest Diagnostics ®
- Quicksilver Scientific ®
- RealTime Labs
- Rocky Mountain Analytical ®
- Rupa Health
- Seeking Health
- SelfDecode
- SpectraCell Laboratories
- Trace Elements Hair Testing
- TrioSmart ®
- US BioTek
- Vibrant Wellness
- ZRT Laboratory

Books

Bone, K. (2007). *The ultimate herbal compendium: A desktop guide for herbal prescribers.* Phytotherapy Press.

Bouchard, C., & Ordovas, J. M. (2012). *Recent advances in nutrigenetics and nutrigenomics.* In *Molecular Biology and Translational Science* (Vol. 108). Elsevier/Academic Press.

Bruton-Seal, J., & Seal, M. (2014). *The herbalist's bible: John Parkinson's lost classic rediscovered.* Skyhorse Publishing.

Burton BT, Foster WR (1988) Human Nutrition. New York, NY: McGraw-Hill.

Jones, D. S. (2006). *Textbook of functional medicine.* Institute for Functional Medicine.

Kapalka, G. M. (2010). *Nutritional and herbal therapies for children and adolescents.* Academic Press.

Knowler, K. (2020). *Blood labs: Lab reference blood test book, and lab values interpretation for fatigue.* Independently published.

Kohlmeier, M. (2013). *Nutrigenetics: Applying the science of personal nutrition.* Academic Press.

Liska, D., & Bland, J. (2004). *Clinical nutrition: A functional approach.* Institute for Functional Medicine.

Lord, R. S., & Bralley, J. A. (2008). *Laboratory evaluations for integrative and functional medicine* (Rev. 2nd ed.). Metametrix.

Lynch, B. (2018). *Dirty genes.* HarperCollins.

Masterjohn, C. (2021). *The vitamins and minerals 101 - Cliff notes.*

Masterjohn, C. (2024). *Testing nutritional status: The ultimate cheat sheet.*

Mills, S., & Bone, K. (2005). *The essential guide to herbal safety.* Churchill Livingstone.

Nelson, R., PhD, MH. *FBC quick start guide: Patterns, systems and interpretation.*

Pagana, K. D., Pagana, T. J., & Pagana, T. N. (2021). *Mosby's diagnostic and laboratory test reference* (15th ed.). Elsevier, Inc.

Patel, V., & Preedy, V. (2018). *Handbook of nutrition, diet, and epigenetics.* Springer.

Pathak, Y. V., & Ardekani, A. M. (2018). *Nutrigenomics and nutraceuticals.* CRC Press.

Pemberton, A. (2021). *Using nutrigenomics within personalized nutrition: A practitioner's guide.* Singing Dragon.

Weatherby, D., & Ferguson, S. (2002). *Blood chemistry and CBC analysis: Clinical laboratory testing from a functional perspective.* Weatherby & Associates, LLC.

Weatherby, R., & Weatherby, D. C. (2000). *Reference guide to blood chemistry analysis.* Weatherby & Associates, LLC.

Williamson, E. M., Driver, S., & Baxter, K. (2010). *Stockley's herbal medicines interactions: A guide to the interactions of herbal medicines, dietary supplements and nutraceuticals with conventional medicines.* Pharmaceutical Press.

Trainings/Teachers/Seminars

- Dr. Brandy Zachary, DC, IFMCP, FMACP - Functional Medicine Academy (FMA) Certification
- Dr. Ben Lynch, ND (Seeking Health) and Elizma Lambert - Your Professional Guide to StrateGene®
- Dr. Dan Kalish, DC, IFMCP - The Kalish Institute - Organic Acids series
- Dr. Kurt Woeller, DO (for Mosaic™ Diagnostics) - Digging Deeper into the Organic Acids Test
- Mark Newman, MS & Dr. Bethany Hays, MD - Precision Analytical (DUTCH ® test) - Interpreting Your DUTCH Plus® Cortisol Results
- Institute for Functional Medicine ® (IFM) - IFMCP Certification program
- Institute for Functional Medicine ® (IFM) - Practitioner Toolkit

Other digital source material

CDC
- https://www.atsdr.cdc.gov/toxprofiles/tp205.pdf
- https://www.atsdr.cdc.gov/toxprofiles/tp205-c3.pdf
- https://www.cdc.gov/aspergillosis/
- https://www.cdc.gov/candidiasis/
- https://www.cdc.gov/dpdx/az.html
- https://www.cdc.gov/dpdx/resources/pdf/benchaids/entamoeba_benchaid.pdf
- https://www.cdc.gov/fungal/diseases/candidiasis/index.html
- https://www.cdc.gov/lyme
- https://www.cdc.gov/mucormycosis/hcp/clinical-overview/index.html
- https://www.cdc.gov/parasites/blastocystis/health_professionals/index.html
- https://www.cdc.gov/parasites/hymenolepis/health_professionals/index.html
- https://www.cdc.gov/parasites/hymenolepis/health_professionals/index.html
- https://www.cdc.gov/parasites/index.html
- https://www.cdc.gov/ringworm/about/index.html

Cyrex ® Laboratories
- https://www.cyrexlabs.com/CyrexTestsArrays/tabid/136/Default.aspx

Dr. Jolene Brighten, NMD, FABNE
- https://drbrighten.com/seed-cycling-menopausal-hormones/

Doctor's Data
- https://s3.amazonaws.com/site-akiajqrf22xmaqzsiz6q/documents/AdrenalDysfunction.pdf
- https://site-akiajqrf22xmaqzsiz6q.s3.amazonaws.com/documents/HPA+Axis+Support.pdf
- https://site-akiajqrf22xmaqzsiz6q.s3.amazonaws.com/DDI+Website/Handouts/DHEA+and+DHEA-S_H-Handout.pdf

DoveMed
- https://www.dovemed.com/diseases-conditions/gold-toxicity

EWG - Environmental Working Group
- https://www.ewg.org/consumer-guides
- https://www.ewg.org/skindeep/

Fullscript ®
- https://fullscript.com/blog/seed-cycling

OTHER DIGITAL SOURCE MATERIAL

GeneCards ®
- https://www.genecards.org/

Genova Diagnostics
- https://www.gdx.net/core/supplemental-education-materials/Parasitic-Organisms-Chart.pdf
- https://www.gdx.net/core/support-guides/Adrenocortex-Stress-Profile-Support-Guide.pdf

GWAS Catalogue
- https://www.ebi.ac.uk/gwas/

Healthmatters.io
- https://healthmatters.io/

Linus Pauling Institute
- https://lpi.oregonstate.edu/mic

Lyme Ontario
- https://lymeontario.com/wp-content/uploads/2020/04/BLP_MISIDSLymeQuestionnaire.pdf

Mosaic™ Diagnostics
- https://mosaicdx.com/resource/8-binders-for-mycotoxins/
- https://mosaicdx.com/resource/clinical-significance-of-the-organic-acids-test-brochure/
- https://mosaicdx.com/resource/more-binders-for-mycotoxins/
- https://mosaicdx.com/resource/organic-acids-detailed-brochure/
- https://mosaicdx.com/resource/part-1-mold-101-mycotox-profile-oat-using-them-to-id-mold-patients/
- https://mosaicdx.com/resource/part-2-mold-102-mycotox-profile-oat-treatments-monitoring-and-additional-insights/
- https://mosaicdx.com/resource/the-evidence-behind-mycotoxins-in-food/
- https://mosaicdx.com/test/mycotox-profile/

MSD Manuals
- https://www.msdmanuals.com/en-gb/professional/infectious-diseases/fungi/phaeohyphomycosis

NCBI Bookshelf

Agnew, U. M., & Slesinger, T. L. (2022, December 11). *Zinc toxicity*. StatPearls - NCBI Bookshelf.
https://www.ncbi.nlm.nih.gov/books/NBK554548

Castano, G., Yarrarapu, S. N. S., & Mada, P. K. (2023, July 24). *Trichosporonosis*. StatPearls - NCBI Bookshelf.
https://www.ncbi.nlm.nih.gov/books/NBK482477

Chen, R. J., & Lee, V. R. (2023, July 29). *Cobalt toxicity*. StatPearls - NCBI Bookshelf.
https://www.ncbi.nlm.nih.gov/books/NBK587403

Eden, R. E., Daley, S. F., & Coviello, J. M. (2023, September 8). *Vitamin K deficiency*. StatPearls - NCBI Bookshelf.
https://www.ncbi.nlm.nih.gov/books/NBK536983

Evans, G. R., & Masullo, L. N. (2023, July 10). *Manganese toxicity*. StatPearls - NCBI Bookshelf. https://www.ncbi.nlm.nih.gov/books/NBK560903

Gates, A., Jakubowski, J. A., & Regina, A. C. (2023, May 20). *Nickel Toxicology*. StatPearls - NCBI Bookshelf. https://www.ncbi.nlm.nih.gov/books/NBK592400

Halmo, L., & Nappe, T. M. (2023, July 4). *Lead toxicity*. StatPearls - NCBI Bookshelf. https://www.ncbi.nlm.nih.gov/books/NBK541097

Imbrescia, K., & Moszczynski, Z. (2023, July 10). *Vitamin K*. StatPearls - NCBI Bookshelf. https://www.ncbi.nlm.nih.gov/books/NBK551578

Koons, A. L., & Rajasurya, V. (2023, August 14). *Cadmium toxicity*. StatPearls - NCBI Bookshelf. https://www.ncbi.nlm.nih.gov/books/NBK536966

Kuivenhoven, M., & Mason, K. (2023, June 12). *Arsenic toxicity*. StatPearls - NCBI Bookshelf. https://www.ncbi.nlm.nih.gov/books/NBK541125

Martel, J. L., Kerndt, C. C., Doshi, H., Sina, R. E., & Franklin, D. S. (2024, January 31). *Vitamin B1 (Thiamine)*. StatPearls - NCBI Bookshelf. https://www.ncbi.nlm.nih.gov/books/NBK482360

Nessel, T. A., & Gupta, V. (2023, April 3). *Selenium*. StatPearls - NCBI Bookshelf. https://www.ncbi.nlm.nih.gov/books/NBK557551

Peechakara, B. V., Sina, R. E., & Gupta, M. (2024, February 1). *Vitamin B2 (Riboflavin)*. StatPearls - NCBI Bookshelf. https://www.ncbi.nlm.nih.gov/books/NBK525977

Posin, S. L., Kong, E. L., & Sharma, S. (2023, August 8). *Mercury toxicity*. StatPearls - NCBI Bookshelf. https://www.ncbi.nlm.nih.gov/books/NBK499935

Reif, B. M., & Murray, B. P. (2024, January 11). *Chromium toxicity*. StatPearls - NCBI Bookshelf. https://www.ncbi.nlm.nih.gov/books/NBK599502

Royer, A., & Sharman, T. (2023, March 27). *Copper toxicity*. StatPearls - NCBI Bookshelf. https://www.ncbi.nlm.nih.gov/books/NBK557456

Stearney, E. R., Jakubowski, J. A., & Regina, A. C. (2023, August 21). *Beryllium toxicity*. StatPearls - NCBI Bookshelf. https://www.ncbi.nlm.nih.gov/books/NBK585042

Tatum R, Pearson-Shaver AL. Borrelia Burgdorferi. [Updated 2022 Jul 18]. In: StatPearls [Internet]. Treasure Island (FL): StatPearls Publishing; 2023 Jan-. Available from: https://www.ncbi.nlm.nih.gov/books/NBK532894/

Walker, B. C., Adhikari, S., & Mittal, S. (2021). Therapeutic potential of curcumin for the treatment of malignant gliomas. In *Exon Publications eBooks* (pp. 139–150). https://doi.org/10.36255/exonpublications.gliomas.2021.chapter8

NCBI Reference Sequence Database

- https://www.ncbi.nlm.nih.gov/refseq/

Precision Analytical (DUTCH ® test)

- https://drive.google.com/file/d/1E8lja2zfxrc_uj8UYcBn6R1jc9Aun52a/view?usp=sharing
- https://dutchtest.com/resources/
- https://dutchtest.com/video/dutch-treatment-guide/

Precision Point Diagnostics

- https://precisionpointdiagnostics.com/test/advanced-barrier-assessment-plasma/

Quest Diagnostics ®

OTHER DIGITAL SOURCE MATERIAL

- https://www.questdiagnostics.com/healthcare-professionals/clinical-education-center/faq/scerevisiae

SelfDecode

- https://selfdecode.com/

SNPedia

- https://www.snpedia.com/

SpectraCell Laboratories

- https://assets.speakcdn.com/assets/2606/306_prescription_depletions_7_19.pdf

Thermo Fisher Scientific

- https://www.thermofisher.com/allergy/us/en/allergen-fact-sheets/mucor-racemosus.html
- https://www.thermofisher.com/phadia/wo/en/resources/allergen-encyclopedia/m10.html
- https://www.thermofisher.com/phadia/wo/en/resources/allergen-encyclopedia/m11.html

UCSFhealth.org

- Hypersensitivity pneumonitis: https://www.ucsfhealth.org/conditions/hypersensitivity-pneumonitis#Treatments

UpToDate ®

- https://www.uptodate.com/contents/treatment-and-prevention-of-fusarium-infection

WHO - World Health Organization

- https://www.who.int/india/home/emergencies/coronavirus-disease-(covid-19)/mucormycosis

ZRT Laboratory

- https://www.zrtlab.com/media/1051/adrenal-stress-booklet.pdf

Drug-Nutrient Interactions and Depletions resources

Natural Medicines Database:

- https://naturalmedicines.therapeuticresearch.com/

MyTavin Drug Nutrient depletion checker:

- https://mytavin.com/

Other:

- https://fullscript.com/blog/nutrient-interactions
- https://integrativepro.com/pages/drug-nutrient-interaction-checker
- https://www.nutriadvanced.co.uk/healthnotes?resource=%2fassets%2fa-z-index%2fa-to-z-index-of-medicines%2f~default
- https://www.pureencapsulationspro.com/drug-nutrient-interactions
- https://www.mskcc.org/cancer-care/diagnosis-treatment/symptom-management/integrative-medicine/herbs/search
- https://naturalmedicines.therapeuticresearch.com/tools/pregnancy-lactation-checker.aspx#G
- https://online.epocrates.com/noFrame/?ICID=eolepocratesheaderbutton
- https://go.drugbank.com/

Unit Conversion Links

- https://thedrz.com/conversion/
- https://unitslab.com/
- https://www.questdiagnostics.com/content/dam/corporate/restricted/documents/test-center/si_units/si_units.pdf
- https://www.questdiagnostics.com/content/dam/corporate/restricted/documents/test-center/units_of_measure_definitions/units_of_measure_definitions.pdf
- https://www.mayocliniclabs.com/order-tests/si-unit-conversion.html
- https://academic.oup.com/amamanualofstyle/si-conversion-calculator
- https://www.labcorp.com/resource/si-unit-conversion-table

Additional Resources

Frequently Ordered Blood Panels: Traditional and Optimal Ranges

Blood Lab Markers: Common Patterns

Examples of Using Lab Analysis by Functional Medicine Practitioners

How to Become a Functional Medicine Practitioner

How to Find a Functional Medicine Practitioner?

How Do I Interpret More Labs in Less Time?

Get LabDx Online Here:

Frequently Ordered Blood Panels: Traditional and Optimal Ranges

CBC with Differential

Name of Marker	Normal Range	Optimal Range
White Blood Cell Count (WBC)	3.4 – 10.8 x10³/µL	5.0 – 7.5 x10³/µL
Red Blood Cell Count (RBC)	**MALE**: 4.2 – 5.8 x10⁶/µL **FEMALE**: 3.8 – 5.1 x10⁶/µL	**MALE**: 4.2 – 4.9 x10⁶/µL **FEMALE**: 3.9 – 4.5 x10⁶/µL
Hemoglobin	**MALE**: 11.1 – 15.9 g/dL **FEMALE**: 11.1 – 15.9 g/dL	**MALE**: 14 – 15 g/dL **FEMALE**: 13.5 – 14.5 g/dL
Hematocrit	**MALE**: 34 – 46.6% **FEMALE**: 34 – 46.6%	**MALE**: 40 – 48% **FEMALE**: 37 – 44%
Mean Corpuscular Volume (MCV)	79 – 97 fL	82.0 – 89.9 fL
Mean Corpuscular Hemoglobin (MCH)	26.6 – 33 pg	28.0 – 31.9 pg
Mean Corpuscular Hemoglobin Concentration (MCHC)	31.5 – 37 g/dL	32.0 – 35.0 g/dL
Red Blood Cell Distribution Width (RDW)	12.3 – 15.4%	12.0 – 13.0%
Platelets	155 – 379 x10³/µL	185 – 385 x10³/µL
Mean Platelet Volume (MPV)	7.5 - 11.5 fL	7.5 - 8.2 fL
Neutrophils	4.0 – 7.4 x10³/µL	4.0 – 6.0 x10³/µL
Lymphocytes	1.4 – 4.6 x10³/µL	2.4 – 4.4 x10³/µL
Monocytes	0.4 – 1.2 x10³/µL	0.4 – 0.7 x10³/µL
Eosinophils	0 – 0.5 x10³/µL	< 0.5 x10³/µL
Basophils	< 0.3 x10³/µL	< 0.3 x10³/µL

CMP (Comprehensive Metabolic Panel)

Name of Marker	Normal Range	Optimal Range
Glucose - Fasting	65 – 99 mg/dL	80 – 100 mg/dL
Glucose - Non-Fasting	65 – 125 mg/dL	80 – 125 mg/dL
Hemoglobin A1C	4.8 – 5.7%	4.1 – 5.3%
Uric Acid	2.5 – 6.8 mg/dL	3.0 – 5.5 mg/dL
BUN (Blood Urea Nitrogen)	8 – 27 mg/dL	10 – 16 mg/dL
Creatinine	0.57 – 1.00 mg/dL	0.8 – 1.0 mg/dL
eGFR (non-African American)	> 59 mL/min/1.73 m²	> 90 mL/min/1.73 m²
eGFR (African American)	> 59 mL/min/1.73 m²	> 90 mL/min/1.73 m²
Sodium	134 - 144 mEq/L	135 - 142 mEq/L
Potassium	3.5 - 5.2 mEq/L	4.0 - 4.5 mEq/L
Chloride	97 - 108 mmol/L	100 - 106 mmol/L
Carbon Dioxide (CO_2)	19 - 28 mmol/L	21 - 26 mmol/L
Calcium	8.6 - 10.2 mg/dL	9.2 - 10.0 mg/dL
Phosphorus	2.5 - 4.5 mEq/L	3.0 - 4.0 mEq/L
Magnesium	1.88 - 2.22 mg/dl	2.0 - 3.0 mg/dl
Protein, Total	6.0 - 8.5 g/dL	6.9 - 7.4 g/dL
Albumin	3.6 - 4.8 g/dL	4.6 - 5.0 g/dL
Globulin	2.2 - 3.5 g/dL	2.8 - 3.0 g/dL
Bilirubin, Total	0.1 - 1.2 mg/dL	0.5 – 0.90 mg/dL
Bilirubin - Direct	0 - 0.2 mg/dL	0.1 - 0.15 mg/dL
Bilirubin - Indirect	0.20 - 1.20 mg/dL	0.40 - 0.75 mg/dL
Alkaline Phosphatase (ALP)	39 - 117 IU/L	70 - 100 IU/L
Lactate Dehydrogenase (LDH)	120 - 240 IU/L	90 - 150 IU/L
Aspartate amino-transferase (AST) (SGOT)	0 - 40 IU/L	10 - 30 IU/L
Alanine amino-transferase (ALT) (SGPT)	0 - 32 IU/L	10 - 30 IU/L

Name of Marker	Normal Range	Optimal Range
Gamma-glutamyl transferase (GGT)	1 - 70 IU/L	20 - 30 IU/L

Lipids

Name of Marker	Normal Range	Optimal Range
Cholesterol	100 - 199 mg/dL	180 - 220 mg/dL
Triglycerides	0 - 149 mg/dL	70 - 100 mg/dL
HDL Cholesterol	> 39 mg/dL	> 55 mg/dL
LDL Cholesterol	65 - 99 mg/dL	80 - 130 mg/dL
Homocysteine	0.0 - 15.0 µmol/L	< 7.2 µmol/L
C-Reactive Protein (hsCRP)	**MALE:** 0 - 3.00 mg/dL **FEMALE:** 0 - 3.00 mg/dL	**MALE:** < 0.6 mg/dL **FEMALE:** < 1.5 mg/dL
Fibrinogen Activity	193 - 507 mg/dL	200 - 300 mg/dL

Thyroid

Name of Marker	Normal Range	Optimal Range
TSH (Thyroid Stimulating Hormone)	0.45 - 4.5 uIU/mL	1.0 - 2.0 uIU/mL
Thyroxine (T4), Total	4.5 - 12 ug/dL	7.5 - 8.1 ug/dL
T3 (Triiodothyronine), Total	71.0 - 180.0 ng/dL	90.0 - 168.0 ng/dL
T4, Free (Direct)	0.82 - 1.77 ng/dL	1.0 - 1.5 ng/dL
T3, Free, Serum	2.0 - 4.4 pg/mL	3.0 - 3.25 pg/mL
TPO Thyroid Peroxidase	0 - 34 IU/mL	0 IU/mL
TGAb Thyroglobulin Antibody	0 - 15 IU/mL	0 IU/mL
T3 Uptake	24-39%	30-35%
Reverse T3	9.2 - 24.1 ng/dL	14.9 - 24.1 ng/dL
Free Thyroxine Index (FTI or T7)	1.2 - 4.9 ng/dL	1.2 - 4.9 ng/dL
Thyroxine Binding Globulin (TBG)	14 - 30 mcg/mL	14 - 28 mcg/mL

Anemia

Name of Marker	Normal Range	Optimal Range
Total Iron Binding Capacity (TIBC)	250 - 450 µg/dL	250 - 350 µg/dL
Unsaturated Iron Binding Capacity (UIBC)	131 - 425 µg/dL	131 - 325 µg/dL
Serum Iron	27 - 159 µg/dL	85 - 130 µg/dL
Iron Saturation (Transferrin Saturation - TSAT)	15 - 55%	25 - 35%
Ferritin, Serum	**MALE**: 30 - 400 ng/mL **FEMALE**: 15 - 150 ng/mL	**MALE**: 33 - 236 ng/mL **FEMALE**: 40 - 122 ng/mL
Hemoglobin	**MALE**: 11.1 - 15.9 g/dL **FEMALE**: 11.1 - 15.9 g/dL	**MALE**: 14 - 15 g/dL **FEMALE**: 13.5 - 14.5 g/dL
Hematocrit	**MALE**: 34 - 46.6% **FEMALE**: 34 - 46.6%	**MALE**: 40 - 48% **FEMALE**: 37 - 44%

Blood Lab Markers: Common Patterns

Indications	Markers Low	Markers High	Comments
Adrenal-related Hyperfunction	Potassium Cholesterol Triglycerides	Sodium Chloride CO2 BUN Estrogen Liver markers	
Adrenal-related Hypofunction	Sodium Chloride Glucose DHEA Cortisol	Potassium Cholesterol Triglycerides	
Signs of alcoholism	ALT / SGPT (chronic) Magnesium Vitamin B6 Vitamin B12 Albumin Platelets Zinc Phosphorus	GGT AST / SGOT ALT / SGPT AST:ALT ratio Alkaline Phos / ALP MCV MCH MCHC Homocysteine Uric Acid Lactate Ammonia Lipids Ferritin Folate Triglycerides	
Anemia - B12/Folate (B9) Deficiency	RBCs Hematocrit Hemoglobin WBCs Neutrophils Uric acid	Homocysteine MCH MCV RDW MCHC Serum iron LDH MMA - methylmalonic acid	
Anemia - Iron Deficiency	Serum iron Ferritin Hemoglobin Hematocrit % Transferrin saturation MCV MCH MCHC Globulin	Transferrin TIBC UIBC Globulin	Globulin high if hypochlorhydria present RBCs (could be normal or low) RDW (could be normal or high)

BLOOD LAB MARKERS: COMMON PATTERNS

Indications	Markers Low	Markers High	Comments
	Phosphorous		
Atherosclerosis	HDL ApoA-1 Calcium	Triglycerides Cholesterol LDL Uric acid Platelets CRP, hs-CRP MPO Lp-Pla2 TMAO Apo-B Fibrinogen	
Cardiovascular Disease Risk	HDL Vitamin D ApoA-1 Calcium Pulse Pressure greater than 40	LDL Cholesterol Triglycerides Fibrinogen Homocysteine CRP, hs-CRP MPO Lp-Pla2 Troponin D-dimer Creatinine kinase TMAO Apo-B Uric Acid (Metabolic Syndrome)	
Dehydration	Phosphorus Potassium (with use of diuretics) Sodium (with use of diuretics)	RBC Albumin Globulin A:G ratio BUN Chloride Sodium Hemoglobin Hematocrit Creatinine Potassium Protein	
Diabetes / Hyperglycemia / Insulin resistance, Dysglycemia (can be early signs for brain health conditions such as depression, dementia, etc)	HDL Adiponectin C-peptide (hypoglycemia)	Fasting Insulin Fasting Blood Glucose HbA1C Cholesterol Triglycerides LDL BUN Creatinine C-Peptide (TIID, dysglycemia)	Elevated fasting insulin is a much earlier indicator of diabetes than fasting glucose

BLOOD LAB MARKERS: COMMON PATTERNS

Indications	Markers Low	Markers High	Comments
		Leptin WBC LDH (and all liver markers - due to fatty liver)	
Digestive issue (ex. hypochlorhydria)	Total protein Albumin Chloride Vitamin B12 Phosphorus	WBC (absent infection) MCV MCH CO2 HDL (H2 blockers) BUN Globulin	
Gallbladder, Liver Dysfunction, and Fatty Liver	ALT / SGPT Albumin HDL	Triglycerides LDL Cholesterol ALT / SGPT (more serious) AST / SGOT LDH GGT Bilirubin Alkaline Phosphatase (ALP) Serum iron Ferritin Uric Acid	
Possible GI issues (digestive, microbiome, parasites, intestinal permeability, etc - further testing needed)	Protein BUN (intestinal hyperpermeability) Hemoglobin (parasites) Vitamin B12	WBC Monocytes Eosinophils Basophils BUN (hypochlorhydria) Creatinine Alkaline Phospatase (ALP) Folate (intestinal hyperpermeability)	
Possible heavy metal burden (additional testing needed)	HDL MCH MCHC TSH Uric Acid Platelets	Ferritin (excess iron consumption) Globulin	
Hemochromatosis (Iron Overload)	Transferrin TIBC UIBC	Serum iron Ferritin % Transferrin saturation	Hemoglobin may be normal Consider genetic testing for HFE SNPs

BLOOD LAB MARKERS: COMMON PATTERNS

Indications	Markers Low	Markers High	Comments
Hypothyroidism	T-3 total or free T-4 total or free T-3 Uptake FTI	TSH Cholesterol Triglycerides rT3	TPO, TBG, TGAb antibodies may indicate auto-immune hypothyroidism in context of symptoms and other thyroid markers
Immune markers (some early signs or chronic low grade infection)	WBC (chronic) Vitamin D Neutrophils (chronic viral infections) Lymphocytes Alkaline Phospatase (Zn def) Iron (bacterial infection, chronic illness) Ferritin Globulin (immune insufficiency) Cholesterol (ex. Chronic autoimmune, heavy metal burden, neuro issues, symptoms of depression or dementia) Platelets TSH (Grave's Dx)	WBC (acute) Neutrophils (acute and chronic bacterial infections) Lymphocytes Monocytes Eosinophils Basophils Iron (viral infection) LDH (viral infection) Globulin (active infection) CRP, hs-CRP Cortisol Alkaline Phospatase (active infection, fatty liver) Cholesterol (ex. MS patients) Triglycerides TSH (Hashimoto's)	
Inflammation and Oxidative Stress	Albumin Lymphocytes Cholesterol	ESR LDH Ferritin CRP, hs-CRP Uric Acid Neutrophils Platelets	
Kidney Insufficiency	eGFR	BUN Creatinine Phosphorus	
Liver Dysfunction	Albumin Total protein BUN Triglycerides	ALT / SGPT AST / SGOT LDH GGT Bilirubin ALP Serum iron Ferritin	

BLOOD LAB MARKERS: COMMON PATTERNS

Indications	Markers Low	Markers High	Comments
Methylation issues	Folic acid, Folate B12 Gluthathione	Homocysteine MMA - methylmalonic acid MCV RBC RDW	Consider genetic testing to check methylation predisposition
Zinc deficiency	Alkaline Phosphatase		ALP is a zinc dependent enzyme

Examples of Using Lab Analysis by Functional Medicine Practitioners

Disclaimer: The following stories were submitted by practitioners and reflect their individual experience with their patient or client base and are not tracked by LabDX. All patient/client names and identifying details have been changed to protect privacy and confidentiality.

Dr. Tracy E. Green DNP, APRN, FNP-BC, CPN, FMACP

Organic Acid Test (OAT) by Mosaic™ Diagnostics: Speech delay and autism behaviors

Child patient is a 4-year-old Hispanic/Italian female with history of speech delay, family history of speech delay in her 2-year-old brother and both parents [resolved in elementary school], behavioral issues, autism behaviors, allergies and frequent URIs requiring antibiotic treatment multiple times per year. She lives with mom, dad and her 2-year-old brother and they have 2 dogs. Spanish, Italian, and English languages are spoken at home. Child patient, however, has unintelligible speech and her parents do not understand or know how to communicate with her most of the time. She was evaluated by her pediatrician at age 2 for autism, but mom refused to have formal evaluation for fear of her being labeled. She, however, did meet criteria for the Early Steps program that allows children with developmental delays to enter the pre-school system early.

Child patient's diet was a standard American diet (SAD) with some organic foods and green smoothies daily with avocado and spinach. She ate fast food/fried food about four times a week which was mostly at school while mom cooked homemade pasta and baked items with unbleached flour. She also consumed about 2-3 servings per day of fruits and veggies and had at least one bread roll daily. She took a daily multivitamin with minerals. Child patient slept on average about eight hours each night but had difficulty getting to sleep, experienced occasional nocturnal enuresis and difficulty waking in the morning.

She currently attends pre-school daily but can only manage to attend for 1-2 hours per day before mom is called to pick her up due to disruptive behavior. During preschool she receives speech and occupational therapy without any improvement in speech and some improvement in fine motor skills. Mom presented with several concerns: speech delay, behavioral issues, autism, frequent URIs/low immunity, and allergies. She was interested in functional medicine testing to find the root cause. Child patient's ROS was significantly positive for the following symptoms of candida that also mimic symptoms of autism spectrum disorder (ASD): inappropriate laughter, sleep disturbances, bedwetting, fatigue, depression," fogginess"/poor cognition, inattentiveness, hyperactivity, increased self-stimulatory (stimming) behavior, high-pitched squealing, increased sensory seeking, defensiveness, climbing/jumping off things, sugar cravings, self-limiting foods and plateauing in skills.

An organic acid test (OAT) by Mosaic™ Diagnostics test was performed that revealed in elevated arabinose level indicating the likelihood of the presence of candida. I devised a plan that included: diet low in sugar and simple carbs, high in vitamin C and healthy fats; Omega Avail Smoothies by Designs for Health ® (DFH), Probiomed Kids by DFH, increased physical activity-Let her wear herself out; create a bedtime routine and stick to a schedule as much as possible; Liposomal NeuroCalm by DFH to help her wind down.

Three months post-implementation of the above plan an amazing report was received from the mom that Child patient only needed the Liposomal calm for about 2 weeks initially and then she stopped it because Child patient was going to sleep on time and staying asleep until time to awake in the morning. She is verbalizing words which she had not done previously even with Speech Therapy. Child patient was playing appropriately with toys and asking to try different foods, and she was able to stay the required length of time at VPK (Voluntary Prekindergarten) which she had never been able to do before working with a functional medicine practitioner.

Lynn Dudley, PAc

Gut health and inflammation: 43 y.o. F with IBS-D

Patient was a 43-year old female who presented with fatigue, joint pain, brain fog, and frequent abdominal pain, bloating, and loose stools. She had been diagnosed with "Irritable Bowel Syndrome". She was frustrated with the lack of effective solutions to help eradicate her symptoms and was looking for a deeper dive into the root cause of her ailments.

We conducted comprehensive functional health testing and the following pertinent findings were revealed:

Blood work:
- Elevated C-reactive protein, cardiac (3.8)
- Elevated uric acid (6.4)
- Low vitamin D3 (25)
- Omega Index (3.8)

Food sensitivity testing (IgG)
- High sensitivity to casein
- High sensitivity to almonds
- High sensitivity to eggs

Stool microbiome testing:
- High secretory IgA and antigliadin Abs
- Low keystone bacteria
- High levels of pseudomonas
- High steatocrit

We advised the patient to remove casein, almonds, and eggs from her diet for 3 months. We also started her on several supplements, including vitamin D3 and fish oil to address those deficiencies. For gut health, we started her on digestive enzymes with meals, probiotics, and a short-term herbal supplement to balance gut bacteria.

After two months, the patient's vitamin D3 (83.7), hsCRP (0.88), and uric acid (5.0) had all normalized. And most importantly, her IBS symptoms had completely resolved! She had more energy than she had in years, and her joint pain and brain fog were gone! She had even lost 15 pounds without trying. She was thrilled with her results and grateful to have uncovered the root cause of her symptoms.

Dr. Tarah Davis, PharmD, MBA

GI-MAP ® to reveal hidden gut issues

PATIENT was a 38 year old male, coming to my practice with complaints of not being able to lose those last 20 lbs. He was active and fit and had no significant medical history except for alcoholism, and he was coming to me 2,000 days sober. As a functional medicine practitioner, I know that holding onto weight is a sign of dis-ease in your body, a larger sign of an underlying cause. So, we began to piece together his unique puzzle.

PATIENT had a diverse diet full of whole foods, healthy meats, and he ate the rainbow. However, he would find himself dreaming about sweet foods, he would gorge himself when he felt like no one was watching, and he would be embarrassed of his behavior the next morning. He had control, until he didn't.

PATIENT was interested in knowing more about what was going on inside of his gut, so I ordered a GI-MAP ®. It was apparent that PATIENT had a candida overgrowth. While he had none of the typical symptoms like chronic diarrhea, skin rashes, athlete's foot, oral thrush, or dandruff. His candida infection was making him crave the foods that yeast thrives on. His yeast wanted to be fed!

So we did the opposite and started a starve 'em out diet. We removed the foods that candida needs to grow. Then we started probiotics and antimicrobial herbs. We eventually added in mucilaginous herbs and foods to heal the mucosal layer. After 21 days on the diet and herbs, we slowly began to add back foods we had removed. Making sure that there were no food sensitivities.

After 90 days, PATIENT had lost 15lbs. He had stopped having vivid dreams about pastries and ice cream, and the joint pain, that he had forgotten to tell me that he frequently had at night, had disappeared too.

The root cause of PATIENT's weight? A yeast infection in his gut caused by over consumption of alcohol all those many years before.

Megan Bliss, FNP-C

The importance of listening and looking beyond "normal" test results

A woman in her late 40s came to me feeling completely defeated. For months, she had been struggling with a range of symptoms that were disrupting her daily life: unpredictable energy levels, trouble sleeping, anxiety, mood swings, irregular cycles, night sweats, breast tenderness, and weight gain that seemed impossible to stop. She told me, "I just know something's wrong with my hormones." But despite numerous visits to her primary care doctor, she wasn't getting any answers. What stood out to me about this patient—and what she ultimately taught me—was the importance of trusting that gut feeling and digging deeper when conventional tests come back "normal."

Her frustration was understandable. She'd been told repeatedly that her symptoms were normal for her age or "probably stress-related." Conventional blood tests for thyroid function, glucose, and cholesterol were all in the normal range, and her doctor had only briefly tested her female hormones, which didn't reveal anything significant. She left each appointment feeling dismissed and unheard, yet she couldn't shake the feeling that something deeper was going on. She was sure her symptoms weren't just from aging or stress. That determination brought her to me—and it was my job to listen.

During our first appointment, it was clear how much she needed validation. She poured out her story, and we talked about how perimenopause—a transitional phase before menopause—can cause a wide range of symptoms, often without showing up clearly on basic lab tests. She taught me the importance of asking the right questions, not just about her symptoms but also about how those symptoms were affecting her life. Together, we decided to take a more comprehensive approach to testing. Instead of just looking at estradiol and FSH, we included progesterone, testosterone, DHEA, and cortisol. I also suggested cycle mapping to track her hormone fluctuations throughout the month.

When the results came back, they told a clear story. Her progesterone levels were low, explaining her irregular cycles, mood swings, and post-ovulation breast tenderness. Her estrogen levels were fluctuating dramatically, which was likely behind the night sweats and stubborn weight gain. Cortisol testing revealed a dysregulated pattern—her levels were too low in the morning and spiked at night, disrupting her sleep and leaving her constantly fatigued. These results confirmed what she had suspected all along: her symptoms weren't random or "just stress." They were directly tied to hormonal and adrenal imbalances.

With this information, we created a personalized plan. We started with bioidentical progesterone cream to support her luteal phase and balance her estrogen levels. I also helped her tweak her lifestyle—adding more protein to her diet, reducing caffeine, and incorporating stress-management techniques to support her adrenal health and regulate her cortisol. We added magnesium and adaptogens to help with sleep and anxiety. She was eager to understand everything, and I made sure to explain how each aspect of the plan was designed to work with her body. This patient reminded me how empowering education can be—when patients understand what's happening in their bodies, they're better equipped to take charge of their health.

Over the next few months, she started seeing real changes. Her sleep improved, and the night sweats disappeared. The anxiety and mood swings that had been overwhelming her became less frequent and less intense. Her cycles became more regular, and the breast tenderness she experienced after ovulation eased. While weight loss was slow, she stopped gaining and felt more in control of her body. More than anything, she felt validated—her gut instinct had been right all along. The labs gave her the clarity she needed to make changes, and for the first time in a long time, she felt hopeful.

This patient taught me an invaluable lesson: the importance of truly listening. Her experience showed me just how often women in perimenopause are dismissed or told to accept their symptoms as "normal." Conventional testing may not always provide the answers, but a deeper, more comprehensive approach can uncover the root issues and help build a path forward. This case reinforced for me that patients know their bodies better than anyone else. When they say something feels off, we need to trust that instinct and dig deeper.

Dr. Juliana Nahas MD, FMACP
Using Lab to Jumpstart a Pediatric Case

This is how viewing lab work from a traditional and functional standpoint helps me to get a better perspective on how to begin working with the pediatric population.

A 9-year-old female presented with ADHD, constipation, and a history of gross motor developmental delays in infancy. Her family history includes Hashimoto's hypothyroidism in her mother and recent recovery from C. difficile and colorectal cancer in her father.

Blood work revealed several key imbalances:
- Low vitamin B12 and vitamin D
- Low copper and zinc
- Elevated liver enzymes
- Increased LDL cholesterol
- Elevated TSH
- HbA1c at 5.5, indicating possible HPA axis and metabolic dysregulation

I suspected hypochlorhydria affecting B12 absorption, we suggested supplementation with digestive enzymes and HCl.

Additional recommendations included:
- Vitamin D3, vitamin C, and a multivitamin containing iron, zinc, and copper
- B12/folate melt
- Probiotics for gut health
- A nutrient-dense diet with lean protein, fruits, vegetables, omega-3 fatty acids, and daily fiber smoothies

These steps aim to optimize her digestion, nutrient absorption, and overall metabolic function.

To gain deeper insight into her gut, metabolism, and neurological function, we recommended:
- A comprehensive thyroid panel (including antibodies)
- GI-MAP ® (gut microbiome analysis)
- Organic Acids Test (OAT)
- Heavy Metal and Mineral Analysis Test
- P88 food sensitivity panel

Dr. Shaina Nolley DC, ACN, FMACP

Case Review: Personalized Care Through GI-MAP ® Testing

A 35-year-old male presented with a multifaceted array of symptoms, including bipolar depression, anxiety, blood sugar dysregulation, poor libido, intense nighttime sugar cravings, bloating, floating and light-colored stools, and IBS-M characterized by alternating diarrhea and constipation. Having served in the Peace Corps in Africa for four years, his history suggested potential exposure to unique pathogens and environmental stressors that could contribute to his chronic health issues. To uncover the root causes, I utilized the GI-MAP ® stool test. The initial results revealed significant dysbiosis, marked by low levels of beneficial bacteria such as Akkermansia muciniphila, Faecalibacterium prausnitzii, and Lactobacillus spp. Additionally, there was an overgrowth of Streptococcus spp., along with the presence of H. pylori, Staphylococcus aureus, Norovirus, and occult blood, indicating both microbial imbalance and compromised gut barrier integrity. Elevated markers of inflammation and immune activation, including Secretory IgA and calprotectin, further confirmed active gut dysfunction.

Leveraging these insights, I developed a tailored six-month treatment plan aimed at restoring microbial balance and enhancing gut health. The interventions included targeted antimicrobial herbs to reduce pathogenic overgrowth, prebiotics and probiotics to support and replenish beneficial bacteria, and dietary modifications to promote gut-healing nutrients. Additionally, supplements were introduced to optimize digestive enzyme activity, improve fat absorption, and address systemic inflammation. Regular monitoring and adjustments to the treatment regimen ensured that interventions remained aligned with the patient's evolving health status.

After six months of dedicated treatment, a follow-up GI-MAP ® test demonstrated remarkable improvements. Beneficial bacteria such as Akkermansia muciniphila reached optimal levels, and markers for Norovirus, H. pylori, Staphylococcus aureus, and occult blood were all resolved. The calprotectin level, a key indicator of gut inflammation, decreased dramatically from 49 to 2, showcasing a substantial reduction in overall inflammation. The patient also no longer exhibited an immune reaction to gluten, and Secretory IgA levels normalized, reflecting enhanced mucosal immunity. Clinically, the patient experienced complete resolution of his IBS symptoms, with regular bowel movements, absence of bloating, and no more floating or light-colored stools. His sugar cravings subsided, mood and energy levels stabilized, and libido returned to normal. Notably, by the end of the six months, he had successfully discontinued his antidepressant medications under his prescribing physician's guidance, a testament to the significant improvements in his mental and emotional health.

The follow-up GI-MAP ® revealed the presence of a parasite, underscoring that despite the significant health improvements achieved, exposure to environmental factors remains a constant challenge. This finding highlights the importance of ongoing health monitoring to promptly address any new imbalances or infections that may arise. It serves as a reminder that maintaining optimal health is a continuous process, requiring vigilance and proactive management.

This case exemplifies the transformative potential of the GI-MAP ® stool test in functional medicine. By precisely identifying microbial imbalances and guiding personalized interventions, the GI-MAP ® enabled the creation of a targeted treatment plan that led to profound improvements in both lab markers and the patient's quality of life. It underscores the essential role of comprehensive lab testing in achieving sustained health outcomes and the necessity of regular monitoring to navigate the ever-present challenges we face every day.

Dr. Rebeccah Shalev, ND

Rapid improvement in quality of life for this active senior after only $30 of basic labs!

Patient is a 76 year old woman, who has been on thyroid medication for Hashimoto's Thyroiditis since her 30's. After helping her to reduce her antibody levels by going gluten-free, I was treating her hypothyroidism with a combination of Levothyroxine and Liothyronine for a handful of years. Then, due to financial reasons, she transferred her thyroid care back to her Medicare PCP a few years ago (I am not a Medicare provider). Her Medicare doctor stopped checking her FT3 levels, took her off Liothyronine and monitored her thyroid levels only through TSH.

Patient came back to me recently with all the classic symptoms of hypothyroidism: Cold all the time (especially hands and feet), low energy, diffusely thinning hair, pain in her muscles and joints, and feeling like her brain just wasn't working as well as it used to. I took a look at her recent Medicare bloodwork (TSH normal, CBC normal), and since I did not want to worry about Medicare rejecting payment, I ordered a small panel through Evexia Diagnostics ® at a significant cash discount. For only $30, we were able to check TSH, FT4, FT3, and a CMP. I didn't really need the CMP to evaluate her thyroid, but it's a cheap test that gives so much useful information, so I generally order it on anyone I'm sending in for bloodwork. I was glad I did!

TSH and FT4 came back WNL, but, not surprisingly, her FT3 was low. So many things can lead to less-than-optimal conversion of the "inactive" FT4 to the "active" FT3, and I had seen this in the past with her as well. In addition, her CMP revealed her slightly elevated liver enzymes (just barely within lab normal range). She's on a lot of pain meds for her arthritis, so I suspect that's the likeliest cause, as she is not a drinker and has no history of hepatitis.

I put her back on Liothyronine, titrating up in tiny doses so her body can get used to the change gradually. Within the very first day, her energy and clarity of mind had increased and her pain level had decreased! Symptoms are continuing to improve as we increase her dosage.

Over the past two years, Patient has been taking liver support herbs containing milk thistle every few days. Milk thistle has recently been discovered to alter thyroid hormone transporters. However, given her elevated liver enzymes, I would not want to discontinue her herbal liver support. Rather, I explained that we will treat it like a medicine, taking the same dose every day, in the evening, away from her thyroid meds, and adjust her thyroid meds accordingly based on her labs. My hope is that as her joint pain levels continue to decrease, we will next be able to start reducing her daily pain meds.

Dr. Angela Davenport DC, FMACP

Diet and lifestyle changes with functional support of the body resulted in a thrilled client

The patient is a 37 year old female with a chief complaint of weight gain, wanting to balance hormones, not feeling good in her body and wanting some insight and guidance in her health journey. During initial consultation, she states that she normally was able to maintain her weight but recently gained at least 20 lbs about 2 years ago and she feels like she cannot lose the weight like she used to with calorie restriction and exercise. She had an egg retrieval 2 years ago and she was taking hormone injections and did gain extra weight around that time. Her current weight is 175 lbs and she desires to be 130 lbs. She is also having her IUD taken out this month after 5 years.

The patient had some basic lab results from her primary doctor over the past couple of years and what stood out most was her rising TSH levels. Both her mother and sister have hypothyroid conditions and are on medication but her levels had not reached the conventional range of hypothyroidism. She had the following history of TSH levels; 1.58 (6/2022), 3.84 (6/2023), and 4.38 (8/2024). Even though she does not fall in the conventional hypothyroid range, her TSH is trending up and functionally her thyroid is underactive and considered primary hypothyroidism. We performed an expanded thyroid panel as TSH simply isn't enough to fully understand how her thyroid is functioning. Her Thyroxine (T4) level was low at 6.5, considered normal conventionally but in functional medicine we know that this can indicate an underactive thyroid. Her T3 uptake was 37 which is considered to be in normal range but optimally this value is high indicating yet again that this patient is suffering from hypothyroidism. Her thyroid antibodies were also performed and negative. Further investigation also revealed insulin resistance as her fasting insulin 13 and optimally, it should be between 4.6-5.5%

It was imperative that the patient needed help with nutrition, lifestyle factors and targeted supplementation. We tried to start slowly by asking the patient to make a couple changes at a time, her biggest fear was starting and feeling like she could never have the things that she wanted again but knew that it was time for a change. Firstly, she stopped her fast food and diet coke habits, and focused on cooking at home, drinking 60-80 ounces of filtered water. Her meal plan recommendation was a gluten free mediterranean diet focusing on good sources of proteins and whole foods of fruits and vegetables. She didn't drink a lot of coffee so she switched to decaffeinated coffee when she wanted coffee and started each day with hot lemon water. She experienced some headaches while she detoxed in the first couple of weeks but she did her best to drink water and keep to the plan. If she felt off track, we would always bring her back to WHY she started. After just a few short weeks, she got into a routine of choosing foods that fit her plan. She also began dairy free on her own as she saw that dairy was affecting her. It was part of her plan once she took out gluten but she become so attuned with her body that she was able to tell what foods were making an impact.

Additionally, lifestyle changes needed to be made in order to help the patient succeed. We focused on sleep quality and quantity. She was falling asleep late while on her phone, scrolling social media, shopping or playing games, so she was encouraged to put her phone away and not keep it on her bedside table to encourage her bedroom for sleeping. It was part of her treatment plan to get 7-9 hours a night of sleep and to be asleep between 10:00-11:00 pm as she was used to going to bed after 11:00 pm and sometimes as late as 1:00 am. She would also sometimes wake up in the middle of the night at 3:00 am and have trouble falling back asleep. One suggestion to her was a calming herbal tea after dinner and a tablespoon of almond butter before bed if she felt hungry or needed a snack. Putting the focus on sleep also really helped her energy levels as before she said she never felt rested in the morning and always dragging through the day. She really started to make sleep a priority and felt so much improvement.

Lastly, we used targeted supplements to help her body function more optimally and work on supporting her thyroid. We started her on a simple regimen of Designs for Health ® supplements; "Thyroid synergy," "B Supreme" and "Digestzymes." Thyroid synergy is a multi-vitamin for the thyroid to help support hormonal balance and optimal functioning. B-Supreme was used to help with her energy levels and work on her adrenals and HPA axis. The digestzymes were added to aid in her digestion, even though it was not a main complaint, her digestion was not optimal so it is a wonderful support option.

Our initial goals of treatment were to help her feel better in her body, naturally and sustainably start to shed weight, balance and support her thyroid after discovering she was hypothyroid. After 3 months of following recommendations to the best of her ability, we did follow-up bloodwork and her TSH had dropped to 2.6 which is a significant improvement. She also lost 13 lbs and she felt that her clothes fit her better and she felt more confident in her body. She was getting good quality sleep and felt rested upon waking and sustained energy throughout the day. She also noted that her hair was healthier and shiner, her skin was clear and glowing and overall she felt significantly better in her body. Her journey did not end after her thyroid started improving and all the benefits that went along with it. She is continuing on her gluten-free, dairy-free mediterranean diet and supplements. She is so thrilled with her results and how her body feels that she has no desire to go back to the way that she was eating before. She has made significant improvements and was successful in her treatment plan.

Melissa Brown

Case Review - Patient, a 75-Year-Old Female with Chronic Symptoms and Misdiagnosis of Muscular Back Pain

Patient, a 75-year-old female, presented with a two-year history of mid-upper back pain, indigestion, frequent colds, and unexplained weight loss. Her primary care physician (PCP) initially diagnosed her with muscular pain and prescribed high-dose NSAIDs and muscle relaxers. However, these treatments provided no relief, and her symptoms persisted. In light of ongoing concerns, she was referred to Cardiology for further evaluation, where a stress test was performed. The results were deemed "normal," and the diagnosis of "muscular back pain" remained unchanged.

Upon presentation at our practice, Patient brought recent blood work, including a CBC and CMP. A thorough review of her lab results revealed iron deficiency anemia, low protein levels, signs of hypochlorhydria, and potential underlying gastrointestinal issues. Given these findings, we ordered a GI MAP test, which revealed hypochlorhydria, dysbiosis, an impaired mucosal lining, compromised immune function, and systemic inflammation.

A comprehensive plan was developed, focusing on repairing the gut lining, restoring immune function, and addressing the underlying inflammation. We implemented foundational healing strategies, including targeted nutrition, sleep optimization, and stress management techniques.

Within two months of beginning the treatment plan, Patient reported complete resolution of both her indigestion and upper back pain. Over the following six months, she experienced significant improvement in her overall symptoms and quality of life. Follow-up lab testing also showed marked improvement in her markers, confirming the success of the intervention.

This case underscores the importance of looking at lab markers through an optimal lens and considering underlying gastrointestinal issues with chronic, unexplained symptoms. With functional wellness and root cause, we were able to provide significant relief and improve Patient's quality of life.

Kelly Jorae Jefferson, FMACC

Improved quality of life through a streamlined targeted approach to symptoms

The client, a 65-year-old woman, presented with significant digestive issues, including chronic constipation, episodes of explosive bowel movements, and bloating after meals. She also experienced nausea, abdominal pain, joint and lower back pain, and challenges maintaining a healthy weight. These symptoms were compounded by a history of diverticulitis, GI bleeding, and UTI, as well as reactions to medications. Her ultimate goal was to improve her digestive health, regain energy and mobility, and feel confident while traveling without fear of digestive distress.

During the initial intake, it was evident that the client felt discouraged by her health limitations but was determined to pursue a holistic approach to healing. She expressed a desire to reduce reliance on medications, establish healthier dietary habits, and regain control over her well-being.

A comprehensive assessment, including a GI Map stool test, revealed elevated bacterial pathogens (H. pylori, E. coli), fungal overgrowth (Candida spp.), and markers of gut inflammation. These findings supported the client's reported symptoms and guided the development of a tailored protocol. LabDx was instrumental in efficiently interpreting and organizing the client's lab results, allowing for clear communication and targeted recommendations. This tool also assisted in identifying appropriate supplements to support gut healing and inflammation reduction.

Initial dietary recommendations focused on eliminating trigger foods, introducing nutrient-dense, gut-friendly options like leafy greens, clean proteins, and green juices, and integrating mindful juicing and fasting practices to reduce digestive burden and support natural healing. Supplement recommendations included targeted probiotics, digestive enzymes, and anti-inflammatory support. Lifestyle guidance centered on hydration with mineral-infused water, stress management through breathwork, and gentle movement practices like swimming.

Over the course of five months, the client experienced remarkable improvements. She reported no further episodes of explosive bowel movements, reduced bloating, significant weight loss, and improved sleep quality. Client specifically said "this is the first time I've ever had daily BMs". Her energy levels increased, and her joint pain subsided, allowing her to move with greater ease and confidence. These improvements also enhanced her ability to travel worry-free, which was a key personal goal. Weekly fitness activity and consistent adherence to her juicing and fasting regimen contributed to her physical and mental well-being. Additionally, she gained an understanding of the importance of premium supplements and established sustainable dietary and lifestyle habits aligned with her goals.

This case reinforced the power of a structured, integrative approach to gut health. Utilizing LabDx for streamlined lab analysis and supplement recommendations allowed me to deliver care more effectively and efficiently. Combining lab insights with bioenergetic findings and personalized care plans led to impactful results for the client. Her dedication and openness to dietary and lifestyle changes played a significant role in her transformation. Moving forward, I plan to continue leveraging advanced tools like LabDx for streamlined care delivery. This case reaffirms the value of functional medicine in creating lasting, meaningful change.

How Do I Become a Functional Medicine Practitioner?

If you're exploring a career in functional medicine or looking to expand your practice, you've likely realized how transformative this approach can be. Functional medicine doesn't just treat symptoms—it dives into the root causes of chronic and acute conditions, offering patients truly personalized care. For many practitioners, this shift is the answer to frustrations with conventional medicine's time constraints and *"one-size-fits-all"* solutions.

But knowing where to start can be daunting. Questions like "Where do I find functional medicine training?", "How do I become a functional medicine doctor?", and "What's involved in starting a functional medicine practice?" often come up. That's why we've created the **first and only comprehensive comparison chart** of functional medicine training programs. This resource breaks down everything you need to know—**price, duration, features, and more**—so you can make an informed decision about your next steps.

You can dive into the chart right away or continue reading through the article:
https://labdx.thedrz.com/fm-chart

Whether you're just beginning your journey or ready to start or grow your own practice, this article will guide you through the essentials of functional medicine training, help you understand the opportunities available, and provide actionable steps to help you achieve your goals. Let's dive in and discover the options that will help you transform your career and your patients' lives.

What is Functional Medicine?

Functional medicine is a **patient-centered approach** to healthcare that focuses on identifying and addressing the root causes of disease rather than simply managing symptoms. Unlike conventional medicine, which relies on standardized treatments for specific diagnoses due to a third-party payer system (health insurance) that necessitates bell-curve care and a predictive model based on "standard of care", functional medicine is built to handle the "outliers" at either end of the bell curve and a **personalized, customized, and individualized** approach for each person that walks through your clinic doors.

Practitioners work in partnership with their patients to focus on "**root-cause care**" and while the preference is for natural means whenever possible, functional medicine is **not** anti-medication or anti-surgery. It's important to not get stuck in any philosophical agenda, but to just give the best treatment possible to that individual patient. The best practitioners use and/or refer to the specialists and tools available to both conventional and functional medicine as needed.

At its core, functional medicine emphasizes the following principles:

- Treating the individual, not just the disease.
- Using evidence-based practices that integrate conventional and alternative therapies.
- Viewing the body as a whole, interconnected system rather than isolated organs.
- Empowering patients to take an active role in their health.

This approach is particularly **effective** for individuals dealing with chronic conditions, complex symptoms, or those seeking a preventative path to long-term health.

The History of Functional Medicine

Functional medicine has its roots in the mid-20th century when healthcare practitioners began exploring holistic and natural approaches to wellness. By the 1980s, doctors started utilizing advanced lab testing to identify imbalances in amino acids, fatty acids, vitamins, and other health markers, focusing on **personalized strategies** to address chronic health issues through nutrition, exercise, and supplementation.

The **term "Functional Medicine"** was officially introduced in 1990 by Jeffrey Bland, Ph.D., a biochemist and researcher known for his groundbreaking work in nutrition and health. He and his wife, Susan, went on to establish the first Functional Medicine Institute in 1991. Their seminars emphasized key areas such as gut health, immune function, hormone balance, and detoxification.

Since then, functional medicine has evolved from being viewed as an "alternative" practice to a ***respected, integrative approach embraced by practitioners worldwide***. With growing patient demand for solutions to complex chronic conditions, functional medicine has gained recognition as a vital complement to conventional healthcare.

There are more schools and universities offering degrees in Functional Medicine and groundbreaking research and partnerships being formed such as the Cleveland Clinic Center for Functional Medicine.

While this is exciting and more to come, the vast majority of Functional Medicine practitioners already have some type of medical license, get certified through advanced training (check out our FM Training Comparison Chart: **https://labdx.thedrz.com/fm-chart**), and operate their own private practice in person, hybrid, or via telemedicine.

Functional Medicine Practitioner Eligibility

Becoming a functional medicine practitioner typically requires a healthcare-related background. The eligibility requirements vary depending on the program, but most certifications and training options are designed for licensed medical professionals.

Eligible professionals typically include:

- Medical Doctors (MD)
- Doctors of Osteopathy (DO)
- Doctors of Chiropractic (DC)
- Naturopathic Doctors (ND)
- Dentists (DDS/DMD)
- Nurse Practitioners (NP)
- Acupuncturists (LAc)
- Pharmacists (PharmD)
- Mental Health Professionals (e.g., Ph.D., Psy.D., LCSW)

Other healthcare providers eligible with specific degrees:

- Physician Assistants (PA)
- Registered Nurses (RN)
- Registered Dietitians (RD)
- Occupational Therapists (OT)
- Physical Therapists (PT)

To qualify for certification programs like those offered by the Institute for Functional Medicine (IFM), or Functional Medicine Academy (FMA), most applicants must have a bachelor's degree or higher in a health-related field.

However, some programs also have a certification for health coaching and nutritionists such as Functional Medicine Academy's FMACC or Institute for Integrative Nutrition's (IIN) coaching certification. These programs offer exposure to the world of Functional Medicine that allows each professional to practice up to their individual scope of practice.

There is room for everyone in Functional Medicine, but it is very important to note that your medical license is what determines your scope. An MD will have access to all the tools in Functional Medicine along with the full breadth of what their license allows in conventional medicine. An NP can set up a private practice using Functional Medicine, but needs to be mindful of the specific license and state regulations which will determine if that NP can practice autonomously or needs a physician supervisor, same with PAs. A DC as a primary point of care chiropractic physician will be able to open a practice and operate independently, but must operate within their scope and won't have access to medications. A health coach can have a Functional Medicine focused practice that is of great service to their clients, but must be mindful to operate within their scope of education and won't diagnose or treat. This article is not designed to provide legal advice and your scope of practice varies state-to-state, please watch our legal training videos and utilize our referral list of attorneys for more information.

While your license or certification determines your "scope of practice", it does *not* determine your success in practice.

We have trained every level of practitioner from a triple-board certified physician to a health coach and every medical license in-between. How you set up your practice, your ability to be coachable and learn new entrepreneurial skills such as marketing will determine if you build a 6-figure, 7-figure, or even 8-figure practice.

Why Doctors, Nurses, PAs, & DCs Are Switching to Functional Medicine

Feeling **burnt out** in your current healthcare role? You're not alone. Studies consistently show that burnout rates among healthcare professionals—especially doctors, nurses, physician assistants (PAs), and chiropractors (DCs)—are alarmingly high. For physicians, nurses, and physician assistants, burnout rates are reported to be over 50%, and in some surveys, they climb as high as 80%. Long hours, high patient loads, and the relentless demands of an overburdened healthcare system leave little room for the meaningful, patient-centered work that most practitioners entered the field to provide. For chiropractors reporting burnout it stems from lower reimbursement rates with insurance, physical demands, high volume practice, and administrative isolation.

At its heart, **healthcare is about helping people heal**, but the current system often prioritizes quick fixes and volume over outcomes. Functional medicine offers an antidote. This approach allows practitioners to dig deeper, addressing the root causes of illness rather than merely treating symptoms. It empowers you to create lasting, transformative results for your patients while rekindling your passion for medicine.

Additionally, functional medicine fosters collaboration, offering a more supportive healthcare model. You're **no longer navigating complex cases alone**—whether through shared knowledge, specialized tools, or a team-based approach, functional medicine provides the resources and environment to truly thrive in your practice. For many professionals, making the switch to functional medicine isn't just about a career change; it's about reclaiming the joy and purpose that brought them into healthcare in the first place.

How to Choose the Right Functional Medicine Training for You

Choosing the right functional medicine training program is more than just picking the best clinical curriculum—it's about finding a program that prepares you for both patient care **and** the business of running a practice. For many healthcare professionals, transitioning into functional medicine is also their first step into entrepreneurship. To succeed, you need training that not only deepens your clinical expertise but also equips you to build and manage a thriving practice.

Here are a few key factors to consider:

- **Comprehensive Clinical Education**
  Look for programs that provide a strong foundation in functional medicine principles, including root cause analysis, personalized treatment planning, and advanced lab interpretation. Ensure the curriculum aligns with your clinical interests and goals.

- **Business and Practice Management Skills**
  Starting and managing a functional medicine practice requires skills in marketing, patient acquisition, and operational efficiency. Prioritize training programs that include modules on building a practice, managing finances, and leveraging technology to streamline your workflow.

- **Flexible Formats**
  As a busy professional, you'll want a program that fits into your schedule. Many programs offer online or hybrid options, allowing you to learn at your own pace while balancing your current work commitments.

- **Support and Resources**
  Choose a program that offers ongoing support, such as mentorship, networking opportunities, and access to practice-building tools. Having a community of like-minded professionals can be invaluable as you grow your practice.

By selecting a program that addresses both clinical expertise and business acumen, you'll be better equipped to deliver transformative care for your patients while creating a sustainable and rewarding career in functional medicine.

Trainings and Certifications in Functional Medicine

Functional Medicine Academy (FMA)

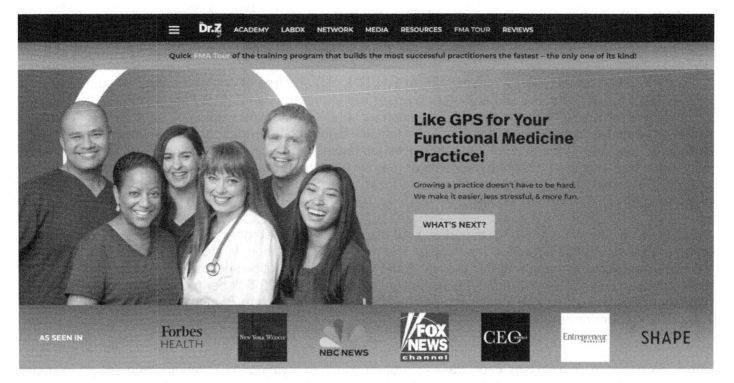

Image source: screenshot TheDrZ.com

Functional Medicine Academy (FMA) launched The Mentorship 3.0 last year which is **unprecedented** in Functional Medicine education - the only comprehensive clinical, practice building, and business growth training of its kind.

FMA was created in response to the lack of practical clinical training, absent marketing education, and confusion about ethical and responsible compliance laws observed by founder Dr. Z in existing functional medicine programs. While they all offered something of benefit, it was her mission to create one program that encompassed everything that was needed for the Functional Medicine practitioner with cutting-edge and contemporary information you could count on.

As a result, Dr. Z has personally invested over $500,000 in education, business training, HIPAA, legal, and financial compliance to make sure FMA is always ahead of the curve for the practitioners they serve.

The Mentorship 3.0 (earn FMACP or FMACC)

The Mentorship 3.0 (TM3.0) has evolved over the years to become your *"one-stop-shop"* for Functional Medicine practice success.

As a practitioner, the clinical training is unparalleled. You will earn your FMACP (Functional Medicine Academy Certified Practitioner) or FMACC (Certified Coach) depending on your current licensure. The training includes comprehensive online education for moving a patient through care, gastrointestinal health, cardiometabolic health, nutrition, weight loss, and functional endocrinology. A case review and certification test must be completed to be certified.

Additional clinical certifications are **included** in the program and may be completed at your pace in Pediatrics (the first comprehensive Functional Medicine Pediatrics certification), Advanced Hormones in Women, Mold Environmental Illness and Detoxification, and Lab Analysis. Upcoming certifications in 2025 include: Psychology, Dermatology, Advanced Hormones in Men, and Peptides. Certifications are included free of charge to current TM3.0 members.

Live Clinical Consults occur **daily** with the clinical staff and include topics such as functional nutrition, supplementation, lab analysis, reviewing patient intake forms, developing treatment protocols, adverse reactions and contraindications, or whatever questions you have clinically.

CE's are included for all types of nurses (NP, APRN, RN, etc) and free of charge for the first quarter of 2025. CME's for MD, DO, PA, DC and other licenses are in progress and eta is February 2025. Clinical tools are also included in the program such as LabDX (the online version of this textbook series) which provides marker definition, therapeutic insight, lifestyle recommendations, and supplementation with dosage for over 60+ of the most popular advanced lab testing in Functional Medicine. The LabDX software is included free of charge to TM3.0 members or may be purchased separately. The intake forms, clinic policy, HIPAA compliance, and patient handouts for your EMR are also provided with substantial savings depending on which EMR you choose.

Practice setup, launch, and growth is part of what places FMA in a category of its own. Doctors and nurses who have never worked outside of the hospital routinely get FM certified, launch their practice, and sign their first new patients through FMA's unique "**Rx5 Formula**" for practice success. FMA practitioners celebrate their first $5-10k per month in new patient signups, then $20-50k per month, and you can watch this recent interview of an FMA client who just had her first $100k month – watch: **https://labdx.thedrz.com/client-interview**.

There are many ways to market and grow your practice and FMA teaches them all - in exacting detail, plus offers more than 20 live classes each week to support you in everything from branding and design to social media and websites to basic marketing and advertising to no charge consults and sales.

FMA is unique in that it includes the FMA Marketing software free of charge to all TM3.0 members - which provides you with website templates, a toll-free phone number, email marketing, texting, social media scheduler and social media content (new each month), automated newsletters by niche, webinar funnels, quiz funnels, a full CRM, analytics and more, plus it is all HIPAA compliant. This marketing and sales software is included free of charge to TM3.0 members or may be purchased separately.

FMA recently launched **SearchFunctionalMedicine.com** (SFM) - the only "find-a-practitioner" search of its kind that showcases the multiple certification you may have earned, allows up to a 2,000 word bio, helps you get found with SEO-friendly links to your website and social media, and the only practitioner search engine that pulls in your Google Reviews as peer evidence is so helpful when the public is choosing a practitioner. They may also use advanced search by location, languages spoken, population served, and treatment specialty. Dr. Z has committed to using her vast knowledge and experience with Facebook advertising to run ads to the consumer public to help practitioners get found - essentially paying for ads for you in 2025. This listing is included free of charge to TM3.0 members or may be purchased separately.

When you are ready for staffing support, FMA has you covered. They have partnered to bring you VA Solutions which are reliable virtual assistant services to help with your tech and admin needs at a very affordable cost that may be purchased as needed, in small blocks, with no long term contracts.

Ready for support in fulfillment on the clinical side? No problem, no long contracts, no onboarding fees, no delays or having to spend months training new staff. FMA has partnered with the leading staffing agency for health coaches and clinical nutritionists. When you are ready, they have staff waiting for you to plug right into your new or existing clinical offerings. All services include a wealth of white-labeled clinical resources (nutrition guides, meal plans, menus and more) and unlimited patient-to-coach messaging all month long.

Legal, financial, and compliance are also at the heart of FMA and something we are uniquely positioned to speak on. While not an attorney or accountant, Dr. Z has worked with all the top Functional Medicine legal firms and can share information and provide valuable referrals (and sometimes discounts) as needed. Having such a varied exposure to every medical license, Dr. Z can present on the safest and most conservative measures to set up your practice so you can be in full compliance, protect your license, and rest easy while still having room to build an amazing practice and impact patient's lives. Her method which she calls "coloring within the legal lines" doesn't stop you from building a hugely successful practice, but does help protect you from the abundance of poor advice and downright illegal methods that show up in most online marketing and other Functional Medicine training. You'll want to watch FMA's legal training, tax/financial training, and utilize our referral list of attorneys, tax specialists, and accountants.

FMA is one of the few Functional Medicine training programs to include 1:1 coaching. You'll be assigned an MSA (Member Success Advisor) for individual, monthly meetings and daily/weekly support in your Slack channel. You'll also have an SA (Strategic Advisor) who helps guide you through assessments (deep dive provided every 90 days and shorter assessment end of each month) to make sure you are on the right growth track - whether you are brand new to FM, in the early stages of your practice, or already well-established and ready to scale) and that you are clear on the next right steps needed to hit your goals. You'll always have two sets of eyes to assist you and monitor your progress - we track everything and take your success seriously.

You'll also have access to your peers in our exclusive TM3.0 Skool community where you'll find recordings of all our current clinical and business training. No one generates more contemporary and current content than FMA. Join Dr. Z live multiple times each month for cutting edge training that impacts Functional Medicine practitioners today. Recent training topics include: Immune Dysregulation and Depression, January Pre-Launch Planning, How to Run a Virtual Marketing Event, How to Create an Online Course, Bredesen/ReCode Cliffnotes & Supplementation Guide, HIPAA Compliance in FM, How to Create a Webinar Outline that Converts, Speak-to-Sell, and Practitioner Tips for Using AI plus What to Avoid.

FMA Duration

90 days and then month to month. A high percentage of practitioners stay with FMA for years due to the unparalleled support and benefits - but that is up to you.

FMA Key Features

A fully comprehensive and "one stop shop" to Functional Medicine training. Whether this is your first FM program or going to be your last one, FMA will have something you need that is missing from the rest of what is currently available. You can read through an overview of FMA: **https://thedrz.com/fma-tour/**

FMA Notes
FMA describes its program as "practical and actionable for practitioners determined to succeed". If curious to learn more, talk to a Practice Advisor: **https://labdx.thedrz.com/book-a-call**

By selecting a program that addresses both clinical expertise and business acumen, you'll be better equipped to deliver transformative care for your patients while creating a sustainable and rewarding career in functional medicine.

Closing

Functional Medicine is an exciting field and one that provides a unique opportunity where all levels - Business Owner, Practitioner, Staff, Patient/Client can benefit and feel good about the impact they are having in their lives and the world around them.

Choosing where to begin (or your next move) in your Functional Medicine training can feel daunting - we know our researchers spend hundreds of hours building the FM Training Comparison Chart!

As we sign off we'll share Top 10 Tips to choosing the right training with the hope that it will be helpful for you.

Top 10 Tips for Choosing Your Mentor aka 10 Criteria Before You Hire

1. Do they understand Functional Medicine clinical **AND** business practices? Have they done it themselves?
2. Do they understand how to market to potential patients **SPECIFIC** to Functional Medicine? Are they aware of FDA and FTC restrictions?
3. Do they have **more than one method** or ability to modify/customize to meet your specific needs?
4. Do they have a **blend** of "doing it yourself", "do it with you", and "done for you" services?
5. What **accountability** and tracking is there in their program so you don't get lost or fall through the cracks?
6. Do they have a **clear map** or method to move through their program and proven systems to get there?
7. Have others **completed** their program and demonstrated success?
8. What kind of **support** do they offer you? 1:1, group coaching, support calls? How often?
9. Do **you like them** and want to learn from them? Do you trust them?
10. Do they **INNOVATE** or are they stagnant? How **dated** is their material? Are they doing this right NOW in the same environment you are? Do they know what to do when things go wrong? What's plan B, C, & D? Are they IN it with you?

DUE DILIGENCE:

Listing in the Functional Medicine Training Comparison Chart does not imply endorsement or validation of any kind. These are some of the online training companies that you will encounter upon performing a Google search and you must perform your own due diligence. Visit the Training Comparison chart **https://labdx.thedrz.com/fm-chart**

How Do I Find a Functional Medicine Practitioner?

Finding the Right Practitioner for You

If you're ready to get to the root cause of your health challenges and experience truly personalized care, finding the right functional medicine practitioner is a crucial step. Functional medicine focuses on identifying and addressing the underlying causes of symptoms, rather than just managing them. Whether you're dealing with chronic issues, hormonal imbalances, digestive concerns, or simply want to optimize your health, a skilled practitioner can guide you toward lasting solutions tailored specifically to your needs.

When searching for a practitioner, consider your goals. Are you looking for someone local for in-person visits, or do you prefer the convenience of virtual care? Do you need someone who specializes in a particular area, such as hormone health, autoimmune conditions, or gut health? A functional medicine practitioner is trained to use advanced lab testing and personalized treatment strategies that integrate natural and conventional approaches, offering benefits like:

- **A whole-person approach** that considers your lifestyle, environment, and genetics.
- **Customized solutions** instead of one-size-fits-all treatments.
- **Proactive health strategies** to help you thrive, not just survive.

To make your search easier, visit **SearchFunctionalMedicine.com**. This no charge online tool allows you to search for practitioners by location, virtual or in-person availability, language preferences, certification, and specialties. With this resource, you can find a practitioner who fits your unique needs and start your journey toward better health.

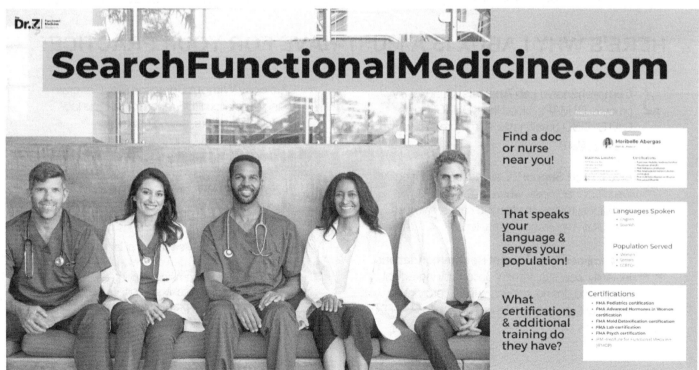

Image source: screenshot SearchFunctionalMedicine.com

Looking for a practitioner? Visit **www.SearchFunctionalMedicine.com**

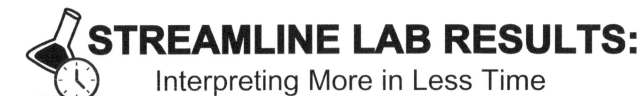

STREAMLINE LAB RESULTS:
Interpreting More in Less Time

LabDX: Transforming Lab Analysis

LabDX combines the trusted insights of your textbooks with powerful technology to streamline your workflow. Save hours of research time and deliver exceptional patient care, all from one easy-access platform.

SCAN THIS CODE TO GET STARTED

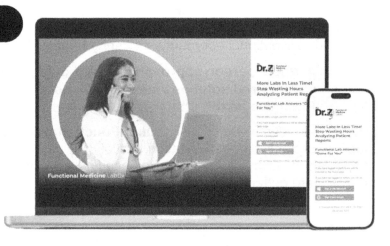

HERE'S WHY LABDX IS A MUST-HAVE FOR YOUR PRACTICE:

 Comprehensive Lab Analysis: Seamlessly process GI MAPs, blood labs, DUTCH tests, OATS, SIBO breath tests, and more—all within a single system.

 Live Expert Support: Gain access to a weekly live clinical lab class, where you can ask questions, review challenging cases, and get consultative guidance in real-time.

 Streamlined Supplement Recommendations: Instantly view supplement options by ingredient, brand, and dosing, making patient care simple and effective - only available in the online LabDX software tool.

 Efficiency Without Compromise: Generate a single, detailed PDF report for multiple labs and/or lab markers, saving hours of preparation without sacrificing quality or accuracy.

 Always Up to Date: Stay ahead in your practice with new tests added monthly, ensuring access to the latest advancements in functional medicine.

 LabDX takes the guesswork out of lab analysis and empowers you to deliver personalized care faster than ever. By combining cutting-edge technology with live weekly support, it's the ultimate tool for elevating your practice and achieving better outcomes for your patients.

Try LabDX FREE for 2 Weeks!
Experience the Difference.

Curious about LabDX? Experience the difference risk-free! For two full weeks, explore all the features with a free trial, or join our exclusive live demo to get your lab analysis questions answered directly by our clinical team. See how **LabDX saves you time, simplifies lab interpretation, and enhances patient care.**

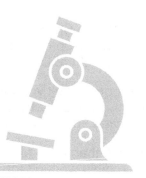

What's Included in Your Free Trial:

- ✓ **Full access to LabDX** - No restrictions, just real-world use.
- ✓ **Seamless lab interpretation** - GI MAPs, blood labs, DUTCH, OATS, and more, effortlessly analyzed.
- ✓ **Automated supplement recommendations** - Instantly view precise ingredient-based options.
- ✓ **Instant PDF reports** - Generate professional, patient-friendly reports in seconds.
- ✓ **Live expert support** - Join our weekly lab Q&A call for expert guidance.
- ✓ **LabDX** is built to make lab analysis faster, easier, and more effective—and now you can see it for yourself!

START YOUR FREE TRIAL TODAY:
www.TheDrZ.com/LabDX

Exclusive LabDX Live Demo - Get Your Lab Questions Answered!

▶ **Live Q&A with Clinical Experts** – Get personalized answers to your toughest lab cases.

▶ **See LabDX in Action** – Watch how it simplifies GI MAPs, DUTCH, OATs, blood labs, and more—all in one system.

▶ **Real-World Case Applications** – See how top practitioners use LabDX to improve patient outcomes.

▶ This isn't just a software walkthrough—it's your chance to sharpen your lab interpretation skills with expert guidance.

CLAIM YOUR SPOT NOW!
tinyurl.com/LabDXSoftwareTraining

LabDx Software Training

We want you to get the most out of LabDX. Join our weekly training class to:
- Experience a live demo of the app.
- Learn more about interpreting labs.
- Submit your own case studies to review together using LabDX.

When: Weekly on Thursdays, 10:00 – 11:30 AM CT
Link to Join: tinyurl.com/LabDxSoftwareTraining

Learn more at www.TheDrZ.com/LabDX

Acknowledgements

Thank you Sharon for finding me through IFM. My sister lab lover from the UK, a data IT geek, nutritional analysis deep dive queen, and so committed to this project. From the early days of initial research to being on the FM LabDX staff to editor - this wouldn't have happened without you.

NP Lorri, thank you for saying "yes" so many times to so many things. Stepping up, serving your patients, testing the lab software, building certifications, leading clinical consults for practitioners - I have always admired your steadfast determination and am grateful to have you on my team.

Angel, thank you for jumping into LabDX, serving as the practitioner liaison for the software and your incredible work on formatting the data for the textbooks. I so appreciate all of your effort and the enthusiastic energy you bring to the project.

Beida, Alder, Tin, Risse, Lovell, Sherie - thank you all for jumping in these last few months from project management to culling data grids to formatting and all the extra hours.

Brandy, my Canadian colleague from the land of cold, thank you for helping to push the LabDX project forward and reminding me I can make anything happen.

Thank you Dr. Burry, Dr. Dufala, Dr. Garvey, Katie, Kelly, Kylene and the many practitioners and staff at my clinic who tested the data and put in the early work serving patients. Thank you Julie for helping with the formulas.

Thank you Dr. Dunham, NP Cari, Dr. Fries, Dr. Wang, Dr. Tina, Dr. Van Wyk, Coach Sarah, and the many practitioners who were early advocates, adopters, and testers - so grateful to you.

Thank you Drs. Nick and Meena Sidhu for writing such a beautiful foreword and caring so deeply for the patients you serve.

To all of the FMA and FML staff - thank you for showing up with such dedication and devotion to the many MD, DO, DC, ND, PA, NP providers we serve and all the allied professionals, nutritionists and health coaches working in this field. You are indeed influencing this profession and the many patient lives impacted by our practitioners. I thank you and am grateful for you every day.

To all the researchers, health professionals, instructors, lab companies, and medical movers and shakers - thank you for your passion for this field. We gather, collect, and build on your work. Thank you for going first. Don't stop.

Thank you to the incredible physicians I consulted from Harvard, Princeton, Stanford and around the world (Australia, Canada, UK, Europe, Latin America) - it has been amazing learning from you. Thank you for asking "why", moving the conversation forward, and digging deeper than anyone else was interested in - I'm glad we found one another.

Dave, thank you for being a phenomenal software developer, so invested in the project, and turning my vision into a reality. I appreciate you so much.

Thank you to the hundreds of practitioners (thousands now!) who have used the LabDX software and data to better help inform your clinical care from a nutritional and functional perspective. If you weren't out there in the trenches doing the work, this project wouldn't have happened.

Susan, thank you for the many years of friendship and patiently witnessing all the behind-the-scenes. I'll never forget you sitting on the couch when I was pacing at a pivotal moment caught in a vortex of "I'll just forget this LabDX thing" and you said "You can't, you've come too far". You were right.

Thank you to my family - David, Nikita, Mom, extended family, home staff team, my friends who check on me when I'm head down in work (thanks Edie & Lynda)- all of whom simultaneously support and tolerate my obsession with making this project happen. "It's a lot" doesn't begin to describe the journey and I am grateful for every one of you.

About the Author

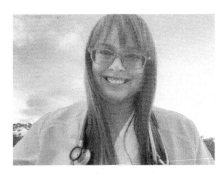

Dr. Brandy Zachary, DC, IFMCP, FMACP ("Dr. Z"), began her Functional Medicine journey after being diagnosed with a rare, incurable primary immunodeficiency. Determined to find answers, she consulted with experts at Princeton, Harvard, and Stanford, transforming her health and igniting her passion for education.

An award-winning entrepreneur and practice owner, Dr. Z founded the Functional Medicine Academy (FMA), achieving 150x growth in one year, and created Functional Medicine LabDX, the first comprehensive lab guide of its kind.

When not immersed in research or work, she's playing with her golden retriever and ever-expanding pack of goldendoodles, enjoying life on the Caribbean Coast. Visit www.TheDrZ.com.

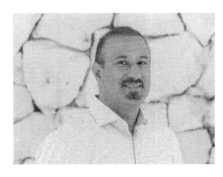

Foreword by: **Dr. Nick Sidhu, M.D., ABIM, ABOM, ABAARM** is a triple board-certified physician with over 30 years of experience in Internal Medicine, Obesity Medicine, and Anti-Aging and Regenerative Medicine. He leads the Advanced Medical and Weight Loss Center in Alpharetta, Georgia, where he helps patients with personalized care for hormone therapy, gut health, thyroid disorders, autoimmune conditions, and weight management. Dr. Sidhu is passionate about Functional Medicine, taking a root-cause approach to prevent and reverse chronic diseases. Known for his expertise and approachable style, he's also an active speaker and a proud supporter of his local community.

Also by the author:

A Practitioner's Guide to Mastering Functional Medicine Lab Values - Gut & Digestion Insights: (Part 2 of 4) Advanced Testing for Gastrointestinal Health, published by Functional Medicine LabDX, Sheridan, WY 2025.

A Practitioner's Guide to Mastering Functional Medicine Lab Values - Hormonal Health & Balance: (Part 3 of 4) Panels for Reproductive, Adrenal, and Thyroid Function, published by Functional Medicine LabDX, Sheridan, WY 2025.

A Practitioner's Guide to Mastering Functional Medicine Lab Values - Metabolic Health & Toxin Testing: (Part 4 of 4) Autoimmunity, Toxins, and Advanced Metabolic Markers, published by Functional Medicine LabDX, Sheridan, WY 2025.

How to Read a Client From Across the Room: Win More Business with the Proven Character Code System, published by McGraw-Hill, NY 2012.

Want to check out LabDX online? Visit **www.TheDrZ.com/LabDX**

Looking for a practitioner? Visit **www.SearchFunctionalMedicine.com**

Made in the USA
Monee, IL
01 April 2025

15006089R00273